THE SINUS NODE

THE SINUS NODE

STRUCTURE, FUNCTION AND CLINICAL RELEVANCE

edited by

FELIX I.M. BONKE

1978

MARTINUS NIJHOFF MEDICAL DIVISION

THE HAGUE/BOSTON/LONDON

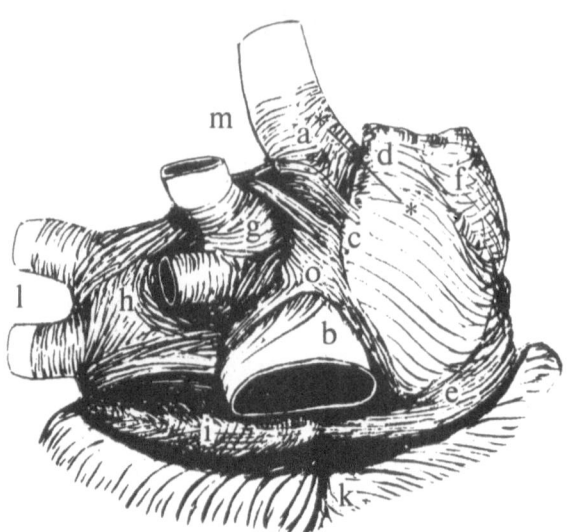

Cover illustration. "The auricular part of the human heart from behind, showing the musculature of the termination of the great veins.

"*a*, superior vena cava surrounded by musculature derived from the sinus; *b*, inferior vena cava; *c*, to the right of the sulcus terminalis, above *c*, sinus fibres cross the sulcus to join auricle proper; *d*, at sino-auricular junction, where peculiar musculature is found most abundantly; *e*, annular fibres of auricle; *f*, appendix; *g*, fibres passing from interauricular septum to vestibule of left auricle between the two left pulmonary veins; *h*, vestibule; *i*, coronary sinus, showing continuity of fibres with right and left auricles; *k*, base of ventricles at interventricular sulcus; *l*, left pulmonary veins; *m*, constant band passing from sinus musculature to vestibule of left auricle; *o*, muscle of auricular canal submerging sinus; ** represent line of section of fig. 6, A."

Source: Keith, A., Flack, M.: The form and nature of the muscular connections between the primary divisions of the vertebrate heart. *J Anat and Physiol* 41 (3rd series, vol 2): 177, 1907.

ISBN-13: 978-94-009-9717-2   e-ISBN-13: 978-94-009-9715-8
DOI: 10.1007/ 978-94-009-9715-8

© 1978 Martinus Nijhoff Medical Division
Softcover reprint of hardcover 1st edition 1978

Photoset in Malta

PREFACE

For the clinician the sinus node is more or less a hidden structure and only by indirect assessment he is able to say something about the function of this center of pacemaker activity.

The morphologist, however, is able to describe the structural microscopic and even electronmicroscopic features of this structure. The only disadvantage is that, as soon as he is coming into the picture, the tissue is dead. The physiologist tries to investigate the electrophysiological behavior of the sinus node. Since there is not a human being willing to give his sinus node for research, he has to do his investigation on isolated preparations of animals.

Though there are a lot of experts in the field of the sinus node they nearly never speak the same 'language'. Therefore, it was my dream to bring all those people – or at least some of them – together on a workshop. I had the feeling that it was important to organize such a meeting without an audience but only with 'experts'.

With the generous help of Astra Pharmaceutica I had the opportunity to invite about forty specialists to come to a workshop on the sinus node. They all immediately accepted my invitation. We organized the Workshop on Sinus Node in Maastricht, The Netherlands, at the end of July, 1977, with an informal program. Nearly all participants gave a presentation and there were very enthusiastic and long discussions about the various topics. We decided to compose a book which would contain all the presentations. We also asked the five chairmen of the various sections to make 'general comments' of the presentations in their sections, not only what they have presented during the session days themselves, but also after having read the manuscripts very carefully. Since they needed some extra time the book will be published belatedly. We think that their contribution might be a great help for the readers. Although all participants will agree that this workshop did not bring the final solution for all the problems around the function, structure, and clinical relevance of the sinus node, we do hope that it has been a step forward.

FELIX I.M. BONKE

ACKNOWLEDGEMENTS

This workshop and therefore also this publication would never have been possible without the enormous help of Astra Pharmaceutica in The Netherlands. The first contact with this company has been made via Prof. dr. H.J.J. Wellens who has been my main advisor in all the organizational problems. I am very happy that we are colleagues at the University of Limburg in Maastricht. This university offered me all possible assistance in the organization of the Workshop.

The secretarial work has been the largest part of this organization, not only before, but also during and especially after the Workshop when the manuscript of this book had to be prepared. This job has been done by Miss Els Geurts and Mrs. Bebby van der Mars-Pastoors. I wish to express my appreciation for all the work they have done.

FELIX I.M. BONKE

CONTENTS

LIST OF CONTRIBUTORS

*Maurits A. Allessie. Dept. of Physiology, Biomedical Center, University of Limburg, Maastricht, The Netherlands.

Fernando Amat-Y-Leon, Abraham Lincoln School of Medicine, University of Illinois, Chicago, Illinois, U.S.A.

*Robert H. Anderson, Dept. of Paediatrics, Cardiothoracic Institute, Brompton Hospital, London, United Kingdom.

*Anton E. Becker, Dept. of Pathology, Wilhelmina Gasthuis, Amsterdam, The Netherlands.

David G. Benditt, Dept. of Medicine, Duke University Medical Center, Durham, North Carolina, U.S.A.

* Wim K. Bleeker, Dept. of Physiology, University of Amsterdam, Jan Swammerdam Institute, Amsterdam. The Netherlands.

* Felix I.M. Bonke, Dept. of Physiology, Biomedical Center, University of Limburg, Maastricht, The Netherlands.

* Lennart N. Bouman, Dept. of Physiology, University of Amsterdam, Jan Swammerdam Institute, Amsterdam, The Netherlands.

Günter Breithardt, First Medical Clinic B, University of Düsseldorf, Germany.

* Hilary Brown, University Laboratory of Physiology, Oxford, United Kingdom.

David J. Browning, Dept. of Medicine, Duke University Medical Center, Durham, North Carolina, U.S.A.

Frans J.L. van Capelle, Dept. of Cardiology and Clinical Physiology, Wilhelmina Gasthuis, The Interuniversity Institute of Cardiology, Amsterdam, The Netherlands.

*Paul F. Cranefield, The Rockefeller University, New York, New York, U.S.A.

Reuben Chuquimia, Division of Cardiology, Dept. of Internal Medicine, Cook County Hospital Veterans Administration Hospital North Chicago, and The Chicago Medical School, Chicago, Illinois, U.S.A.

* Anthony N. Damato, Cardiovascular Program, U.S. Public Health Service Hospital, Staten Island, New York, U.S.A.

Pablo Denes, Abraham Lincoln School of Medicine, University of Illinois, Chicago, Illinois, U.S.A.

Ramesh C. Dhingra, Abraham Lincoln School of Medicine, University of Illinois, Chicago, Illinois, U.S.A.

Renzo Dianda, Dept. of Cardiology, General Hospital, Lucca, Italy.

* D. Fleischmann, First Medical Division, Rheinisch-Westfälische Technische Hochschule, Aachen, Germany.

Wayne Giles, Center for Bioengineering, University of Washington, Seattle, Washington, U.S.A.

John A. Gosling, Dept. of Anatomy, University of Manchester, Manchester, United Kingdom.

D. Gros, Laboratory of Zoology and Cellular Biology, Poitiers, France.

Noel Goupil, Laboratoire de Physiologie Animale, Bâtiment P, Université de Poitiers, Poitiers, France.

* Aya Irisawa, Dept. of Physiology, School of Medicine, Hiroshima University, Hiroshima, Japan.

*Hiroshi Irisawa, Dept. of Physiology, School of Medicine, Hiroshima University, Hiroshima, Japan.

*Michiel J. Janse, Dept. of Cardiology and Clinical Physiology, Wilhelmina Gasthuis, The Interuniversity Institute of Cardiology, Amsterdam, The Netherlands.

*Jay L. Jordan, Dept. of Cardiology, Cedars-Sinai Medical Center, Los Angeles, California, U.S.A.

André G. Kléber, Dept. of Cardiology and Clinical Physiology, Wilhelmina Gasthuis, The Interuniversity Institute of Cardiology, Amsterdam, The Netherlands.

*Danielle Kreitner, Laboratoire de Physiologie Comparée et de Physiologie Cellulaire associé au CNRS, Université de Paris XI, Orsay, France.

An LaBarre, Dept. of Medicine, Duke University Medical Center, Durham, North Carolina, U.S.A.

*Wim J.E.P. Lammers, Dept. of Physiology, Biomedical Center, University of Limburg, Maastricht, The Netherlands.

*Jacques Lenfant, Laboratoire de Physiologie Animale, Bâtiment P, Université de Poitiers, Poitiers, France.

Christian Leuner, First Medical Clinic B, University of Düsseldorf, Düsseldorf, Germany.

Joseph W. Linhart, Division of Cardiology, Dept. of Internal Medicine, Cook County Hospital, Veterans Administration Hospital North Chicago, and The Chicago Medical School, Chicago, Illinois, U.S.A.

Stephen L. Lipsius, Dept. of Physiology and Biophysics, University of Vermont, College of Medicine, Burlington, Vermont, U.S.A.

*Berndt Lüderitz, Dept. of Medicine, University of Munich, Medical Clinic I, Klinikum Grosshadern, Munich, Germany.

*Albert J. C. Mackaay, Dept. of Physiology, University of Amsterdam, Jan Swammerdam Institute, Amsterdam, The Netherlands.

*William J. Mandel, Dept. of Cardiology, Cedars-Sinai Medical Center, Los Angeles, California, U.S.A.

*Giuseppe Masini, Dept. of Cardiology, General Hospital, Lucca, Italy.

*Mireille Masson-Pévet, Dept. of Physiology, University of Amsterdam, Jan Swammerdam Institute, Amsterdam, The Netherlands.

*Onkar S. Narula, Division of Cardiology, Dept. of Medicine, The Chicago Medical School, University of Health Sciences, Chicago, Illinois, U.S.A.

*C. Naumann d'Alnoncourt, Dept. of Medicine, University of Munich, Medical Clinic I, Klinikum Grosshadern, Munich, Germany.

*Susan Noble, University Laboratory of Physiology, Oxford, United Kingdom.

*Akinori Noma, Dept. of Physiology, School of Medicine, Hiroshima University, Hiroshima, Japan.

*Gerald H. Pollack, Depts. of Anesthesiology and Bioengineering, University of Washington, Seattle, Washington, U.S.A.

*T. Pop, First Medical Division, Rheinisch-Westfälische Technische Hochschule. Aachen, Germany.

*Kenneth M. Rosen, Abraham Lincoln School of Medicine, University of Illinois, Chicago, Illinois, U.S.A.

W. Rosenberger, Dept. of Medicine, University of Munich, Medical Clinic I, Klinikum Grosshadern, Munich, Germany.

Melvin M. Scheinman, Medical Service, San Francisco General Hospital Medical Center, University of California, San Francisco, California, U.S.A.

*Ludger Seipel, First Medical Clinic B, University of Düsseldorf, Düsseldorf, Germany.

*Issei Seyama, Dept. of Physiology, School of Medicine, Hiroshima University, Hiroshima, Japan.

Naràsimhan Shantha, Division of Cardiology, Dept. of Internal Medicine, Cook County Hospital, Veterans Administration Hospital North Chicago, and The Chicago Medical School, Chicago, Illinois, U.S.A.

*Gerhard Steinbeck, Dept. of Medicine, University of Munich, Medical Clinic I, Klinikum Grosshadern, Munich, Germany.

*Harold C. Strauss, Dept. of Medicine and Pharmacology, Duke University Medical Center, Durham, North Carolina, U.S.A.

William D. Towne, Division of Cardiology, Dept. of Internal Medicine, Cook County Hospital, Veterans Administration Hospital North Chicago, and The Chicago Medical School, Chicago, Illinois, U.S.A.

*Jørgen Tranum-Jensen, Anatomy Dept. C, University of Copenhagen, Copenhagen, Denmark.

*Wolfgang Trautwein, Institute of Physiology, University of Saarland, Homburg/Saar, Germany.

Miguel Vasquez, Division of Cardiology, Dept of Internal Medicine, Cook County Hospital, Veterans Administration Hospital North Chicago, and The Chicago Medical School, Chicago, Illinois, U.S.A.

*Mario Vassalle, Dept. of Physiology, Downstate Medical Center, State University of New York, Brooklyn, New York, U.S.A.

Andrew G. Wallace, Dept. of Medicine, Duke University Medical Center, Durham, North Carolina, U.S.A.

*Hein J. J. Wellens, Dept. of Cardiology, Medical Faculty, University of Limburg, St. Annadal Hospital, Maastricht, The Netherlands.

Thomas L. Wenger, Dept. of Medicine, Duke University Medical Center, Durham, North Carolina, U.S.A.

Eberhard Wiebringhaus, First Medical Clinic B, University of Düsseldorf, Düsseldorf, Germany.

Delon Wu, Abraham Lincoln School of Medicine, University of Illinois, Chicago, Illinois, U.S.A.

Christopher Wyndham, Abraham Lincoln School of Medicine, University of Illinois, Chicago, Illinois, U.S.A.

Kaoru Yanagihara, Dept. of Physiology, School of Medicine, Hiroshima University, Hiroshima, Japan.

*Iwao Yamaguchi, Dept. of Cardiology, Cedars-Sinai Medical Center, Los Angeles, California, U.S.A.

Ho Siew Yen, Dept. of Paediatrics, Cardiothoracic Institute, Brompton Hospital, London, United Kingdom.

* active participants of the workshop

SECTION ONE

FUNCTION AND DYSFUNCTION OF THE SINUS NODE

FUNCTION AND DYSFUNCTION OF THE SINUS NODE: CLINICAL STUDIES IN THE EVALUATION OF SINUS NODE FUNCTION*

JAY L. JORDAN, IWAO YAMAGUCHI, AND WILLIAM J. MANDEL**

The sick sinus syndrome is a descriptive term coined by Lown (1966) and popularized by Ferrer (1968), referring to a constellation of clinical signs, symptoms, and electrocardiographic (ECG) criteria defining sinus node dysfunction. The syndrome is characterized by syncope or other manifestations of cerebral dysfunction in association with sinus brady-cardia, sinus arrest, sinoatrial block, alternating bradyarrhythmias and tachyarrhythmias and/or carotid hypersensitivity. Clinical signs and symptoms, however, result from failure of escape pacemaker function not from sinus node malfunction per se (Mandel and Laks, 1974); thus, the sick sinus syndrome may represent a generalized disorder of the conduction system.

The incidence of sinus node dysfunction is unknown. Limited information suggests that in cardiac patients, the incidence of sinus node dysfunction is approximately 3 in 5000 (Kulbertus et al., 1973). Between 6.3% and 24% of all patients with permanent pacemakers being followed in pacemaker clinics have sinus node disease (Rasmussen, 1971; Conde et al., 1973; Sigurd et al., 1973; Rokseth and Hatle, 1974; Radford and Julian, 1974; Sowton 1974; Hartel and Talvensaari, 1975). However, in the past five years, abnormalities of sinus node function may have been the primary indication for permanent pacing in as many as 50% of permanently paced patients. Men and women appear to be equally affected by disturbances of sinus node function (Rubenstein et al., 1972). Age distribution is bimodal with peaks occurring in the third and fourth decades of life and again in the sixties and seventies (Rubenstein et al., 1972). The majority of patients in the older age group have co-existing hypertensive or coronary heart disease (Rubenstein et al., 1972; Wan et al., 1972; Moss and Davis, 1974).

Many etiologic factors have been implicated in the sick sinus syndrome; (Cohn and Lewis, 1912, 1913; James, 1961; Fraser et al., 1964; Ward, 1964; Barks et al., 1964; Spellberg, 1971; Metzger et al., 1971; Davies and Pomerance, 1972; Kaplin et al., 1973; Rockseth and Hatle, 1974). The most frequent anatomic findings in sick sinus patients are coronary atherosclerosis, atrial amyloidosis and diffuse fibrosis. The syndrome has also been described in association with other infiltrative disorders, collagen-vascular diseases, infectious processes, as a familial pattern and in pericardial disease. Drug-induced abnormalities of sinus node function are frequently recognized. Perhaps the most common form of the sick sinus syndrome is the idiopathic variety.

* This work was supported in part by NIH Grant no. 17651.
** Milly Factor Clinical Investigator of the Western Cardiac Foundation.

ATRIAL OVERDRIVE

Transient arrest of spontaneous sinus node activity follows cessation of overdrive atrial pacing as an apparent physiologic event. In general, patients with sinus node dysfunction demonstrate longer periods of sinus arrest than do normals (Figure 1A). The mechanism(s) by which overdrive pacing suppresses pacemaker automaticity has been the subject of much speculation. Two general hypotheses have been promulgated: 1) suppression is mediated by the release of autonomic neurotransmitters and/or; 2) overdrive pacing directly disrupts intrinsic mechanisms of pacemaker automaticity (Lange, 1965; Scher et al., 1959; Amory and West, 1962; Vincenzi and West, 1963; Lu et al., 1965; Jordan et al., 1977d).

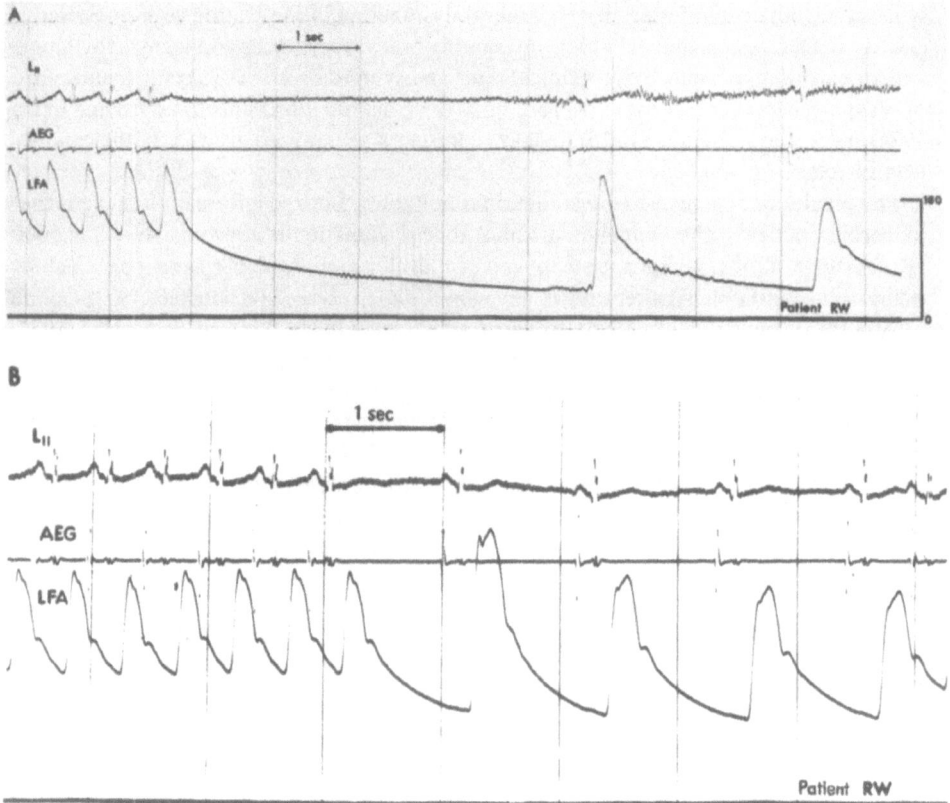

Figure 1. Panel A demonstrates the effect of high right atrial overdrive on sinus node function. The traces are, from above downward: a lead II electrocardiogram, an atrial electrogram and the left femoral artery blood pressure with its calibrations seen to the right of the panel. Four driven beats at a rate of 130 per minute are seen to the left of the panel. Following termination of the pacing, a greater than 5 second electrical arrest is noted which is terminated by a sinus beat (the sinus node recovery time) and subsequent marked sinus bradycardia.

Panel B shows the same patient following the intravenous administration of atropine. The traces are identical to panel A. Six driven beats are seen followed by termination of the pacing. Now a pause just in excess of one second is noted with restoration of sinus rhythm at a rate of 55 per minute.

Atrial overdrive does result in a release of autonomic neurotransmitters from storage sites within myocardial tissue and nerve endings (Amory and West, 1962; Vincenzi and West, 1963; Furchgott et al., 1959). Assuming that there is a net release of a negative chronotropic neurotransmitter, presumably acetycholine, suppression of sinus node automaticity may indeed be mediated by this neurohumoral agent. Vagal stimulation or acetycholine administration do infact prolong sinus node recovery (Brooks and Lu, 1972).

Catecholamine release may play a role in post-overdrive electrophysiologic events as suggested by the observation that the often-seen post-overdrive acceleration of sinus rate can be abolished by reserpine or propranolol pre-treatment (Lu et al., 1965; Brooks and Lu, 1972): this phase is not seen with subsidiary pacemakers (Jordan et al., 1977b). More-over, isoproterenol infusion results in a predictable shortening of the sinus node recovery time (Brooks and Lu, 1972). Nevertheless, in the intact human heart, overdrive suppression takes place in the milieu of extrinsic autonomic tone as well as under the influence of locally released autonomic neurotransmitters.

Intracardiac pacing is performed in the cardiac catheterization laboratory in the fasting state. All cardiac drugs and medications known to interfere with sinus node or autonomic neural function are withdrawn 48 hours or 2 half-lives prior to the study. Mild sedation is achieved with Seconal 100 mg orally given 30 minutes in advance of the procedure. After local anesthesia has been achieved, a quadripolar pacing catheter is positioned at the high right atrium. Electrocardiographic leads I, II and III, as well as an intra-atrial electrogram are monitored on a photographic oscillographic recorder. Atrial pacing is performed at a milliamperage two times the diastolic threshold. An initial intra-atrial pacing rate of approximately 20 beats/minute faster than the patient's resting heart rate is chosen with increments of 20 beats/minute in succeeding pacing trials up to a rate of 170 beats/minute. Pacing is continued for 30, 60 and 180 seconds at each pacing rate and abruptly terminated; sixty second is allowed to elapse between each pacing trial. The sinus node recovery time (SNRT) is measured in milliseconds as the time elapsing from the last paced P-wave to the first spontaneous depolarization on the intra-atrial electrogram. The shape of the P-wave is noted to confirm that the complex ending the sinus pause is indeed sinoatrial in origin. Furthermore, the sinus node recovery time is corrected for the spontaneous sinus cycle length (SCL): CSNRT = SNRT − SCL (Chadda et al., 1975).

Reported SNRT values for normals include: 1400 msec, (Rosen et al., 1971); 1040 ± 56 msec (M ± SEM) (Mandel et al., 1971). Reported normal CSNRT values range from 450 msec (Jordan et al., 1977a) to 525 msec (Narula et al., 1972).

In man and animals SNRT increases only slightly as the pacing rate increases. However, at rapid rates (> 130 beats/min) SNRT decreases somewhat (Mandel et al., 1971) (Figure 2A). This phenomenon is thought to be a consequence of sino-atrial entrace block (Goldreyer and Damato, 1971). This finding supports the theory that overdrive pacing exerts an effect on pacemaker automaticity by direct disruption of intrinsic mechanisms and emphasizes the importance of pacing at multiple rates (Strauss et al., 1976b). In contrast, subsidiary pacemakers demonstrate significant proportional increases in recovery time with increasing pacing rates (Jordan et al., 1977b) (Figure 2B).

Most normals demonstrate little correlation between duration of pacing and SNRT. The correlation in sick sinus patients is variable. Subsidiary pacemakers generally show a positive correlation between pacing duration and recovery time (Jordan et al., 1977b): this finding may reflect different mechanisms mediating overdrive suppression in different pacemaker sites.

The proximity of the pacing catheter to the intrinsic pacemaker being studied appears

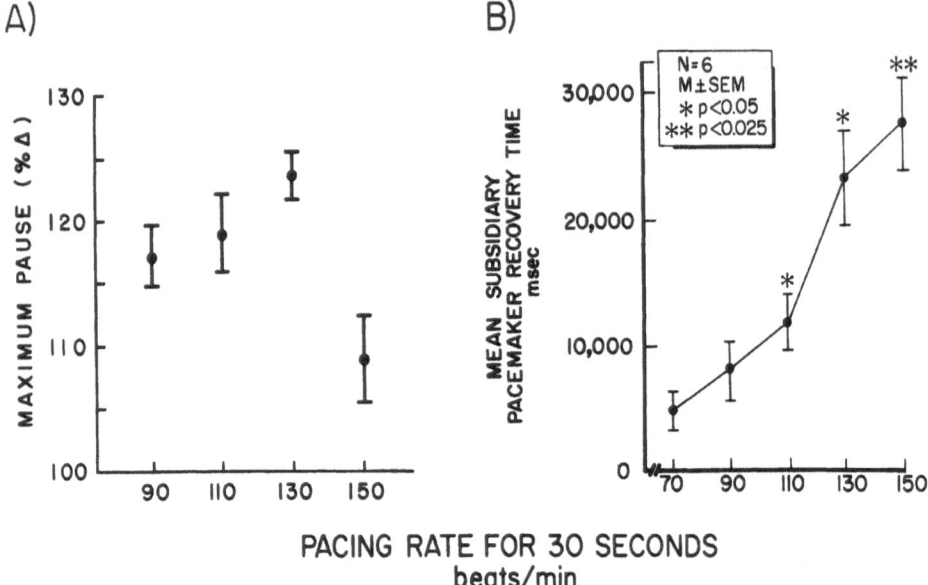

Figure 2. The effect of pacing rate on sinus node recovery time. In panel A, the effects of overdrive pacing for 30 seconds at rates of 90, 110, 130, and 150 per minute on sinus node recovery time are shown. Recovery times increased at rates of 90 to 130 with a sharp fall off seen at 150 per minute. This latter finding may, in part, be related to sino-atrial entrance block due to rapid pacing rates.

In panel B, subsidiary pacemakers were subjected to overdrive using rates from 70 to 150 per minute. In these studies, a progressive increase in the recovery time was observed with increasing driving rates.

to be an important determinant of the magnitude of the overdrive suppression. Ventricular pacing results in less depression of AV junctional pacemakers than does atrial pacing and even less suppression of the sinus node (Lange, 1965); suppression of Purkinje fiber automaticity is best achieved by ventricular pacing (Brooks and Lu, 1972). Variations in pacing amperage effect no significant change in SNRT or CSNRT (Mandel et al., 1971; Chadda et al., 1975).

In normal subjects, the uncorrected sinus node recovery time prolongs in a linear fashion with longer resting sinus cycle lengths. However, at abnormally slow heart rates, the recovery time generally becomes disproportionately prolonged (Mandel et al., 1971; Kulbertus et al., 1975) (Figure 3).

It has been shown that the sinus node recovery time in children and in elderly normals is not significantly different from mean values in the general population (Kulbertus et al., 1975; Okimoto et al., 1976; Yabek et al., 1976). The pacing rate at which there is a sudden decrease in SNRT seems to be slower in elderly individuals, suggesting that sinoatrial entrance block occurs at a slower rate (Kulbertus et al., 1975). This phenomenon may represent differential aging of the perinodal zone.

Generally, sick sinus patients with marked sinus arrest (five seconds or longer) and CNS symptoms have relatively longer CSNRT than asymptomatic patients with sinus arrest of lesser magnitude. However, frequent exceptions suggest that there is no linear relationship between the magnitude of sinus bradycardia or sinus arrest and the duration of CSNRT.

Furthermore, relationships between SA block or the bradycardia-tachycardia syndrome

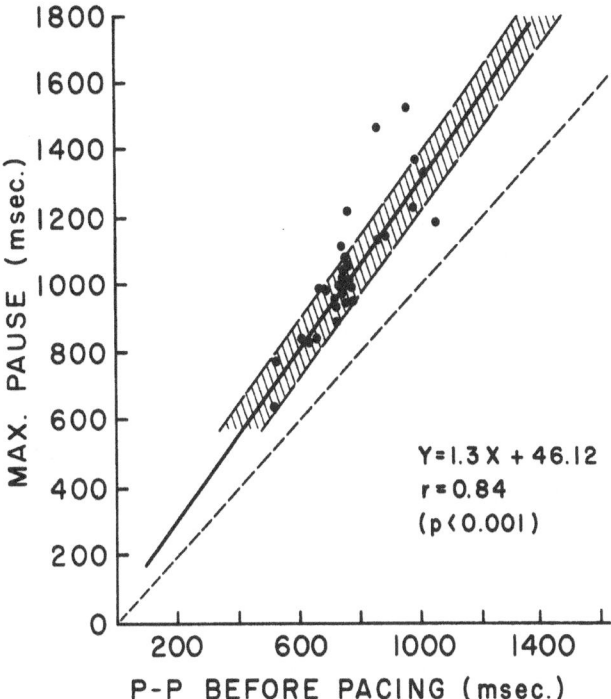

Figure 3. The effect of sinus rate on sinus node recovery time. The horizontal axis identified the basic sinus cycle length and the vertical axis identifies the sinus node recovery time in milliseconds (maximum pause). Note that a linear relationship exist between the sinus cycle length and the maximum pause with slight deviation seen from the regression line at the longest sinus cycle length.

and SNRT abnormalities have been disputed (Okimoto et al., 1976). Atherosclerosis of the sinus node artery is not associated with abnormalities of sinus node recovery time (Engel et al., 1975). SNRT and CSNRT have been shown to be reproducible whether pacing is performed on consecutive days or at an interval of many months (Narula et al., 1972; Chadda et al., 1975; Okimoto et al., 1976). Limited information suggests that sick sinus patients with abnormalities of AV nodal or intraventricular conduction may have a greater incidence of abnormal SNRT than patients without distal conduction abnormalities (Okimoto et al., 1976; Rosen et al., 1971).

Little information exists on the effect of antiarrhythmic drugs and other cardioactive agents on sinus node recovery time. Interpretation of results, however, must be made with the recognition that acute drug administration may have different effects than chronic oral therapy.

Acute ouabain administration has been observed to shorten SNRT in normals and in sick sinus patients (Engel and Schaal, 1973; Dhingra et al., 1975b). On the other hand, in denervated transplanted human hearts, Goodman et al. (1975) found that ouabain prolonged SNRT in three of six cases and had no effect in the remainder.

Strauss et al. (1976a) found that propranolol 0.1 mg/kg had no significant effect on CSNRT in the sick sinus syndrome.

Verapamil causes a prolongation of the corrected sinus node recovery time in isolated atrial preparations (Konisai, 1976). The effect of Verapamil on sinus node response to intra-atrial pacing in man has not yet been examined.

Seipel et al. (1974) reported that intravenous injections of the following drugs resulted in statistically significant prolongation of the uncorrected sinus node recovery time: Sparteine 3–4 mg/kg (13% prolongation); Ajmaline 1–1.5 mg/kg (15%); Antazoline 2-3 mg/kg (13%); Aprindine 1.5–2.5 mg/kg (16%).

Recently, the value of the sinus node recovery time as a diagnostic tool in the sick sinus syndrome has been questioned. Specifically, not all sick sinus patients demonstrate abnormal prolongation of the sinus node recovery time (Gupta et al., 1974). However, to expect the sinus node recovery time to be prolonged in all cases of the sick sinus syndrome, presupposes that overdrive pacing tests a common underlying pathophysiologic mechanism. Based on our knowledge of the large number of potential determinants of sinus node automaticity and overdrive suppression, it is unlikely that the sick sinus syndrome is a homogeneous entity in terms of pathophysiologic mechanisms.

Normal sinus node function is dependent upon a complex and delicately balanced interaction between intrinsic sinus node electrophysiologic properties, sinoatrial conduction properties and factors extrinsic to the sinoatrial region. Among the extrinsic factors, the role of the autonomic nervous system is perhaps most important. Considering that abnormalities of different intrinsic electrophysiologic properties of sinus node automaticity may be differentially influenced directly by overdrive pacing and that pacing takes place at different levels of autonomic activity, it is not surprising that all patients with the sick sinus syndrome do not demonstrate abnormal prolongation of the sinus node recovery time.

Based on observations that many sick sinus patients have blunted sinus rate acceleration to the administration of atropine and that atropine shortens the sinus node recovery time in normals, this drug has been employed to distinguish sick sinus patients with intrinsic sinus node disease from those with abnormally exaggerated parasympathetic influences, (Dhingra et al., 1976b). The effects of atropine on the sinus node recovery time is variable in sick sinus patients, shortening it in some, having no effect in others and paradoxically prolonging it in a small number (Figure 1B) (Bashour et al., 1973; Reiffel et al., 1975; Dhingra et al., 1976b). These different results may represent differences in residual parasympathetic tone which must be accounted for before comparing the effect of parasympathetic blockade on sinus node recovery time in different individuals. Differences in resting sympathetic tone, now unopposed in the post-atropine state, also must be taken into account.

The problems associated with determining normal values for post-propranolol SNRT are similar to those discussed for atropine. Standards for completeness of sympathetic blockade must be established. Differences in unopposed parasympathetic tone must be taken into account.

Most of the disadvantages of separate atropine and propranolol administration can be overcome by their simultaneous administration and determination of intrinsic heart rate at the time of overdrive pacing. Complete autonomic blockade can be achieved utilizing a modification of the protocol of Jose and Collison (1970). Propranolol 0.2 mg/kg is administered intravenously at a rate of 1 mg/min. Ten minutes thereafter, atropine sulfate 0.04 mg/kg is administered intravenously over two minutes. The resultant sinus rate is the observed intrinsic heart rate (IHR). The dose of propranolol used abolishes the positive beta-adrenergic effects of large doses of isoproterenol for approximately 20 minutes. After atropine has been administered, the intrinsic heart rate remains stable for approximately 30 minutes. Therefore, within the physiologic range, functional autonomic blockade appears to be complete.

Utilizing the technique of intrinsic heart rate determination, sick sinus patients with intrinsic sinus node dysfunction can be distinguished from those patients with disturbed autonomic regulation of sinus node function. Since the observed intrinsic heart rate is theoretically dependent upon only intrinsic electrophysiologic properties of sinus node automaticity, an abnormal IHR reflects an abnormality of one or more of these intrinsic properties. In contrast, when the heart rate is normal after autonomic blockade, it follows that disturbed autonomic regulation is most likely the underlying mechanism responsible for the manifestations of sinus node dysfunction.

In our unit, intrinsic heart rates have been determined in 17 patients with symptomatic sinus bradycardia. Overdrive pacing was performed before and following autonomic blockade. These studies indicate that: 1) sick sinus patients demonstrating normal sinus node recovery times (< 450 msec) adjusted for the magnitude and direction of autonomic chronotropy consistently have normal intrinsic heart rates and, therefore, abnormalities of autonomic regulation of sinus node function; 2) sick sinus patients demonstrating abnormal sinus node recovery times consistently have abnormal intrinsic heart rates and, therefore, abnormalities of intrinsic sinus node function. Exceptions to these results may be proven to exist in the future. However, the technique does improve the sensitivity and specificity of the sinus node recovery time as well as clarify mechanisms of sinus node dysfunction in the sick sinus syndrome.

In patients with normal intrinsic heart rates, there does not appear to be a correlation between the duration of overdrive pacing and the magnitude of CSNRT (Jordan et al., 1977b). However, preliminary observations suggest that patients with abnormal intrinsic heart rates may show progressively longer recovery times with longer durations of pacing. Recognizing this phenomenon as an abnormal response to overdrive pacing could potentially further increase the sensitivity of the technique.

In the normal patient, the sinus cycles following the first recovery sinus beat are either shorter (secondary acceleration) or initially longer than the basic sinus cycle with gradual but progressive return to the basic sinus cycle length. In some sick sinus patients, the P-P interval immediately following cessation of pacing is not the longest, nor even abnormally prolonged, but is followed by longer P-P intervals (Figure 4). This secondary suppression may persist for 10 to 20 beats or more. Instances of secondary suppression have been occasionally reported in sick sinus patients but not in normal patients. Secondary suppression should properly be considered an abnormal sinus node response to overdrive pacing (Strauss et al., 1976; Okimoto et al., 1976), and another observation that could potentially increase the sensitivity of the technique in the diagnosis of sinus node dysfunction.

PREMATURE ATRIAL STIMULATION

Analysis of sinus node responses to premature atrial depolarizations has revealed important electrophysiologic features of normal and abnormal sinus node function and sinoatrial conduction (Bonke et al., 1969 and 1971; Klein et al., 1973; Strauss et al., 1973). Utilizing methods similar to that described in the section on sinus node recovery times, premature atrial stimuli are introduced in late diastole during spontaneous sinus rhythm after every eighth beat at progressively decreasing coupling intervals (in 10 msec increments). In this fashion, the sinus cycle length is scanned until atrial capture is lost.

Four types of sinus node responses to atrial premature depolarizations (APD), dependent on the timing of the APD in the sinus cycle (A_1 -A_1) and whether the APD retrogradely

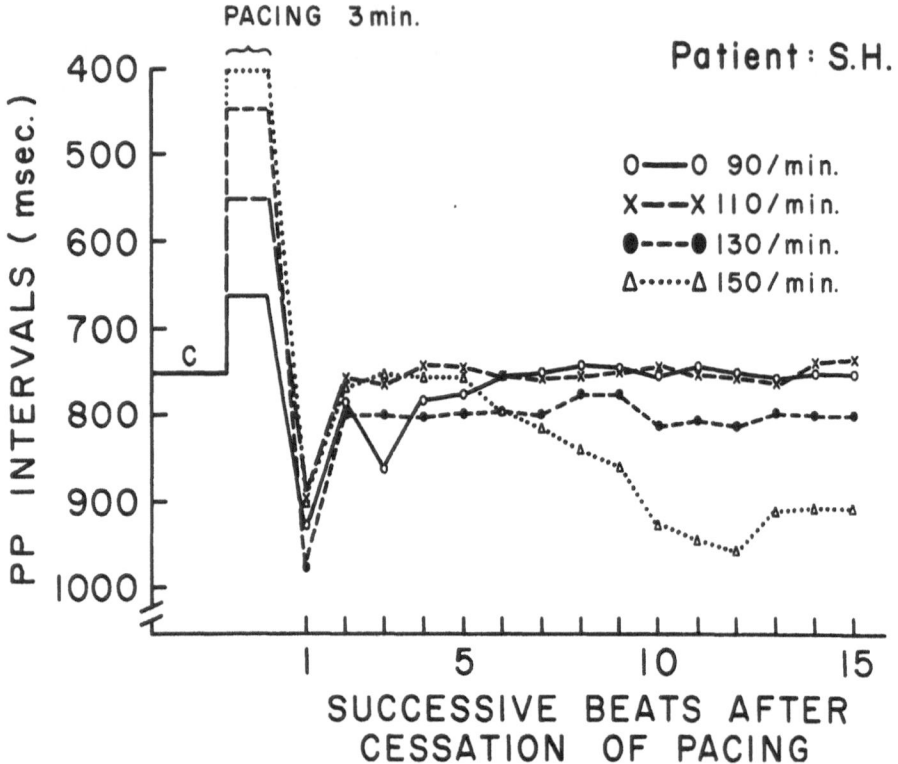

Figure 4. Secondary pauses observed following overdrive pacing. The horizontal axis illustrates successive beats following termination of pacing. The vertical axis illustrates the PP intervals in milliseconds. Overdrive pacing was performed at rates of 90, 110, 130 and 150 per minute for 3 minute periods. Although sinus node recovery times were within the normal range, subsequent prominent sinus bradycardia was observed following pacing at a rate of 150 per minute (secondary suppression).

penetrates the sinus node, have been identified: 1) Compensation resulting from a late diastolic extrastimulus that fails to depolarize the sinus node because of collision with the normal sinus depolarization; 2) reset, reproduced by premature depolarization of the sinus node by the extrastimulus resulting in an A_2-A_3 interval of shorter duration than a compensatory pause; 3) interpolation, produced by failure of the extrastimulus to enter the sinus node, but not causing a barrier to conduction to the atrium of the next sinus impulse; 4) reentry which results from reflection of the extrasystole, producing an early "sinus" depolarization (Figures 5, 6).

Identification of a perinodal zone of tissue in the right atrium of the rabbit by Strauss and Bigger (1972), has contributed significantly to our understanding of the above events. The perinodal cells have electrophysiologic characteristics distinct from atrial muscle and sinus node cells and may represent a potential conduction barrier.

The fibers of the sinoatrial node and perinodal zone share some electrophysiologic properties with AV junctional tissue. Specifically, the depolarization velocity of the action potential of an APD progressively slows as the extrasystole is delivered earlier in diastole, exhibiting decremental conduction (Pasmooij et al., 1976; Hoffman and Cranefield, 1960).

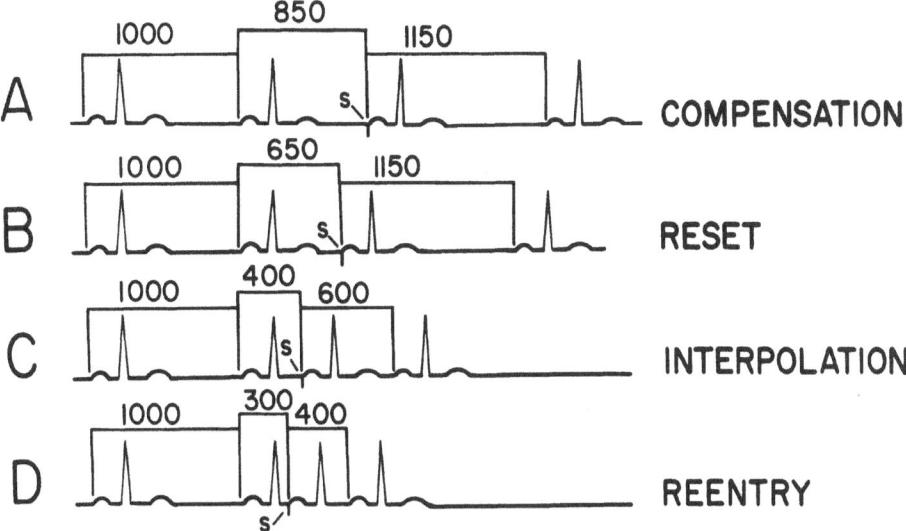

Figure 5. The types of sinus node response to atrial premature depolarizations. In panel A, the effect of a late diastolic extrasystole is seen. The basic sinus cycle length is 1000 msec. The premature beat occurs at a coupling interval of 850 msec (85% of control) and is followed by a sinus beat after a pause of 1150 msec (115% of control). The atrial extrasystole did not depolarize the sinus node and the next sinus beat occurred on time. Therefore, 850 + 1150 = 2000 msec, or two times the basic sinus cycle length. In panel B, the more frequently observed phenomenon of sinus node reset following atrial premature systoles is demonstrated. Here the atrial extrasystole is initiated at coupling interval of 650 msec (65% of control). The next sinus beat occurs, as in panel A, after 1150 msec (115% of control). However, the two intervals add up to less than two spontaneous sinus cycles (650 + 1150 = 1800 msec). Therefore, the sinus node has been depolarized by the extrasystole causing the next spontaneous sinus depolarization to occur earlier. In panel C, an even earlier premature depolarization is demonstrated (400 msec: 40% of control). The next sinus beat occurs very early (600 msec). However, the two intervals (400 + 600 msec) add up to a normal spontaneous sinus cycle indicating that the extrasystole did not alter the normal sinus discharge rate. Therefore, the extrasystole was interpolated. In panel D, the most unusual situation is depicted. A very early atrial extrasystole is initiated (300 msec: 30% of control) and is followed by an early spontaneous discharge. Note that the sum of two intervals (300 + 400 msec) is less than the spontaneous sinus cycle length. Furthermore, the first beat after the extrasystole has a normal P wave morphology. This phenomenon is considered to represent reentry of the extrastimulus utilizing the perinodal zone, i.e., a sinus node echo.

Moreover, an APD may be completely blocked in the retrograde direction within the perinodal zone or within the sinoatrial node if it encounters these tissues in the absolute refractory period of excitability (Goldreyer and Damato, 1971; Bonke et al., 1971; Klein et al., 1973; Strauss and Bigger, 1972).

The phenomenon of the compensatory pause seen when APD's are introduced late in the sinus cycle may be attributed to the electrophysiologic properties of the perinodal zone because the APD does not penetrate or disturb the sinus node and the subsequent sinus beat occurs on time. If the perinodal zone is abnormal, as might be the case in the sick sinus syndrome, the zone of compensation may be expected to occupy a greater percentage of the sinus cycle than in patients with normal perinodal tissue. Thus, even earlier APD's would encounter the exiting sinus beat in the perinodal zone. These events form the electrophysiologic basis of first degree sinoatrial block, a common manifestation of the sick sinus syndrome (Scherf, 1969; Rasmussen 1971, (Figure 7).

During a portion of the zone of sinus node reset, the postextrasystolic pause (A_2-A_3)

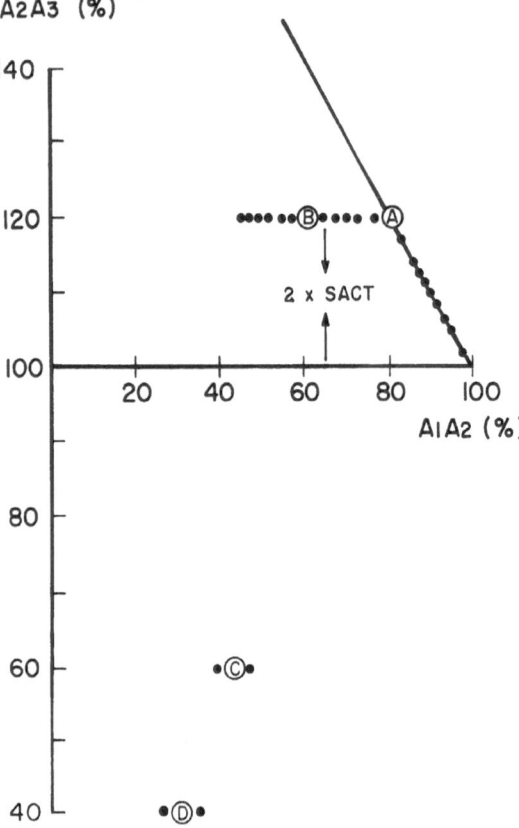

Figure 6. The effect of progressively premature atrial depolarizations on sinus function. This figure shows, on the horizontal axis, a plot of the A_1-A_2 intervals (test cycle length) expressed as a percentage of the basal heart rate (A_1-A_1 interval). On the vertical axis is plotted the A_2-A_3 interval (return cycle) again as a percentage of the basal heart rate. The oblique line to the right of the figure identifies the line which would represent a compensatory response. Point A demonstrates the effect of a late diastolic atrial premature depolarization with the coupling interval of 85% of control. The resultant return cycle would be fully compensatory. Point B demonstrates the effect of earlier premature atrial depolarization at 65% of the control sinus rate. This point identifies a zone in which premature atrial depolarizations will cause sinus node reset; the resultant A_3 will be less than compensatory. Point C identifies a short coupling interval, i.e., 40% of the control sinus cycle length. The return cycle length occurs at the time a normal sinus P would occur; the premature depolarization was interpolated. Point D indicates a very short coupling interval, i.e., 30% with a resultant return cycle that is *less than* that expected for an interpolated response. This is consistent with sinus node reentry (see Figure 5). Sino-atrial conduction time can be calculated from measurements of the A_2-A_3 responses during the early period of reset (see text).

lengthens progressively as the premature beat is elicited earlier in the midportion of the atrial cycle. Three mechanisms of this lengthening have been proposed: 1) a progressive slowing of the conduction velocity of the premature impulse and/or 2) a temporary depression of rhythmicity of sinus node pacemaker cells, (Bonke et al., 1969; Klein et al., 1973; Strauss et al., 1973; Engel et al., 1976); and 3) intra-SA nodal pacemaker shifts (Bonke et al., 1969). In patients with abnormalities of sinoatrial conduction, the zone of reset theoretically occupies less of the sinus cycle than in normals, (Masini et al., 1975) (Figure 7).

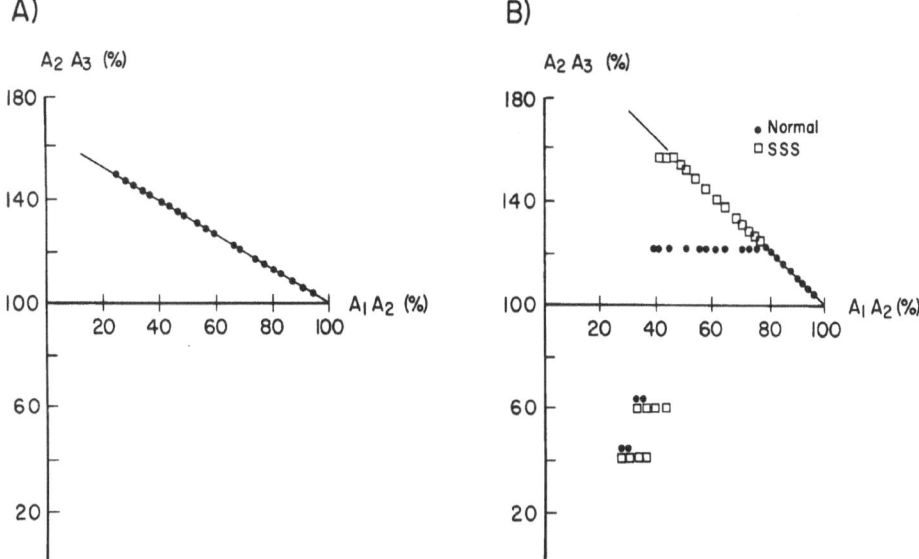

Figure 7. Hypothetical responses anticipated in patients with sinus node dysfunction. Panel A showed a plot of series of atrial premature depolarizations (horizontal axis) which persistently result in points which fall along the line of identity, i.e., compensatory-like responses. This would identify a patient with first degree SA block.

In panel B, the open squares identify responses which might be anticipated in the sinus node disease patients whereas the filled circles identify the normal response (see Figure 6). In the sinus node dysfunction patients, a marked prolongation of the zone of compensation indicates entrance delay. A shortened zone of reset with a marked increase in SA conduction time is associated with a longer zone of interpolation and reentry (see Figure 6).

Very early APD's may find a portion of the perinodal zone and sinus node recovered sufficiently from the previous spontaneous sinus beat to enter these tissues. However, retrograde conduction would be markedly slowed, allowing other portions of the sinus node and perinodal zone to recovery excitability. Such an electrophysiologic circumstance would allow for sinus node reentry. Theoretically, abnormalities of the sinoatrial region should increase the probability of sinus node reentry (Figure 7) and the occurrence of atrial arrhythmias (Han et al., 1968; Childers et al., 1973; Paulay et al., 1973a and b; Paritsky et al., 1974; Strauss et al., 1974, Narula, 1974). These events may be the underlying electrophysiologic bases for the observed increased frequency of occurrence of supraventricular tachyarrhythmias in the sick sinus syndrome.

In 1962, Langendorf and co-workers, deduced some of the functional characteristics of conduction between the sinoatrial node and the atrium from an analysis of the surface electrocardiogram in a patient with atrial parasystole. Based on their clinical observations and the experimental observations of Bonke and co-workers (1969), Strauss et al. (1973) described a technique of assessing sinoatrial conduction utilizing programmed atrial stimulation. The calculation of the sino-atrial conduction time (SACT) assumes that the difference between the mean return cycle length (A_2-A_3) in the zone of sinus node reset and the spontaneous sinus cycle length (A_1-A_1) is equal to the time required for the APD to retrogradely conduct through the perinodal zone plus the time required for the reset sinus impulse to traverse the perinodal zone antegradely and enter the atrium. An abnormally prolonged SACT is compatable with first degree sinoatrial block, a characteristic of some patients with sick sinus syndrome (Strauss et al., 1973 and 1976a; Scheinman et al., 1973; Bigger, 1974; Hirschfeld et al., 1975; Mandel et al., 1975; Dhingra et al., 1977; Breithardt et al., 1977) (Figure 7).

However, this method requires certain assumptions: 1) all APD's resulting in a post-extrasystolic pause that is less than compensatory must reset the sinus node, 2) APD's must not depress sinus node automaticity, an event that would cause an overestimation of SACT, 3) antegrade and retrograde conduction must be equally influenced by an APD, 4) SACT must be independent of variations in spontaneous sinus rate, a phenomenon common to many patients with sinus node dysfunction, 5) the velocity of retrograde sinoatrial conduction must be independent of the site of atrial stimulation.

In isolated tissue, Miller and Strauss (1974), demonstrated that the transition between compensatory and less than compensatory postextrasystolic pauses included APD's that did not penetrate and reset the sinus node. Shortening of the sinus node return cycle in these cases was due to a shortening of the sinus node action potential by electrotonic inter-action between sinus node and adjacent cells during repolarization. This artifactual shortening of the return cycle resulted in underestimation of the actual sinoatrial conduction time.

APD's delivered in the middle of the sinus cycle in animal hearts may depress sinus node automaticity and cause pacemaker shifts (Bonke et al., 1969). However, differences of opinion do exist concerning the magnitude of the influence of depressed pacemaker auto-maticity on estimated SACT in man (Engel et al., 1976; Breithardt and Seipel, 1976).

Miller and Strauss (1974) noted that measured antegrade and retrograde conduction times are not equal, retrograde conduction usually being faster than antegrade conduction. In addition, SACT appears to vary as a function of the spontaneous sinus cycle length (Denes et al., 1974; Reiffel et al., 1974); at slower heart rates estimated SACT is shorter than at faster heart rates.

Finally, Yamaguchi and Mandel (1977), have recently demonstrated that the speed of retrograde conduction of an APD does depend on the site of atrial stimulation (Table 1). This observation may relate to the existence of specialized functional pathways of conduction between the sinus node and the atrium (Sano and Yamagishi, 1965).

Despite these inherent problems, the method of Strauss et al., has proven itself to be a valuable addition to the diagnostic modalities available for evaluation of sinus node dysfunction. Differentiation between abnormalities of sinus node generator function and impulse conduction is now potentially possible.

Reported ranges of normal values for calculated sinoatrial conduction time in patients without apparent sinus node dysfunction include: 56 ± 22 msec (Steinbeck and Lüderitz, 1975), 70 ± 30 msec (Masini et al., 1975), 82 ± 19.2 msec (Breithardt et al., 1977), 84.5 ± 26 msec (Engel et al., 1976), 88 ± 7 msec (Jordan et al., 1977c) and 92 ± 60 msec (Dhingra et al., 1975a). However, many of these patients had evidence of organic heart disease, some with abnormalities of the distal conduction system, many with ischemic heart disease and others with valvular abnormalities. Jordan and co-workers (1977c) reported that patients with atherosclerotic involvement of the sinus node artery and no clinical or electrocardio-graphic evidence for sinus node dysfunction have significantly longer (although "normal") SACT values than coronary artery disease patients without such lesions. Similar differences in SACT may eventually be found in patients without apparent sinus node dysfunction dependent on other underlying pathologic processes. The important point is that pro-gression of sinoatrial disease to the stage of overt clinical and electrocardiographic mani-festations may be a dynamic, but gradual process.

Table 1. Sinoatrial conduction times and transition points during crista terminalis, coronary sinus and atrial septal stimulation.

	Crista terminalis	Coronary sinus	Atrial septum
Retrograde conduction time msec	19.7 ± 1.1	18.6 ± 1.6	15.7 ± 1.0***
Antegrade conduction time msec	$32.5 \pm 2.6^{\Delta\Delta\Delta}$	$33.5 \pm 2.6^{\Delta\Delta\Delta}$	$34.7 \pm 2.8^{\Delta\Delta\Delta}$*
Total measured conduction time msec	52.2 ± 3.3	52.1 ± 4.1	50.4 ± 3.0
Estimated conduction time msec	57.8 ± 6.3	66.4 ± 10.7	43.6 ± 4.8**
Transition point %	83.6 ± 1.2	83.0 ± 1.9	88.7 ± 0.9

Values are: Mean $\pm$ SEM.
N = 18.
* = significantly different from crista terminalis stimulation.
Δ = significantly different from retrograde conduction time.
$^\Delta$ *p < 0.05.
$^{\Delta\Delta}$ **p < 0.01.
$^{\Delta\Delta\Delta}$ ***p < 0.005.

Furthermore, as sinus node recovery time may be influenced by differences in autonomic tone, so may SACT be modified by changes in autonomic activity. Bonke et al. (1969) and Klein et al. (1973), could demonstrate no effect of atropine on sinoatrial conduction. Miller and Strauss (1974) found that shortening of the sinus node action potential by APD's was not affected by atropine or propranolol. However, in 17 normal human subjects, Dhingra et al. (1976a), reported a significant shortening of calculated SACT following 1–2 mg of atropine (from 103 ± 5.7 msec to 58 ± 3.9 msec) as well as a shortening of the zone of non-rest.

That SACT is shortened in man by atropine independent of any change in heart rate is suggested by the observation that the return cycle following an APD shortened to a greater extent than did the sinus cycle length (Dhingra et al., 1976a). In keeping with a hypothesis that atropine facilitates perinodal conduction, this drug has been shown to eliminate interpolation and echo responses in some individuals (Dhingra et al., 1976a). Techniques for lengthening the perinodal refractory period, such as pacing the atrium at a rate faster than the sinus rate, have been shown to increase the number of normals with zones of interpolation and reentry (Dhingra et al., 1975a).

The effect of atropine on SACT in patients with sinus node dysfunction is variable. Some sick sinus patients have marked shortening of SACT following atropine while others have only minimal shortening (Dhingra et al., 1976b; Breithardt et al., 1976). The mean pre- and post-atropine SACT in 21 sick sinus patients was not significantly different than the mean post-atropine SACT in 17 patients without evidence for sinus node dysfunction (Dhingra et al., 1976a and b). Individual sick sinus patients who do show significant shortening of SACT following atropine may have lower levels of resting parasympathetic activity and therefore less residual parasympathetic tone following similar doses of atropine. Alternatively, these patients may have greater resting sympathetic activity than patients failing to demonstrate SACT shortening. Finally, these patients may have no abnormalities of intrinsic electrophysiologic properties of sinoatrial conduction, their sinus node dysfunction being primarily a manifestation of abnormal autonomic control of sinoatrial conduction.

Dhingra et al. (1976b) did not find an overall shortening of the zone of non-reset following atropine nor a lengthening of the zone of sinus reset in sick sinus patients. Similarly, interpolation and echo responses were unaffected by atropine in these patients.

Strauss et al. (1976a) found that propranolol (1 mg/kg) significantly lengthened SACT in sick sinus patients, however, effects on sinus node automaticity may have contributed to this finding.

The incidence of abnormal prolongation of calculated SACT in 418 patients without evidence of sinus node dysfunction was found to be 2% by Dhingra et al. (1977). However, these investigators used an SACT of 152 msec as their criterium for abnormal, a figure considerably greater than other investigators have used. Therefore, their number of "false positives" may be spuriously low. This high cutoff value for normals may also explain their low incidence of abnormal SACT found in suspected cases of sinus node dysfunction (29% of 52 cases). Breithardt et al. (1977) reported that 45% of 41 patients with a variety of manifestations of sinus dysfunction had prolonged SACT when 120 msec was used as the upper limit of normal. Utilizing a normal value of 215 msec for total antegrade plus retrograde conduction, Strauss et al. (1976) reported that 38% of 16 patients with sinus node dysfunction demonstrated an abnormally long total SACT.

Recently, Breithardt et al. (1977) attempted to correlate prolongation of SACT and SNRT with specific electrocardiographic abnormalities in sick sinus patients. Patients with asymptomatic sinus bradycardia did not have significantly longer CSNRT or SACT values than controls, whereas patients with symptoms did. Patients with the bradycardia-tachycardia syndrome and/or episodic sinoatrial block demonstrated significantly longer SNRT values than controls, although SACT in the bradycardia-tachycardia group did not differ from controls. SNRT was found to be a somewhat more sensitive measure than SACT, showing fewer false negative results in patients with sinus node dysfunction. Nonetheless, SACT determination proved to be a better method of distinguishing sick sinus patients from normals than had previously been reported (Narula et al., 1972; Strauss et al., 1974).

Studies on the effects of antiarrhythmic agents and other cardioactive drugs on sinoatrial conduction have been limited. Yamaguchi et al. studied the effects of lidocaine (1×10^{-5} M), procaine amide (1.1×10^{-4} M) and ouabain (3×10^{-7} M) on sinoatrial conduction in isolated tissue. Lidocaine produced a significant shortening of retrograde conduction without any alteration in antegrade conduction. Procaine amide produced significant lengthening of antegrade conduction without significant alteration in retrograde conduction. Neither drug produced significant changes in estimated conduction time. Although ouabain did not significantly prolong either antegrade or retrograde conduction time, it did prolong total measured sinoatrial conduction time (Table 2). Interestingly, estimated conduction time was more prolonged than measured conduction time because sinus node reset occurred even with APD's that fell on the compensatory line. This latter finding suggests that falsely prolonged estimated conduction times may be obtained during clinical studies in patients taking digitalis preparations. Clinically, digitalis has been noted to have variable effects on sinus node function in man (Hoffman and Singer, 1964; Fisch et al., 1964; Toda and West, 1966; Ten Eick and Hoffman, 1969; Scherlag et al., 1971; Szekeres and Papp, 1971; Bond and Engel, 1974; Rosen et al., 1975; Dhingra et al., 1975; Goodman et al., 1975).

ECG MONITORING

1) Exercise Testing – Exercise testing assesses the ability of the sinus node to accelerate in an appropriate fashion to internal physiologic chronotropic stimuli. Although a patient

Table 2. Effect of drugs on measured and estimated SACT.

	Total measured msec	Retrograde msec	Antegrade msec	Estimated msec
Control	52.5 ± 5.8	21.0 ± 2.3	31.5 ± 4.0	53.0 ± 9.4
			NS	NS
Lidocaine	43.1** ± 4.7	11.1** ± 1.9	32.0 ± 3.7	42.0 ± 5.6
Control	50.6 ± 7.1	20.0 ± 2.1	31.0 ± 3.9	51.0 ± 7.5
		NS		NS
Procaine amide	63.5* ± 5.3	23.5 ± 2.9	40.0* ± 3.3	58.0 ± 3.7
Control	54.0 ± 4.8	21.0 ± 2.3	33.0 ± 2.9	49.1 ± 7.8
		NS	NS	
Ouabain	58.5* ± 3.3	22.5 ± 1.9	36.0 ± 2.4	80.0*** ± 7.1

M ± SEM.
N = 5.
*p < 0.05.
**p < 0.01.
***p < 0.005.

may have no evidence of sinus node dysfunction in the resting electrocardiogram, abnormal sinus node responses to stress may be uncovered by treadmill testing. Established norms for standard stress testing protocols for age and sex are available (Balke and Ware, 1959; Goldberg et al., 1970).

Although some investigators have found that mean oxygen consumption at maximum stress was significantly lower for sick sinus patients compared with predicted maximum oxygen consumption for controls (Abbott et al., 1974; Scheinman et al., 1974), a recent report indicates that maximal oxygen consumption may not differ between the two groups (Holden et al., 1976). Thus, a normal O_2 consumption in the presence of a reduced heart rate response to exercise may separate sick sinus patients from age matched "normals" with autonomic chronotropic incompetence secondary to myocardial disease (Ellestad, 1975). Also, patients with sinus node dysfunction as a consequence of heightened vagal tone appear to have normal heart rate responses to exercise compared to patients with intrinsic sinus node disease (Arguss et al., 1972).

2) Holter Monitoring – Ambulatory monitoring during normal daily activities (Corday et al., 1965; Crook et al., 1973) may detect bradyarrhythmias and tachyarrhythmias in the sick sinus syndrome which are missed on a routine electrocardiogram. Furthermore, ambulatory monitoring is diagnostic if the simultaneous occurrence of symptoms and sinus dysrhythmia is documented. More recent technical advances have enabled a patient to carry a device to be used only when symptoms occur, transmitting his ECG to a central station via telephone or record his ECG on a portable recorder. "Intelligent recorders" are being developed that attempt to record the ECG only when abnormalities of rate or rhythm occur.

TESTING THE SINUS NODE-AUTONOMIC NERVOUS SYSTEM AXIS

1) Tests of Sinus Node Responsiveness to Autonomic Activity – The signs, symptoms and ECG features of the sick sinus syndrome may be secondary to sinus node over- or under-responsiveness to appropriate autonomic activity. Arguss et al. (1972) have demonstrated that the well-established phenomenon of slowing of the sinus rate with age may be, in part, secondary to increased parasympathetic tone. In some patients, sinoatrial block may be

mediated by abnormal autonomic tone (Brasil, 1955; Dighton, 1975), and sinus arrhythmia is often produced primarily by periodic alterations in parasympathetic efferent cardiac activity (Hamlin et al., 1966). Finally, patients with myocardial dysfunction have been shown to have profound abnormalities of parasympathetic and sympathetic control of heart rate (Covell et al., 1966; Beiser et al., 1968; Eckberg et al., 1971; Goldstein et al., 1975).

The importance of the autonomic nervous system to intrinsic sinus node function suggests that heart rate response to sympathomimetic (isoproterenol), sympatholytic (propranolol) vagotonic (bethanechol or edrophonium) and vagolytic (atropine) drugs be employed routinely in the clinical evaluation of the sick sinus syndrome (Mandel et al., 1975; Bigger, 1977). Unfortunately, no standardized or systematic protocols have been described for administration of these agents (Strauss et al., 1976; Dauchat and Gravenstein, 1974; George et al., 1972), and dose response curves in normals must be described for comparative purposes. Patients with intrinsic sinus node dysfunction may exhibit all, some or various combinations of the following abnormal responses: 1) A blunted heart rate acceleration with isoproterenol administration, suggesting sinus node unresponsiveness to appropriate beta-adrenergic stimulation, 2) a blunted acceleration response to atropine, suggesting that sinus node dysfunction is not due to oversensitivity to parasympathetic tone nor to the presence of excessive parasympathetic tone, 3) an exaggerated response to atropine, indicating an oversensitivity to parasympathetic tone, 4) an exaggerated slowing response to bethanechol or edrephonium, indicating oversensitivity to parasympathetic stimulation.

2) Testing the Integrity of the Autonomic Nervous System – A characteristic clinical presentation of the sick sinus syndrome may result from primary dysfunction of the auto-nomic nervous system. Carotid massage, the performance of the Valsalva maneuver or phenylephrine-induced hypertension should normally produce slowing of the heart rate by reflex responses to the autonomic nervous system. In contrast, lowering the blood pressure by titrated nitroprusside infusion should normally result in a reflex increase in heart rate. Regretably, blood pressure heart rate response curves are not available for normals.

Utilizing the combined results of studies designed to test the integrity of sinus node response to direct autonomic stimulation and inhibition and studies testing the integrity of the autonomic nervous system, the status of autonomic regulation of sinus node function can be completely characterized. Recently, Dighton (1974), suggested that individuals with symptomatic sinus bradycardia are more likely to have normal sinus rate responses to autonomic stimulation and inhibition than are asympatomatic patients.

REFERENCES

Abbott, J.P., Kunkel, F., Hirschfeld, D.S., Scheinman, M.M.: Effects of cardiac pacing and heart rate accelera-tion on exercise-induced symptoms in patients with sick sinus syndrome. *Circulation* 49 and 50: 111–119, 1974

Amory, D.W., West, T.C.: Chronotropic response following direct electrical stimulation of the isolated sinoatrial node: A pharmacological evaluation. *J Pharmacol Exptl Therap* 137: 14, 1962

Arguss, N.S., Rosin, E.Y., Adolph, A.J., Fowler, N.O.: Significance of chronic sinus bradycardia in elderly people. *Circulation* 46: 924, 1972

Balke, B., Ware, R.W.: An experimental study of physical fitness of air force personnel. *U.S. Armed Forces Med J* 10: 675, 1959

Barks, J.B., Bosman, C.K., Cochrane, J.W.C.: Congenital cardiac arrhythmias. *Lancet* 2: 531, 1964

Bashour, T., Hemb, R., Wickramesekaran, R., Strauss, H.C., Bigger, J.T., Jr.: An unusual effect of atropine on overdrive suppression. *Circulation* 48: 911, 1973

Beiser, G.D., Epstein, S.E., Stampfer, M., Goldstein, R.E.: Impaired heart rate response to sympathetic nerve stimulation in patients with cardiac decompensation. *Circulation* 38: VI–40, 1968

Bigger, J.T.: A simple, rapid method for the diagnosis of first-degree sinoatrial block in man. *Am Heart J* 87: 731, 1974

Bigger, J.T.: The sick sinus syndrome. *Prac Cardiol* 3: 66, 1977

Bond, R.C., Engel, T.R., Schaal, S.F.: Effect of digitalis on sinoatrial conduction in man (abstract). *Am J Cardiol* 33: 128, 1974

Bonke, F.I.M., Bouman, L.N., Van Rijn H.E.: Change of cardiac rhythm in the rabbit after an atrial premature beat. *Circ Res* 24: 533, 1969

Bonke, F.I.M., Bouman, L.N., Schopman, F.J.G.: Effect of an early atrial premature beat on activity of the sinoatrial node and atrial rhythm in the rabbit. *Circ Res* 24: 704, 1971

Brasil, A.: Autonomic sinoatrial block. A new disturbance of the heart mechanism. Arquivos Brasileiras de Cardiologia 8: 159, 1955

Breithardt, G., Seipel, L.: The effect of premature atrial depolarization on sinus node automaticity in man. *Circulation* 53: 920, 1976

Breithardt, G., Seipel, L., Both, A., Loogen, F.: The effect of atropine of calculated sinoatrial conduction time in man. *Eur J Cardiol* 4: 49, 1976

Breithardt, G., Seipel, L., Loogen, F.: Sinus node recovery time and calculated sinoatrial conduction time in normal subjects and patients with sinus node dysfunction. *Circulation* 56: 43, 1977

Brooks, C./McC., Lu, H.-H.: The sinoatrial pacemaker of the heart. Charles C. Thomas, Publishing Co., Springfield, Illinois, p. 109–110, 1972

Chadda, K.D., Banke, V.S., Bodenheimer, M.M., Helfant, R.H.: Corrected sinus node recovery time: Experimental, physiological and pathologic determinents. *Circulation* 51: 797, 1975

Childers, R.W., Arnsdorf, M.F., de la Fuente, D.J., Gambetta, M., Svenson, R.: Sinus node echoes. *Am J Cardiol* 31: 220, 1973

Cohen, A.E., Lewis, T.: Auricular fibrillation and complete heart block: A description of a case of Adams-Stokes syndrome including the postmortem examination. *Heart* 4: 15, 1912

Cohn, A.E., Lewis, T.: Auricular fibrillation and complete heart block. A description of a case of Adams-Stokes syndrome including the postmortem examination. *Heart* 4: 15, 1913

Conde, C., Leppo, J., Lipski, J., Stimmel, B., Litwak, R., Donoso, E., Dack, S.: Effectiveness of pacemaker treatment in the bradycardiatachycardia syndrome. *Am J Cardiol* 32: 209, 1973

Corday, E., Bazika, V., Lang, T.W., Pappelbaum, S., Gold, H., Berstein, H.: Detection of phantom arrhythmias and evanescent ECG abnormalities. *JAMA* 193: 417, 1965

Covell, J.W., Chidsey, C.A., Braunwald, E.: Reduction of the cardiac responses to postganglionic sympathetic nerve stimulation in patients with cardiac decompensation. *Circ Res* 19: 51, 1966

Crook, B.R.M., Cashman, P.M.M., Stott, F.D., Raftery, E.B.: Tape monitoring of the electrocardiogram in ambulant patients with sinoatrial disease. *Br Heart J* 35: 1009, 1973

Dauchat, P., Gravenstein, J.S.: Effects of atropine on the electrocardiogram in different age groups. *Clin Pharmacol Therap* 12: 274, 1974

Davies, M.J., Pomerance, A.: Quantitative study of aging changes in the human sinoatrial node and internodal tracts. *Br Heart J* 34: 150, 1972

Denes, P., Delon, W., Dhingra, R.: The effects of cycle length on cardiac refractory periods in man. *Circulation* 49: 32, 1974

Dhingra, R.C., Wyndham, C., Amat-y-Leon, F., Denes, P., Wu, D., Rosen, K.M.: Sinus nodal responses to atrial extra stimuli in patients without apparent sinus node disease. *Am J Cardiol* 36: 445, 1975a

Dhingra, R.C., Amat-y-Leon, F., Wyndam, C., Denes, P., Wu, D, Pouget, J.M., Rosen, K.M.: Electrophysiologic effects of atropine on human sinus node and atrium. *Am J Cardiol* 38: 429, 1976a

Dhingra, R.C., Amat-y-Leon, F., Wyndham, C., Wu, D., Denes, P., Rosen, K.M.: The electrophysiological effects of ouabain on sinus node and atrium in man. *J Clin Invest*, 56: 555, 1975b

Dhingra, R.C., Amat-y-Leon, F., Wyndham, C., Denes, P., Wu, D., Miller, R.H., Rosen, K.M.: Electrophysiologic effects of atropine on sinus node and atrium in patients with sinus node dysfunction. *Am J Cardiol* 38: 848, 1976b

Dhingra, R.C., Amat-y-Leon, F., Wyndham, C., Deedwania, P.C., Wu, D., Denes, P., Rosen, K.: Clinical significance of prolonged sinoatrial conduction time. *Circulation* 55: 8, 1977

Dighton, D.H.: Sinus bradycardia: Autonomic influences and clinical assessment. *Br Heart J* 36: 791, 1974

Dighton, D.H.: Sinoatrial block: Autonomic influences and clinical assessment. *Br Heart J* 37: 321, 1975

Eckberg, D.L., Drabinsky, M., Braunwald, E.: Defective cardiac parasympathetic control in patients with heart disease. *New Engl J Med* 285: 877, 1971

Ellestad M.H.: Stress testing: Principles and practice. F.A. Davis, Publishing Co., Philadelphia Penn., p. 38, 1975

Engel, T.R., Schaal, S.F.: Digitalis in the sick sinus syndrome: The effects of digitalis on sinoatrial automaticity and atrioventricular conduction. *Circulation* 48: 1201, 1973

Engel, T.R., Meister, S.G., Feitosa, G.S., Fisher H.A., Frankl, W.S.: Appraisal of sinus node artery disease. *Circulation* 52: 286, 1975

Engel, T.R., Bond, R.C., Schaal, S.F.: First-degree sinoatrial heart block: Sinoatrial block in the sick sinus syndrome. *Am Heart J* 91: 303, 1976

Ferrer, M.I.: The sick sinus syndrome in atrial disease. *JAMA* 206: 645, 1968

Fisch, C., Greenspan, K., Knobel, S.B., Feigenbaum, H.: Effect of digitalis on conduction of the heart. *Prog Cardiovasc Dis* 6: 343, 1964

Furchgott, R.F., De Gubaroff, T., Grossman, A.: Release of autonomic mediators in cardiac tissue by supra-threshold stimulation. *Science* 129: 328, 1959

Fraser, G.R., Froggatt, P., James, T.N.: Congenital deafness associated with electrocardiographic abnormalities, fainting attacks and sudden death: A recessive syndrome. *Quart J Med* 33: 361, 1964

George, C.F., Conolly, M.E., Briant, F., Dollery, C.T.: Intravenously administered isoproterenol sulfate: Dose-response curves in man. *Arch Int Med* 30: 361, 1972

Goldberg, A.N., Moran, J.F., Resnekov, L.: Multistage electrocardiographic tests. *Am J Cardiol* 26: 84, 1970

Goldreyer, B.N., Damato, A.N.: Sinoatrial node entrance block. *Circulation* 44: 789, 1971

Goldstein, R.E., Beiser, D.G., Stampfer, M., Epstein, S.E.: Impairment of autonomically mediated heart rate control in patients with cardiac dysfunction. *Circ Res* 36: 571, 1975

Goodman, D.J., Rosen, R.M., Ingham, R., Rider, A.K., Harrison, D.C.: Sinus node function in the deverated human heart. Effect of digitalis. *Br Heart J* 37: 612, 1975

Gupta, P.K., Lichstein, E., Chadda, K.D., Baduri, E.: Appraisal of sinus nodal recovery time in patients with sick sinus syndrome. *Am J Cardiol* 34: 265, 1974

Hamlin, R.L., Smith, C.R., Smetzer, D.L.: Sinus arrhythmia in the dog. *Am J Physiol* 210: 321, 1966

Han, J.H., Malozzi, A.M., Moe, G.K.: Sino-atrial reciprocation in the isolated rabbit heart. *Circ Res* 22: 355, 1968

Hartel, G., Talvensaari, T.: Treatment of sinoatrial syndrome with permanent cardiac pacing in 90 patients. *Acta Med Scan* 198: 341, 1975

Hirschfeld, D.S., Peters, R., Kunkel, F., Scheinman, M.M.: Sinoatrial conduction time (SACT) and abnormal perinodal refractoriness in patients with sinus node disease (SND). *Circulation* 52: II–112, 1975

Hoffman, B.F., Cranefield, P.F.: Electrophysiology of the heart. New York, McGraw-Hill, 1960

Hoffman, B.F., Singer D.H.: Effects of digitalis on electrical activity of cardiac fibers. *Prog Cardiovasc Dis* 7: 226, 1964

Holden, W., McAnullty, J., Rahimtoola, S.: Inadequate heart rate response to exercise in the sick sinus syndrome. *Circulation* 53 and 54: II–146, 1976

James, T.N.: Myocardial infarction and atrial arrhythmias. *Circulation* 24: 761, 1961

Jordan, J.L., Yamaguchi, I., Mandel, W.J.: The sick sinus syndrome: Pathophysiology, significance and treatment. *Cardiol Dig* 12: 11, 1977a

Jordan, J., Yamaguchi, I., Mandel, W.J., McCullen, A.E.: Comparative effects of overdrive on sinus and subsidiary pacemaker function. *Am Heart J* 93: 367, 1977b

Jordan, J.L., Yamaguchi, I., Mandel, W.J.: Characteristics of sinoatrial conduction in patients with coronary artery disease. *Circulation* 55: 569, 1977c

Jordan, J.L., Yamaguchi, I., Mandel, W.J.: Studies on the mechanism of sinus node dysfunction in the sick sinus syndrome. *Circulation*, 1977d (in press)

Jose, A.D., Collison, D.: The normal range and determinants of the intrinsic heart rate in man. *Cardiovasc Res* 4: 160, 1970

Kaplin, B.M., Langendorf, R., Lev, M., Pick, A.: Tachycardiabradycardia syndrome (so-called "sick sinus syndrome"). Pathology, mechanisms and treatment. *Am J Cardiol* 31: 497, 1973

Klein, H.O., Singer, D.H., Hoffman, B.F.: Effects of atrial premature systoles on sinus rhythm in the rabbit. *Circ Res* 32: 480, 1973

Konisai, T.: Electrophysiologic consideration on sick sinus syndrome. *Japan Circ J* 40: 194, 1976

Kulbertus, H.E., Leval-Rutten, F. de, Demoulin, J.C.: Sino-atrial disease: A report on 13 cases. *J Electrocardiol* 6: 303, 1973

Kulbertus, H.E., Leval-Rutten, F. de, Mary, L., Casters, P.: Sinus node recovery time in the elderly. *Br Heart J* 37: 420, 1975

Lange, G.: Action of driving stimuli from intrinsic and extrinsic sources on in situ cardiac pacemaker tissues. *Circ Res* 17: 449, 1965

Langendorf, R., Lesser, M.E., Plotkin, P., Levin, B.D.: Atrial parasystole with interpolation: Observations on prolonged sinoatrial conduction. *Am Heart J* 63: 649, 1962

Lown, B.: *In* 14th Hahnemann symposium on mechanisms and therapy of cardiac arrhythmias, Edited by Dreifus, L., Likoff, W., Moyer, J., Philadelphia, Grune Stratton, 1966, p. 185

Lu, H.H., Lange, G., Brooks, C.McC.: Factors controlling pacemaker action in cells of the sinoatrial node. *Circ Res* 17: 460, 1965

Mandel, W.J., Hayakawa, H., Danzig, R., Marcus, H.S.: Evaluation of sino-atrial node function in man by overdrive suppression. *Circulation* 44: 59, 1971

Mandel, W.J., Laks M.M.: Overview of the sick sinus syndrome. *Chest* 66: 223, 1974

Mandel, W.J., Laks, M.M., Obayashi, K.: Sinus node function: Evaluation in patients with and without sinus node disease. *Arch Int Med* 135: 388, 1975

Masini, G., Dianda, R., Grazina, A.: Analysis of sinoatrial conduction in man using premature atrial stimulation. *Cardiovasc Res* 9: 498, 1975

Metzger, A.L., Goldberg, A.N., Hunter, R.L.: Sick sinus node syndrome as the presenting manifestation of reticulum cell sarcoma. *Chest* 60: 602, 1971

Miller, H.C., Strauss, H.C.: Measurement of sinoatrial conduction time by premature atrial stimulation in the rabbit. *Circ Res* 35: 935, 1974

Moss, A.J., Davis, R.J.: Brady-tachy syndrome. *Prog Cardiovasc Dis* 16: 439, 1974

Narula, O.S.: Sinus node reentry. A mechanism for supraventricular tachycardia. *Circulation* 50: 114, 1974

Narula, O.S., Samet, P., Javier, R.P.: Significance of the sinus node recovery time. *Circulation* 45: 140, 1972

Okimoto, T., Veda, K., Kamata, C., Yoshida, H., Ohkawa, S., Hiracka, K., Kuwajima, I., Sugiura, M., Murakami, M., Matsuo, H.: Sinus node recovery time and abnormal post-pacing phase in the aged patients with sick sinus syndrome. *Japan Heart J* 17: 290, 1976

Paritsky, Z., Obayashi, K., Mandel, W.J.: Atrial tachycardia secondary to sino-atrial node reentry. *Chest* 66: 526, 1974

Pasmooij, J.H., Van Enst G.C., Bouman, L.N., Allessie, M.A., Bonke, F.I.M.: The effect of heart rate on the membrane responsiveness of rabbit atrial muscle. *Pflügers Arch* 366: 223, 1976

Paulay, K.L., Varghese, P.J., Damato, A.N.: Atrial rhythms in response to an early atrial premature depolarization in man. *Am Heart J* 85: 323, 1973a.

Paulay, K.L., Varghese, P.J., Damato, A.N.: Sinus node reentry: An in vivo demonstration in the dog. *Circ Res* 32: 455, 1973b

Radford, D.J., Julian, D.G.: Sick sinus syndrome: Experience of a cardiac pacemaker clinic. *Br Med J* 3: 504, 1974

Rasmussen, K.: Chronic sinoatrial heart block. *Am Heart J* 81: 38, 1971

Reiffel, J.A., Bigger, J.T., Konstam, M.A.: The relationship between sinoatrial conduction time and sinus cycle length during spontaneous sinus arrhythmia in adults. *Circulation* 50: 924, 1974

Reiffel, J.P., Bigger, J.T., Giardina, E.-G.V.: "Paradoxical" prolongation of sinus nodal recovery time after atropine in the sick sinus syndrome. *Am J Cardiol* 36: 98, 1975

Rokseth, R., Hatle, L.: Prospective study on the occurrence and management of chronic sinoatrial disease with follow-up. *Br Heart J* 36: 582, 1974

Rosen, K.M., Loeb, H.S., Sinno, M.Z., Rahimtoola, S.H., Gunnar, R.M.: Cardiac conduction in patients with symptomatic sinus node disease. *Circulation* 43: 836, 1971.

Rosen, M.R., Wit, A.L., Hoffman, B.F.: Electrophysiology and pharmacology of cardiac arrhythmias. IV. Cardiac antiarrhythmic and toxic effects of digitalis. *Am Heart J* 89: 391, 1975

Rubenstein, J.J., Schulman, C.L., Yurchack, P.M., et al.: Clinical spectrum of the sick sinus syndrome. *Circulation* 46: 5, 1972

Sano, T., Yamagishi, S.: Spread of excitation from the sinus node. *Circ Res* 16: 423, 1965

Saroff, A., Strauss, H.C., Bigger, J.T., Steiner, C., Giardina, E.-G.V.: Evaluation of sinus node function in patients with sinus bradycardia. *Circulation* 44: II–97, 1971

Scheinman, M.M., Kunkel, F.W., Peter, R.W., Schoenfeld, P.L., Abbott, J.A.: Sino-atrial function and atrial refractoriness in patients with sick sinus syndrome. *Circulation* 48: IV–215, 1973

Scheinman, M.M., Peter, R., Hirschfeld, D.S., Abbott, J.A., Kunkel, F.W.: The sick sinus and failing atrium. *West J Med* 121: 473, 1974

Scher, A.M., Rodrigues, M.I., Lukane, J., Young, A.C.: The mechanism of atrio-ventricular conduction. *Circ Res* 7: 54, 1959

Scherf, D.: The mechanisms of sinoatrial block. *Am J Cardiol* 23: 769, 1969

Scherlag, B.J., Abelleira, J.L., Narula, O.S., Samet, P.: The differential effects of ouabain on sinus, AV nodal, His bundle and idioventricular rhythms. *Am Heart J* 81: 227, 1971

Seipel, L., Both, A., Breithardt, G., Gleichman, U., Loogen, F.: Action of antiarrhythmic drugs on His bundle electrogram and sinus node function. *Acta Cardiol* XVIII: 251, 1974

Sigurd, B., Jensen, G., Meibom, J., Sandoe, E.: Adams-Stokes syndrome caused by sinoatrial block. *Br Heart J* 35: 1002, 1973

Sowton, E., Hendrix, G., Roy, P.: Ten-year survey of treatment with implanted cardiac pacemaker. *Brit Med J* 3: 155, 1974

Spellberg, R.D.: Familial sinus node disease. *Chest* 60: 246, 1971

Steinbeck, G., Luderitz, B.: Comparative study of sinoatrial conduction time and sinus node recovery time. *Br Heart J* 37: 956, 1975

Strauss, H.C., Bigger, J.T.: Electrophysiological properties of the rabbit sinoatrial perinodal fibers. *Circ Res* 31: 490, 1972

Strauss, H.C., Saroff, A.L., Bigger, J.T., Giardina E.-G.V.: Premature atrial stimulation as a key to the understanding of sinoatrial conduction in man. Presentation of data and cirtical review of the literature. *Circulation* 47: 86, 1973

Strauss, H.C., Saroff, A.L., Bigger, J.T.: Slowed conduction, block and reentry in perinodal fibers. *Circulation* 43 and 44, suppl. II, 1974

Strauss, H.C., Gilbert, M., Svenson, R., Miller, H.C., Wallace, A.G.: Electrophysiologic effects of propranolol on sinus node function in patients with sinus node dysfunction. *Circulation* 54: 452, 1976a

Strauss, H.C., Bigger, J.T., Saroff, A.L., Giardina, E.-G.V.: Electrophysiologic evaluation of sinus node function in patients with sinus node dysfunction. *Circulation* 53: 763, 1976b

Szekeres, L., Papp, G.J.: Experimental cardiac arrhythmias and antiarrhythmic drugs. Budapest, Akademiai Kiado, 1971

Ten Eick, R.E., Hoffman, B.F.: Chronotropic effect on cardiac glycosides in dogs, cats, and rabbits. *Circ Res* 25: 365, 1969

Toda, N., West, T.C.: Influence of ouabain on chalinergic responses in sonoatrial node. *J. Pharmacol Exp Ther* 153: 104, 1966

Vincenzi, F.F., West, T.C.: Release of autonomic mediators in cardiac tissue by direct subthreshold electrical stimulation. *J Pharmacol Exp Ther* 141: 185, 1963

Wan, S.H., Lee, G.S., Ton, C.S.: The sick sinus syndrome. A study of 15 cases. *Br Heart J* 34: 942, 1972

Ward, P.C.: A new familial cardiac syndrome in children. *J Irish Med Assoc* 54: 103, 1964

Yabek, S.M., Jarmakani, J.M., Robert, N.K.: Sinus node function in children. Factors influencing its evaluation. *Circ* 53: 28, 1976

Yamaguchi, I., Mandel, W.J.: The effect of stimulation site on electrophysiologic features of the sinus node. *Am J Cardiol* 41: 374, 1978

2

MEASUREMENT OF SINUS NODE RECOVERY TIME AFTER ATRIAL PACING

T. POP AND D. FLEISCHMANN

Until now the selective recording of sinus potentials in man is not yet possible. Therefore, information about the sinus node function can only be obtained by means of indirect methods. One of these methods is the measurement of the so-called sinus node recovery time (Mandel et al., 1971; and Mandel et al., 1972). This method is based upon the known electrophysiological phenomenon of postdrive or overdrive suppression.

The purpose of this paper is to review our knowledge of this phenomenon in the human heart, in healthy subjects as well as in patients with diseases of the sinus node. Before proceeding with the data obtained in man, we briefly will review the knowledge on this phenomenon in the experimental animal.

SINUS NODE POSTDRIVE SUPPRESSION IN THE EXPERIMENTAL ANIMAL

As early as 1884, Gaskel found that pacemaker activity of the tortoise heart tissue is inhibited by tetanic stimuli. Studies performed with isolated sinus node tissue have shown that after repetitive electrical stimulation a period of depression of the sinus node pacemaker activity is manifested by a slower sinus rate (West, 1961; Amory and West, 1962; Vincenzi and West, 1963; Lu et al., 1965). This depression is caused by a membrane hyperpolarization (West, 1961; Lu et al., 1965). Because the same phenomenon can be seen after vagal stimulation (Hutter and Trautwein, 1956) it was assumed that the postdrive suppression of the sinus node is of cholinergic nature (Amory and West, 1962). The finding that atropine reduces postdrive supression but does not abolish it, led Lu et al. (1965) to the conclusion that factors other than acetylcholine release are involved in this process. Such factors could be an augmented K^+ efflux, a pacemaker shift within the sinus node or a failure of conduction within the sinus node (Lu et al., 1965).

The phenomenon of postdrive suppression was also found and extensively investigated in the in situ dog heart (Lange, 1965; Paulay and Damato, 1973; Chadda et al., 1975).

There are several factors which influence the duration and the degree of postdrive suppression:

1. The rate of the drive. After a driving rate of less than 10–15% above the control rate one generally observes an acceleration of the sinus rhythm (Lange, 1965). Driving at rates more than 20% above the control rate results in an initial slowing down of the sinus rate (Lange, 1965). The intensity and duration of this slowing down are greater when the rates of the drive are increased (Lange, 1965; Chadda et al., 1975). This trend is reversed at very high rates (Lange, 1965), so that then the first escape cycle can become shorter than at lower rates (Ticzon et al., 1975). After pacing the sinus rhythm is initially slow, but it accelerates progressively. The interval between the last paced atrial beat and the first sinus P wave is generally the longest (Lange, 1965).

At the cessation of the electrical drive the sinus rhythm is promptly resumed. An ectopic pacemaker escape is rarely seen after electrical stimulation (Chadda et al., 1975) because the junctional pacemaker is much more readily depressed than the sinus nodal pacemaker under similar conditions (Lange, 1965; Jordan et al., 1977).

2. The duration of the electrical drive. The intensity and duration of the slowing down of the sinus rate augment with increased duration of the drive (Lange, 1965). Nevertheless there are no significant variations when atrial pacing duration is increased from 1 to 5 min (Chadda et al., 1975) respectively to 6 min (Ticzon et al., 1975).

3. The site of the drive. The degree of the slowing down is greater when the driving is performed near the sinus node than when it is performed within the left atrium (Lange, 1965). This difference is explained by the amount of released acetylcholine which influences the sinus node directly. The closer the stimulating electrode is located to the sinus node, the greater will be the amount of released acetylcholine, which finally will slow down the sinus rate (Lange, 1965).

When changing the pacing site from the right atrium to the right ventricle, slowing down of the sinus rate is minimal (Lange, 1965) or there is an acceleration of the sinus rhythm (Paulay and Damato, 1973). This response pattern is explained by the action of positive chronotropic reflexes, which are induced by the haemodynamic events resulting from the disturbed AV conduction sequence (Paulay and Damato, 1973).

4. The stimulus strength. Variation from 2 to 10 mA has no significant influence on the postdrive suppression (Chadda et al., 1975).

5. Similarly, minimal variations were encountered when the studies were performed on consecutive days, but in the same animal (Chadda et al., 1975).

6. The autonomic nervous system plays a crucial role as far as the duration and intensity of the postdrive suppression are concerned. Vagal stimulation and sympatholysis prolong and augment the slowing down of the postdrive sinus rate (Lange, 1965; Chadda et al., 1975). On the other hand, adrenergic stimulation and vagolysis minimize postdrive suppression without abolishing it (Lange, 1965; Chadda et al., 1975). Section of the vagi has no effect on this phenomenon (Lange, 1965). Therefore, Lange (1965) assumed, as did West et al. (1962; 1963) in isolated tissue, that the postdrive suppression is due – at least partly – to the release of acetylcholine from the nerve endings.

7. Infusions of potassium chloride increase postdrive suppression (Lange, 1965). Thus, beside the release of acetylcholine, it is assumed that a potassium release or a potassium efflux built up by the driving stimuli is responsible for this phenomenon.

Beside the two factors mentioned before – release of acetylcholine and/or potassium –, the degree and intensity of postdrive suppression are also dependent upon the anatomic integrity of the sinus node. After acute sinus node injury the postdrive slowing down of the sinus rate is more prolonged and more severe than before injury (Chadda et al., 1975).

SINUS NODE POSTDRIVE SUPPRESSION IN THE HEALTHY MAN

In healthy subjects as well as in animals atrial driving induces a dperession of the sinus node automaticity, manifested by a slowing down of the postdrive heart rate or, in other words, a lengthening of the postdrive P-P intervals (Mandel et al., 1971). Generally the interval between the last driven P wave and the first sinus P wave is the longest and its value is referred to as the sinus node recovery time (Mandel et al., 1972) (Figure 1). The

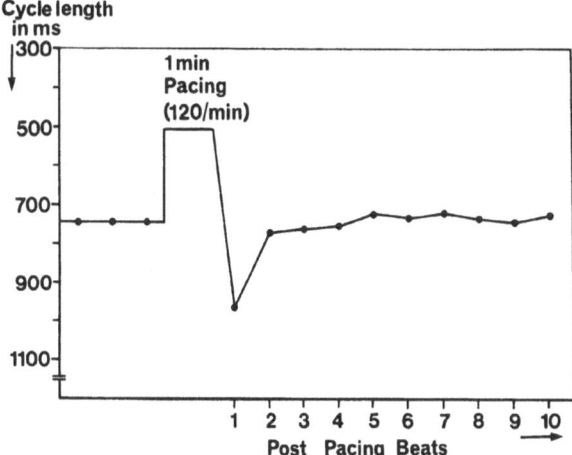

Figure 1. Cycle length duration in a healthy subject before (at the left) and after 1 min atrial pacing at a rate of 120/min (at the right). The first post pacing cycle is the longest and is followed by a progressive shortening of the subsequent ones to reach quickly the prepacing cycle length.

so-called corrected sinus node recovery time (Narula et al., 1972) is obtained by subtracting the mean cycle length before pacing from the sinus node recovery time.

As in the case with the experimental animal, the postdrive pause ends generally with a sinus beat (Rich et al., 1971). It is rarely a junctional, a ventricular (Kulbertus et al., 1975) or an atrial escape beat (Yabek et al., 1976). This is explained by the fact that the subsidiary pacemakers are more readily depressed during the atrial drive than the sinus node (Jordan et al., 1977).

At the cessation of pacing the sinus rate accelerates progressively to reach the initial heart rate (Mandel et al., 1971) (Figure 1). After faster rates of driving (150/min or more) a phenomenon of secondary depression can occasionally be seen in some subjects occurring after a few faster beats (Mandel et al., 1971; Kulbertus et al., 1975; Benditt et al., 1976). Sometimes, after cessation of pacing, a pacemaker acceleration can be observed (Yabek et al., 1976). This might be explained by a local release of catecholamines (Amory and West, 1962) or by induction of a short living sinus node reentrant tachycardia (Narula, 1974; Wu et al., 1974; Weisfogel et al., 1975).

As discussed above, postdrive suppression of the sinus node may be influenced by several factors: (1) the rate or (2) the duration oft he drive, (3) the site of the drive within the right atrium, (4) the stimulus strength, (5) the control rate of the sinus rhythm, (6) the autonomic nervous system and (7) the age of the patient.

ad 1. When the drive rate is increased there is a parallel prolongation of the sinus node recovery time. However, maximal value is reached at a rate of 120–130/min (Mandel et al., 1971; Kulbertus et al., 1975; Yabek et al., 1976). When speaking of the sinus node recovery time, this maximal value is generally meant. However, the pacing rate at which the longest value of the sinus node recovery time is reached, varies from subject to subject. Investigating 110 patients without sinus node dysfunction or conduction disturbances, we observed that it was reached at rates as low as 90/min in some subjects or at rates as high as 170/min in others. The mean value was 118 ± 23.4 beats/min.

The duration of the sinus node recovery time tends to decline at faster rates (Mandel et al., 1971). This decline is probably the result of enhanced sympathetic discharge (Mandel et al., 1971). An other explanation is the occurrence of a second degree retrograde sinoatrial block (Goldreyer and Damato, 1971), leading to a slower discharge of the sinus node (Bigger and Strauss, 1973).

When we compared the sinus node recovery times at various rates in the same patient, the difference between them was generally no longer than 0.5 sec.

It is interesting to observe that in contrast to animal studies, in man a driving rate of less than 10–15% above the control rate does not induce a sinus node acceleration. Only a slowing down of the sinus node is seen.

ad 2. Studies performed with atrial pacing for 15–180 sec showed no statistically significant differences in the duration of the sinus node recovery time (Mandel et al., 1971). Narula et al. (1972) came to the same conclusion when pacing for 2 respectively 5 min.

ad 3. The site of the drive in the right atrium does not influence the value of the corrected sinus node recovery time (Narula et al., 1972). When the right atrium and the right ventricle are alternatively paced at the same rate and for the same duration, longer recovery times are observed with right atrial stimulation. Thus, investigating 10 patients we found that the mean recovery time after atrial pacing was 1015 ± 209.5 msec while after ventricular pacing it reached only 829 ± 140 msec (p < 0.05).

ad 4. The stimulus strength has no influence on the duration of the corrected sinus node recovery time (Narula et al., 1972).

ad 5. The control rate plays an important role when determining the maximun duration of the sinus node recovery time. The maean cycle length before pacing shows a positive correlation with the maximal duration of the sinus node recovery time. Mandel et al., (1971) found a correlation coefficient of 0.84 when studying 31 patients. In 110 subjects without sinus node dysfunction or conduction defects we found a value of 0.886 (p < 0.001). There was also a positive correlation between the mean cycle length before pacing and the corrected sinus node recovery time (r = 0.465; p < 0.001), The correlation between the prepacing cycle length and the sinus node recovery time is also present in the denervated human heart (Goodman et al., 1975), showing that it is independent of central nervous influences.

ad 6. The influence of the autonomic nervous system on the sinus node recovery time in the healthy human subjects can only be tested indirectly. While beta-adrenergic stimulation with isoproterenol shortens the sinus node recovery time, beta-adrenergic blockade with propranolol prolongs it (Rich et al., 1971). Vagolysis with atropine shortens the pause after overdrive pacing, without abolishing it (Mandel et al., 1971; Rich et al., 1971; Yabek et al., 1976; Dhingra et al., 1976a).

ad 7. Concerning the age of the patient Yabek et al. (1976) found in children a similar degree of sinus node depression, expressed as a percentage of the basic P-P interval, as did Narula et al. (1972) in normal adults. Kulbertus et al. (1975) found similar absolute values of sinus node recovery time in patients over 50 years of age as did other investigators in heterogeneous groups. Okimoto et al. (1976) found longer absolute values in 10 patients over 69 years of age.

We investigated 110 patients without sinus node dysfunction and with normal AV and intraventricular conduction times and observed a tendency of prolongation for both sinus node recovery time as well as for corrected sinus node recovery time with increasing age (Figure 2). The prepacing control cycle length curve shows the same behavior as the two recovery times. Its lengthening with increasing age is a well-known phenomenon

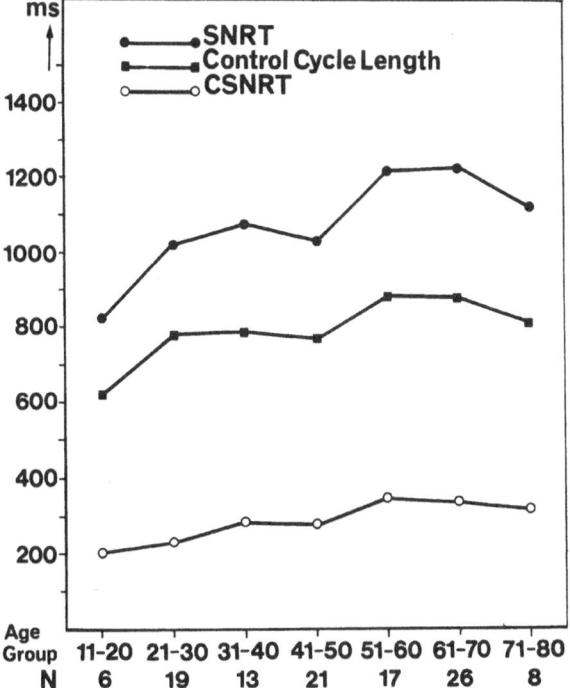

Figure 2. Relationship of age – on the abscissa – to mean values of control cycle length, sinus node recovery time (SNRT) and corrected sinus node recovery time (CSNRT) which are plotted on the ordinate. All three parameters show a tendency to increase with age. Note the parallel course of sinus node recovery times to the control cycle length curve. The SD was omitted for purposes of clarity.

(Brandfonbrenner et al., 1955). Because there is a positive correlation between the control cycle length and the two sinus node recovery times, we assume that the progressive prolongation of the sinus node recovery times with increase in age is secondary to the longer prepacing cycle length in elderly people.

In the age group of 71–80 years (Figure 2) a slight decline of both sinus node recovery times and control cycle length can be seen. It is difficult to say whether this decline is a real one, because the age group of 71–80 years comprises only 8 patients.

Summing up, one can assume that in man as well as in animals, the sinus node recovery time depends primarily upon the state of the autonomic nervous system and the amount of extracellular potassium, but also upon the individual prepacing sinus rate.

Although there are many studies concerning the sinus node recovery time in healthy subjects, there still persists, some uncertainty regarding its normal limits. There are two different ways in which the normal duration of the sinus node recovery time is given: as an absolute value or by taking into account the control cycle length.

For the upper limit of the sinus node recovery time three different values can be found in literature: 1400 msec (Rosen et al., 1971), 1500 msec (Kulbertus et al., 1975) and 1680 msec (Dhingra et al., 1973).

Keeping in mind the correlation between the duration of the sinus node recovery time and the basic cycle length, a correction for the prepacing cycle length seems to be preferable. There are three possibilities:

a. The corrected sinus node recovery time is the result of the subtraction of control cycle length from the sinus node recovery time (Narula et al., 1972). Its normal value is equal to or less than 525 msec.

b. The percentual form giving the sinus node recovery time as a percentage of the control cycle length. Benditt et al. (1976) found that the upper limit of the sinus node recovery time for a control cycle length of less than 800 msec is 183% of the prepacing sinus cycle length. For a control cycle length of more than 800 msec this value is only 161%.

c. Strauss et al. (1976b) use a formula which gives the upper limit of the sinus node recovery time as a function of the prepacing cycle length, namely:

$$SNRT = 1.3 \times \text{control cycle length} + 156$$

A critical discussion of these different ways to evaluate the upper limit of the sinus node recovery time will follow later.

SINUS NODE POSTDRIVE SUPPRESSION IN PATIENTS WITH SICK SINUS SYNDROME

The patients with sick sinus syndrome (Ferrer, 1968; Ferrer, 1973) generally respond to atrial pacing with a greater postdrive suppression than healthy subjects (Mandel et al., 1971; Mandel et al., 1972; Narula et al., 1972) (Figure 3). The postdrive pause respectively the sinus node recovery time is frequently found to be prolonged and the sinus rhythm is markedly slower than before pacing (Mandel et al., 1971; Mandel et al., 1972; Narula et al., 1972). In contrast to healthy subjects, in patients with sick sinus syndrome, at the end of driving the first beat is frequently an escape beat of ectopic origin (Rosen et al., 1971; Narula et al., 1972; Engel et al., 1973; Scheinmann et al., 1976). In most cases the ectopic

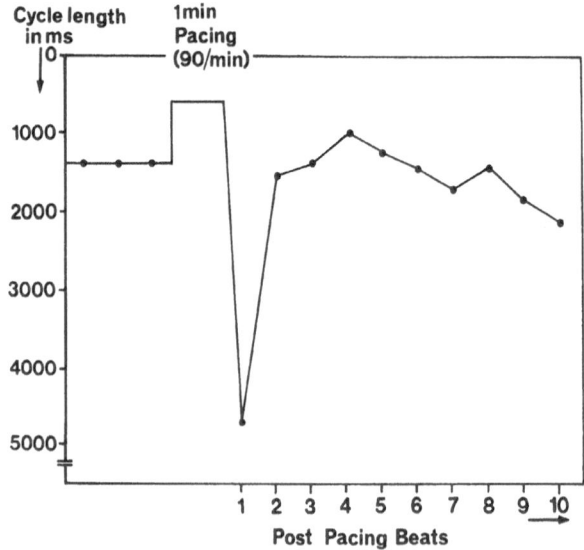

Figure 3. Cycle length duration in a subject with sick sinus syndrome before (at the left) and after 1 min atrial pacing at a rate of 90/min (at the right). Note the long duration of the first post pacing cycle.

beat is a junctional escape (Narula et al., 1972; Engel et al., 1973; Gupta et al., 1974; Reiffel et al., 1975; Scheinmann et al., 1976) and, more rarely, an atrial one (Rosen et al., 1971; Rich et al., 1971; Rios et al., 1972; Scheinmann et al., 1976).

Another feature of the postdrive suppression of the sinus node in patients with sick sinus syndrome is the fact that the prepacing rate is reached at a greater delay than in normal subjects (Schwarz et al., 1975; Delius et al., 1975).

With the increase of the rate of atrial stimulation there is a gradual prolongation of the sinus node recovery time (Ferrer, 1973; Seipel et al., 1975). A maximum value is reached at rates between 90/min (Strauss et al., 1976a) and 140/min (Seipel et al., 1975). In 67 patients with sinus node dysfunction, we found that the maximum value of the sinus node recovery time was reached at a mean driving rate of 114 ± 25 beats/min. This value does not differ significantly from the one we observed in our patients without sinus node dysfunction: 118 ± 23.4 beats/min.

At higher driving rates a shortening of the duration of the sinus node recovery time takes place (Seipel et al., 1975; Delius et al., 1975). This shortening is explained by the same mechanisms as those discussed with regard to the healthy subjects.

When a patient with sick sinus syndrome is paced at several driving rates, the difference between the longest and the shortest post pacing pause often exceeds 0.5 sec; it sometimes reaches several seconds.

There are contradictory reports about the effect of the duration of the drive on the sinus node recovery time. While Narula et al. (1972) observed a parallel increase of the postdrive suppression with the duration of pacing, Schwarz et al. (1975) found that the duration of stimulation has no influence on the value of the sinus node recovery time.

The control rate plays a crucial role in the duration of the maximum value of the sinus node recovery time in healthy subjects. In patients with sick sinus syndrome this correlation is lost. In our 67 patients with sinus node dysfunction, we have found a nonsignificant correlation coefficient of 0.111 between these two parameters.

In patients with sick sinus syndrome the influence of the autonomic nervous system on the sinus node recovery time is not as constant as in healthy subjects. After administering beta-adrenergic blocking agents as propranolol, some prolongation of the sinus node recovery time is seen, however this effect is not significant (Strauss et al., 1976b). Vagolysis with atropine has a variable effect on the duration of the sinus node recovery time. Generally a shortening is seen (Mandel et al., 1971; Mandel et al., 1972; Engel et al., 1973; Seipel et al., 1975; Delius et al., 1975; Steinbeck and Lüderitz, 1975; Dhingra et al., 1976b; Steinbeck and Lüderitz, 1976). Thus the sinus node recovery time can remain prolonged or can attain normal values (Mandel et al., 1971; Mandel et al., 1972; Narula et al., 1972; Delius et al., 1975; Engel et al., 1975). On the other hand, a prolongation of the sinus node recovery time can occasionally be encountered after administering atropine (Bashour et al., 1973; Narula et al., 1972; Seipel et al., 1975; Reiffel et al., 1975; Delius et al., 1975; Steinbeck and Lüderitz, 1976). This phenomenon is explained by a better conduction of the electrical impulse from the atrium to the sinus node which is induced by atropine (Breithardt et al., 1976). This allows more driven atrial stimuli to penetrate in the sinus node inducing a greater depression (Bashour et al., 1973; Reiffel et al., 1975; Steinbeck and Lüderitz, 1976). An argument in favor of this hypothesis is the observation that after administering atropine the rate at which the maximum value of the sinus node recovery time occurs tends to increase (Steinbeck and Lüderitz, 1975; Delius et al., 1975).

Another effect of atropine is the more frequent occurrence of junctional escape beats following atrial pacing than before its administration (Gupta et al., 1974; Narula et al., 1972; Delius et al., 1975).

In contrast to healthy subjects, the sinus node recovery time in patients with a sick sinus syndrome is often prolonged. Both depression of sinus node automaticity and impairement of antegrade sinoatrial conduction account for this prolongation (Steinbeck and Lüderitz, 1975).

The proportion with which the recovery time is found to be prolonged in patients with a sick sinus syndrome varies between 35% (Gupta et al., 1974) and 100% (Simonin et al., 1975). These differences can partly be explained by the different criteria used by the various investigators to define the normal limit of the sinus node recovery time. These criteria have been mentioned and explained above.

We have investigated the predictive value of these six different criteria testing these criteria for sensitivity and specificity. Table 1 gives the sensitivity (per cent of all 67 patients with a sick sinus syndrome who manifested a prolonged sinus node recovery time) and the specificity (per cent of normal sinus node recovery time in the 110 normal subjects) for each of the six criteria to define the normal value of the sinus node recovery time. Two facts are easily recognized: firstly, the sensitivity varies greatly between 56.7% and 80.6%. Secondly there is an inverse correlation between sensitivity and specificity for each of the six used criteria. The more specific the criterium the less sensitive it is and vice-versa. This finding can be explained by an overlapping of the sinus node recovery time values at the upper limit of the normal group and the lower limit of the sick sinus syndrome group. In other words, a part of the patients with sinus node dysfunction has a sinus node recovery time within the normal limits for a given criterium. The clinical implication of this finding is that there does not exist an ideal criterium for defining the upper limit of the normal value of the sinus node recovery time.

Table 2 shows the percentual repartition of the cases with prolonged sinus node recovery time depending on the used criterium in the four main forms of sick sinus syndrome, namely: sinoatrial block, persistent sinus bradycardia, bradycardia-tachycardia syndrome and sinoatrial arrest. It can be seen that, – except for the first criterium SNRT $\leq$ 1400 msec – a prolonged sinus node recovery time is most often encountered in the group with sinoatrial block. The proportion of the occurrence of a prolonged sinus node recovery time in the patients with sinoatrial block is significantly greater than in the group with sinoatrial arrest when criterium no. 3 – SNRT $\leq$ 1680 msec – and criterium no. 5 – SNRT expressed as a percentage of the control cycle length – are used. When the latter criterium is used, there is also a significant difference between the group with sinoatrial block and the group with persistent bradycardia.

The sinus node recovery time fails tosshow a correlation with the spontaneous pauses observed in the group of patients with sinoatrial block or arrest (Figure 4).

Narula et al. (1972) found in a patient with sick sinus syndrome a sinus node recovery time being almost identical to the pause observed occurring after termination of a spontaneous atrial tachycardia. In 8 patients with bradycardia-tachycardia syndrome we fortuitously induced an episode of atrial flutter or fibrillation during the electrophysiologic study. The episodes lasted for ½–24 min. The end of the flutter or fibrillation phase could be recorded in all patients. The pause that preceded the first sinus node beat was longer than the sinus node recovery time in 4 patients, shorter in one patient and almost equal in the other 3 patients. However, a good correlation between these two parameters could be found (r = 0.7735; p < 0.05) (Figure 5).

From this finding it can be said that the sinus node recovery time reflects only the

Table 1. Predictive value of six different sinus node recovery time criteria.

Criterium		SNRT ≤ 1400 msec	SNRT ≤ 1500 msec	SNRT ≤ 1680 msec	CSNRT ≤ 525 msec	SNRT % CCL	Regression equation
Sensitivity n = 67	%	80.6	73.1	64.2	68.7	56.7	74.6
Specificity n = 110	%	90.9	96.3	100	98.2	100	76.4

Table 2. Comparative analysis of the incidence of prolonged sinus node recovery time in the four main forms of sick sinus syndrome when six different criteria are used.

Criterium Clinical form		SNRT ≤ 1400 msec	SNRT ≤ 1500 msec	SNRT ≤ 1680 msec	CSNRT ≤ 525 msec	SNRT % CCL	Regression equation
SA-Block n = 27	%	85.2	81.5	77.8	81.5	77.8	77.8
Sinus bradycardia n = 15	%	86.7	73.3	53.3	53.3	26.7**	73.3
Brady-Tachy syndrome n = 22	%	77.3	68.2	63.6	68.2	59.1	72.7
Sinus arrest n = 3	%	33.3	33.3	0*	33.3	0*	66.6

* p < 0.05 when compared with the SA-block group.
** p < 0.01 when compared with the SA-block group.

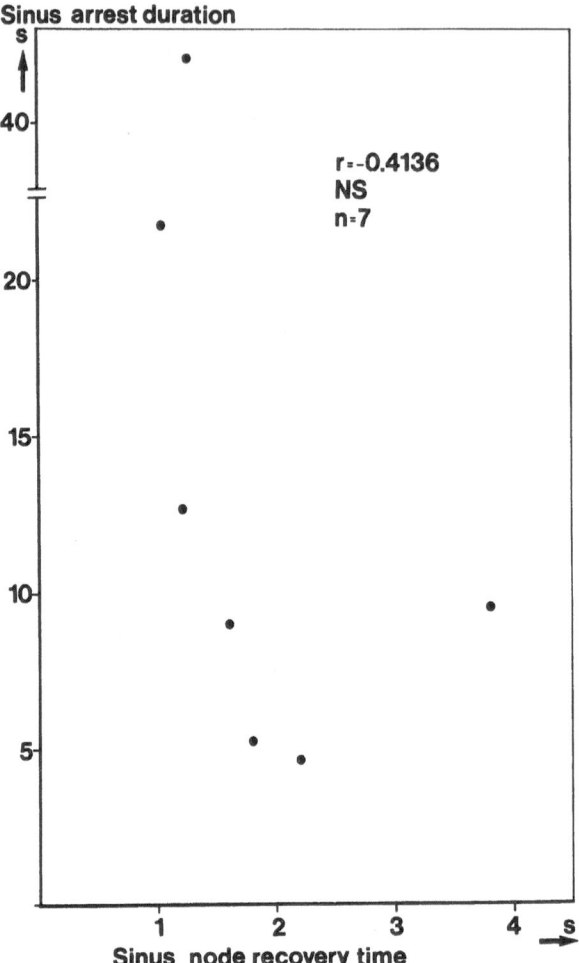

Figure 4. Plot of sinus node recovery time (on the abscissa) against sinus arrest duration (on the ordinate) in 7 patients with sick sinus syndrome. There was a lack of correlation between these two parameters.

degree of sinoatrial depression induced by a spontaneously occurring or artificially provoked atrial tachycardia. It does not correlate with the intrinsic spontaneous dysfunction in automaticity or conduction responsible for the occurrence of sinus arrest or pauses.

Controls of the duration of sinus node recovery time performed after several months showed either no significant change (Gupta et al., 1974) or a prolongation (Narula et al., 1972;.Okimoto et al., 1976).

In patients with a sick sinus syndrome prolongation of cycle length subsequent to the first postdriving cycle are seen occasionally (Narula et al., 1972; Bigger and Strauss, 1973; Margolis et al., 1975; Schwarz et al., 1975; Steinbeck and Lüderitz, 1975; Bleifeld et al., 1975; Okimoto et al., 1976; Strauss et al., 1976a; Beneditt et al., 1976). They have been named secondary pauses (Bigger and Strauss, 1973; Strauss et al., 1976a; Benditt et al., 1976). These pauses can be preceded by a normal (Steinbeck and Lüderitz, 1975; Okimoto et al., 1976; Strauss et al., 1976a; Benditt et al., 1976) or by a prolonged first postdriving cycle (Steinbeck and Lüderitz, 1975; Strauss et al., 1976a).

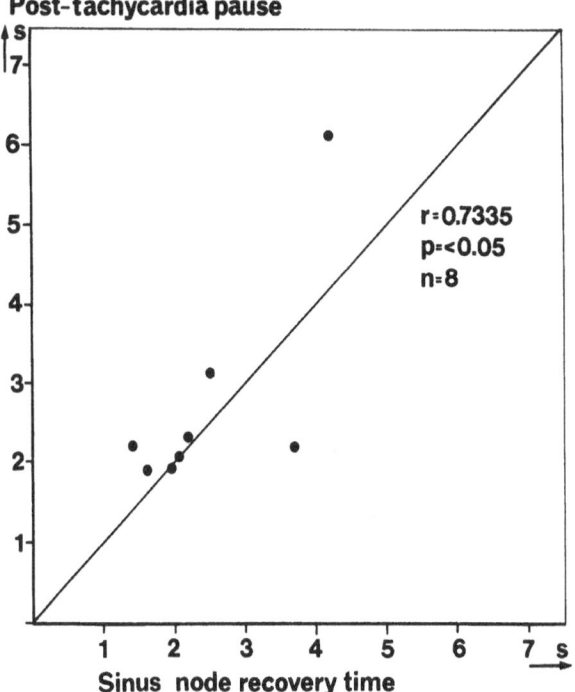

Figure 5. The relationship between the sinus node recovery time – on the abscissa – and the post-tachycardia pause – on the ordinate – observed after fortuitously induced atrial fibrillation or flutter in 8 patients with sick sinus syndrome. The straight line is the line of identity. There was a good correlation between the two parameters (r = 0.7335; p < 0.05).

Benditt et al. (1976) described two types of secondary pauses. Type I shows an abrupt prolongation of cycle length subsequent to the first postdriving cycle. Type II of secondary pause shows a sustained prolongation of the postdrive cycle for more than three cycles following termination of pacing. The secondary pauses are interpreted as the result of both depression of automaticity and of conduction (Benditt et al., 1976). They occur more frequently at pacing rates higher than those at which the maximum value of sinus node recovery time is reached (Bigger and Strauss, 1973).

Benditt et al. (1976) found that the secondary pauses occur more frequently in patients with sinoatrial block than in patients with other forms of sick sinus syndrome. Our results are in agreement with this observation (Table 3).

Table 3. Incidence of secondary pauses in patients with sick sinus syndrome.

Clinical form		% of cases	Sinus arrest	Statistical analysis Brady-Tachy syndrome	Sinus bradycardia
SA-Block	n = 27	85.2	p < 0.01	p < 0.05	p < 0.01
Sinus bradycardia	n = 15	40	NS	NS	
Brady-Tachy syndrome	n = 22	50	NS		
Sinus arrest	n = 3	0			

CONCLUSION

The atrial pacing is an useful method to demask or to confirm the presence of a sick sinus syndrome, disclosing a disturbed sinoatrial response. This disturbed pattern of response is expressed among other things by a prolonged sinus node recovery time. However, the main limitation of this method is the relatively great incidence of either false negative or false positive results, depending upon the used criterium which sets the upper limit of the normal value of the sinus node recovery time. When the chosen criterium is rather specific a greater per cent of false negative results is to be expected. When one uses a more sensitive criterium, the number of false positive cases will prevail. A prolongation of the sinus node recovery time is encountered most often in the group of patients with sinoatrial block. This group of patients also shows a higher incidence of secondary pauses. A prolongation of the sinus node recovery time is rarely seen in patients with persistent sinus bradycardia or bradycardia-tachycardia syndrome. However, in this latter group the prolongation of the SNRT has a predictive value which correlates well with the pauses that occur after cessation of a run of atrial tachycardia.

REFERENCES

1. Amory, D.A., West, T.C.: Chronotropic response following direct electrical stimulation of the isolated sinoatrial node: a pharmacologic evaluation. *J Pharmacol Exp. Ther* 137: 14, 1962
2. Bashour, T.: An unusual effect of atropine on overdrive suppression. *Circulation* 48: 911, 1973
3. Benditt, D.G., Strauss, H.C., Scheinmann, M.M., Behar, U.S., Wallace, A.G.: Analysis of secondary pauses following termination of rapid atrial pacing in man. *Circulation* 54: 436, 1976
4. Bigger, J.T., Strauss, H.C.: The evaluation of sinoatrial node function in man. *Med Coll Virg Quart* 9: 79, 1973
5. Bleifeld, W., Rupp, M., Fleischmann, D., Effert, S.: Syndrom des kranken Sinusknotens ("Sick-Sinus"-Syndrom). *Dtsch Med Wochenschr* 99: 795, 1974
6. Brandfonbrener, M., Landowne, M., Shock, N.W.: Changes in cardiac output with age. *Circulation* 12: 557, 1955
7. Breithardt, G., Seipel, L., Both, A., Loogen, F.: The effect of atropine on calculated sinoatrial conduction time in man. *Eur J Cardiol* 4: 49, 1976
8. Chadda, K.D., Banka, V.S., Bodenheimer, M.M., Helfant, R.H.: Corrected sinus node recovery time. Experimental physiologic and pathologic determinants. *Circulation* 51: 797, 1975
9. Delius, W., Wirtzfeld, A., Sebening, H., Blömer, H.: Bedeutung der Sinusknotenerholungszeit beim Sinusknotensyndrom. *Dtsch Med Wochenschr* 100: 2305, 1975
10. Dhingra, R.C., Rosen, K.M., Rahimtoola, S.H.: Normal conduction intervals and responses in sixty-one patients using His bundle recording and atrial pacing. *Chest* 64: 55, 1973
11. Dhingra, R.C., Amat-y-Leon, F., Wyndham, C., Denes, P., Wu, D., Pouget, J.M., Rosen, K.M.: Electrophysiologic effects of atropine on human sinus node and atrium. *Am J Cardiol* 38: 429, 1976a
12. Dhingra, R.C., Amat-y-Leon, F., Wyndham, C., Denes, P., Wu, D., Miller, R.H., Rosen, K.M.: Electrophysiologic effects of atropine on sinus node and atrium in patients with sinus nodal disfunction. *Am J Cardiol* 38: 848, 1976b
13. Engel, T.R., Schaal, S.F.: Digitalis in the sick sinus syndrome. The effects of digitalis on sinoatrial automaticity and atrioventricular conduction. *Circulation* 48: 1201, 1973
14. Ferrer, M.I.: The sick sinus syndrome in atrial disease. *JAMA* 206: 645, 1968
15. Ferrer, M.I.: The sick sinus syndrome. *Circulation* 47: 635, 1973
16. Gaskell, W.H.: On the innervation of the heart with especial reference to the heart of the tortoise. *J Physiol (London)* 4: 43, 1884
17. Goldreyer, B.N., Damato, A.N.: Sinoatrial-node entrance block. *Circulation* 44: 789, 1971
18. Goodman, D.J., Rossen, R.M., Ingham, R., Rider, A.K., Harrison, D.C.: Sinus node function in the denervated human heart. Effect of digitalis. *Br Heart J* 37: 612, 1975
19. Gupta, P.K., Lichstein, E., Chadda, K.D., Badui, E.: Appraisal of sinus nodal recovery time in patients with sick sinus syndrome. *Am J Cardiol* 34: 265, 1974
20. Hutter, O.F., Trautwein, W.: Vagal and sympathetic effects on the pacemaker fibers in the sinus venosus of the heart. *J Gen Physiol* 39: 715, 1956

21. Jordan, J., Yamaguchi, I., Mandel, W.J., McCullen, A.E.: Comparative effects of overdrive on sinus and subsidiary pacemaker function. *Am Heart J* 93: 367, 1977
22. Kulbertus, H.E., De Leval-Rutten, F., Mary, L., Casters, P.: Sinus node recovery time in the elderly. *Br Heart J* 37: 420, 1975
23. Lange, G.: Action of driving stimuli from intrinsic and extrinsic sources on in situ cardiac pacemaker tissues. *Circ Res* 17: 449, 1965
24. Lu, H.H., Lange, G., McC. Brooks, C.: Factors controlling pacemaker action in cells of the sinoatrial node. *Circ Res* 17: 460, 1965
25. Mandel, W., Hayakawa, H., Danzig, R., Marcus, H.S.: Evaluation of sinoatrial node function in man by overdrive suppression. *Circulation* 44: 59, 1971
26. Mandel, W.J., Hayakawa, H., Allen, H.N., Danzig, R., Kermaier, A.I.: Assessment of sinus node function in patients with sick sinus syndrome. *Circulation* 46: 761, 1972
27. Margolis, J.R., Strauss, H.C., Miller, H.C., Gilbert, M., Wallace, A.G.: Digitalis and the sick sinus syndrome. Clinical and electrophysiologic documentation of a severe toxic effect on sinus node function. *Circulation* 52: 162, 1975
28. Narula, O.S., Samet, P., Javier, R.P.: Significance of the sinus-node recovery time. *Circulation* 45: 140, 1972
29. Narula, O.S.: Sinus node re-entry. A mechanism for supraventricular tachycardia. *Circulation* 50: 1114, 1974
30. Okimoto, T., Ueda, K., Kamata, C., Yoshida, H., Ohkawa, S., Hirooka, K., Kuwajima, I., Sugiura, M., Murakami, M., Matsuo, H.: Sinus node recovery time and abnormal postpacing phase in the aged patients with sick sinus syndrome. *Jpn Heart J* 17: 290, 1976
31. Paulay, K.L., Damato, A.N.: Comparison of atrial and ventricular drive on sinus nodal function in dog. *Am J Cardiol* 31: 41, 1973
32. Reiffel, J.A., Bigger, J.T., Giardina, E.G.V.: "Paradoxical" prolongation of sinus nodal recovery time after atropine in the sick sinus syndrome. *Am J Cardiol* 36: 98, 1975
33. Rich, J.M., Meisner, M.H., Fontana, M.E., Wooley, C.F.: Electrophysiologic stress tests in man: sinoatrial node suppression and recovery. (Abstract). *J Lab Clin Med* 78: 805, 1971
34. Rios, J.C., Bashour, T., Cheng, T.O., Motomiya, T.: Atrial pacing in sick sinus node syndrome. (Abstract). *Circulation* 45–46: suppl. II–211, 1972
35. Rosen, K.M., Loeb, H.S., Sinno, M.Z., Rahimtoola, S.H., Gunnar, R.M.: Cardiac conduction in patients with symptomatic sinus node disease. *Circulation* 43: 836, 1971
36. Scheinman, M.M., Kunkel, F.W., Peters, R.W., Hirschfeld, D.S., Schoenfeld, P.L., Abbott, J.A., Modin, G.: Atrial pacing in patients with sinus node dysfunction. *Am J Med* 61: 641, 1976
37. Schwarz, F., Thormann, J., Zimmermann, H.: Vagaler Einfluss auf Sinusknotenfrequenz und AV-Überleitung bei hypersensitivem Karotissinusreflex und "Sick-Sinus-Syndrome". *Schweiz Med Wochenschr* 105: 240, 1975
38. Seipel, L., Breithardt, G., Both, A., Loogen, F.: Diagnostische Probleme beim Sinusknotensyndrom. *Z Kardiol* 64: 1, 1975
39. Simonin, P., Niederhauser, H.U., Duchosal, P.W.: Contribution de l'exploration électrique endocavitaire à l'etude de la dysrythmie auriculaire. *Arch Mal Coeur* 69: 341, 1976
40. Steinbeck, G., Lüderitz, B.: Comparative study of sinoatrial conduction time and sinus node recovery time. *Br Heart J* 37: 956, 1975
41. Steinbeck, G., Lüderitz, B.: Sinus node recovery time and sinoatrial conduction time. In: Lüderitz, B.: Cardiac Pacing. Diagnostic and Therapeutic Tools. Springer-Verlag, Berlin, Heidelberg, New York, 1976, p. 45
42. Strauss, H.C., Bigger, J.T., Saroff, A.L., Giardina, E.G.V.: Electrophysiologic evaluation of sinus node function in patients with sinus node dysfunction. *Circulation* 53: 763, 1976a
43. Strauss, H.C., Gilbert, M., Svenson, R.H., Miller, H.C., Wallace, A.G.: Electrophysiologic effects of propranolol on sinus node function in patients with sinus node dysfunction. *Circulation* 54: 452, 1976b
44. Ticzon, A.R., Strauss, H.C., Gallagher, J.J., Wallace, A.G.: Sinus nodal function in the intact dog heart evaluated by premature atrial stimulation and atrial pacing. *Am J Cardiol* 35: 492, 1975
45. Vincenzi, F.F., West, T.C.: Release of autonomic mediators in cardiac tissue by direct subthreshold electrical stimulation. *J Pharmacol Exp Ther* 141: 185, 1963
46. Weisfogel, G.M., Batsford, W.P., Raulay, K.L., Josephson, M.F., Ogunkelu, J.B., Akhtar, M., Seides, S.F., Damato, A.N.: Sinus node re-entrant tachycardia in man. *Am Heart J* 90: 295, 1975
47. West, T.C.: Effects of chronotropic influences on subthreshold oscillations in the sino-atrial node. In: The Specialized Tissues of the Heart, edited by Paes De Carvalho, A., De Mello, W.C. and Hoffman, B.F. Elsevier Publishing Company. Amsterdam, London, New York, Princeton, 1961, p. 81
48. Wu, D., Amat-y-Leon, F., Denes, P., Dhingra, R.C., Pietras, R.J., Rosen, K.M.: Demonstration of sustained sinus and atrial re-entry as a mechanism of paroxysmal supraventricular tachycardia. *Circulation* 51: 234, 1975
49. Yabek, S,M., Jarmakani, J.M., Roberts, N.K.: Sinus node function in children. Factors influencing its evaluation. *Circulation* 53: 28, 1976

3

PROGRAMMED ATRIAL STIMULATION USED FOR THE CALCULATION OF SINO-ATRIAL CONDUCTION TIME (SACT) IN MAN*

LUDGER SEIPEL, GUENTER BREITHARDT, AND CHRISTIAN LEUNER

A direct recording of sinus node activity has not yet been accomplished in man. Therefore, indirect methods for estimation of sinus node activity and sino-atrial conduction have been used. In addition to high rate test, programmed atrial stimulation was introduced for assessing sinus node function (Goldreyer and Damato, 1971; Saroff et al., 1971; Narula et al., 1972). In 1973 Strauss et al. used this technique for calculation of sino-atrial conduction time in man. Since then many clinical investigators have published their experiences with this method (Seipel et al., 1974; Steinbeck et al., 1974; Dhingra et al., 1975; Goodman et al., 1975; Mandel et al., 1975; Masini et al., 1975; Medvedowsky et al., 1975; Engel et al., 1976; Scheinman et al., 1976; Strauss et al., 1976; Breithardt et al., 1977; Crook et al., 1977; Dhingra et al., 1977; Jordan et al., 1977; Steinbeck and Lüderitz, 1977; Ueda et al., 1977). However, experimental and clinical data have shown that this method is burdened by unresolved methodological problems (Miki and Rothberger, 1922; Eccles and Hoff, 1934; Langendorf et al., 1962; Bonke et al., 1969, 1971; Strauss and Bigger, 1972; Fleischman, 1973; Klein et al., 1973; Miller and Strauss, 1974; Reiffel et al., 1974, 1975; Seipel and Breithardt, 1975; Ticzon et al., 1975; Breithardt and Seipel, 1976; Strauss and Wallace, 1976). In addition, the clinical relevance of the method is an unanswered question. Therefore, we performed programmed atrial stimulation in different groups of patients with and without sinus node dysfunction in order to correlate SACT with other clinical data.

METHOD AND MATERIAL

A quadripolar electrode catheter was introduced into the high right atrium (HRA) via the femoral route. The distal pair of electrodes at the tip of the catheter was connected with a battery-powered pacemaker. (Medtronic 5325). The pacer has an output for connection to the recorder which enables the registration of the atrial signal (HRA_2) from the pacemaker electrodes during sensing mode. If pacing, the output to the recorder is short-circuited with a stimulus artifact appearing on the record (Figure 1, 2). An additional bipolar atrial electrogram (HRA_1) was recorded by the proximal pair of electrodes. The intracardiac signals entered a modified 8-channel ink ejection paper recorder (Siemens Cardirex) via a current limiting selector (Elema). A beat-to-beat interval counter (H. Mescher, IFD) was used for measuring the A-A intervals from the lead HRA_1. To control the accuracy of triggering, every triggered A wave was marked by the counter on the original record (Figure 2). The automatically measured A-A intervals were on-line

* Supported in part by Landesamt für Forschung NRW.

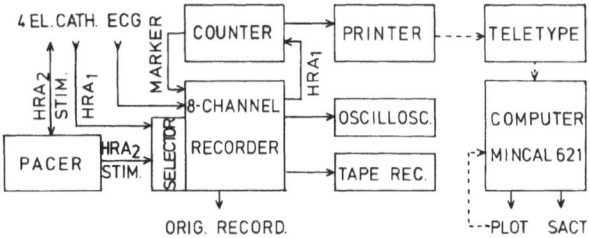

Figure 1. Diagram of pacing and recording equipment for measurement of SNRT and SACT. For explanation see text.

printed out by a digital printer (Kienzle). The data obtained during premature atrial stimulation were given into a computer (Dietz Mincal 621) via a teletype. The computer was used for plotting the return and postreturn cycles normalized for the spontaneous cycle length (Figure 3). After the zone of reset responses (plateau) has been marked as the area of

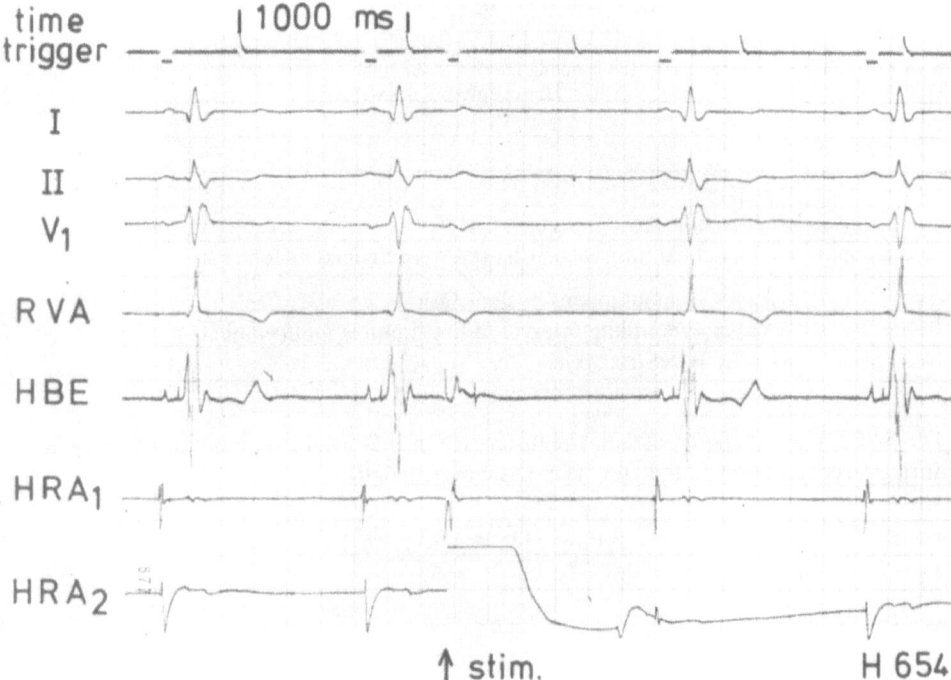

Figure 2. Original record during programmed atrial stimulation. From top to bottom: time mark and trigger impuls of the counter (rectangle), lead I, II, V$_1$, electrogram from the right ventricular apex (RVA), His bundle electrogram (HBE), high right atrial electrogram from the proximal pair of electrodes (HRA$_1$), high right atrial electrogram from the distal electrodes via the pacemaker (HRA$_2$), Stim. = stimulus artifact.

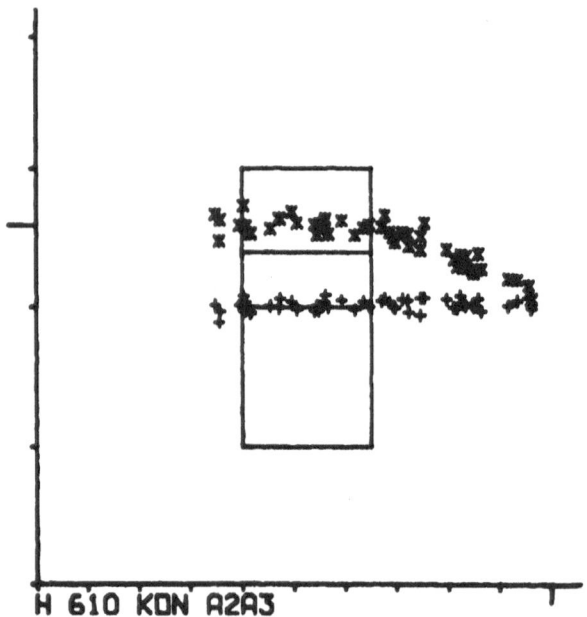

H 610 KON A2A3

Figure 3. Original computer plot of the return cycles (A_2-A_3/A_1-A_1) (∗) and the postreturn cycles (A_3-A_4/ A_1-A_1) (+) on the ordinate against the coupling interval of the stimulus (A_1-A_2/A_1-A_1) on the abscissa. The upper rectangle marks the "points of interest" for calculation of SACT.

interest on an oscilloscopic storage screen, SACT was calculated from the selected points by the computer. The atrial intervals measured were defined as follows:

A_1-A_1 = spontaneous cycle length
A_1-A_2 = coupling interval of the stimulus-induced beat
A_2-A_3 = return cycle
A_3-A_4 = postreturn cycle

The SACT was calculated as half the difference of the mean length of the return cycles during reset responses minus the mean basic cycle length.

$$SACT = \frac{\overline{(A_2\text{-}A_3)} - \overline{(A_1\text{-}A_1)}}{2}$$

Sinus node recovery time (SNRT) after high rate test was also measured automatically by the counter. SNRT was corrected for the spontaneous cycle length (CSNRT) by calculating the difference between both according to Narula et al. (1972). All clinical and electrophysiological data were stored in a computer (Telefunken TR 445) using version 6 of the SPSS program (Statistical Package for the Social Sciences).

Statistical evaluation was done by use of Student's t-test for unpaired data. For variance analysis within the single groups the F-test was used.

Altogether 202 patients were studied. The patients were devided into three groups (Table 1):

Table 1. Clinical and electrophysiological findings in 202 patients studied by programmed and high rate atrial stimulation. A_1-A_1 = basic sinus cycle length during the study. SNRT = sinus node recovery time. SACT = calculated sino-atrial conduction time. SN = sinus node.

group	patients	n	age (y)	A_1-A_1 (msec)	SNRT (msec)	SACT (msec)	p <
1	normal persons	30	32.1 ± 13.3	759.6 ± 136.2	1040.6 ± 194.3	87.3 ± 20.2	0.002
2	patients without SN dysfunction	106	47.1 ± 15.5	785.0 ± 158.7	1140.0 ± 158.8	104.8 ± 28.8	0.004
3	patients with SN dysfunction	66	55.2 ± 14.4	1041.6 ± 239.0	1967.0 ± 1086.7	126.3 ± 51.8*	

0.0001 (group 1 vs 3)

* n = 58, 9 pts. CP

1. Normal persons (n = 30) in whom programmed atrial stimulation was performed during heart catheterization to exclude an atrial septal defect etc.
2. Patients without clinical signs of sinus node disease (n = 106) in whom His bundle study was done for evaluation of atrioventricular or intraventricular conduction defects etc. Many of these patients had coronary heart disease.
3. Patients with sinus node dysfunction (n = 66) as defined by constant or intermittent sinus bradycardia with or without either intermittent atrial tachycardia, especially atrial fibrillation or intermittent sinus pauses during long-term tape recording.

RESULTS

The normals were younger (mean age 32.1 years) than the patients with sinus node dysfunction (mean age 55.2 years) and had a shorter basis cycle length during the study (759.6 ± 136.2 msec vs. 1041 ± 239.0 msec) (Table 1). In the normals and in the group of patients without sinus node dysfunction there was no correlation between SACT and age. In the group of patients with sinus node dysfunction the longest values for SACT were found in the older age (Figure 4). No correlation could be found plotting SACT versus basic cycle length during the study in the group of patients with sinus node dysfunction. In the patients without sinus node disease, there was a trend to longer values of SACT with increasing cycle length. However, the correlation coefficiency was insufficient (r = 0.35, p < 0.0001, Figure 5).

The SACT in normals (87.3 ± 20.2 msec) was significantly shorter than in the group of patients with sinus node dysfunction (126.3 ± 51.8 msec) (p < 0.0001). The SACT in patients without signs of sinus node disease (group 2) was between those of group 1 and 3 (104.8 ± 28.8 msec) with significant differences between this group and the two other groups (Table 1). In some of the patients of group 2 the calculated SACT was very abnormal (Figure 6). In 9 patients with sinus node dysfunction (group 3) a "chaotic pattern" of the return cycles was found, i.e. there was no correlation between the coupling interval of the stimulus (A_1-A_2) and the length of the return cycle (A_2-A_3). In this situation no

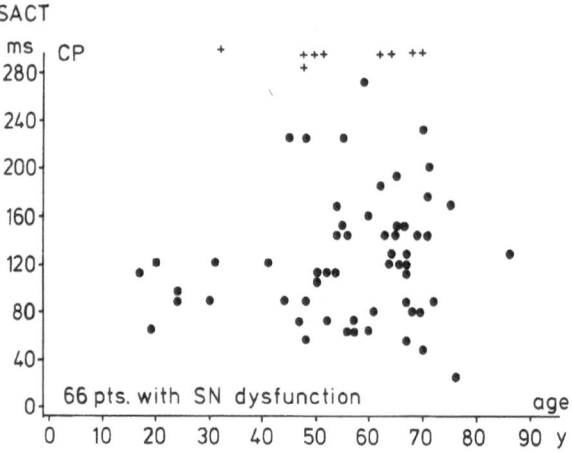

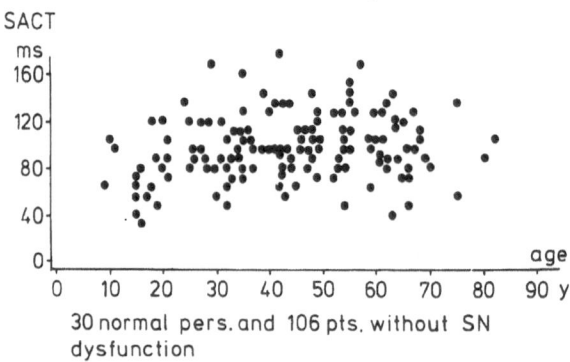

Figure 4. Plot of SACT versus age in patients with sinus node dysfunction (group 3) as well as in normals and patients without sinus node disease (group 1 and 2). CP = chaotic pattern of the return cycles.

calculation of SACT was possible. This pattern was only seen in patients with sinus node dysfunction.

Plotting SACT versus CSNRT a poor correlation was found in patients with and without sinus node dysfunction. In 15 of the 106 patients without signs of sinus node disease (group 2) SACT was abnormal whereas CSNRT was within the normal range of 525 msec. In the group of patients with sinus node dysfunction 10 of 66 cases had a prolonged SACT or a chaotic pattern of the return cycles with a normal CSNRT. Almost the same number of patients had a normal SACT and a prolonged CSNRT (Figure 6).

In the group of patients with sinus node dysfunction no correlation could be found between calculated SACT and the symptoms (syncope-like events). The same was true for SNRT (Figure 7).

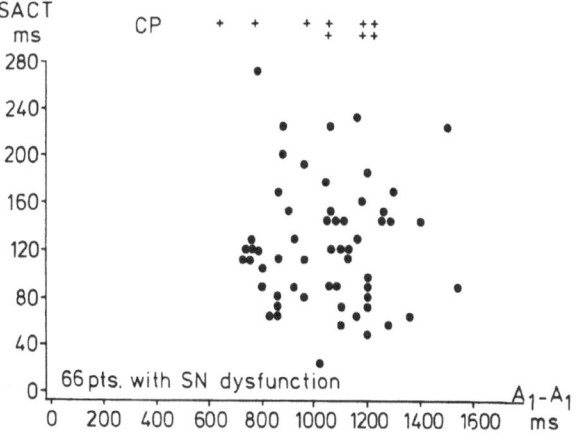

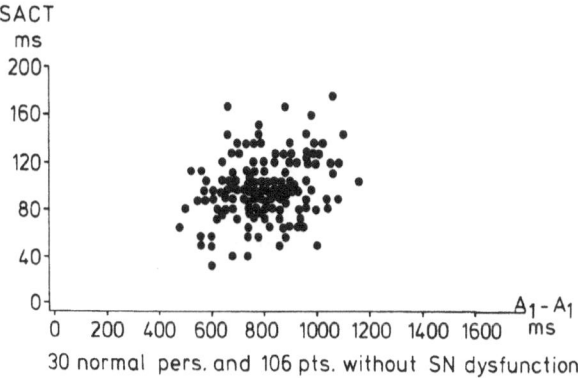

Figure 5. Plot of SACT versus mean basic cycle length (A_1-A_1) during the study in normals and in patients without sinus node disease (group 1 and 2) as well as in patients with sinus node dysfunction (group 3).

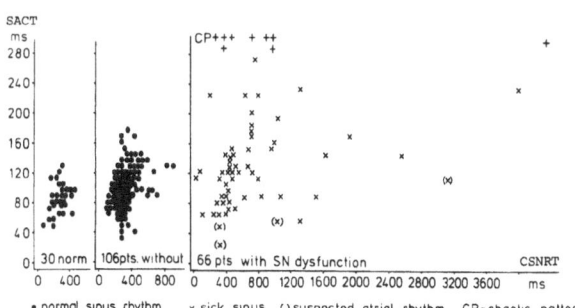

Figure 6. Plot of SACT versus CSNRT in normals, patients without sinus node disease and patients with sinus node dysfunction.

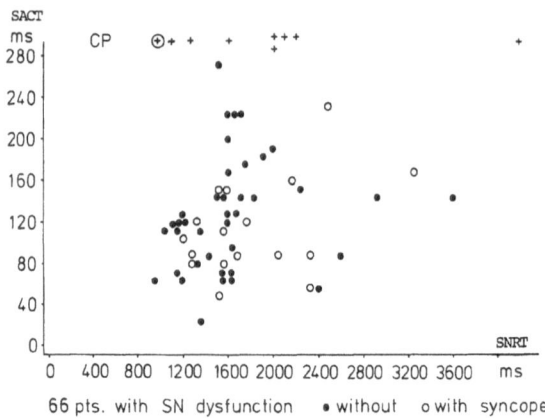

Figure 7. Plot of SACT versus SNRT in patients with sinus node dysfunction with and without a history of syncope-like events.

DISCUSSION

Many clinical investigators have calculated SACT in patients with and without sinus node disease. The results are not uniform in all studies. Some authors found that calculation of SACT is a useful clinical tool for the differentiation of patients with normal and abnormal sinus node function (Mandel et al., 1975; Masini et al., 1975; Engel et al., 1976; Strauss et al., 1976; Breithardt et al., 1977; Dhingra et al., 1977; Jordan et al., 1977; Steinbeck and Lüderitz, 1977). Other investigators concluded from their results that programmed atrial stimulation is not of great clinical value (Narula et al., 1972; Scheinman et al., 1976; Crook et al., 1977; Ueda et al., 1977).

The differences may in part be due to the selection of patients. The first problem is to get real normal values. Patients with intraventricular conduction defects, for example, are not normal even if they have no signs of sinus node disease. Figure 6 shows that many patients with A-V or intraventricular conduction defects have a prolonged sino-atrial conduction time. The findings would suggest that in some patients a disease of the entire conduction system may exist which has been described as "panconductional disease" (Rasmussen, 1971).

A second problem is whether or not we are allowed to compare the data in normals with the findings in patients with sinus node dysfunction. Our normals are relatively young in comparison to the patients with sinus node dysfunction. However, as far as our data indicate, age does not play an important role. There is no trend to higher values of SACT in the older group of patients without clinical signs of sinus node dysfunction (Figure 4). In the patients with sinus node disease the highest values for SACT were found in the older age group. One can only speculate that this may indicate a progressive involvement of the sinus node in the underlying pathologic process with increasing age. The normals had a shorter cycle length during the study than patients with sinus node dysfunction. Plotting mean SACT versus mean sinus cycle length during the study showed no correlation in the group of patients with sinus node dysfunction. In the patients without sinus node disease, there was a slight trend to longer values of SACT with increasing cycle length without a close correlation between these two parameters (Figure 5). The same was found by Ueda et al. (1977). Using another approach, Reiffel et al. (1974) and Seipel and Breithardt (1975) found an inverse relationship between the length of the preceding sinus cycle and the SACT calculated from the following return cycle in patients with sinus arrhythmia. Possibly, these changes in the length of the return cycles are only due to phasic changes in sinus node automaticity and have nothing to do with sino-atrial conduction. In spite of these problems, the different groups of patients seem to be comparable as far as SACT is concerned.

The third problem is how to define sinus node disease. We feel that there are at least four different subgroups of patients who are sometimes taken together. Patients with hypersensitive carotid sinus syndrome, patients with isolated sinus bradycardia, patients with bradycardia-tachycardia syndrome and those with intermittent sinus pauses. In a former study (Breithardt et al., 1977) we found significant differences between SACT in patients with isolated sinus bradycardia without other rhythm disturbances and in those with sinus bradycardia and different atrial dysrhythmias in addition. The SACT in asymptomatic patients with isolated sinus bradycardia was not significantly different from the SACT of our normal group. This explains why within the group of patients with sinus node dysfunction (group 3) many cases had normal values for SACT (Figure 6). In addition, an abnormal behaviour of the return cycles (chaotic pattern) was seldom found in patients with isolated sinus bradycardia in contrast to the group with "typical" sick sinus syndrome. From these findings we concluded that sinus bradycardia and sick sinus syndrome are different entities or that both represent different stages of the same disease. Performing the high rate test Masini and Dianda (1977) found normal values in most of their patients who were classified as "functional sinus bradycardia". Another approach to this problem was made by Dighton (1974) who found a different response to atropine and autonomic reflex manoeuvres in patients with sick sinus and "bradycardia of physiological origin."

There was no correlation between the SACT and the symptoms of the patients. The same was true for the SNRT (Figure 7). The problem is that in most of the patients we do not know the mechanisms of syncope. During our long-term tape recordings we found that in some patients the symptoms are not related to rhythm disturbances. The same was reported by others (DeSilva and Shubrooks 1977). In this situation one would not expect any correlation between the complaints of the patients and the result of the electrophysiological studies.

The most important question is whether or not programmed atrial stimulation gives an additional information to high rate test in patients with sinus node dysfunction. Figure 6 shows that in all normals CSNRT is in the normal range of 525 msec according to Narula et al. (1972). In the group without sinus node dysfunction (group 2) some patients had a prolonged SACT whereas CSNRT was normal. In these patients programmed atrial stimulation seems to be a more sensitive indicator for sinus node dysfunction than high rate test. The same was found by Jordan et al. (1977) in patients with coronary heart disease without clinical signs of sick sinus syndrome. However, nearly the same number of cases showed a normal SACT whereas CSNRT was abnormal. Even in the group of patients with sinus node dysfunction the same number of cases had a prolonged SACT whereas CSNRT was normal and vice versa. That means that the calculation of SACT has the same diagnostic value as the measurement of SNRT as far as the characterization of sinus node dysfunction is concerned. However, if therapeutical consequences as pacemaker indication or possible side effects of antiarrhythmic treatment are under discussion, high rate test is of greater importance. In this situation, calculation of SACT gives no additional information for taking the decision.

These conclusions invite a final comment on the clinical significance of programmed atrial stimulation. Calculations of SACT enables a characterization of sinus node function in the majority of patients with and without sinus node disease. This is not only true for the differentiation between normals and patients with typical sick sinus syndrome but also for the separation between the last group and patients with isolated sinus brady-cardia. Therefore, calculation of SACT is a useful clinical tool in addition to other inter-ventions. However, there are only a few cases in which programmed atrial stimulation gives an additional information to high rate test. In contrast to the measurement of sinus node recovery time after overdrive suppression, the calculation of sino-atrial conduction time has no practical consequences for the management of the patients. From this point of view, programmed atrial stimulation is of limited clinical value.

REFERENCES

Bonke, F.I.M., Bouman, L.N., van Rijn, H.E.: Change of cardiac rhythm in the rabbit after an atrial pre-mature beat. *Circulation Res* 24: 533, 1969

Bonke, F.I.M., Bouman, L.N., Schopman, F.J.G.: Effect of an early atrial premature beat on activity of the sinoatrial node and atrial rhythm in the rabbit. *Circulation Res* 29: 704, 1971

Breithardt, G., Seipel, L.: The effect of premature atrial depolarization on sinus node automaticity in man. *Circulation* 53: 920–925, 1976

Breithardt, G., Seipel, L., Loogen, F.: Sinus node recovery time and calculated sinoatrial conduction time in normal subjects and patients with sinus node dysfunction. *Circulation* 56: 43, 1977

Crook, B., Kitson, D., McComish, M., Jewitt, D.: Indirect measurement of sinoatrial conduction time in patients with sinoatrial disease. *Brit Heart J* 39: 771, 1977

DeSilva, R.A., Shubrocks, S.J.: Mitral valve prolaps with atrioventricular and sinoatrial node abnormalities of long duration. *Amer Heart J* 93: 772, 1977

Dhingra, R.C., Wyndham, C., Amat-y-Leon, F., Denes, P., Wu, D., Rosen, K.M.: Sinus nodal responses to atrial extrastimuli in patients without apparent sinus node disease. *Amer J Cardiol* 36: 445, 1975

Dhingra, R.C., Amat-y-Leon, F., Wyndham, C., Deedwania, P.C., Wu, D., Denes, P., Rosen, K.M.: Clinical significance of prolonged sinoatrial conduction time. *Circulation* 55: 8, 1977

Dighton, D.H.: Sinus bradycardia. Autonomic influences and clinical assessment. *Brit Heart J* 36: 791, 1974

Eccles, J.C., Hoff, H.E.: Rhythm of heart beat; II. Disturbance of rhythm produced by late premature beats. *Proc R Soc Lond (Biol)* 115: 327, 1934

Engel, T.R., Bond, R.C., Schaal, S.F.: First-degree sinoatrial heart block: Sinoatrial block in the sick sinus syndroms. *Amer Heart J* 91: 303, 1976

Fleischman, P.: Sinoatrial node entrance block (letter). *Circulation* 47: 210, 1973

Goldreyer, B.N., Damato, A.N.: Sinoatrial-node entrance block. *Circulation* 44: 789, 1971

Goodman, D.J., Rossen, R.H., Ingham, R., Rider, A.K., Harrison, D.C.: Sinus node function in the de-nervated human heart. Effect of digitalis. *Brit Heart J* 37: 612, 1975

Jordan, J., Yamaguchi, I., Mandel, W.J.: Characteristics of sinoatrial conduction in patients with coronary artery disease. *Circulation* 55: 569, 1977

Klein, H.O., Singer, D.H., Hoffman, B.F.: Effects of atrial premature systoles on sinus rhythm in the rabbit. *Circulation Res* 32: 480, 1973

Langendorf, R., Lesser, M.E., Plotkin, P., Levin, B.D.: Atrial parasystole with interpolation: Observations on prolonged sinoatrial conduction. *Amer Heart J* 63: 649, 1962

Mandel, W.J., Laks, M.M., Obayashi, K.: Sinus node function. *Arch Intern Med* 135: 386, 1975

Masini, G., Dianda, R.: Rilievi clinici ed elettrofisiologici in pazienti con bradicardia sinusale. *G Ital Cardiol* 7; 325, 1977

Masini, G., Dianda, R., Graziina, A.: Analysis of sino-atrial conduction in man using premature atrial stimulation. *Cardiovasc Res* 9: 498, 1975

Medvedowsky, J.L., Barney, C., Delaage, M., Nicolai, P., Chostakoff, F.: Étude de la fonction sinusale. *Arch Mal Coeur* 68: 225, 1975

Miki, Y., Rothberger, C.J.: Experimentelle Untersuchungen über die Pause nach Vorhofextrasystolen. *Z ges exper Med* 30: 347, 1922

Miller, H.C. Strauss, H.C.: Measurement of sinoatrial conduction time by premature atrial stimulation in the rabbit. *Circulation Res* 35: 935, 1974

Narula, O.S., Samet, P., Javier, R.P.: Significance of the sinus-node recovery time. *Circulation* 45: 140, 1972

Rasmussen, K.: Chronic sinoatrial heart block. *Amer Heart J* 81: 38, 1971

Reiffel, J.A., Bigger, J.T., Konstam, M.A.: The relationship between sinoatrial conduction time and sinus cycle length during spontaneous sinus arrhythmia in adults. *Circulation* 50: 924, 1974

Reiffel, J.A., Reid, D.S., Bigger, J.Th.: Holter monitoring and functional testing for sinus node dysfunction. *Circulation Suppl* 52/II: 111, 1975

Saroff, A.L., Strauss, H.C., Bigger, J.T., Steiner, C., Giardina, E.G.V.: Evaluation of sinus node function in patients with sinus bradycardia. *Circulation Suppl* 43–44/II: 97, 1971

Scheinman, M.M., Kunkel, F.W., Peters, R.W., Hirschfeld, D.S., Schoenfeld, P.L., Abbott, J.A., Modin, G.: Atrial pacing in patients with sinus node dysfunction. *Amer J Med* 61: 641, 1976

Seipel, L., Breithardt, G.: Sinusknotenautomatie und sinu-atriale Leitung. *Z Kardiol* 64: 1014, 1975

Seipel, L., Breithardt, G., Both, A., Loogen, F.: Messung der "sinuatrialen Leitungszeit" mittels vorzeitiger Vorhofstimulation beim Menschen. *Dtsch Med Wschr* 99: 1895, 1974

Steinbeck, G., Lüderitz, B.: Störungen der Sinusknotenfunktion. Diagnostik und klinische Bedeutung. *Dtsch Med Wschr* 102: 33, 1977

Steinbeck, G., Körber, H.J., Lüderitz, B.: Die Bestimmung der sinuatrialen Leitungszeit beim Menschen durch gekoppelte atriale Einzelstimulation. *Klin Wschr* 52: 1151, 1974

Strauss, H.C., Bigger, J.T.: Electrophysiological properties of the rabbit sinoatrial perinodal fibers. *Circulation Res* 31: 490, 1972

Strauss, H.C., Wallace, A.G.: Direct and indirect techniques in the evaluation of sinus node function. In: The conduction system of the heart, edited by Wellens, H.J.H., Lie, K.I., Janse, M.J., Stenfert Kroese, Leiden, 1976, p. 227

Strauss, H.C., Saroff, A.L., Bigger, J.T., Giardina, E.G.V.: Premature atrial stimulation as a key to the understanding of sinoatrial conduction in man. *Circulation* 47: 86, 1973

Strauss, H.C., Bigger, J.T., Saroff, A.L., Giardina, E.G.V.: Electrophysiologic evaluation of sinus node function in patients with sinus node dysfunction. *Circulation* 53: 763, 1976

Ticzon, A.R., Strauss, H.C., Gallagher, J.J., Wallace, A.G.: Sinus nodal function in the intact dog heart evaluated by premature atrial stimulation and atrial pacing. *Amer J Cardiol* 35: 492, 1975

Ueda, K., Kamata, C., Matsuo, H., Ohkawa, S., Okimoto, T., Sugiura, M.: A study on sinoatrial conduction in the aged. *Jap Heart J* 18: 143, 1977

4

THE PATTERN OF THE FIRST AND SECOND RETURN CYCLE AFTER PREMATURE ATRIAL STIMULATION

GIUSEPPE MASINI AND RENZO DIANDA

Several investigators (Han et al., 1968; Bonke et al., 1969, 1971; Goldreyer and Damato, 1971; Strauss and Bigger, 1972; Klein et al., 1973; Pauley et al., 1973a,b; Strauss et al., 1973; Childers et al., 1973; Miller and Strauss, 1974; Narula, 1974; Ticzon et al., 1975; Masini et al., 1975; Steinbeck and Lüderitz, 1975; Breithardt and Seipel, 1976; Engel et al., 1976; Dhingra et al., 1976; Strauss and Wallace, 1976; Strauss et al., 1976) have studied the effects of premature atrial stimulation on sinoatrial node function. Depending on the prematurity of the atrial stimulation, different types of response were observed. Premature atrial stimulations elicited in the last part of the atrial cycle, induce return cycles (or postextrasystolic cycles) longer than the basal one, making compensatory pauses. When premature atrial stimulations are introduced earlier, return cycles of almost the same length occur ("plateau" effect). In other cases, return cycles shorter than the basal ones may occur when premature atrial stimulations are introduced early in the atrial cycle, shortly after atrial refractoriness is ended.

The purpose of this report is to present the sinus node response to premature atrial stimulation observed in 137 patients, particularly concerning the pattern of the first and second return cycle.

MATERIALS AND METHOD

137 patients, ranging in age from 26 to 87 years, were studied. In these patients the electrophysiological study was performed because previous ECG had pointed out 1) sinoatrial dysfunction, 2) AV or intraventricular conduction defects, 3) ventricular pre-excitation. In some patients the study was performed during cardiac catheterization designed to evaluate chest pain not diagnostic of angina pectoris. In all patients sinus rhythm was present at the time of the examination. They were studied in the post-absorptive state, non sedated and none of them had received cardioactive medication for a week at least. The design and objective of the investigation was explained to each patient and signed informed consent obtained. A 6F bipolar pacing electrode catheter (with ring electrodes 1 mm wide and 1 cm apart) was introduced percutaneously via a femoral vein and placed across the septal leaflet of the tricuspid valve in the His bundle (HB) region, to record the His bundle electrogram (HBE). One quadripolar (7F) or two bipolar (4F) catheters were introduced via an antecubital vein and positioned against the high lateral wall of the right atrium in the region of the sinus node, for recording (HRA) and stimulation purposes. Bipolar electrograms displayed at frequency settings of 40–500 Hz were recorded from HRA and HB regions simultaneously with two or three standard ECG leads (I, II, III) and sometimes with an additional precordial lead (VI). All recordings were made on a multichannel photographic recorder at a paper speed of 50 or 100 mm/sec.

The right atrium was paced with a battery operated pacemaker (Programmable Pacing System CD-6) delivering rectangular stimuli 1 msec in duration and twice the diastolic threshold. Premature atrial stimulation (PAS)* was introduced after every 8th sinus cycle at least, starting very late in atrial diastole. The entire atrial cycle was scanned with 10–20 msec steps until the atrial refractory period was reached.

Then atrial pacing was performed at different rates ranging from 90 to 150 beats/min for periods of two minutes at each rate, to measure the sinus node recovery time (SNRT).

The following events were measured in milliseconds (msec) during each study:

1. Average sinus cycle: the mean value calculated from 20 sinus cycles immediately before eliciting a premature atrial stimulation;
2. A_1A_1 or basic cycle: the spontaneous sinus cycle length immediately preceding the introduction of the premature atrial stimulus;
3. A_1A_2 or test cycle (TC): the coupling interval measured from the last spontaneous beat (A_1) to the premature atrial complex (A_2);
4. A_2A_3 or first return cycle (RC): the interval measured from the premature atrial complex (A_2) to the subsequent atrial beat (A_3);
5. A_3A_4 or second or post return cycle (PRC): the interval between the first atrial beat of sinus origin (A_3) and the subsequent one (A_4);
6. $A_1A_2 + A_2A_3$: the sum of the test cycle and the return cycle;
7. Atrial effective refractory period (atrial ERP): the longest coupling interval between the sinus beat (A_1) and the stimulus at which A_2 failed to occur.

In each patient, the effects of premature atrial stimulation on the return cycle and the post return cycle at various coupling intervals were analysed. A plot was made, in which the test cycle (TC) expressed as $[(A_1A_1 - A_1A_2)/(A_1A_1)] \times 100$, was plotted on the ordinate, and the return cycle (RC) and the post return cycle (PRC), expressed as $[(A_2A_3 - A_1A_1)/(A_1A_1)] \times 100$, and as $[(A_3A_4 - A_1A_1)/(A_1A_1)] \times 100$ respectively, on the abscissa.

RESULTS

FIRST RETURN CYCLE (RC)

Plotting the return cycle as a function of the test cycle, no particular disposition of data points (chaotic pattern) was recognized in 5 (3.7%) out of 137 studied patients. In the remaining 132 patients, the distribution of data points was rather regular, permitting further analysis. Depending on the prematurity of atrial stimulation, different types of response have been observed.

Zone I (compensatory zone, no-reset-zone)
When premature atrial stimuli were elicited late in atrial diastole the return cycle (RC) was fully compensatory, i.e. $A_1A_2 + A_2A_3 = 2A_1A_1$. Plotting RC as function of the test cycle (TC) these points fell on the line of identity (compensatory line) (Figure 1, panel A). The shortest coupling interval of a premature atrial stimulation followed by a compensatory return cycle represents the inner limit of zone I or the "no-reset limit". In normal subjects the no-reset limit usually occurred after premature atrial stimuli introduced in

* Other authors are using the terminology of APD or "atrial premature depolarization".

the last 12–22% of the atrial cycle. Only in 3 normal subjects the no-reset limit occurred in the last 10% of the atrial cycle (Figure 1, panel B). In patients with sinoatrial conduction disturbances, the inner limit of zone I was observed after premature atrial stimuli introduced earlier in the atrial cycle (24–39%) (Figure 1, panel C). In five patients, all with serious dysfunction of the sinus node, a particular pattern was demonstrated. After the phase of fully compensatory return cycles, the premature atrial beats elicited earlier in the atrial cycle, were followed by return cycles that were more than compensatory (Figure 2).

Zone II (non-compensatory zone, reset zone)

An increasing prematurity of the atrial stimulation generally coincided with the appearance of less than compensatory return cycles, that is $A_1 A_2 + A_2 A_3 < 2 A_1 A_1$. This type of response defined the outer limit of zone II or reset-zone. The transition from zone I to zone II was rather sharp and easily identified in half of the patients; in other half, a slow and prolonged divergence from the compensatory line occurred prior to the beginning of zone II.

During zone II, the return cycles had usually the same length tending to a so-called "plateau" (Figure 3, panel A). A slight divergence to the left or the right (usually less than 5%) has been often observed. A more than 5% progressive divergence of data points towards the left in 5 (3.7%) normal subjects (Figure 3, panel B) and towards the right in 16

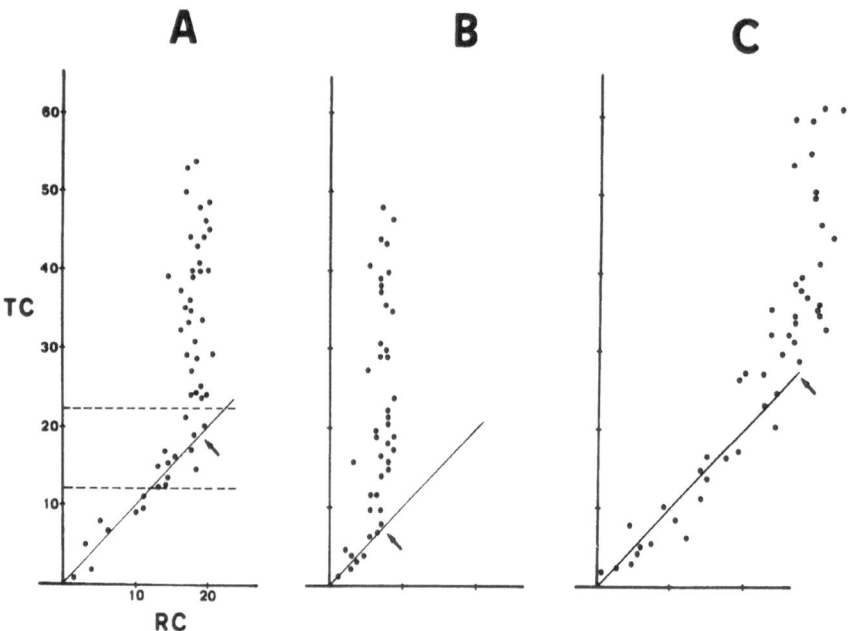

Figure 1. The return cycle (RC) expressed as $\left[(A_2 A_3 - A_1 A_1)/(A_1 A_1)\right] \times 100$ (on the abscissa) is plotted as a function of the test cycle (TC), expressed as $\left[(A_1 A_1 - A_1 A_2)/(A_1 A_1)\right] \times 100$ (on the ordinate).

In most normal subjects the no-reset limit ($\nwarrow$), representing the inner limit of zone I, occurred after premature atrial stimuli that were introduced in the last 12–22% of the atrial cycle (panel A). Only in three normal subjects the no-reset limit occurred after premature atrial beats, elicited in the last 10% of the atrial cycle (panel B), whereas in patients with sinoatrial conduction disturbances, the no-reset limit was often observed after premature atrial beats, introduced earlier in the atrial cycle (24–39%) (panel C).

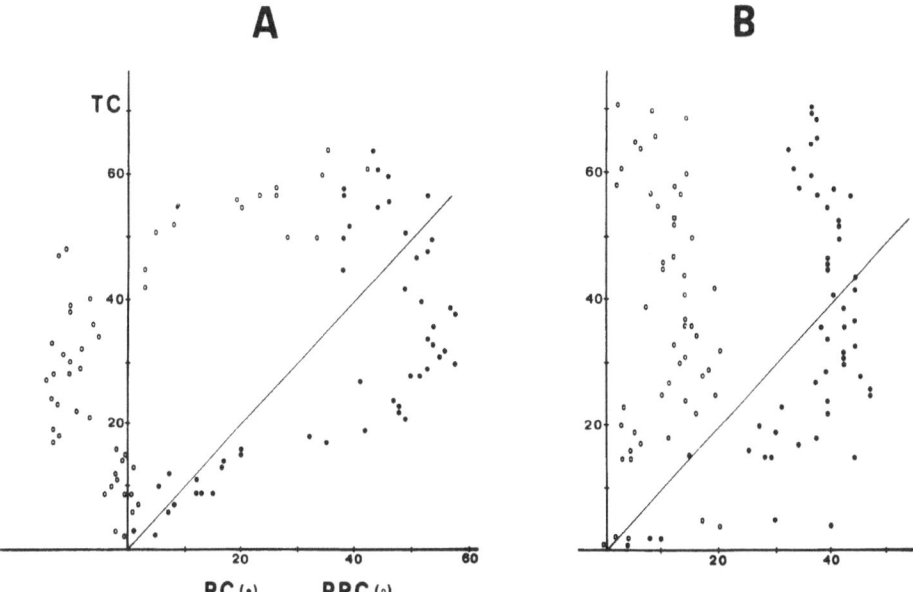

Figure 2. Pattern of the return cycle of RC (●) and the post return cycle or PRC (○). The RC, expressed as in Figure 1, and the PRC, expressed as $[(A_3A_4 - A_1A_1)/(A_1A_1)] \times 100$ (both represented on the abscissa), are plotted as a function of the test cycle (TC), expressed as in Figure 1 (on the ordinate).

In five patients with severe sinus node dysfunction, the RC, after a compensatory phase, suddenly lengthened; then it became relatively constant, forming a "plateau" (panel A, B). The PRC was in four patients longer (panel A) and in the other patient significantly shorter (panel B) than the basic cycle.

(11.7%) patients with sinoatrial conduction defects (Figure 3, panel C) could be demonstrated.

In the group of subjects with a normal function of the sinus node, the return cycle in the first 5% of zone II was between 80–220 msec (mean value: 168 ± 33 msec) longer than the basic cycle length.

Zone III
In 96 (70%) out of 132 patients, the reset-zone (zone II) outlasted until the atrial refractoriness was reached. In the remaining 41 cases (30%), an evident variation of the return cycle was observed when early premature beats were introduced. A progressive prolongation of the return cycle, that is a deviation of data points to the right, occurred in 6 subjects (4.4%) (Figure 4); whereas a shortening of the return cycle, that is a deviation of data points to the left, occurred in 35 patients (25.5%), most of them with normal sinus nodal function (Figure 5). In these cases the polarity and the shape of the P wave of the beat following the atrial premature beat, were almost identical in the surface ECG leads (I, II, III and VI) to that of the control sinus beat, and the intra-atrial conduction times and the sequence of atrial activation were similar. Analysing these short return cycles, three types of response have been identified. In 34 out of the 35 patients, after premature atrial stimuli, elicited in the range of 48.1–36.5% of the basic cycle length, the return cycle was shorter than the basic cycle but the sum of the test cycle and return cycle was longer than the basic cycle ("incomplete interpolation"); in 6 patients this sum was found to be equal or nearly equal to the basic cycle, after premature atrial stimuli that were elicited in a

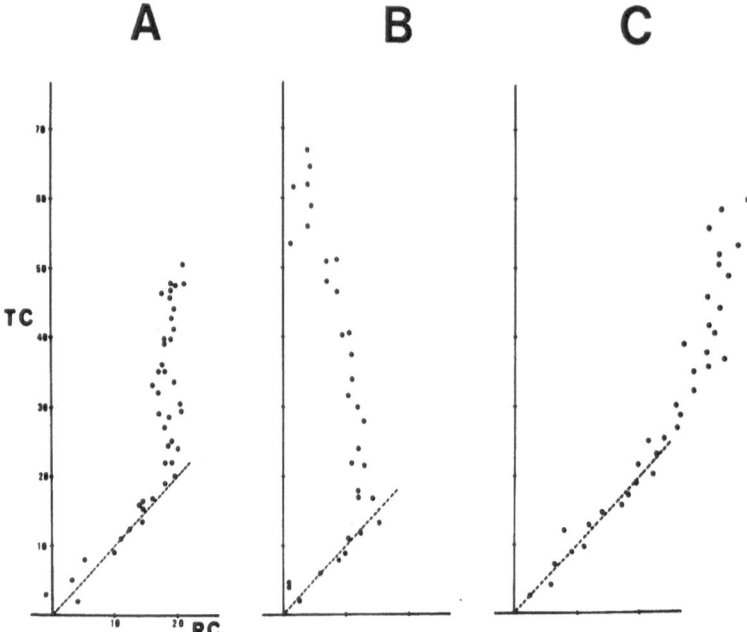

Figure 3. The test cycle (TC) and the return cycle (RC) are expressed as in Figure 1. During zone II, the return cycles have almost the same length ("plateau" effect) (panel A). In some patients, however, a significant and progressive shortening (panel B) or lengthening (panel C) of the return cycle has been observed in reaction on premature atrial beats elicited earlier in the atrial cycle.

range between 43.8–40.1% of the basic cycle ("complete interpolation") whereas in 10 patients, after premature atrial stimuli elicited in a range of 38.7–32.7% (m.v.) of the basic cycle, the sum of the test cycle and the return cycle was shorter than the basic cycle ("sinus echoes"). Sinus echoes always occurred in association with the other types of response, except in one patient. The incomplete interpolation was found as single phenomenon in 24 patients, associated with complete interpolation in 1 patient and with sinus echoes in 4. In 5 patients all three phenomena were observed.

Zone of atrial vulnerability
In some patients, premature atrial stimuli elicited very early in the atrial cycle, induced a progressive prolongation of the atrial latency. These atrial premature beats did cause sometimes a single or a short run of atrial re-entry beats (because of the different morphology of the P wave and different sequence of atrial activation). The atrial cycle was usually very short (about 280–300 msec) during these atrial tachycardias.

SECOND RETURN CYCLE (PRC)

During the zone of no-reset (zone I), the post return cycle usually equal or slightly longer than the basic cycle. The mean value of the post return cycle, calculated on the whole group, was +1.7% longer than the basic cycle. During the reset-zone (zone II), in most patients (76%) the post return cycle was identical or differred only to a small degree from

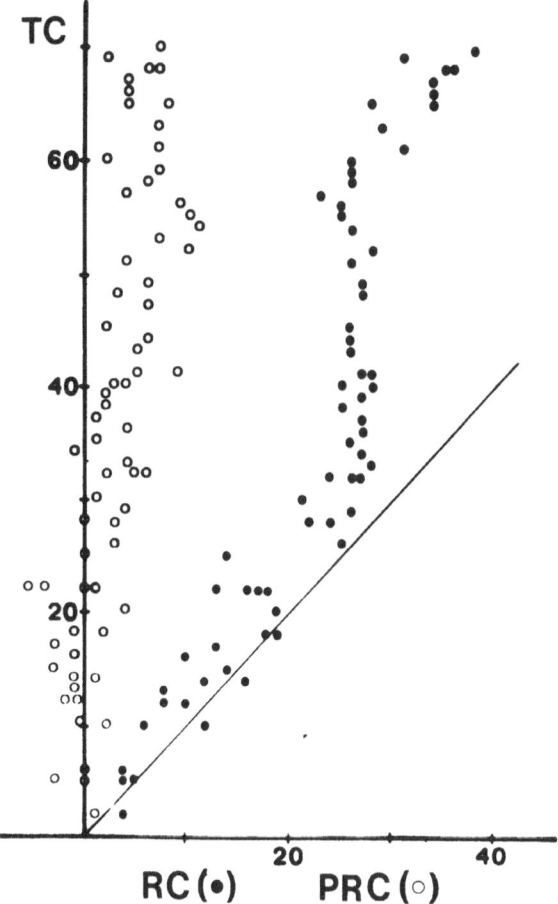

Figure 4. A prolongation of the return cycle (that is, a deviation of data points to the right) occurred after premature atrial stimuli introduced very early in the atrial cycle. Beyond about 40% shortening of the atrial cycle, the post return cycle (open circle) is obviously longer than the basic cycle.

the basic cycle. In the 5 patients with severe sinoatrial node dysfunction, in whom the "overcompensatory" return cycles occurred (Figure 2A,B), a different response was observed. In 4 of them, the post return cycle was significantly longer (mean value $+29\%$) (Figure 2, panel B) and in the remaining case shorter (-11.8%) than the basic cycle (Figure 2, panel A).

DISCUSSION

In man, the electrical activity of the sinus node has not yet been recorded. In addition, the electrophysiological properties of the sinus node are very complex and they may at any moment change in the presence of various interventions. For these reasons the interpretation of the sinus node response to premature atrial stimuli is still discussed.

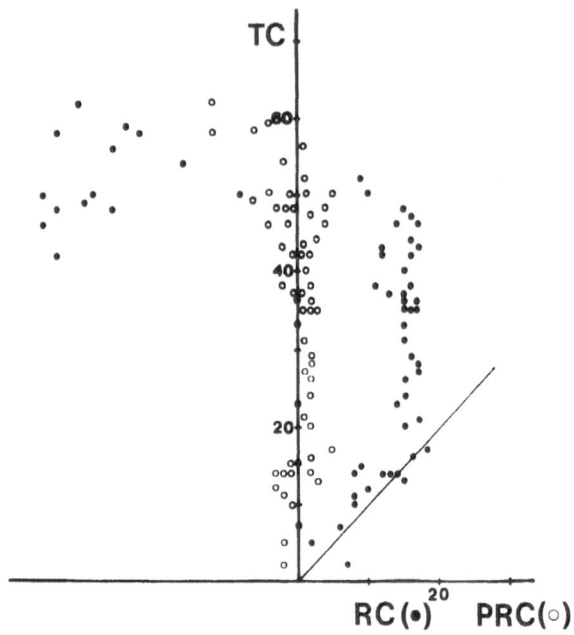

Figure 5. Early premature beats – more than about 50% shortening of the atrial cycle – are followed in this case by return cycles that are shorter than the normal interval. Note that the post return cycle (open circle) has almost not changed.

In most patients, after premature atrial stimuli introduced late in the cycle, fully compensatory return cycles are observed (zone I). This is explained by the fact that the premature atrial impulse collides with the emerging sinus impulse somewhere in the border of the sinus node (Bonke et al., 1969; Strauss et al., 1973). When premature atrial stimuli are introduced earlier, the return cycles often have nearly the same length (zone II); these premature atrial beats do reset the pacemaker in the sinus node. The transition from zone I to zone II (transitional zone) may occur either abrupt or not. The reset-point, that is the outer limit of zone II, is usually observed after premature atrial stimuli given in the last 12–22% of the atrial cycle. However, in some patients, the reset-point may occur earlier or later. In the first case it might be possible that the dominant pacemaker is located at the periphery of the sinus node in the neighbourhood of the crista terminalis; in the second case a delay in the conduction through the sinoatrial border might be suggested. In rare occasions, especially in patients with severe, sinus node dysfunction, the return cycle after the compensatory phase lengthens suddenly and becomes then relatively constant. Such a lengthening of the return cycle could be explained assuming the occurrence of a lengthening of the sinus node cycle due to perhaps acetylcholine release (Strauss et al., 1976) or a block of the impulse of the dominant pacemaker (intrasinusal block), followed by an escape of another pacemaker with slower automaticity.

During zone II the return cycle usually remains relatively constant until atrial refractoriness is reached. In some patients, however, significant variations of the return cycle such as a progressive shortening or lengthening may be observed. Several factors could be involved as electrotonic influences on the sinus node action potential prior to sinus node capture (Miller and Strauss, 1974), variation in sinus node cycle length depending on either shifting of the sinus pacemaker (Bonke et al., 1969) or depression of the sinus node automaticity (Ticzon et al., 1975) and variation of the sinoatrial conduction time (Miller and Strauss, 1974). At present, there are no satisfactory techniques to differentiate between these possibilities in human studies (Strauss and Wallace, 1976).

In a group of patients, especially with a short atrial effective refractory period the return cycle may be prolonged considerably after premature atrial beats elicited early in the atrial cycle; this prolongation might be related to a decrease in sinoatrial conduction velocity. These responses should not necessarily be interpreted as pathological. In some cases the early premature atrial beats are followed by a return cycle that is considerably shorter than the basic cycle. In these circumstances, the almost identical polarity and shape of the P wave between the postextrasystolic and sinus beat, the same intra-atrial conduction time from high right atrium to low right atrium and the same sequence of atrial activation, made it likely that the postextrasystolic premature beat originated from the high right atrium and that the sinus node might be the site of impulse formation. The sum of the test cycle (TC) and the return cycle (RC) is longer (incomplete interpolation phenomenon), equal or almost equal (complete interpolation phenomenon) or shorter (sinus echoes) than the basic cycle. Sometimes, in the same patient, two and even three types of response could be observed. In the 5 patients of our series, in whom all three types were present, sinus echoes were usually observed after complete interpolated beats, i.e. when the coupling interval was further shortened.

Some investigators (Bonke et al., 1971; Goldreyer and Damato, 1971; Strauss and Bigger, 1972; Childers et al., 1973; Ticzon et al., 1975) explain the interpolation phenomenon by suggesting that the atrial premature beat fails to discharge the sinus pacemaker and that only partial penetration through the sinoatrial junction occurs (sinoatrial entrance block). In our opinion, this explanation is not compatible with the occurrence of sinus echoes, since the premature atrial impulse elicited with a coupling interval that is shorter than in case of the complete interpolation, never will find an entrance into the sinus node.

An alternate explanation might be that all early premature beats cause sinus node re-entry (Klein et al., 1973; Pauley et al., 1973; Narula, 1974; Masini and Dianda, 1977) and that the completely interpolated beat is also a sinus re-entry, occurring at an appropriate interval. The slow impulse transmission (Han et al., 1968; Bonke et al., 1969; Strauss and Bigger, 1972) and the fact that the functional refractory period of the sinus node exceeds that of the surrounding atrial tissue (Goldreyer and Damato, 1971; Narula, et al., 1972) are essential to assure that an early premature beat induces a sinus re-entry.

In most subjects the post return cycle is usually similar to or slightly longer than the basic cycle during both zone I and zone II.

In a small group of patients the post return cycle lengthens during zone II. This might be explained by a depressant effect on sinus node automaticity (Bonke et al., 1969; Strauss et al., 1976; Breithardt and Seipel, 1976). Considering that in the calculation of SACT it is assumed that changes in the sinus node cycle do not occur, the depressant effect of premature atrial stimuli on sinus node automaticity tends to overestimate the true SACT. In order to take this possible error into account, some investigators (Strauss et al., 1976; Breithardt and Seipel, 1976) proposed to use the length of the post return cycle instead of the cycle immediately preceding the test cycle, for the calculation of SACT. The observation that the lengthening of the post return cycle may occur in patients with normal or abnormal sinus node function as well as the lack of correlation between the lengthening of the post return cycle and the degree of sinus node dysfunction (Masini and Dianda, 1977) made it clear that this phenomenon is based upon a more complex mechanism (shifting of sinus pacemaker, humoral or haemodynamic interventions, autonomic reflex influences). Therefore, the proposal to use the post return cycle instead of the basic cycle for the calculation of SACT, does not seem satisfactory.

In the group of patients in whom, after very early premature atrial beats the return cycle is shorter than the basic cycle, a particular response of the post return cycle was not observed. Therefore, the analysis of the post return cycle does not seem to be useful in evaluating this type of response, as suggested by Ticzon et al. (1975).

At the occurrence of sinus echoes the post return cycle sometimes was found longer than the basic cycle, suggesting a reset of the sinus node pacemaker by the sinus re-entry beat. However, on many other occasions, the post return cycle (and sometimes the subsequent cycles) were shorter than the basic cycle.

In conclusion, a variety of different responses of the sinus node after premature atrial stimuli may be observed. Because of the lack of an accurate knowledge of the electrophysiological properties of the sinus node in man, the underlying electrophysiological mechanism of some responses remains unknown.

REFERENCES

1. Bonke, F.I.M., Bouman, L.N., van Rijn, H.E.: Change of cardiac rhythm in rabbit after an atrial premature beat. *Circ Res* 24: 533, 1969
2. Bonke, F.I.M., Bouman, L.N., Schopman, F.J.G.: Effect of an early atrial premature beat on activity of the sino-atrial node and atrial rhythm in the rabbit. *Circ Res* 29: 704, 1971
3. Breithardt, G., Seipel, L.: The effect of premature atrial depolarization on sinus node automaticity in man. *Circulation* 53: 920, 1976
4. Childers, R.W., Arnsdorf, M.F., de la Fuente, D.J., Gambetta, M., Svenson, R.: Sinus nodal echoes. Clinical case report and canine studies. *Am J Cardiol* 31: 220, 1973
5. Dhingra, R.C., Amat-Y-Leon, F., Wyndham, C., Denes, P., Wu, D., Pouget, J.M., Rosen, K.M.: The electrophysiologic effects of atropine on human sinus node and atrium. *Am J Cardiol* 38: 429, 1976
6. Engel, T.R., Bond, R.C., Schaal, S.F.: First-degree sino-atrial heart block: sino atrial block in the sick sinus syndrome. *Am Heart J* 91: 303, 1976
7. Goldreyer, B.N., Damato, A.N.: Sino-atrial node entrance block. *Circulation* 44: 789, 1971
8. Han, J., Malozzi, A.N., Moe, G.K.: Sino-atrial reciprocation in the isolated rabbit heart. *Circ Res* 22: 355, 1968
9. Klein, H.O., Singer, D.H., Hoffman, B.F.: Effects of atrial premature systoles on sinus rhythm in the rabbit. *Circ Res* 32: 480, 1973
10. Masini, G., Dianda, R., Graziina, A.: Analysis of sino-atrial conduction in man using premature atrial stimulation. *Cardiovascular Res* 9: 498, 1975
11. Masini, G., Dianda, R.: Analysis of the interpolation phenomenon in man evaluated by premature atrial stimulation. *Cardiovascular Res* 11: 334, 1977
12. Miller, H.C., Strauss, H.C.: Measurement of sino atrial conduction time by premature atrial stimulation in the rabbit. *Circ Res* 35: 935, 1974
13. Narula, O.S.: Sinus node re-entry. A mechanism for supraventricular tachycardia. *Circulation* 50: 1114, 1974
14. Pauley, K.L., Varghese, J.P., Damato, A.N.: Atrial rhythms in response to an early atrial premature depolarization in man. *Am Heart J* 84: 323, 1973a
15. Pauley, K.L., Varghese, J.P., Damato, A.N.: Sinus node re-entry: an in vivo demonstration in the dog. *Circ Res* 32: 455, 1973b
16. Steinbeck, G., Luderitz, B.: Comparison of sinoatrial conduction time and sinus recovery time. *Brit Heart J* 37: 956, 1975

17. Strauss, H.C., Bigger, J.T.: Electrophysiological properties of the rabbit sino-atrial perinodal fibres. *Circ Res* 31: 490, 1972
18. Strauss, H.C., Saroff, A.L., Bigger, J.T. Jr., Giardina, E.G.V.: Premature atrial stimulation as a key to the understanding of sino atrial conduction in man. *Circulation* 47: 86, 1973
19. Strauss, H.C., Wallace, A.G.: Direct and indirect techniques in the evaluation of sinus node function. The conduction System of the heart. Wellens, Lie, Janse, eds., Leiden, 1976
20. Strauss, H.C., Bigger, J.T., Saroff, A.L., Giardina, E.G.V.: Electrophysiologic evaluation of sinus node function in patients with sinus node dysfunction. *Circulation* 53: 763, 1976
21. Ticzon, A.R., Strauss, H.C., Gallagher, J.J., Wallace, A.G.: Sinus nodal function in the intact dog heart evaluated by premature atrial stimulation and atrial pacing. *Am J Cardiol* 35: 492, 1975

5

PROGRAMMED ATRIAL STIMULATION AND RAPID ATRIAL PACING IN PATIENTS WITH SINUS PAUSES AND SINOATRIAL EXIT BLOCK*

HAROLD C. STRAUSS, MELVIN M. SCHEINMAN, AN LaBARRE,
DAVID J. BROWNING, DAVID G. BENDITT, AND ANDREW G. WALLACE

Although Eyster and Evans (1915) and Levine (1916) described second-degree sinoatrial block in ECG recordings many years ago they realized that other possible sinoatrial conduction disturbances eluded analysis, primarily because electrical activity in the sinus node cannot be directly recorded in vivo. In 1973, Strauss et al. proposed that the premature atrial stimulation technique could be used to derive the sinoatrial conduction time. In the application of this technique a programmable stimulator is used to elicit variably coupled atrial premature depolarizations during spontaneous sinus rhythm. The last undisturbed spontaneous sinus cycle (A_1A_1), premature cycle (A_1A_2) and return cycle (A_2A_3) are analyzed and the normalized return cycles (A_2A_3/A_1A_1) are plotted as a function of the normalized premature cycles (A_1A_2/A_1A_1) (Figure 1). Late atrial premature cycles are followed by compensatory return cycles. Atrial premature depolarizations elicited earlier in atrial diastole are followed by less than compensatory return cycles. The duration of the less than compensatory A_2A_3 cycle is determined by the retrograde conduction time from the atrium to the sinus node (A_2SAN_2), the sinus node return cycle (SAN_2SAN_3) and the antegrade sinoatrial conduction time (SAN_3A_3). The estimation of the sinoatrial conduction time is based on the assumption that the sinus node return cycle (SAN_2SAN_3) equals the spontaneous sinus node cycle (SAN_1SAN_1) or the corresponding spontaneous atrial cycle (A_1A_1) (Figure 1). Hence, the difference between the atrial return cycle (A_2A_3) and the spontaneous atrial cycle (A_1A_1) should equal the retrograde conduction time (A_2SAN_2) for A_2 and the antegrade conduction time (SAN_3A_3) for the subsequent sinus node depolarization (SAN_3). The difference between A_2A_3 and A_1A_1 computed for atrial premature depolarizations falling in the latest third of the reset zone (zone II) is used to derive a mean value for the estimated antegrade and retrograde sinoatrial conduction time ($SACT_{A+R}$) (Strauss et al., 1976). It is also assumed that the sum of the A_2SAN_2 + SAN_3A_3 equals a value that is twice the normal antegrade sinoatrial conduction time (SAN_1A_1). For this reason many investigators have divided $SACT_{A+R}$ by 2 to obtain a value that approximates the antegrade sinoatrial conduction (Dhingra et al., 1975; Breithardt et al., 1976; Jordan et al., 1977). Since antegrade and retrograde conduction times may not be equal, (Bonke et al., 1969; Klein et al., 1973; Miller and Strauss, 1974) we have chosen to express our sinoatrial conduction times as the total value, i.e. $SACT_{A+R}$.

Because estimating $SACT_{A+R}$ is indirect, validation of the hypotheses underlying the method requires an experimental technique that permits direct measurement of the sino-

* Supported in part by the U.S. Public Health Service Grants HL 19216, 05736, 15190, 07101, 01613 and RR 30 from the General Clinical Research Centers Program of the Division of Research Resources, National Institutes of Health, and by a Research Career Development Award (1-K04-HL-00268) to Dr. Strauss, by an American Heart Association Teaching Scholar Award to Dr. Scheinman, and by a Medical Research Council of Canada, Fellowship Award to Dr. Benditt.

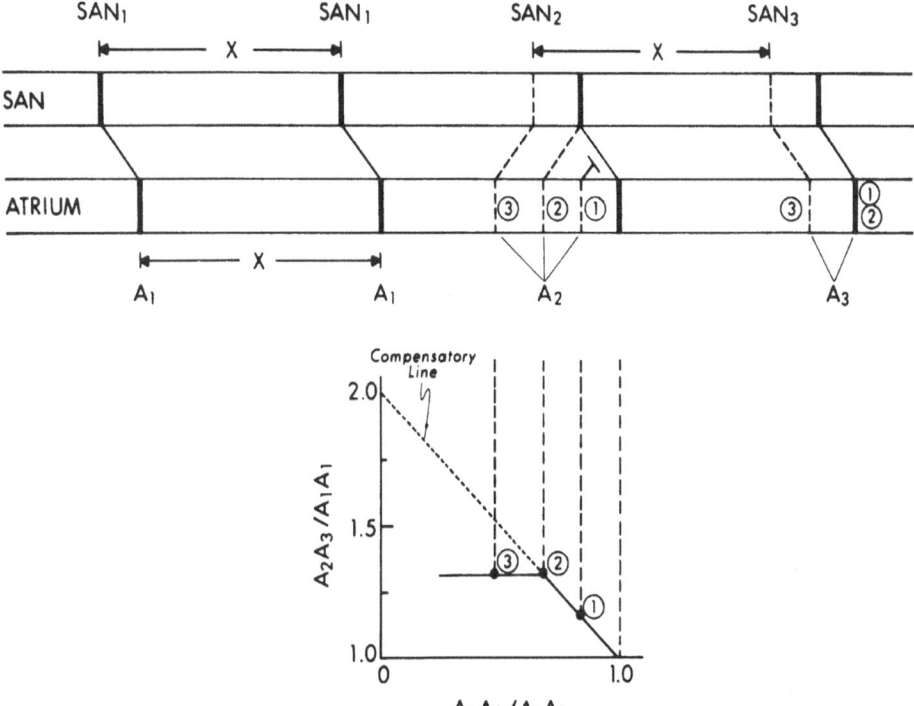

Figure 1. Derivation of $SACT_{A+R}$. A_1A_1 = spontaneous cycle length. A_2 = atrial premature depolarization. A_2A_3 = atrial return cycle. This technique is based on the assumption that $SAN_1SAN_1 = A_1A_1 = SAN_2SAN_3$. Therefore the difference between A_2A_3 and A_1A_1 is the antegrade and retrograde sinoatrial conduction time (between atrium and SAN and SAN and atrium).

The graph shows A_2A_3/A_1A_1 – plotted against A_1A_2/A_1A_1. A late APD (point 1) is followed by a compensatory response, where $A_1A_3 = 2A_1A_1$, which falls on the compensatory line. An early APD (point 3) is followed by a less than compensatory response which falls on the plateau below the compensatory line. Point 2 marks the transition between compensatory and less than compensatory responses.

atrial conduction time. Miller and Strauss (1974) performed a series of experiments in isolated superfused rabbit right atrial preparations in which the measured and estimated sinoatrial conduction times were compared. They demonstrated that late atrial premature depolarizations shortens the sinus node action potential and the subsequent sinus node return cycle, causing the technique to underestimate the measured sinoatrial conduction time (Miller and Strauss, 1974). In addition, intra-atrial conduction delays, sinus arrhythmia, changes in sinus node automaticity and differences between retrograde and antegrade sinoatrial conduction times could decrease the accuracy of the premature atrial stimulation technique in the estimation of the SACT too and hence further impair its usefulness in the analysis of sinoatrial conduction disturbances (Strauss and Wallace, 1976a; Strauss and Wallace, 1976b).

Despite the experimental limitations, most investigators still believe that the premature atrial stimulation technique is currently the best available for characterizing sinoatrial conduction disturbances. Whether or not this belief is justified depends on the answers to the following questions: First, is the premature atrial stimulation technique more sensitive than other available techniques in revealing sinoatrial conduction disturbances? Second, does the technique add to the sensitivity of other techniques in diagnosing sinoatrial conduction disturbances? Third, can the technique be of diagnostic importance in a group of symptomatic patients (e.g., syncope) with intermittent sinoatrial conduction disturbances when other techniques fail? Fourth, does the technique shed light on underlying pathophysiology, so that, for example, adverse drug reactions can be predicted? We will confine ourselves here to some observations on the first question concerning the respective sensitivities of the premature atrial stimulation and rapid atrial pacing techniques in a group of patients with sinus pauses and/or sinoatrial exit block in whom a high prevalence of sinoatrial conduction disturbances is anticipated.

Thirty consecutive symptomatic patients with electrocardiographically documented episodes of sinus pauses and/or sinoatrial exit block were studied (Scheinman et al.). Cardioactive drugs were discontinued for a period exceeding 3 drug half-lives prior to study in all but one patient, who was maintained on diphenylhydantoin sodium (to prevent seizures).

Studies were performed in the resting, nonsedated, post-absorptive state in a catheterization laboratory. A quadripolar electrode catheter was inserted into a peripheral vein and passed to the right atrium where it was positioned against the high lateral right atrial wall for the purpose of recording the atrial electrogram and stimulating the atrium.

Programmed premature atrial stimuli were introduced following every eighth spontaneous sinus cycle and the estimated sinoatrial conduction time was computed as previously described (Strauss et al., 1973; Strauss et al., 1976). $SACT_{A+R}$ was considered abnormal if it exceeded 206 msec (M + 2SD) (Scheinman et al., 1976). After a stabilization period, control recordings were obtained in each patient. Rapid atrial pacing was then performed as previously described (Benditt et al., 1976; Scheinman et al.).

Mean spontaneous cycle length ($\overline{SCL}$) and standard deviation (SD) were computed using 20 consecutive cycles recorded during the control period. If sinus pauses or sinoatrial exit block occurred during the control period, then these cycles were excluded from analysis of $\overline{SCL}$ and SD. The duration of each of the first 10 post-pacing cycles was divided by $\overline{SCL}$.

The maximum normalized cycle length for each of the 10 post-pacing cycles was compared to a previously described nomogram derived from the study of 44 control subjects. Any post-pacing cycle was defined as abnormally prolonged it it exceeded two SDs above the mean control value of maximum cycle length computed for that post-pacing cycle (Benditt et al., 1976).

The estimated $SACT_{A+R}$ in patients with sinoatrial block and/or sinus pauses was analyzed and depicted in the histogram illustrated in Figure 2. $SACT_{A+R}$ exceeded 206 msec in 4/11 (36%) patients with sinoatrial block and in 12/19 (63%) patients with sinus pauses. The occurrence of abnormal responses is surprisingly low in this group of patients in whom one would have anticipated a high incidence of sinoatrial conduction disturbances.

The low prevalence of abnormal responses to premature atrial stimulation may depend on the value selected to represent the upper limit of normal for $SACT_{A+R}$. If one selects the Mean + 2SD to represent the upper limit of normal for $SACT_{A+R}$, values of 198, 226, 240, 260 and 304 msec can be calculated from the data of Masini et al. (1975), Jordan et al. (1977), Breithardt et al. (1977), Engel et al. (1976), and Dhingra et al. (1975). A variety of factors could explain this range in values. First, the presence of moderate to severe coronary artery stenosis proximal to the sinus node artery has been implicated as a factor that may lengthen $SACT_{A+R}$ (Jordan et al., 1977). Second, the presence of atrial disease and slow intra-atrial conduction may increase the value of $SACT_{A+R}$ (Strauss and Wallace,

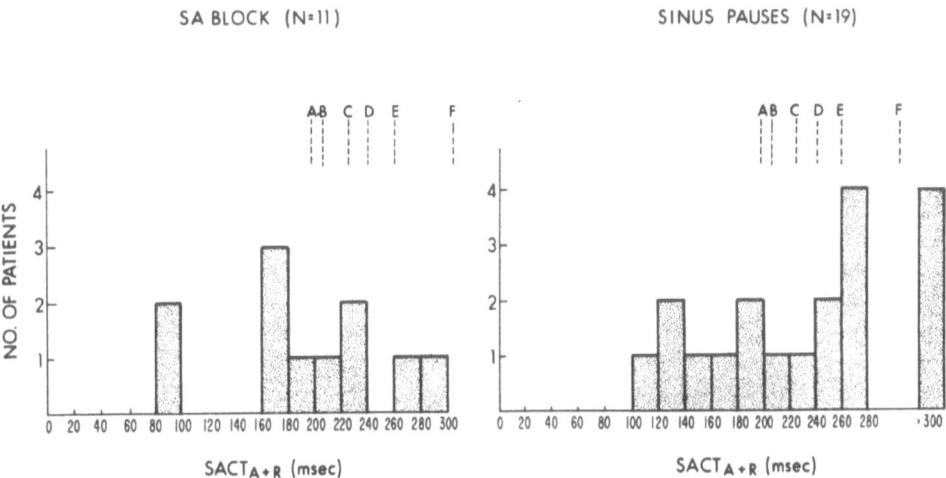

Figure 2. Distribution of sino-atrial conduction times in 11 patients with sino-atrial block (left) and 19 patients with sinus pauses (right). Lines A–F represent values for the upper limit of normal SACT$_{A+R}$ derived from different investigators' data. If one selects the Mean + 2SD to represent the upper limit of normal for SACT$_{A+R}$, values of 198 msec – A, 206 msec – B, 226 msec – C, 240 msec – D, 260 msec – E and 304 msec – F can be calculated from the data of Masini et al., 1975; Scheinman et al., 1976; Jordan et al., 1977; Breithardt et al., 1977; Engel et al., 1977; and Dhingra et al., 1975.

1976a). Third, patients identified as control subjects may nonetheless have sufficient occult sinus node dysfunction and disturbance of sinoatrial conduction to cause elevated SACT$_{A+R}$ values. Fourth, the SACT might also depend on the spontaneous cycle length (Reiffel et al., 1974). Fifth, the stress of the catheterization procedure may blunt the diagnostic accuracy of the premature atrial stimulation technique (Strauss et al., 1976c). Finally, the use of A$_2$A$_3$ cycles that fall in the early part of zone II in the calculation of SACT may increase the value of SACT, since the slope of the line drawn through the data points (A$_2$A$_3$ vs. A$_1$A$_2$) may be negative, approaching values as large as -0.5 (Strauss and Wallace, 1976b).

When a value of 198 msec was used as the upper limit of normal for SACT$_{A+R}$ the premature atrial stimulation technique identified abnormal responses in 5/11 (45%) patients with SA block and 12/19 (63%) patients with sinus pauses. When a value of 304 msec was used as the upper limit of normal for SACT$_{A+R}$, the premature atrial stimulation technique identified abnormal responses in 0/11 (0%) patients with SA block and 4/19 (21%) patients with sinus pauses.

The range of values reported for the upper limits of normal for SACT$_{A+R}$, 198–304 msec, is wide and selection of a particular value will undoubtedly affect the specificity and sensitivity of the technique in detecting abnormalities of sinoatrial conduction. In the absence of any evidence clearly favoring one value over another, we have chosen 206 msec to represent the upper limit of normal for SACT$_{A+R}$. Using this value of 206 msec only 16/30 (53%) patients with sinoatrial block and/or sinus pauses demonstrated an abnormal response to premature atrial stimulation. Apart from the difficulty in selecting an appropriate range of normal values for SACT$_{A+R}$ and the inaccuracies of the premature atrial stimulation technique, other factors should be considered to explain the low occurrence of abnormal responses. First, the relatively large dimensions of the sinus node would seem to be able to accommodate many functioning pacemaker units and shifts of pacemaker site have been demonstrated to occur when the sinus rate changes (Lu, 1970; West, 1972; Bonke, 1973; Strauss et al., 1977). If a shift of pacemaker site toward the crista terminalis occurs in patients with extensive damage to the sinus node, this might result in a relatively normal sinoatrial conduction time. Second, sinus pauses and/or sinoatrial exit block could also result from subthreshold oscillations which occur occasionally without detectable abnormalities in sinoatrial conduction time.

At this time it is clear that in our hands the premature atrial technique is unable to identify abnormal responses in all of the patients expected to have a high prevalence of sinoatrial conduction disturbances. This may be due to the limitations of the technique, the underlying pathophysiology or the difficulty in identifying an appropriate range of normal values for $SACT_{A+R}$. The use of the premature atrial stimulation technique in identifying abnormal responses in the two groups of patients needs to be clarified by establishing a range of normal values for $SACT_{A+R}$ and only then can the specificity and sensitivity of the method be appropriately analyzed.

We now address ourselves to the second problem, namely the comparison of abnormal responses to premature atrial stimulation and rapid atrial pacing in the two groups of patients. Responses to rapid atrial pacing were also analyzed using previously described criteria (Benditt et al., 1976) in the two groups of patients (Figure 3). The maximal value

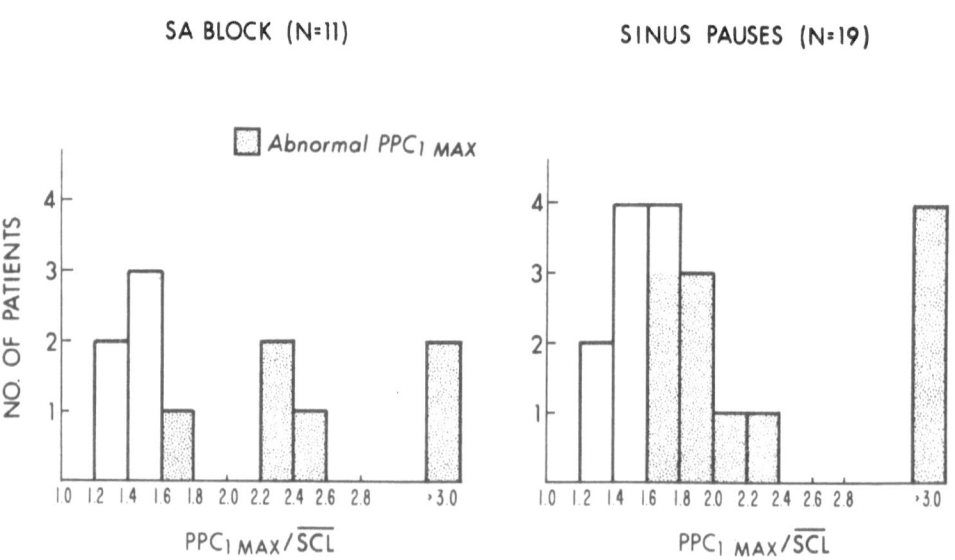

Figure 3. Distribution of values for the maxmum length of the first cycle following pacing (max PPC_1) normalized by the individual's own spontaneous cycle length ($\overline{SCL}$) in 11 patients with sinoatrial block (left) and 19 patients with sinus pauses (right). The max PPC_1 was abnormal in 6/11 (55%) (indicated by stippling) of patients with sinoatrial block and in 12/19 (63%) of patients with sinus pauses.

of the first post-pacing cycle (max PPC_1) was abnormally prolonged in 6/11 (55%) patients with SA block and 12/19 (63%) patients with sinus pauses. Abnormalities in the subsequent (2–10) post-pacing cycles or secondary pauses occurred in 9/11 (82%) patients with sinoatrial block and 14/19 (74%) patients with sinus pauses (Figure 4). Abnormal responses to pacing (abnormal max PPC_1 and/or secondary pauses) occurred in 10/11 (91%) patients with sinoatrial block and 14/19 (74%) patients with sinus pauses. Thus, in contrast to the premature atrial stimulation technique, which identified abnormal responses in 16/30 (53%) patients the rapid atrial pacing technique identified abnormal responses in 24/30 (80%) of such patients (Figure 5). This difference was statistically significant (p < .005). Although the majority of patients demonstrated more than one type of abnormal response, three patients had secondary pauses alone, another had a prolonged maximum first post-pacing cycle alone and one other had isolated prolongation of the sinoatrial conduction time.

Abnormal prolongation of any of the post-pacing cycles was seen in 80% of our patients suggesting a close association between the prevalence of electrocardiographically documented episodes of spontaneous sinoatrial block and/or sinus pauses and abnormalities in the post-pacing period. These data suggest that the rapid atrial pacing technique may be

MAX PPC_1 AND SECONDARY PAUSES

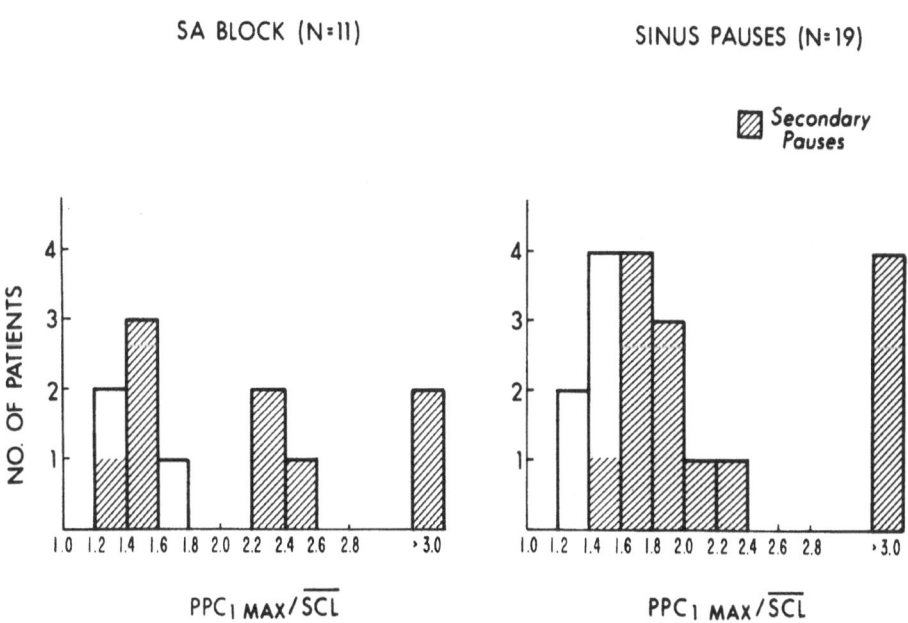

Figure 4. Demonstration of the value of analyzing both maximum first post-pacing cycle length (max PPC_1 – indicated by bars) and secondary pauses (secondary pauses – indicated by presence of shading within the bars) in 11 patients with sinoatrial block (left) and in 19 patients with sinus pauses (right). Secondary pauses were present in 9/11 (82%) of patients with sinoatrial block and 14/19 (74%) of patients with sinus pauses. Abnormal responses to pacing (abnormal max PPC_1 and/or secondary pauses) were present in 10/11 (91%) of patients with sinoatrial block and 14/19 (74%) of patients with sinus pauses.

SACT$_{A+R}$ AND ABNORMAL RESPONSES TO PACING

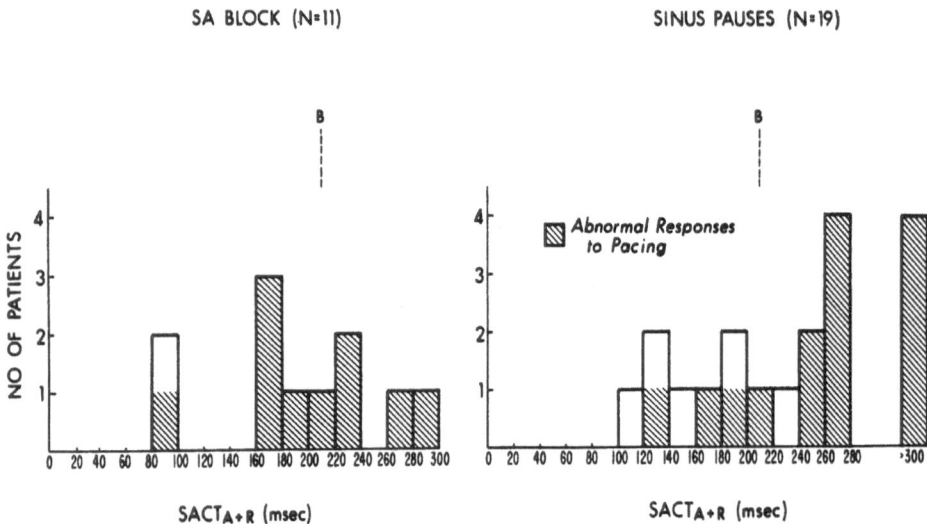

Figure 5. Comparison of premature atrial stimulation and rapid atrial pacing techniques. Values of SACT$_{A+R}$ are indicated by bars (dashed line indicates our upper limit of normal) and occurrence of abnormal response to pacing is indicated by shading within bars. SACT$_{A+R}$ was abnormal in 4/11 (36%) of patients with SA block and 12/19 (63%) of patients with sinus pauses. Pacing responses were abnormal in 10/11 (91%) and 14/19 (74%), respectively.

able to unmask disturbances of sinoatrial conduction. The pathophysiologic basis of post-pacing abnormalities remains unknown, but certain experimental observations suggest that disturbances of automaticity and/or conduction (Both sinoatrial and intranodal) as well as the occurrence of subthreshold oscillations could explain the prolonged post-pacing cycles (Lu, 1965; West, 1972).

It should also be noted that we were unable to detect abnormal responses to either premature atrial stimulation and/or rapid atrial pacing in 5/30 (17%) patients. Since electrophysiologic testing was performed in patients with overt electrocardiographic abnormalities, the absence of abnormal responses in 5 patients is disconcerting. This finding may be explained by the limitations of the testing procedure (Strauss et al., 1976c; Benditt et al., 1976) or by the episodic nature of the electrocardiographic disturbance and presumably underlying electrophysiologic disturbance (Strauss et al., 1976c; Scheinman et al.). Negative findings in five patients, however, do not preclude the usefulness of the rapid atrial pacing technique as a screening test for the evaluation of symptomatic patients with intermittent sinus pauses and/or sinoatrial exit block.

In summary, we have shown that patients with documented episodes of sinus pauses and/or sinoatrial exit block more frequently have abnormal responses to rapid atrial pacing than to premature atrial stimulation. Whether or not electrophysiologic testing can detect abnormalities of sinus node function that appear very infrequently and prove to be of diagnostic importance can only be determined by a larger prospective study.

ACKNOWLEDGEMENT

We would like to express our thanks to Laura Cook and Don Kopp for their help in the electrophysiology laboratory during the studies, to Don Powell for the art work, to Dave Hugett for the photography and to Marilyn McIntosh for her aid in typing the manuscript.

REFERENCES

1. Benditt, D.G., Strauss, H.C., Scheinman, M.M., Behar, V.S., Wallace, A.G.: Analysis of secondary pauses following termination of rapid atrial pacing in man. *Circulation* 54: 436, 1976
2. Bonke, F.I.M., Bouman, L.N., Van Rijn, H.E.: Change of cardiac rhythm in the rabbit after an atrial premature beat. *Circ Res* 24: 533, 1969
3. Bonke, F.I.M.: Electrotonic spread in the sinoatrial node of the rabbit heart. *Pflügers Arch* 339: 17, 1973
4. Breithardt, G., Seipel, L.: The effect of premature atrial depolarizations on sinus node automaticity in man. *Circulation* 53: 920, 1976
5. Breithardt, G., Seipel, L., Loogen, F.: Sinus node recovery time and calculated sinoatrial conduction time in normal subjects and patients with sinus node dysfunction. *Circulation* 56: 43, 1977
6. Dhingra, R.C., Wyndham, C., Amat-y-Leon, F., Denes, P., Wu, D., Rosen, K.M.: Sinus nodal responses to atrial extra-stimuli in patients without apparent sinus node disease. *Am J Cardiol* 36: 445, 1975
7. Eyster, J.A.E., Evans, J.S.: Sino-auricular heart block: with report of a case in man. *Arch Intern Med (Chicago)* 10: 832, 1915
8. Engel, T.R., Bond, R.C., Schaal, S.F.: First-degree sinoatrial heart block: Sinoatrial block in the sick sinus syndrome. *Am Heart J* 91: 303, 1976
9. Ferrer, M.I.: The Sick Sinus Syndrome. Futura. Mount Kisco, New York, 1974
10. Jordan, J., Yamaguchi, I., Mandel, W.J.: Characteristics of sinoatrial conduction in patients with coronary artery disease. *Circulation* 55: 569, 1977
11. Klein, H.O., Singer, D.H., Hoffman, B.F.: Effects of atrial premature systoles on sinus rhythm in the rabbit. *Circ Res* 32: 480, 1973
12. Levine, S.A.: Observations on sino-auricular heart block. *Arch Intern Med (Chicago)* 17: 153, 1916
13. Lu, H.H., Lange, G., McBrooks, C.: Factors controlling pace-maker action in cells of the sinoatrial node. *Circ Res* 17: 460, 1965
14. Lu, H.H.: Shifts in pacemaker dominance within the sinoatrial region of cat and rabbit hearts resulting from increase of extracellular potassium. *Circ Res* 27: 339, 1970
15. Mandel, W., Hayakawa, H., Danzig, R., Marcus, H.S.: Evaluation of sino-atrial node function in man by overdrive suppression. *Circulation* 44: 59, 1971
16. Masini, G., Dianda, R., Graziina, A.: Analysis of sino-atrial conduction in man using premature atrial stimulation. *Cardiovasc Res* 9: 498, 1975
17. Miller, H.C., Strauss, H.C.: Measurement of sinoatrial conduction time by premature atrial stimulation in the rabbit. *Circ Res* 35: 935, 1974
18. Narula, O.S., Samet, P., Javier, R.P.: Significance of the sinus-node recovery time. *Circulation* 45: 140, 1972.
19. Reiffel, J.A., Bigger, J.T. Jr., Konstam, M.A.: The relationship between sinoatrial conduction time and sinus cycle length during spontaneous sinus arrhythmia in adults. *Circulation* 50: 924, 1974
20. Scheinman, M.M., Kunkel, F.W., Peters, R.W.: Atrial pacing in patients with sinus node dysfunction. *Am J Med* 61: 641, 1976
21. Scheinman, M.M., Strauss, H.C., Abbott, J.A., Evans, G.T., Peters, R.W., Benditt, D.G., Wallace, A.G.: Electrophysiologic testing in patients with sinus pauses and/or sinoatrial exit block. (Eur J Cardiol, in press)
22. Strauss, H. C., Saroff, A.L., Bigger, J.T. Jr., Giardina, E.G.C.: Premature atrial stimulation as a key to understanding of sinoatrial conduction in man. *Circulation* 47: 86, 1973
23. Strauss, H.C., Bigger, J.T. Jr., Saroff, A.L., Giardina, E.G.V.: Electrophysiologic evaluation of sinus node function in patients with sinus node dysfunction. *Circulation* 53: 763, 1976
24. Strauss, H.C., Wallace, A.G.: Direct and indirect techniques in the evaluation of sinus node function. In, the Conduction System of the Heart: Structure, Function, and Clinical Implications (Wellens, H.J.J., Lie, K.I., Janse, M.J., eds.). Leiden, Stenfert Kroese B.V., 1976a, p. 227
25. Strauss, H.C., Wallace, A.G.: Premature atrial stimulation for evaluation of sinoatrial conduction in man. In, Cardiac Pacing. Diagnostic and Therapeutic Tools (Lüdertiz, B., ed.), New York, Springer-Verlag, 1976b, p. 33

26. Strauss, H.C., Gilbert, M., Svenson, R.H., Miller, H.C., Wallace, A.G.: Electrophysiologic effects of propranolol on sinus node function in patients with sinus node dysfunction. *Circulation* 54: 452, 1976c
27. Strauss, H.C., Prystowsky, E.N., Scheinman, M.M.: Sino-atrial and atrial electrogenesis. *Prog Cardiovasc Dis* 19: 385, 1977
28. West, T.C.: Electrophysiology of the sinoatrial node, in DeMello, W.C. (ed.): Electrical Phenomena in the Heart. New York, Academic Press, 1972, p. 191

6

A NEW TECHNIQUE FOR MEASUREMENT OF SINOATRIAL CONDUCTION TIME*

ONKAR S. NARULA

INTRODUCTION

In 1973 Strauss and co-workers had proposed the use of programmed atrial premature stimulation to estimate the sino-atrial conduction time (SACT). During the last four years a large number of reports have appeared utilizing the premature atrial stimulation technique for estimation of SACT, but the experience gained over these years indicates several problems with this technique (Narula, 1975). Recently Strauss and Wallace (1976) have also agreed to the problems with their technique.

In view of this, our efforts were directed to devise an alternative means for measurement of SACT. The purpose of this study is to report our preliminary experience with a new approach which utilizes regular atrial pacing for estimation of SACT.

MATERIALS AND METHODS

Electrophysiological evaluation of sinus node function was performed in 15 patients. In ten patients (group A) the sinus node function was normal on the basis of clinical findings, ECG or holter recordings and electrophysiological testing of sinus node function. In 5 patients (group B) the sinus node function was documented to be abnormal either on the ECG, Holter recordings and/or electrophysiological testing of sinus node function. All patients were studied in the post absorptive state and were premedicated with 100 mg Nembutal, administered intramuscularly 30 minutes prior to the study. In each patient an informed consent was obtained.

A quadripolar electrode catheter (with ring electrodes 10 mm apart) was placed in the right atrium, so that the proximal electrode pair was located in the region of the sinus node for recording high right atrial electrograms and the distal pair was used for atrial stimulation. Another bipolar electrode catheter was placed in the His bundle (BH) region for recording BH electrograms. All recordings were made at paper speeds of 50–100 mm/sec. Multiple ECG leads representing the three planes of the ECG were recorded simultaneous with intra-atrial electrograms. Atrial stimulation studies were performed at double the diastolic threshold with stimuli 2 msec in duration.

Programmed premature atrial beats were introduced during normal sinus rhythm for estimation of SACT as previously described by Strauss et al. (1973).

Responses to premature atrial beats in the latter third of the zone II (zone of reset) provided the mean A_2A_3 interval which was used for estimation of SACT. Mean cycle length

---

* From The Division of Cardiology, Department of Medicine, The Chicago Medical School, University of Health Sciences, Chicago, Illinois.

(A_1A_1) was calculated on the basis of 10 consecutive cycles recorded during the control period, immediately preceeding the introduction of the premature atrial beats. The SACT was calculated according to the most recently described criteria of Strauss et al. (1976) (SACT = A_2A_3-A_1A_1).

The interval thus obtained represents the sum total of the conduction time into and out of the sinus node.

Sinus rhythm was observed for a period of two minutes without any interventions. The last ten cycles were recorded to obtain a new mean cycle length so as to detect any changes that might have occurred. This mean cycle length was used to calculate SACT by the proposed new method. In each patient regular atrial pacing was performed at a rate slightly faster ($\leq$ 5–10 beats/min) than the control sinus rhythm for a chain of eight or 16 consecutive beats (Figure 1). Pacing was performed for a chain of 16 beats when the pacing rate

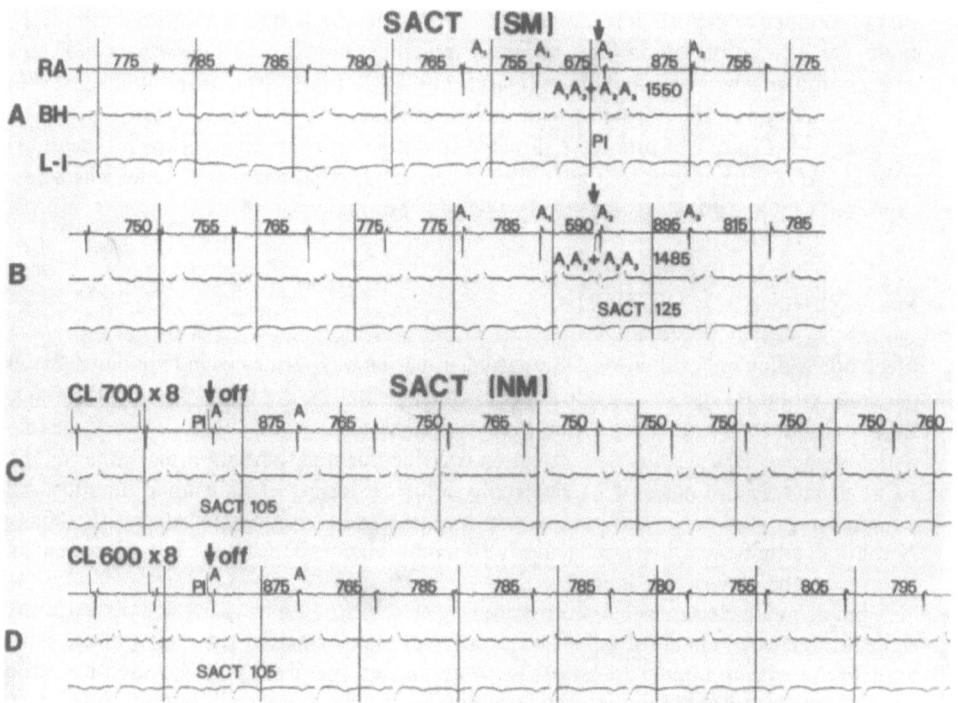

Figure 1. Estimation of the sinoatrial conduction time (SACT) by the two methods i.e. Strauss et al (SM) and the new method (NM).

A. During sinus rhythm an induced (PI) premature atrial beat at an A_1A_2 coupling interval of 675 msec is followed by a fully compensatory pause.

B. A premature beat at a shorter A_1A_2 interval (590 msec) is followed by a return cycle (A_2A_3) which is less than fully compensatory. The SACT with SM is 895 − 770 = 125 msec.

C. The new method shows termination of atrial pacing (AP) after 8 beats at a cycle length (CL) of 700 msec. The interval between the last paced A wave and the first spontaneous escape A wave of sinus origin is 875 msec. The SACT is calculated by deducting the mean spontaneous cycle length from the latter interval (875 − 770 = 105 msec).

D. Despite a decrease in AP cycle length to 600 msec, the estimated SACT (105 msec) is similar to that noted at a slower rate. PI = pacing impulse. A = atrial electrogram. Time lines on this and subsequent figures are at one second intervals.

was faster than the spontaneous sinus by ≤ 5 beats/min. When the pacing rates were faster by more than 5 beats/min, pacing was performed for eight beats. After a chain of 8 or 16 paced beats, pacing was terminated and recordings were continued for the subsequent 8 or more spontaneous cycles. This procedure was repeated 4 to 5 times with the same pacing rate. Similarly atrial pacing was performed at two or more additional pacing rates with increments in steps of 10 beats/min so as to assess the effect of pacing rate on the data obtained.

The SACT by the new method (NM) was calculated by deducting tne mean sinus cycle length from the interval between the last paced atrial electrogram and the first escape sinus cycle. This represents the sum total of the conduction time into and out of the sinus node if there is no sinus node depression. The measurements of SACT during several repeat observations at the same pacing rate provided the range of variation in reproducibility and were used to calculate the mean SACT. The mean SACT obtained in this fashion was compared with that obtained by the Strauss's method (SM). In addition, eight subsequent spontaneous SN cycles were also analyzed. The study of SACT by both the techniques was generally completed within 15 minutes.

Another variation of this new technique was also used during the same studies. After a basic drive for eight beats at a rate faster by ≤ 10 beats/min than the spontaneous sinus rate an extra-stimulus (S_2) was induced to scan the last 25% of the basic driving cycle ($S_1 S_1$). Following the extrastimulus (S_2) eight to ten spontaneous cycles were recorded (Figure 2). In addition, in each patient sinus node recovery time (SNRT*) and corrected sinus node recovery time (CSNRT) were measured, as previously described by Narula (1972). These measurements were obtained to confirm or rule out sinus node entrance block.

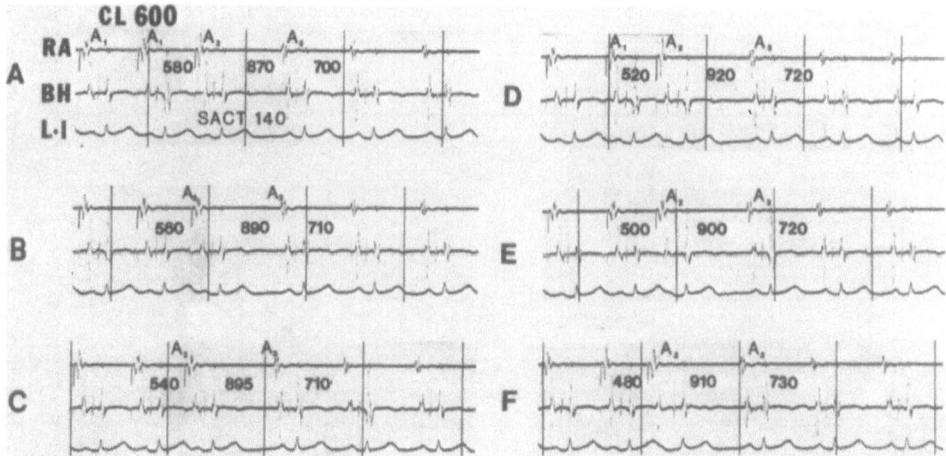

Figure 2. Shows a variation of the new technique. After a chain of 8 basic driving stimuli at CL of 600 msec an extrastimulus (A_2) is induced with a progressively increasing prematurity to scan the last 25% of the basic ($A_1 A_1$) cycle length. The $A_2 A_3$ interval is utilized to calculate the SACT, which progressively lengthens (panels A to F) as the $A_2 A_3$ interval lengthens. This figure shows that a minimal increase in prematurity may artificially lengthen the estimation of SACT.

*The author introduced in 1972 the abbreviation SRT for sinus node recovery time; the editor has chosen for SNRT for reasons of uniformity of the different chapters.

RESULTS

GROUP A

The SACT was calculated by both techniques and the results were generally comparable. In some the method of Strauss gave slightly longer values (8–60 msec), whereas in others the new method showed longer values (6–46 msec). In group A the two methods differed in a range of 6 to 50 msec (mean 27 msec): the mean SACT of the new method was 18 msec shorter compared to those by the   Strauss   method. In one of the group A patients, the SACT could not be calculated by the method of Strauss as the onset of the zone of reset (zone II) was not clearly definable: all A_2A_3 intervals were almost fully compensatory. In addition, at identical coupling intervals (A_1A_2) markedly different A_2A_3 intervals were obtained, so there was a scatter of the data (Figure 3). In this patient with the new method the SACT was measured 198 msec. The possibility of sino atrial entrance block as underlying mechanism for the inability to reset the sinus node by premature atrial beats, is very unlikely since the corrected sinus node recovery time in this patient was 430 msec.

GROUP B

The SACT's in the group B patients by the two methods were generally comparable. In four of these patients the mean SACT with the NM was 33 msec shorter than with the SM. In

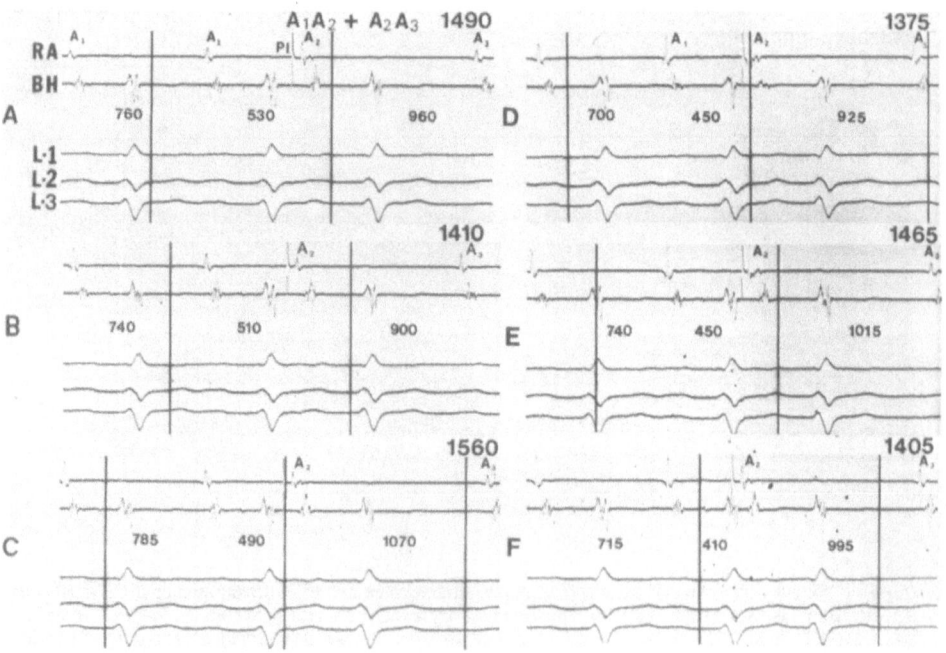

Figure 3. Shows that SACT with the premature atrial stimulation technique could not be calculated in this patient as the zone of reset was not definable. The sum total of A_1A_2 and A_2A_3 is listed on top of each panel. This figure also shows that a markedly variable A_2A_3 intervals may result from premature atrial beats at a constant A_1A_2 coupling interval (panels D and E). The mean A_1A_1 interval was 755 msec.

the fifth patient the SACT could not be calculated by the Strauss method as the onset of zone II responses could not be defined (Figure 4). The SACT by the new method was determined to be 350 msec (Figure 5).

In the group A patients the repeated measurements of SACT with the new method at a constant pacing rate, exhibited reproducible results. The fluctuations were in a range of 0–140 msec (mean 57 msec). These fluctuations were comparable with those of the spontaneous cycle length of the sinus node, namely 0–160 msec (mean 70 msec). During estimation of SACT with the method of Strauss, the A_2A_3 intervals, clearly definable to be

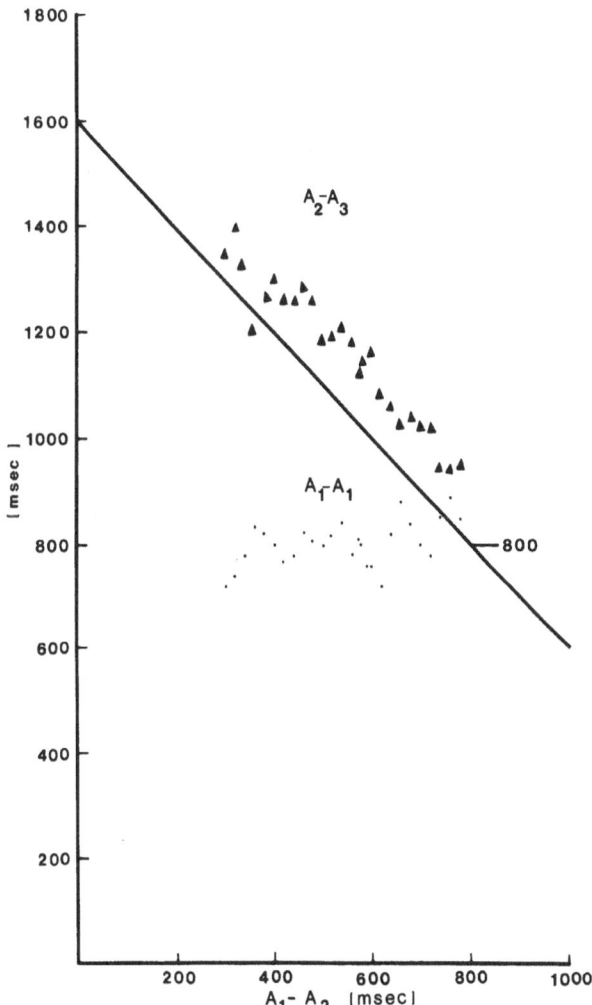

Figure 4. A plotting of A_1A_2 (Horizontal axis) and A_2A_3 sinus node (vertical axis) intervals in a patient with SA block and sinus node dysfunction demonstrates that the reset never occurred as all the A_2A_3 points (triangles) fell to the right of the diagonal line.

This indicates first degree or third degree sinus node entrance block. The SACT could not be measured. The A_1A_1 intervals are also plotted to show the fluctuations in spontaneous sinus cycles (small circular dots).

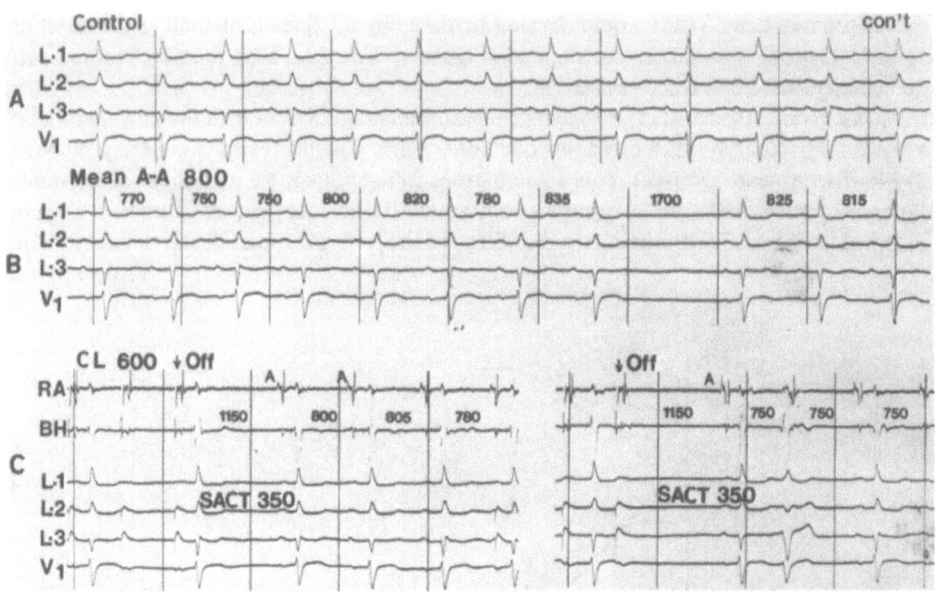

Figure 5. Recordings in the same patient as in Figure 4. The SACT was 350 msec after atrial pacing at a cycle-length of 600 msec for 8 beats (panel C). Spontaneous sinus rhythm with an occassional period of S-A block is shown by continuous recordings in panels A and B.

in the last third of the zone of reset responses and therefore used for the estimation of SACT, showed fluctuations in a range of 20 to 240 msec (mean 70 msec).

POST PACING CYCLES

On cessation of the atrial pacing procedure, the subsequent eight spontaneous cycles following the first escape cycle, were also analyzed. In group A patients the second post pacing cycle was similar to the control mean cycle length when the atrial pacing rate was no higher than the spontaneous rate by ≤ 5 beats/min. When the atrial pacing rate was faster by more than 10 beats/min than the spontaneous rate, the second post pacing cycle was slightly longer (2.8%) than the control mean cycle length. Similarly during measurement of SACT with the method of Strauss the A_3A_4 were also slightly longer (3%) than the mean A_1A_1. The remaining post pacing cycles (3 to 8) were almost similar to the control sinus cycles.

EFFECT OF PACING RATE ON SACT

With the new method in group A patients the SACT remained similar at all pacing rates if no faster than the normal sinus rate by ≤ 10 beats/min. Frequently, no appreciable differences in SACT were noted even when the atrial pacing rates were faster by ≥ 20 beats/min than the normal sinus rate, however, most of these patients exhibited a minimal lengthening of SACT ranging from 10–30 msec. These increments usually became apparent only if mean values of repeated reproductions of SACT measurement after atrial pacing at a faster rate were compared with those at a comparatively slower rate. In addition, at faster atrial pacing rates the increase in SACT was associated with a slight but obvious prolongation of the lengths of the post pacing sinus cycles (4–5%) which gradually returned to control levels by 6th or 7th spontaneous cycles. The observations in group B patients were parallel to those of group A. However, the prolongation of SACT with faster atrial pacing rates was more pronounced in group B patients. In addition, the prolongation of the post pacing cycles lasted at times for more than 5–beats if the pacing rates were high.

DISCUSSION

The method described by Strauss et al. (1973) for estimation of SACT is based on artificial depolarization and reset of the sinus node. For the new method, it was reasoned that it may be possible to artificially depolarize and reset the sinus node by utilizing regular atrial pacing instead of the premature atrial stimulation. It was further deduced that the data thus obtained may be utilized to calculate SACT, if it could be demonstrated that atrial pacing does not depress the automaticity of the sinus node. Accordingly it was decided to utilize pacing rates preferably ≤ 5 beats/min or ≤ 10 beats/min higher than the spontaneous sinus rhythm for a chain of 8 or 16 consecutive beats. The number of eight beats was arbitrarily chosen for the following reasons: a) It was realized that as the atrial pacing rates were almost similar to the sinus rhythm, several paced beats would be needed to capture the sinus node; b) Furthermore, if the sinus node was initially captured prematurely, during early diastole, an additional number of paced beats would be required to return the sinus node to near control levels. Now it is obvious from our data that most of the time with pacing rates faster by 5–10 beats/min, eight paced beats are sufficient. When the pacing rates are faster than the sinus rhythm by ≤ 5 beats/min usually a larger number of paced beats, i.e. 16, are necessary to capture the sinus node.

The results of our study clearly demonstrate the feasibility and reproducibility of the new method for estimation of SACT. The SACT's estimated with this method 1) are comparable to those with the method of Strauss (SM), both in patients with normal and abnormal sinus node function; 2) do not exhibit a depression of sinus node automaticity as the subsequent post pacing cycles were comparable to those of control when atrial pacing rates were higher by ≤ 5 beats/min. (At times the second post pacing cycle was slightly longer (2.8%) than the mean sinus cycle length, when pacing rates were faster by ≤ 10 beats/min); 3) could be obtained in all cases as opposed to a failure to accomplish this goal in two patients with the method of Strauss; 4) at a constant pacing cycle length, showed fluctuations which were on the whole lesser than those noted during spontaneous sinus cycles or in the A_2A_3 utilized with the Strauss method.

In 1973, at the time of the original description of their method for estimation of SACT, Strauss et al had stated "Linear regression analysis of points falling in the last 3rd of zone II adjacent to zone I gave a slope not significantly different from zero, indicating the remarkable constancy of the return cycle." Experience over the past four years has exhibited major problems and revealed that the return cycles often are not remarkably constant as expected, in 1973.

Major additional problems exist in estimating SACT by the Strauss method. Some of the problems with the method of Strauss for estimation of SACT are revealed by a review of the normal values for SACT reported by different groups of investigators. (Steinbeck and Lüderitz, 1975; Dhingra et al., 1975; Masini et al., 1975; Strauss et al., 1976). These studies show a large variation in the upper limit of normal SACT's. Furthermore, the normal range for SACT from any given laboratory is very wide and the lower limits at times are almost 1/5 of the upper limits. Of course, some of these variations may be explained on the basis of differences in patient population or due to differences in resting autonomic tone from individual to individual. However, in my opinion the range of normal values is significantly affected by the technical problems inherent in the use of premature atrial stimulation for estimation of the SACT.

With the introduction of premature atrial beats, a lack of sinus node reset has been termed as first degree sinus node entrance block with interference (Strauss et al., 1973). However, there are two problems with this interpretation: a) as not only a first degree delay may prevent sinus node reset but it may also be due to complete sinus node entrance block. Therefore, such a response always cannot be interpreted to be indicative of only 1° sinoatrial block. b) Findings in the present study reveal that sinus node entrance block may be fallaciously misinterpreted when premature atrial beats are utilized for evaluation of SACT. This is demonstrated by the observations in two patients in whom the zone of reset could not be defined by the premature atrial beats. With the method of Strauss all A_2A_3 intervals were fully compensatory (Figures 3, 4). However, SACT's were obtained with the new method. In these two patients, additional evidence of sinus node penetration was demonstrated by a longer CSNRT. The reason for failure to define zone II or reset of the sinus node with the premature atrial beats is probably an inherent problem in the use of premature atrial beats as: a) in some patients with an increase in prematurity, the atrio-sinus conduction time may be proportionately lengthened and thus the premature impulse may never reach the dominant pacemaker in the sinus node (Figure 6), and b) it is possible that the premature impulse in reality may reach and reset the sinus node, however, it may not be obvious from the A_2A_3 intervals if the conduction times are disproportionally longer on either limb (conduction into or out of the sinus node). In spite of sinus node reset such a marked degree of conduction delay may result in A_2A_3 intervals which are fully compensatory. Similar mechanisms may explain the cases in which the SACT cannot be defined. A difficulty in defining SACT's with the method of Strauss is quite frequent as was reported in a recent study where in 5 out of 17 cases zone II responses could not be defined (Breithardt et al., 1977). Our experience is parallel to the recently reported study.

Studies in isolated tissue have demonstrated some other problems in using premature atrial stimulation for estimation of SACT: a) the retrograde and antegrade conduction times usually are not equal; the retrograde time is shorter than the antegrade time. b) the estimated SACT is generally shorter than those obtained by direct measurements, possibly due to a shortening of the postextrasystolic cycle of the sinus node fibers produced by the premature depolarization. c) Late premature atrial beats, which fail to capture the sinus node, shorten the sinus node potential. d) With an increase in prematurity the retrograde time may gradually lengthen. In view of the above facts a valid comparison of total SACT between patients with normal and abnormal SACT is further complicated.

Additional following problems exist in estimating SACT by using the premature atrial stimulation technique: 1) the calculated SACT contains a segment of intra-atrial conduction time from the site of atrial stimulation to the border of the sinus node; 2) a shortening of the post extrasystolic sinus node cycle cannot be detected from A_2A_3 intervals; 3) with shorter A_1A_2 coupling intervals the retrograde time into the sinus node may lengthen and result in longer A_2A_3 intervals and an erroneous misinterpretation of sinus node entrance block; 4) the transition from compensatory to the "constant" and less than compensatory A_2A_3 cycle is gradual. This adds a significant margin of error in estimation of SACT. The

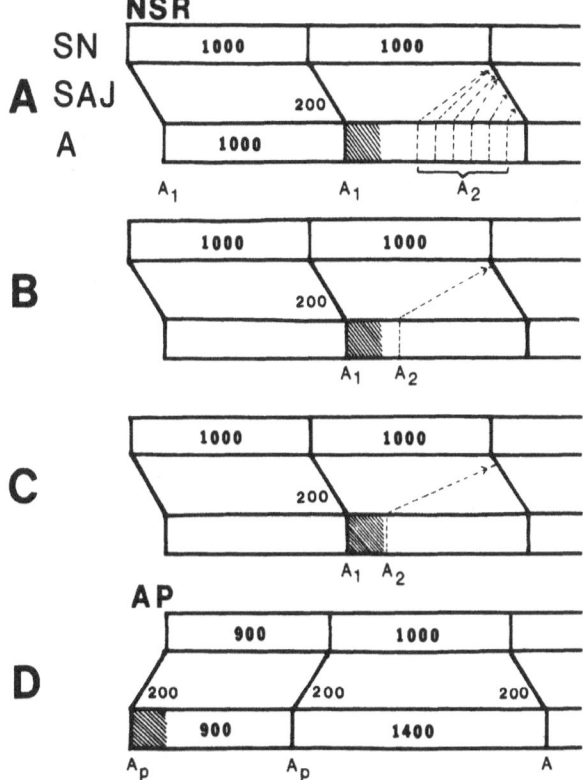

Figure 6. The ladder diagram shows how a premature atrial beat (A_2) with progressively shorter A_1A_2 intervals may never reach the sinus node (SN) if the conduction through the sinoatrial junction (SAJ) is disproportionately slowed with an increase in prematurity(panels A, B, C). The shaded area is indicative of atrial effective refractory period.

NSR = normal sinus rhythm.

The utilization of atrial pacing (AP) (panel D) permits atrial impulses to reach the sinus node without incurring increasing delays and thereby permit measurement of SACT with the new method which was not possible with the method of Strauss.

A = atrial electrogram. Ap = atrial paced atrial electrogram.

defining of onset of zone II responses is further complicated by the spontaneous fluctuations in the spontaneous cycle length (Figure 7). 5) Although Strauss (1976) has stated that SACT is more accurate at short spontaneous cycle lengths and least accurate at long cycle lengths, this is not always true as in one of our cases with a short cycle length the onset of zone II responses could not be defined (Figure 3). 6) estimation of SACT with premature atrial stimulation is cumbersome and requires a large number of measurements. This has lead some investigators to devise a computer program for the analysis of SACT. In addition it requires the use of a special programmable stimulator; 7) however remote, there is a theoretical and to some degree a real concern for inducing atrial arrhythmias during estimation of SACT by the premature stimuli.

It appears that the new method cannot rectify all the problems inherent in indirect measurements of SACT. For example problem number one (as discussed above) cannot be deleted with the new method as the intra-atrial segment of conduction is again incor-

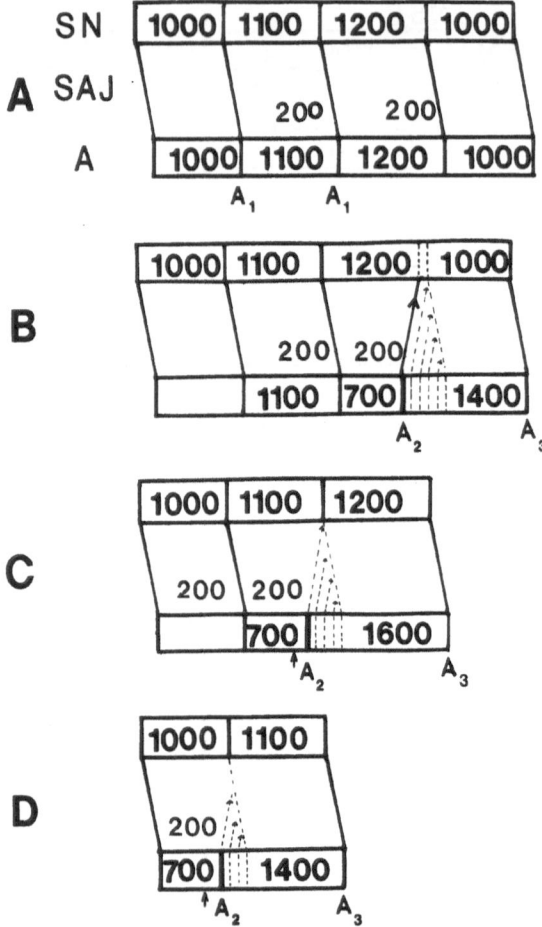

Figure 7. This ladder diagram shows possible problems with Strauss's method in defining the onset of the zone of sinus node reset or zone II responses. In panel A the control situation is given.

A constant A_1A_2 interval (700 msec) may (panel B) or may not (panel C and D) result in sinus node reset due to fluctuations in spontaneous sinus node cycles.

SN = sinus node. SA = sinoatrial junction. A = atrium.

porated into the calculations. However, other problems namely 2–5 (listed above) should be remedied by the new method, as they are a consequence of the use of premature atrial stimulations. Problems number 6 and 7 are also solved as only a few beats need be measured and any ordinary pulse generator should suffice.

The magnitude of fluctuations in A_2A_3 intervals used for estimation of SACT cannot be fully detected and appreciated from the results of the studies published by others. The point of transition between zone I and II responses cannot be always precisely demarcated. Therefore, during the present study, the A_2A_3 intervals at the point of transition or at the very onset of zone II were not utilized in calculating SACT by the SM. Only those A_2A_3 intervals which could not be confused and were clearly defineable to be less than fully compensatory, within the zone II, were utilized to calculate SACT. Therefore, the range of fluctuations in A_2A_3 intervals with the Strauss method has been artificially minimized.

The true magnitude of these fluctuations cannot be assessed as they are inherent in the use of premature atrial stimuli and to a great degree are artificially eliminated simply to permit estimation of SACT. The nature of this problem is illustrated by recordings in Figure 3.

On the other hand with the new method there is no difficulty in defining the range of fluctuations as none of the measured responses were eliminated. Several repeat responses following atrial pacing at a constant cycle length were used to determine the range and the magnitude of fluctuations and to calculate the SACT. [The new method should minimise the possible error in estimating SACT], which is incurred with the method of Strauss by arbitrarily eliminating transitional A_2A_3 intervals which in turn is compared with a mean of A_1A_1. [With the new method the mean of first post pacing escape sinus cycles provides a valid comparison with the mean of spontaneous sinus cycles. In this fashion the influence of fluctuations in both of these intervals used in calculations should be negated in a realistic fashion.] In some patients the subsequent post pacing cycles were slightly longer when the atrium was paced at rates 10–15 beats/min higher than the spontaneous rhythm. This suggests that in these cases the sinus node automaticity is affected. In view of these observations it is recommended that for estimation of SACT with the new method, preferably the atrial pacing rates should be no more than 5 beats/min and at the most 10 beats/min higher than the spontaneous sinus rates. This consideration should be given special importance when SACT is being analyzed in patients with sick sinus node syndrome.

In summary this study describes a new method for estimation of SACT. The preliminary data appear promising. This study provides an alternative approach which is simpler, quicker, and possibly better. It is to be cautioned at this time that only the test of time will indicate its proper role in clinical cardiology. It is hoped that this approach will stimulate experimental studies in isolated tissues to test its pitfalls and advantages. The results of such experimental studies may provide some refinements of the present protocol which are also being investigated in our clinical laboratory.

ACKNOWLEDGEMENTS

The author is extremely indebted to Mrs. Jackie Porter for her superb secretarial assistance in the preparation of this manuscript. We also express our thanks to Ms. Erna Braun, Mr. Jack deBruin and the Photography Section of The Chicago Medical School for the preparation of illustrations.

REFERENCES

1. Breithardt, G., Seipel, L., Loogen, F.: Sinus node recovery time and calculated sino-atrial conduction time in normal subjects and patients with sinus node dysfunction. *Circulation* 57: 43, 1977
2. Dhingra, R.C., Wyndham, C., Amat-y-Leon, F., Denes, P., Wu, D., Rosen, K.M.: Sinus nodal responses to atrial extra-stimuli in patients without apparent sinus node disease. *Am J Cardiol* 36: 445, 1975
3. Masini, G., Dianda, A.: Analysis of sinoatrial conduction in man using premature atrial stimulation. *Cardiovasc Res* 9: 498, 1975
4. Miller, H.C., Strauss, H.C.: Measurement of sinoatrial conduction time by premature atrial stimulation. *Circ Res* 35: 935, 1974
5. Narula, O.S.: Disorders of sinus node function: electrophysiologic evaluation. In: The His Bundle Electro-

cardiography and Clinical Electrophysiology, edited by Narula, O.S., Davis, F.A., Philadelphia, 1975, p. 275

6. Narula, O.S., Samet, P., Javier, R.P.: Significance of the sinus node recovery time. *Circulation* 45: 140, 1972

7. Steinbeck, G., Lüderitz, B.: Comparative study of sinoatrial conduction time and sinus node recovery time. *Br Heart J* 37: 956, 1975

8. Steinbeck, G., Allessie, M.A., Bonke, F.I.M., Lammers, W.J.E.P.: The response of the sinus node to premature stimulation of the atrium studied with microelectrodes in isolated atrial preparations of the rabbit heart. This book, 1978

9. Straus,, H.C., Saroff, A.L., Bigger, J.T. Jr., Giardina, E.G.V.: Premature atrial stimulation as a key to the understanding of sinoatrial conduction in man. *Circulation* 47: 86, 1973

10. Strauss, H.C., Bigger, J.T. Jr., Saroff, A.L. Giardina, E.G.V.: Electrophysiologic evaluation of sinus node function in patients with sinus node dysfunction. *Circulation* 53: 763, 1976

11. Strauss, H.C., Wallace, A.G.: Direct and indirect techniques in the evaluation of sinus node function. In the conduction system of the heart. Structure, function and clinical implications, edited by Wellens, H.J.J., Lie, K.I., Janse, M.J., Leiden, Stenfert Kroese B.V., 1976, p. 227

7

RELEVANCE OF DIAGNOSTIC ATRIAL STIMULATION FOR PACEMAKER TREATMENT IN SINOATRIAL DISEASE*

BERNDT LÜDERITZ, GERHARD STEINBECK, CHRISTOPH NAUMANN
d'ALNONCOURT, AND WERNER ROSENBERGER

INTRODUCTION

Recognition of the clinical importance of sinoatrial disease is growing. Impaired sinus node function in sinoatrial disease including sinus bradycardia, sinus arrest, sinoatrial block and the bradycardia-tachycardia syndrome cannot easily be assessed, especially when rhythm disturbances are occurring intermittently, as the recording of electrical activity of sinus node pacemaker cells is not available in man. The analysis of atrial activity in the surface electrocardiogram permits only an overall estimation of sinus node function. This involves the ability to act as an impulse generator and includes the conduction of the impulse from the pacemaker site to the atrium. Therefore, methods of provocative atrial stimulation have been developed which are thought to allow indirect estimation of sinus node automaticity and sinoatrial conduction in man.

The method of rapid atrial stimulation was established to measure sinus node recovery time which is assumed to permit the evaluation of sinus node automaticity. When sinus node recovery time was prolonged in patients with sinoatrial disease, this has been interpreted as a sign of disturbed sinus node automaticity (Narula et al., 1972; Mandel et al., 1972).

In 1973 Strauss et al. described a way of determining sinoatrial conduction time in man by using the premature atrial stimulation technique. Thus, with both provocative atrial pacing methods a discrimination between sinus node automaticity and sinoatrial conduction seemed to be possible (Steinbeck and Lüderitz, 1975). In respect to the methodical limitations of each of these atrial stimulation procedures (Miller and Strauss, 1974; Seipel et al., 1975; Steinbeck and Lüderitz, 1976) we recommended the measurement of both sinoatrial conduction time and sinus node recovery time for the estimation of sinus node function in sinoatrial disease (Steinbeck and Lüderitz, 1975, 1977). In this study, the results of rapid atrial stimulation as well as premature atrial stimulation are correlated with clinical data in the same patients in whom sinoatrial disease was supposed to be present. The aim was to examine the diagnostic value of atrial stimulation in patients who may require a pacemaker implantation.

PATIENTS AND METHODS

Definition: Atrial arrhythmias and conduction disorders were diagnosed using standard electrocardiographic criteria (Katz and Pick, 1956). Sinus bradycardia was defined as a mean sinus rate of less than 60 beats per minute. Our study included initial clinical

*Supported by the Deutsche Forschungsgemeinschaft.

evaluation of patients, namely history, physical examination, chest-X-ray, serial electro-cardiograms (routine-ECG, electrocardiographic 24 hour tape monitoring), carotid sinus massage and evaluation of the response to atropine. – Electrocardiographic abnormalities encountered with sinoatrial disease were: sinus bradycardia, sinoatrial block, sinus arrest with or without escape beats or rhythm, atrial tachycardia, atrial flutter and atrial fibril-lation. The following clinical symptoms were regarded as possible indicators of sino-atrial disease: syncope, dizziness, congestive heart failure, angina pectoris and palpitations.

In 1976 and 1977, 110 patients underwent diagnostic electrophysiological studies in our catheter laboratory for different reasons. Suspected sinus node disease was the indica-tion for the study in 64 patients. In 40 of them both rapid atrial pacing and premature atrial stimulation were applied. 20 of this group were kept on conventional drug therapy (group A) and the other 20 required pacemaker implantation (group B). 13 patients without clinical or electrocardiographic evidence of sinoatrial disease represent the control group in this study (group C).

All patients gave informed written consent for evaluation of sinus node function. They were studied in the cardiac catheterization laboratory in the nonsedated state and did not receive any cardioactive drugs. In all patients sinus rhythm was present during the study. A quadripolar electrode catheter was inserted via the right basilic vein or the femoral vein, and the tip placed at the lateral wall of the right atrium. The caudal-distal pair of electrodes (interelectrode distance 8 mm) was always used for stimulation. From the proximal pair of electrodes, lying closer to the sinus node, a high right atrial electro-gram was simultaneously recorded with a standard electrocardiogram at a paper speed of 100 mm/sec. An additional bipolar electrode catheter was passed percutaneously by way of the right femoral vein to the right atrium to lie across the tricuspid valve for recording of a His bundle electrogram by use of a previously described technique (Scherlag et al., 1969).

The sinus node recovery time is defined as the time interval between the last paced atrial activation and the first spontaneous beat of sinus origin after cessation of rapid atrial stimulation. Sinus node recovery time was measured after stimulation with rates slightly higher than sinus rhythm. The pacing rate was then increased by steps of 10 beats/min up to a maximal rate of 160 or 170 beats/min, and corresponding sinus node recovery time was measured. Each pacing period lasted one minute. The maximal sinus node recovery time (SNRT) is the longest time interval seen at any of the pacing rates.

Applying the premature atrial stimulation technique, premature depolarizations were elicited after every eighth spontaneous activation of sinus origin by use of a program-mable stimulator. For that purpose, the bipolar atrial electrogram was used as trigger signal. Electrical stimuli passed an isolation unit, were rectangular in shape, twice di-astolic threshold, and 2 msec in duration. Thus, the entire atrial cycle was scanned except for the refractory period.

The following time intervals were measured:

1. the interval between the last two spontaneous atrial depolarizations preceding the stimulation (a_1-a_1);
2. the interval between the last atrial depolarization and the stimulus-induced atrial excitation (so-called curtailed cycle, a_1-a_2);
3. the interval between the stimulus-induced atrial excitation and the next spontaneous atrial depolarization (so-called postextrasystolic cycle, a_2-a_3);
4. the interval of the subsequent spontaneous atrial cycle (so-called post-postextra-systolic cycle, a_3-a_4).

The postextrasystolic cycle a_2-a_3 is plotted in a diagram as a function of the curtailed cycle a_1-a_2, both values expressed as a percentage of the spontaneous atrial cycle a_1-a_1. For calculation of sinoatrial conduction time, the postextrasystolic cycle following the longest curtailed cycle which was followed by a non-compensatory pause was taken (see Figure 1). Hence we used the transition from the compensatory to the non-compensatory pause (for further discussion about this method see Steinbeck and Lüderitz, 1976). SNRT and SACT were regarded as prolonged when they exceed the mean plus single standard deviation of the values measured in the control group. The significance of the differences was checked according to Fisher's t-test.

RESULTS

Controls

In 13 patients without sinus node dysfunction SNRT was 1172 msec $\pm$ 200 ($\pm$SD), and SACT was 66 ms $\pm$ 17 ($\pm$SD) (Table 1). Concerning SACT our normal values range between 40 and 95 msec which is understood as half the conduction time into and out of the sinus node. With respect to SNRT we obtained results similar to other authors (Narula et al, 1972; Gupta et al., 1974; Kulbertus et al., 1975). Concerning SACT, different values were reported by Seipel et al. (1974) and Dhingra et al. (1975, 1977), as these authors used the non-compensatory phase for indirect calculation of SACT (for discussion see Steinbeck and Lüderitz, 1976). In contrast, in animal studies experimentally determined

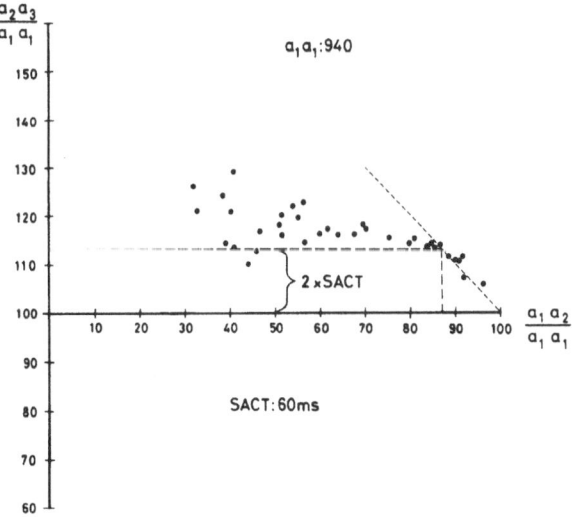

Figure 1. Postextrasystolic cycle a_2-a_3 as a function of the curtailed cycle a_1-a_2. Both values are related to the preceding a_1-a_1 interval: a_1-a_1 interval = 940 msec $\pm$ 55 ($\pm$SD) (n = 36). Transition from compensatory to noncompensatory a_2-a_3 interval occurs at a curtailed cycle of 87% of the a_1-a_1 interval. Postextrasystolic interval a_2-a_3 at this borderline (113%) minus the spontaneous atrial cycle a_1-a_1 (= 100%) represents conduction time into and out of the sinus node: i.e. the sum of conduction time from atrium to the sinus node plus from sinus node to atrium. Half of the total sum of conduction time gives the sinoatrial conduction time; in this case = 60 msec (see Steinbeck et al., 1974).

SACT was found to be much shorter (Sano and Yamagishi, 1965; Strauss and Bigger, 1972; West, 1972 and Steinbeck et al., 1978).

Sinoatrial disease

In a total of 40 patients with clinical and electrocardiographic evidence of sinoatrial disease values of SNRT and SACT are both increased (Table 1). The maximum sinus node recovery time ranged between 880 and 5880 msec with a mean of 1859 msec $\pm$ 1068 ($\pm$SD) and SACT ranged from 45 to 165 with a mean of 110 msec $\pm$ 31 ($\pm$SD) (n = 34). The results of SNRT agree with those of other authors (Narula et al., 1972; Mandel et al., 1972; Seipel et al., 1975; Delius and Wirtzfeld, 1976). Using a method of SACT determination similar to ours, a mean value of 126.5 msec was reported in 7 patients with sinoatrial block (Masini et al., 1975). When, however, the non-compensatory pause is taken for SACT estimation, much larger values have been reported (Breithardt and Seipel, 1976; Strauss and Wallace, 1976).

The correlation between clinical data and parameters obtained invasively in patients with sinoatrial disease is shown in Figure 2. Clinical symptoms were present in all patients. Pathological electrocardiographic findings were observed in 38 patients (95%); SACT was prolonged in 26 patients (65%). In 6 patients (15%) exact calculation of SACT was not possible because of severe sinus arrhythmia. A prolonged sinus node recovery time was seen in 23 patients (57.5%).

20 out of a total of 40 patients with sinoatrial disease were kept on conventional drug treatment (group A) and 20 (50%) required pacemaker therapy (group B). The differentiation of clinical symptoms in both groups was scrutinized (Figure 3). No clear cut changes could be seen concerning dizziness, syncope and palpitation. However, congestive heart failure and angina pectoris was more frequently observed in the pacemaker group. The profile of clinical signs, i.e. single or combined occurrence of different symptoms in group A and B, is evaluated in Table 2.

The incidence of electrocardiographic abnormalities in group A and B is shown in Figure 4. (For evaluation of each patient in detail see Table 3). Only two patients of group A do not reveal any electrocardiographic symptoms at all. Sinus bradycardia is much more frequent in the pacemaker group (16 patients = 80%) than in the no-pacemaker group (9 patients = 45%). Only small differences exist between both groups

Table 1. Results of atrial stimulation studies in 13 control patients and in 40 patients with sinoatrial disease.

Diagnostic atrial stimulation	Max. sinus node recovery time [msec]	Sinoatrial conduction time [msec]
Control	1172 $\pm$ 200 n = 13	66 $\pm$ 17 n = 13
p	<0.001	<0.001
Sinoatrial disease	1859 $\pm$ 1068 n = 40	110 $\pm$ 31 n = 34*

* No SACT calculation in 6 patients because of severe sinus arrhythmia.

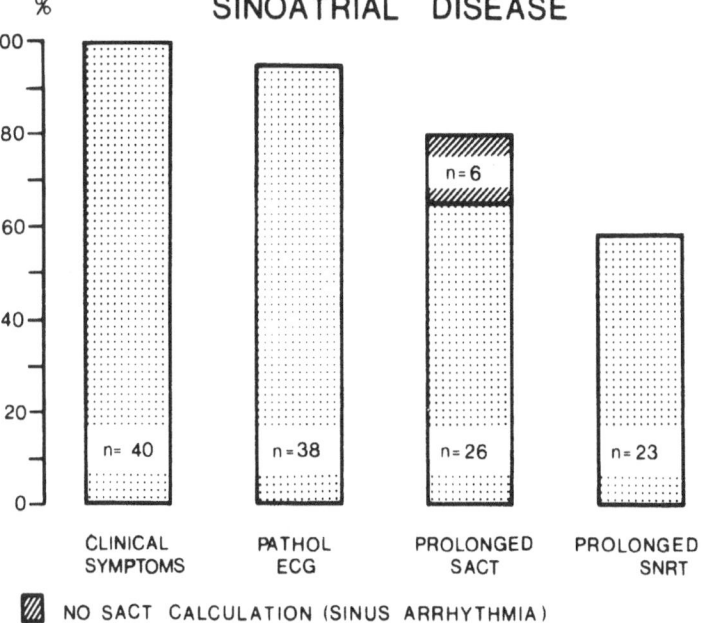

Figure 2. Correlation between clinical data and results of atrial stimulation studies in 40 patients with sinoatrial disease (40 = 100%).

concerning sinus arrest, atrial tachycardia, atrial fibrillation and atrial flutter. Sinoatrial disease was associated with atrio-ventricular conduction disease in 9 cases of the pace-maker group and in 5 cases (25%) of the no-pacemaker-patients.

The electrophysiological data of the no-pacemaker (A) and the pacemaker group (B) were compared with those of the control group (Figure 5). The sinus rate was markedly decreased in patients who required pacemaker implantation. However, no significant changes were observed between controls and the no-pacemaker group. A similar pattern was observed for the maximal sinus node recovery time. SNRT is conspicuously pro-longed in those cases needing pacemaker therapy. Patients without pacemaker require-ment revealed no prolongation of SNRT when compared with the control group. The feature of calculated sinoatrial conduction time was completely different. Patients with sinoatrial disease showed significantly prolonged SACT values in comparison with the control group. However, there was no difference between the no-pacemaker and the pacemaker group. After administering atropine (1 mg i.v.) an increase of sinus rate was observed in the no-pacemaker group (A) from 67/min $\pm$ 13 ($\pm$SD) up to 91/min $\pm$ 16 ($\pm$SD) (n = 11). On the other hand the pacemaker group (B) showed an elevation of sinus rate from 55/min $\pm$ 12 ($\pm$SD) up to 77/min $\pm$ 11 ($\pm$SD) with atropine. The shortening of SNRT following application of atropine was much more pronounced in group A than in the B-group.

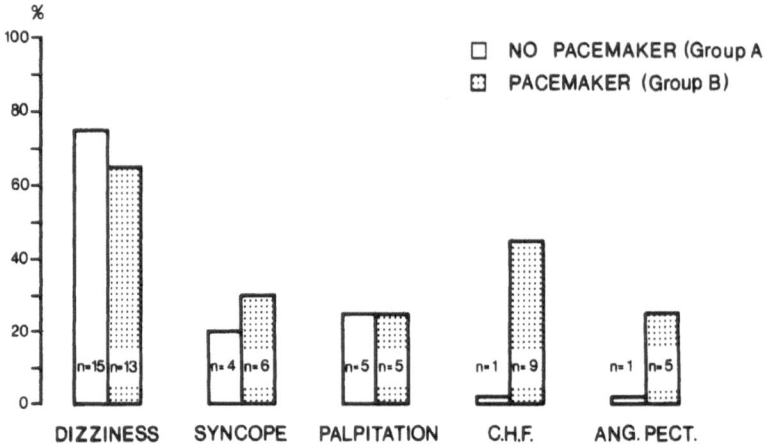

Figure 3. Differentiation of clinical symptoms in 40 patients suffering from sinoatrial disease without (20 patients) and with (20 patients) requirement of pacemaker therapy. 20 = 100% in each column. (C.H.F. = Congestive heart failure; Ang.pect. = angina pectoris).

DISCUSSION

The therapy of symptomatic sinoatrial disease is still under discussion. Theoretically, cases with severe bradycardia should be treated with drugs inducing an acceleration of heart rate. Clinical experience including our own, however, revealed that except in very mild cases neither belladonna preparations nor sympathico-mimetic agents are able to maintain an increased heart rate or to prevent severe clinical complications (Rubenstein et al., 1972; Wan et al., 1972; Sigurd et al., 1973; Kulbertus et al., 1973; Rokseth and Hatle, 1974; Blömer et al., 1975; Gurtner et al., 1976). The effect of digitalis in sinoatrial disease is not yet sufficiently clarified (Engel and Schaal, 1973; Steinbeck et al., 1976). As a whole, the conservative management remained disappointing and cardiac pacemaker treatment became more and more the therapy of choice. The combination of implanted pacemaker and appropriate antiarrhythmic agents especially in the bradycardia-tachycardia-syndrome provided an almost complete control of clinical symptoms and severe arrhythmias (Moss and Davis, 1974; Lüderitz and Steinbeck, 1976).

However, the selection of patients suffering from sinoatrial disease for pacemaker therapy has proved especially difficult. Since no recording of electrical activity of the sinus node can be obtained from the body surface, analysis of electrocardiograms does not allow appropriate interpretation of sinus node behaviour. Several invasive electrophysiologic techniques have been developed to characterize or to unmask the disturbances of sinus node automaticity and sinoatrial conduction (Rosen et al., 1971, Mandel et al.,

Table 2. Clinical features in patients without and with pacemaker requirement in sinoatrial disease.

Group A (no pacemaker)

No.	Sex, age	Dizzi- ness	CHF	Syn- cope	Angina pect.	Palpita- tion
1	F 57	⊕	–	–	–	–
2	F 66	⊕	–	–	–	–
3	M20	⊕	–	⊕	–	–
4	M33	–	–	–	–	⊕
5	M37	⊕	–	–	⊕	–
6	M69	⊕	–	⊕	–	–
7	F 45	⊕	–	⊕	–	–
8	M75	⊕	–	–	–	–
9	M50	⊕	–	⊕	–	⊕
10	M28	⊕	–	–	–	–
11	F 49	⊕	–	–	–	–
12	F 60	⊕	–	–	–	–
13	M17	⊕	–	⊕	–	–
14	F 20	–	–	–	–	–
15	M35	⊕	–	–	–	⊕
16	F 53	–	–	–	–	⊕
17	M57	–	⊕	–	–	–
18	F 50	–	–	–	–	–
19	M63	⊕	–	–	–	⊕
20	M64	–	–	–	–	⊕

Group B (pacemaker)

No.	Sex, age	Dizzi- ness	CHF	Syn- cope	Angina pect.	Palpita- tion
1	M74	⊕	–	–	–	–
2	M53	⊕	–	–	⊕	–
3	F 62	⊕	⊕	–	–	–
4	F 41	⊕	–	–	–	⊕
5	F 67	–	–	–	–	–
6	F 57	–	⊕	–	⊕	⊕
7	M63	–	⊕	–	⊕	–
8	M71	–	–	–	–	⊕
9	F 59	⊕	⊕	⊕	–	–
10	M55	⊕	–	–	–	⊕
11	M64	⊕	⊕	–	⊕	–
12	F 70	⊕	–	–	–	–
13	F 48	⊕	⊕	–	–	–
14	M50	–	–	–	–	–
15	M55	⊕	⊕	⊕	⊕	⊕
16	F 58	–	⊕	⊕	–	–
17	F 75	–	–	⊕	–	⊕
18	F 61	⊕	⊕	⊕	–	–
19	F 69	⊕	⊕	⊕	–	⊕
20	M71	⊕	–	⊕	⊕	–

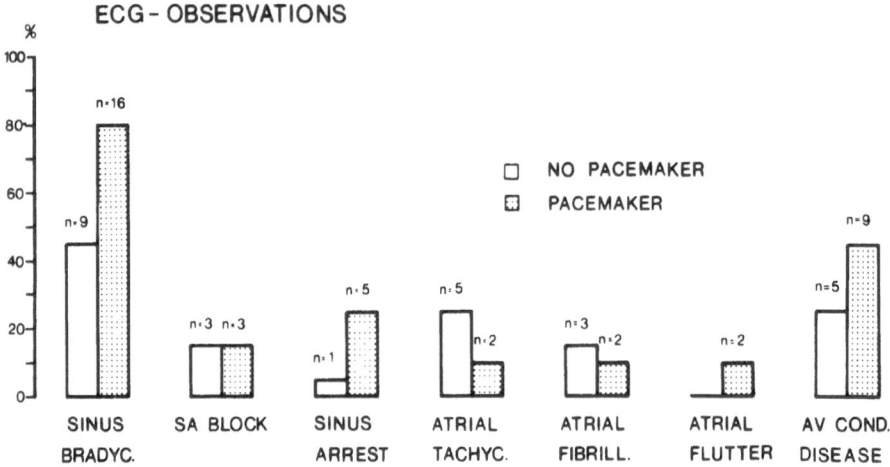

Figure 4. Frequency of pathologic electrocardiographic findings in 40 patients with sinoatrial disease in relation to pacemaker requirement. For each column: 20 = 100% (sa block = sinoatrial block; av cond. disease = atrioventricular conduction disease).

1971, Strauss et al., 1973, 1977). The purpose of this study was to discuss the relevance of rapid pacing technique and premature atrial stimulation for evaluation of sinus node function in respect to pacemaker treatment.

Sinoatrial disease can be characterized by clinical *and* electrocardiographic findings despite the lack of detailed information about sinus node function. ECG-abnormalities were missing in 2 cases: group A no. 15 and 20. In patient no. 15 SACT was prolonged by 107 msec, patient no. 20 revealed SNRT of 2060 msec as possible sign of mild sinoatrial disease. SACT was prolonged in most cases studied (82.5%). It should be mentioned, however, that exact calculation of SACT is sometimes impossible because of severe sinus bradycardia (15%). SNRT is prolonged in about half of the cases (23/40). Patients suffering from severe sinoatrial disease who required pacmaker treatment were characterized predominantly by major clinical symptoms as syncope, congestive heart failure and angina pectoris.

In 4 cases mentioned in Figure 3, the history of syncope was not related to obvious sinoatrial dysfunction (see Table 2). The same was assumed in 15 patients of group A with dizziness (Table 2). The severe forms of sinoatrial disease demanding cardiac pacemaker treatment were closely correlated with predominating sinus bradycardia, which has to be regarded as symptomatic (16/20). Sinus arrest was seen in 5/20 and atrio-ventricular conduction disease in 9/20 cases. Atrio-ventricular conduction disease associated with sinoatrial disease caused clinical symptoms in 3 cases and demanded permanent pacemaker treatment (Table 2, group B, no. 1, 14, 17). Carotid sinus hypersensitivity was present in 3/20 cases. Prolongation of SNRT agrees well with the clinical severity of sinoatrial disease. Sinus node recovery time of those patients who needed pacemaker treatment was markedly prolonged (Figure 5). In cases of moderate sinoatrial disease

Table 3. Frequency of pathologic electrocardiographic findings in group A (no pacemaker) and group B (pacemaker).

Group A (no pacemaker)

No.	Sex, age	Sinus bradyc.	SA block	Sinus arrest	Atrial tachyc.	Atrial fibrill.	Atrial flutter	AV-cond disease
1	F 57	–	⊕	–	⊕	⊕	–	–
2	F 66	⊕	–	–	–	–	–	⊕
3	M20	–	–	–	–	–	–	⊕
4	M33	⊕	–	–	⊕	⊕	⊕	–
5	M37	–	⊕	–	–	–	–	–
6	M64	–	–	–	–	–	–	–
7	M69	⊕	–	–	⊕	–	–	⊕*
8	F 45	⊕	–	–	⊕	–	–	⊕
9	M75	⊕	–	–	–	–	–	⊕
10	M50	⊕	–	–	–	⊕	–	⊕
11	M28	–	–	–	–	–	–	–
12	F 49	⊕	⊕	–	–	–	–	–
13	F 60	–	–	⊕	–	–	–	–
14	M17	–	–	–	–	–	⊕	–
15	F 20	–	–	–	–	–	–	–
16	M35	–	–	–	⊕	–	–	–
17	F 53	⊕	–	–	–	–	–	–
18	M57	⊕	–	–	–	–	⊕	–
19	F 50	⊕	–	–	⊕	–	–	–
20	M63	–	–	–	–	–	–	–

Group B (pacemaker)

No.	Sex, age	Sinus bradyc.	SA block	Sinus arrest	Atrial tachyc.	Atrial fibrill.	Atrial flutter	AV-cond. disease
1	M74	–	–	–	–	–	–	⊕*
2	M53	⊕	–	–	–	–	–	⊕
3	F 62	⊕	–	–	–	–	–	–
4	F 41	⊕	–	–	–	–	–	⊕
5	F 67	⊕	–	⊕	–	–	–	⊕
6	F 57	⊕	–	–	⊕	⊕	–	–
7	M63	⊕	–	–	⊕	⊕	–	–
8	M71	⊕	–	⊕	–	–	–	⊕
9	F 59	–	–	⊕	⊕	–	–	–
10	M55	–	–	–	–	–	–	–
11	M64	⊕	–	–	–	–	–	⊕
12	F 70	⊕	⊕	–	–	–	–	⊕
13	F 48	⊕	⊕	–	–	–	–	–
14	M50	–	–	–	–	–	–	⊕
15	M55	⊕	–	⊕	–	–	–	⊕
16	F 58	⊕	–	⊕	–	–	–	–
17	F 75	–	⊕	–	–	–	–	⊕*
18	F 61	⊕	–	⊕	–	–	–	–
19	F 69	⊕	–	–	–	–	–	⊕
20	M71	⊕	–	–	–	–	–	–

* Carotid Sinus Hypersensitivity

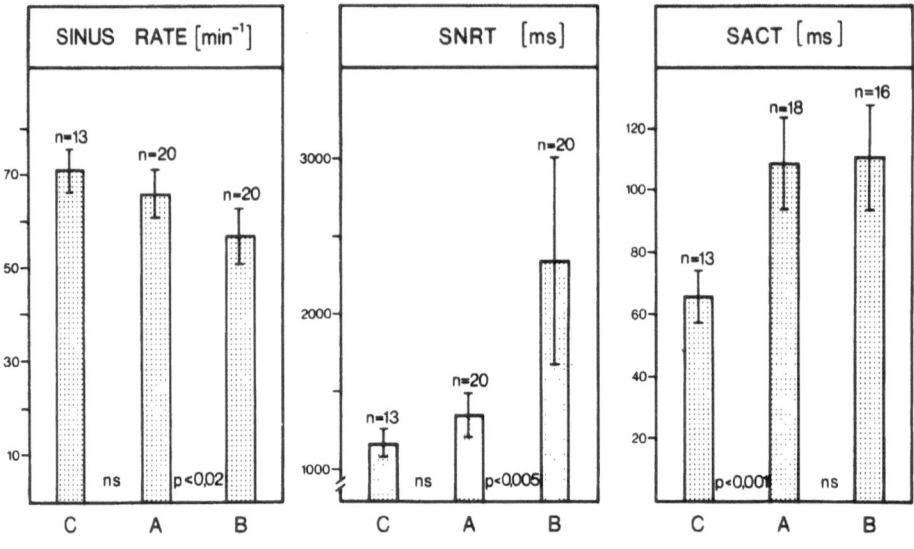

C CONTROL; A NO PACEMAKER; B PACEMAKER;

Figure 5. Electrophysiological data of sinus node function for all patients studied by diagnostic atrial stimulation. Control group (C), and patients with sinoatrial disease; A = no pacemaker requirement, B = pacemaker requirement (ns = no significant difference).

SNRT was not significantly different from the control values. While determination of SNRT seems to be useful for the additional differentiation between severe and mild cases of sinoatrial disease, calculation of SACT fails in this respect. Sinoatrial conduction time is conspicuously prolonged in the whole group of patients with sinoatrial disease; however, no difference between severe and mild forms could be detected (Figure 5). Patient follow-up over a 6–12 months period consisting of periodical visits of the patient revealed a marked improvement of all patients in group B (pacemaker implantation). No patient died until now. Persisting severe symptoms in patients of group A were not related to sinoatrial disease.

In conclusion: the decision for pacemaker treatment in sinoatrial disease is largely determined by the particular symptoms which are troublesome and correlated with electrocardiographic and electrophysiological abnormalities. Prolonged SNRT was associated with a high incidence of clinically severe sinoatrial disease in patients requiring pacemaker therapy. The calculation of SACT seems to be helpful for the diagnosis rather than for the estimation of the severity in sinoatrial disease. In our opinion moderate prolongation of SNRT or SACT in the absence of clinical symptoms is not an indication for (prophylactic) pacemaker implantation.

REFERENCES

Blömer, H., Wirtzfeld, A., Delius, W., Sebening, H.: Das Sinusknoten-Syndrom. *Z. Kardiol* 64: 697, 1975
Breithardt, G., Seipel, L.: The influence of drugs on sinoatrial conduction time in man. In: Cardiac Pacing, Diagnostic and Therapeutic Tools, edited by Lüderitz, B., Springer Berlin, Heidelberg, New York, 1976

Delius, W., Wirtzfeld, A.: Significance of the sinus node recovery time. In: Cardiac Pacing, Diagnostic and Therapeutic Tools, edited by Lüderitz, B., Springer Berlin, Heidelberg, New York, 1976

Dhingra, R.C., Wyndham, C., Amat-y-Leon, F., Denes, P., Wu, D., Rosen, K.M.: Sinus nodal responses to atrial extrastimuli in patients without apparent sinus node disease. Am J Cardiol 36: 445, 1975

Dhingra, R.C., Amat-y-Leon, F., Wyndham, C., Deedwania, P.C., Wu, D., Denes, P., Rosen, K.M.: Clinical significance of prolonged sinoatrial conduction time. Circulation 55: 8, 1977

Engel, T.R., Schaal, S.F.: Digitalis in the sick-sinus-syndrome. The effects of digitalis on sinoatrial automaticity and atrioventricular conduction. Circulation 48: 1201, 1973

Gupta, P.K., Lichstein, E., Chadda, K.D., Badui, E.: Appraisal of sinus nodal recovery time in patients with sick sinus syndrome. Am J Cardiol 34: 265, 1974

Gurtner, H.P., Lenzinger, H.R., Dolder, M.: Clinical aspects of sick sinus syndrome. In: Cardiac Pacing, Diagnostic and Therapeutic Tools, edited by Lüderitz, B., Springer Berlin, Heidelberg, New York, 1976.

Katz, L.N., Pick, A.: The arrhythmias. In: Clinical Electrocardiography, Part I, Philadelphia, Lea and Febiger, 1956

Kulbertus, H.E., De Leval-Rutten, F., Demoulin, J.C.: Sino-atrial disease: A report on 13 cases. J Electrocardiol 6: 303, 1973

Lüderitz, B., Steinbeck, G.: The use of programmed rate related premature stimulation in managing tachyarrhythmias. In: Cardiac Pacing, Diagnostic and Therapeutic Tools, edited by Lüderitz, B., Springer Berlin, Heidelberg, New York, 1976

Mandel, W.J., Hayakawa, H., Danzig, R., Marcus, H.S.: Evaluation of sino-atrial node function in man by overdrive suppression. Circulation 44: 59, 1971

Mandel, W.J., Hayakawa, H., Allen, H.N., Danzig, R., Kermaier, A.I.: Assessment of sinus node function in patients with the sick sinus syndrome. Circulation 46: 761, 1972

Masini, G., Dianda, R., Graziina, A.: Analysis of sino-atrial conduction in man using premature atrial stimulation. Cardiovasc Res 9: 498, 1975

Moss, A.J., Davis, R.J.: Brady-tachy syndrome. Progr cardiovasc Dis 16: 439, 1974

Narula, O.S., Samet, P., Javier, R.P.: Significance of the sinusnode recovery time. Circulation 45: 140, 1972

Rokseth, R., Hatle, L.: Prospective study on the occurrence and management of chronic sinoatrial disease, with follow-up. Brit Heart J 36: 582, 1974

Rosen, K.M., Loeb, H.S., Sinno, M.Z., Rahimtooia, S.H., Gunnar, R.M.: Cardiac conduction in patients with symptomatic sinus node disease. Circulation 43: 836, 1971

Rubenstein, J.J., Schulman, C.L., Yurchak, P.M., DeSanctis, R.W.: Clnical spectrum of the sick sinus syndrome. Circulation 46: 5, 1972

Sano, T., Yamagishi, S.: Spread of excitation from the sinus node. Circulat Res 16: 423, 1965

Scherlag, B.J., Lau, S.H., Helfant, R.H., Berkowitz, W.D., Stein, E., Damato, A.N.: Catheter technique for recording His bundle activity in man. Circulation 39: 13, 1969

Seipel, L., Breithardt, A., Both, A., Loogen, F.: Messung der sinuatrialen Leitungszeit mittels vorzeitiger Vorhofstimulation beim Menschen. Dtsch med Wschr 99: 1895, 1974

Seipel, L., Breithardt, G., Both, A., Loogen, F.: Diagnostische Probleme beim Sinusknotensyndrom. Z Kardiol 64: 1, 1975

Sigurd, B., Jensen, G., Meibom, J., Sandoe, E.: Adams-Stokes-syndrome caused by sinoatrial block. Brit Heart J 35: 1002, 1973

Steinbeck, G., Körber, H.-J., Lüderitz, B.: Untersuchungen zur Sinusknotenfunktion beim Bradykardie-Tachykardie-Syndrom. Verh dtsch Ges inn Med 80: 1126, 1974

Steinbeck, G., Lüderitz, B.: Comparative study of sinoatrial conduction time and sinus node recovery time. Brit Heart J 37: 956, 1975

Steinbeck, G., Naumann d'Alnoncourt, C., Lüderitz, B.: Digitalis und Sinusknotenfunktion. Z Kardiol Suppl. 3, 135, 1976

Steinbeck, G., Lüderitz, B.: Sinus node recovery time and sinoatrial conduction time. In: Cardiac Pacing, Diagnostic and Therapeutic Tools, edited by Lüderitz, B., Springer Berlin, Heidelberg, New York, 1976

Steinbeck, G., Lüderitz, B.: Störungen der Sinusknotenfunktion, Diagnostik und klinische Bedeutung. Dtsch med Wschr 102: 35, 1977

Steinbeck, G., Allessie, M.A., Bonke, F.I.M., Lammers, W.J.E.P.: The response of the sinus node to premature stimulation on the atrium studied with microelectrodes in isolated atrial preparations of the rabbit heart. This book, Chapter 8, 1978

Strauss, H.C., Bigger, J., J.T.: Electrophysiological properties of the rabbit sinoatrial perinodal fibers. Circ Res 31: 490, 1972

Strauss, H.C., Saroff, A.L., Bigger, J.T., Giardina, E.G.V.: Premature atrial stimulation as a key to the understanding of sinoatrial conduction in man. Circulation 47: 88, 1973

Strauss, H.C., Wallace, A.G.: Premature atrial stimulation for evaluation of sinoatrial conduction in man. In: Cardiac Pacing, Diagnostic and Therapeutic Tools, edited by Lüderitz, B., Springer Berlin, Heidelberg, New York, 1976

Strauss, H.C., Prystowsky, E.N., Scheinmann, M.M.: Sinoatrial and atrial electrogenesis. *Progr cardiovasc Dis* 19: 385, 1977

Wan, S.H., Lee, G.S., Toh, C.C.S.: The sick sinus syndrome. A study of 15 cases. *Brit Heart J* 34: 942, 1972

West, T.C.: Electrophysiology of the sinoatrial node. In: Electrical Phenomena in the Heart, edited by de Mello, W.C., (ed.) New York and London: Academic Press, 1972, p. 191

8

THE RESPONSE OF THE SINUS NODE TO PREMATURE STIMULATION OF THE ATRIUM STUDIED WITH MICROELECTRODES IN ISOLATED ATRIAL PREPARATIONS OF THE RABBIT HEART*

GERHARD STEINBECK, MAURITS A. ALLESSIE, FELIX I.M. BONKE, AND WIM J.E.P. LAMMERS

INTRODUCTION

The effect of ectopic atrial beats on the natural pacemaker of the heart has been discussed among electrophysiologists since a long time (Engelmann, 1897; Cushny and Matthews, 1897; Wenckebach, 1903). The advent of the microelectrode technique made it possible to study the response of single sinoatrial pacemaker cells to premature atrial beats (Bonke et al., 1969 and 1971; Klein et al., 1973; Miller and Strauss, 1974). Recently, Strauss et al. (1973) suggested that the premature atrial stimulation technique may be used for indirect assessment of sinoatrial conduction time in man. This method takes advantage of the fact that the length of the atrial cycle following an ectopic beat, which occurs early enough to discharge the sinus node, is determined by the sum of: (1) retrograde conduction time of the premature impulse from the atrium to the pacemaker center in the sinus node, (2) postextrasystolic pacemaker cycle, and (3) antegrade conduction time from the pacemaker center to the atrium. If there occurs no pacemaker shift within the sinus node and if the rate of pacemaker discharge is not influenced by the premature beat, the difference between the postextrasystolic atrial interval and the basic atrial cycle can be attributed to the sum of retrograde and antegrade sinoatrial conduction time. If one further assumes that antegrade and retrograde sinoatrial conduction velocities are equal, half of this time will give a calculated value for unidirectional sinoatrial conduction time.

Regarding the validity of this method and its possible clinical relevance, the key question is whether the assumptions given above, are valid. For instance, if the intrinsic rate of the sinus node pacemaker is affected by the premature beat, the calculation will be erroneous. Another uncertainty relates to possible discrepancies between antegrade and retrograde sinoatrial conduction time. Experimental studies undertaken to test the validity of the above-mentioned assumptions at the cellular level are not consistent. Klein et al. (1973) pointed out that a premature beat initiated during the middle of the atrial cycle always captured the sinus node, and usually resulted in a postextrasystolic pacemaker cycle which was either unchanged or prolonged. In contrast, shortening of the pacemaker cycle following capture was the prevailing finding in a consecutive study (Miller and Strauss, 1974).

Inherent to all electrophysiologic studies hitherto being reported on this subject is the tentative assumption that the cell under investigation is representative for the group of dominant pacemaker fibers, and will truly reflect the behaviour of the sinus node as a whole. Since we believe that the function of the sinus node as a whole is not adequately described by the study of only a single fiber out of the total population, we decided to reinvestigate the matter.

* Supported by a grant of the "Deutsche Forschungsgemeinschaft" (Ste 257/1 and Ste 257/2) to G. Steinbeck.

The responses to premature atrial stimulation of at least 45 fibers of each sinus node preparation were investigated. In this way, spread of activation of the total pacemaker area could be mapped both during spontaneous beating and induction of single ectopic beats of different prematurity. This resulted in a clear image of the response of the sinus node as a whole to premature atrial stimulation. With these data the method of calculation of sinoatrial conduction time could be reevaluated.

METHODS

Young rabbits were anesthetized with a mixture of fluanison and fentanyl (Hypnorm[R]) (1 mg/kg i.m.), and given heparin, 1500 IU, intravenously. While under artificial endotracheal respiration, the thorax was opened and the heart rapidly removed. The right atrium including the superior vena cava and the right atrial appendage, but without the AV node, was isolated and fixed in a tissue bath with its endocardial surface uppermost. The perfusion fluid contained (in mM): NaCl 130, KCl 5.6, $CaCl_2$ 2.2, $MgCl_2$ 1.7, $NaHCO_3$ 24, NaH_2PO_4 1.2, glucose 11, and saccharose 13. The pH was kept at 7.35 ± 0.05 and temperature at 37 ± 0.1°C. The fluid, oxygenated by bubbling with a gas mixture containing 95% O_2 and 5% CO_2, entered the tissue bath at the bottom, and was sucked off from the surface at a rate of 100 ml/min. The preparations were allowed to beat spontaneously, the basic cycle length varying from preparation to preparation between 350 and 450 milliseconds. To record a bipolar surface electrogram, a pair of teflon-coated silver wires was placed on crista terminalis. A second pair of teflon-coated silver wire placed on the right atrial appendage was used for stimulation (see Figure 1). A programmable stimulator was used which, after fifteen spontaneous beats, delivered a premature stimulus (rectangular in shape, 2 msec in duration, and twofold diastolic threshold) via an isolation unit. The last 100 msec of the spontaneous atrial cycle were scanned by premature atrial depolarizations in 5 msec steps.

Transmembrane potentials of fibers in the sinus node area were recorded by glass microelectrodes filled with 2.7 M KCl and 2.0 mM K-citrate. Electrical resistances ranged from 10–35 megohm. The microelectrode was connected by a chlorided silver wire to a high-impedance input, capacitance neutralizing amplifier. An Ag-AgCl plate served as indifferent electrode. The microelectrode was rigidly mounted on a micromanipulator provided with an electrode steering device; horizontal movement of the microelectrode was possible in an area of 25 times 25 mm with an accuracy of 10 micron (Schreurs et al., 1974). When enough meàsurements of a single fiber were obtained, the microelectrode was redrawn and moved to another place. Thus, the whole pacemaker area was consecutively studied by one microelectrode, using an at random mapping procedure. Mostly, superficial endocardial layers of fibers were impaled only; however, if this was not possible at some locations, the microelectrode was penetrated to deeper layers. Steps between neighbouring places were chosen between 0.25 and 1.0 mm, the small ones in the vicinity of the pacemaker center, and the larger ones far away from it. With this method it was possible to analyze the responses to premature stimulation of 45 to 60 sinus node fibers within 3–4 hours. The nomenclature of cycles is illustrated in Figure 1. As moment of activation the 50% amplitude level of the transmembrane potential during depolarization and the intrinsic deflection of the surface electrogram were taken. Time intervals were measured by feeding the signals into a time interval counter (HP 5300 B Measuring System). Following digital-analog conversion, the curve relating curtailed to postextrasystolic cycle of a nodal cell was plotted on-line by an XY-plotter. All signals were stored on magnetic tape for

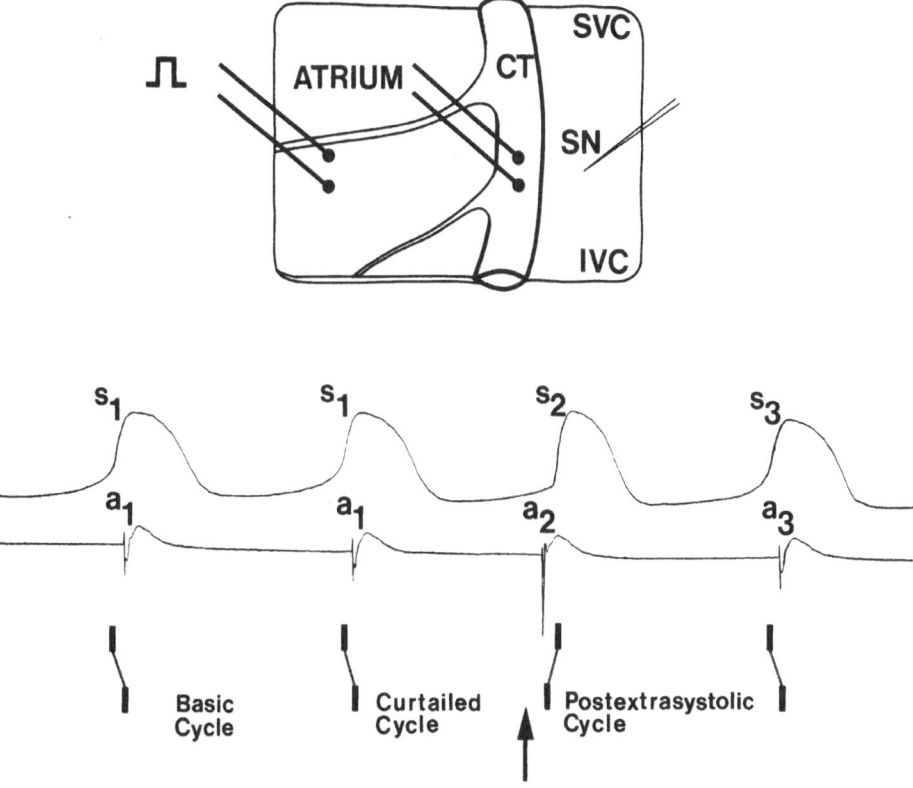

Figure 1. Above: Sketch of the isolated right atrium of the rabbit. CT = crista terminalis. SN = pacemaker area of the sinus node. SVC = superior vena cava. IVC = inferior vena cava. A surface electrogram was recorded from crista terminalis, single premature stimuli were applied to the right atrial appendage. Intracellular recordings were obtained from the sinus node.

Below: Microelectrode recordings of a sinus node pacemaker fiber (upper trace), a surface electrogram (lower trace). The preparation was allowed to beat spontaneously and after a series of fifteen spontaneous beats of which the last two are shown, a premature stimulus is given. The moment of stimulation is indicated by the arrow. Basic beats are indicated by a_1 or s_1, the premature beat by a_2 or s_2, and the postextrasystolic beat by a_3 or s_3. Consequently the cycles are indicated by: basic cycle a_1-a_1 or s_1-s_1, curtailed cycle a_1-a_2 or s_1-s_2, and the postextrasystolic cycle a_2-a_3 or s_2-s_3. The sequence of activation across the sinoatrial junction is illustrated by a ladder diagram below the tracings.

(With permission of the American Heart Association.)

subsequent additional analysis (Ampex PR 2200; tape speed 15 inches/s). Although there are usually small changes of spontaneous cycle length during the course of an experiment, we assume that the pacemaker location and the spread of impulse propagation remained the same. This is based upon the following observations:

1. Reevaluation of the same places, especially at the pacemaker center, yielded reproducible results at different stages of the experiment.
2. The configuration of the electrogram recorded from the reference electrode on the crista terminalis, was constant throughout the experiment.
3. No sudden changes of spontaneous rhythm were observed during impalement of a sinus node fiber or withdrawal of the microelectrode.
4. The relationship between atrial curtailed and postextrasystolic cycle – determined as

control during every fiber evaluation – was essentially unchanged during the course of the experiment.

Hence, for the experiments to be described in detail, we feel justified to combine the results obtained at different times and locations as if they were recorded simultaneously.

RESULTS AND DISCUSSION

We did a series of experiments, but in six experiments we were able to make a complete study of the activation pattern having more than 45 different sites of impalement in the sinus node. We will discuss the results of one single experiment in detail in the following figures. The results of the other experiments are in complete agreement with the one shown in the figures.

Figure 2 shows a surface electrogram (A) and three action potential recordings (B, C, and D) obtained from one sinus node preparation. The places of recording are indicated in the sketch above. Fiber D discharges earliest during spontaneous rhythm, followed by C and B. After two spontaneous beats, a premature one (curtailed atrial cycle 389 msec) is induced on the auricle. The sequence of discharge is now from A to D as schematically indicated by the arrow. Whereas the moment of the premature stimulus is identical in all records, the curtailed $(s_1$-$s_2)$ and postextrasystolic $(s_2$-$s_3)$ cycles differ markedly at the different recording sites: a_2-a_3 rp. s_2-s_3 gets continuously shorter from A to D, in D being shorter than a_1-a_1. This figure therefore demonstrates that – in one and the same sinus node preparation – the postextrasystolic cycle can be either prolonged, unchanged, or shortened in different fibers.

Figure 3 depicts the whole set of data from the atrial and the three nodal recording sites as given in Figure 2. In each panel, the curtailed and postextrasystolic cycles are plotted against the coupling interval (time between the last spontaneous atrial complex and the moment the stimulus is given). In A, the well-known atrial response to premature stimuli is shown exhibiting a compensatory pause with late premature beats, and a non-compensatory pause with earlier premature beats. The atrial "reference" response in A is repeated as stippled lines in diagrams B, C, and D. s_1-s_2 becomes longer than a_1-a_2, and s_2-s_3 becomes shorter than a_2-a_3 from diagram B over C to D, the difference between corresponding cycles being most marked in diagram D. Thus, three main types of fiber responses to premature atrial stimulation can be distinguished: prolongation of s_2-s_3 (diagram B), constancy of s_2-s_3 (diagram C), and shortening of s_2-s_3 (diagram D), when compared with s_1-s_1.

In Figure 4, these three types of responses were correlated with their spatial distribution within the sinus node. Fibers along the sinoatrial border show a prolongation of s_2-s_3 (open circles), whereas the fibers exhibiting a shortening of the postextrasystolic cycle are located in the center of the node or behind it (filled circles). Between these areas, fibers are found exhibiting a constancy of s_2-s_3 (crosses).

MECHANISM OF SHORTENING OF POSTEXTRASYSTOLIC CYCLE OF DOMINANT PACEMAKER FIBERS

In Figure 5 the course of the transmembrane potential of the dominant pacemaker fiber is shown during a premature beat with a coupling interval of 380 msec (left) and 330 msec (right). In all panels the postextrasystolic cycle is superimposed on the normal cycle,

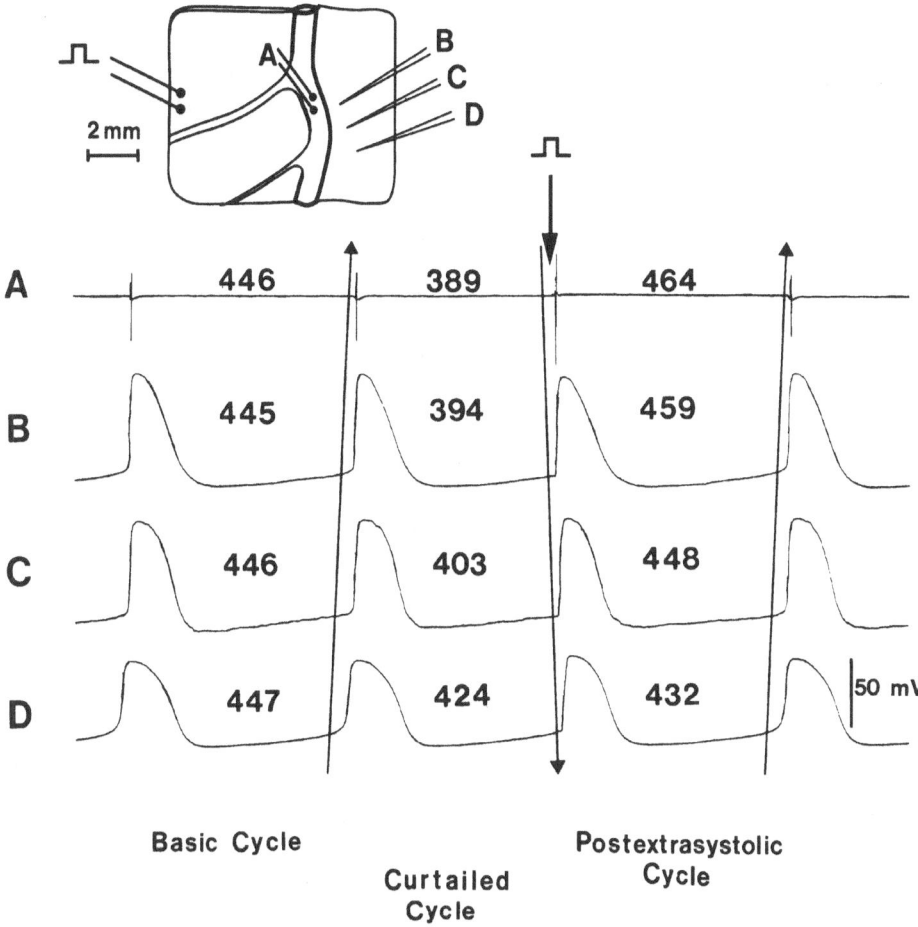

Figure 2. Composite figure including surface electrogram (A) and the transmembrane potential of three different sinus node fibers (B, C, and D). The sinus node action potentials were recorded subsequently and time aligned using the atrial complex as a reference. In all records the stimulus is delivered at the same moment (see arrow). The places of recording and stimulation are indicated in the sketch. The durations of basic cycle, curtailed cycle, and postextrasystolic cycle at the different recording sites are given in the tracings in milliseconds. See text for further discussion.

(With permission of the American Heart Association.)

the course of the transmembrane potential during the postextrasystolic cycle being stippled. From this composition it followed that the duration of the action potential of the dominant pacemaker is shortened as consequence of an atrial premature beat. In case of a relatively late premature beat which just did not capture the dominant pacemaker fiber, this shortening of the action potential duration is caused exclusively by an acceleration of the repolarization. In case of capture of the dominant pacemaker fiber the action potential is shortened both by an acceleration of the upstroke of the action potential and by an acceleration of the repolarization. In the lower panels the diastolic depolarization of the fiber during the normal cycle and the postextrasystolic cycle are superimposed. It is obvious that the process underlying diastolic depolarization is not affected (at least in

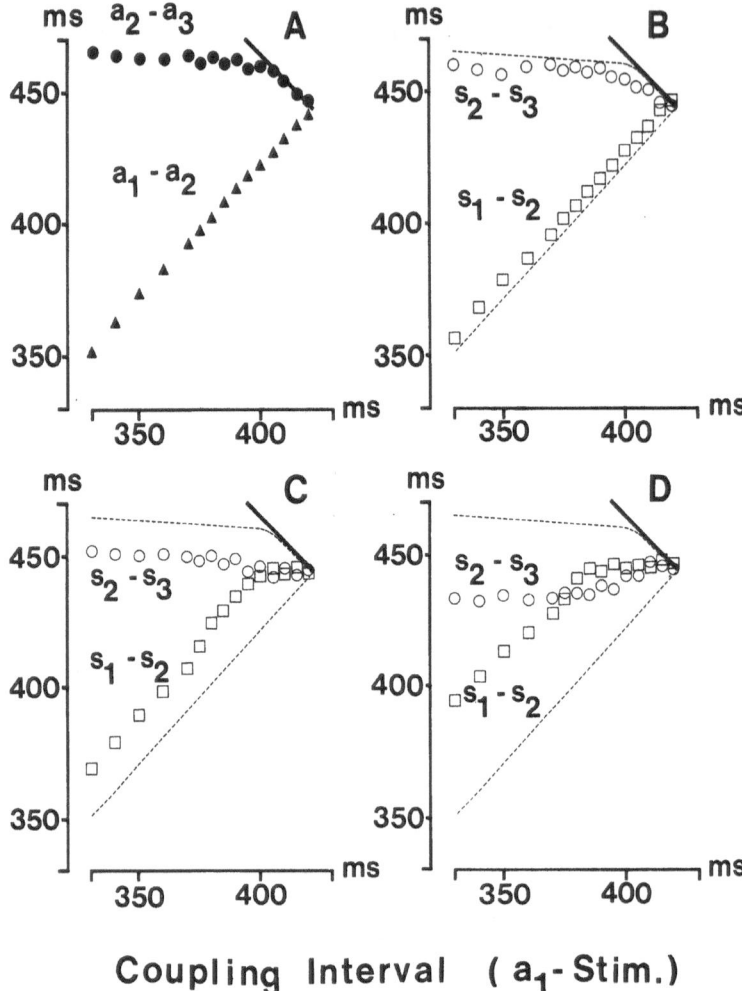

Coupling Interval (a₁- Stim.)

Figure 3. Relation between the degree of prematurity of stimulation and the curtailed and postextrasystolic cycle. On the abscissa: the coupling interval between the last spontaneous atrial complex and the moment of stimulation. On the ordinate: the duration of curtailed and postextrasystolic cycle. All values are expressed in milliseconds.

In panel A the response of the atrium is shown. Panels B, C, and D give the responses of the same three sinus node fibers as in Figure 2. In all panels the compensatory line is given. For comparison the atrial response, as plotted in panel A, is given by stippled lines in the remaining panels. See text for further description.

(With permission of the American Heart Association.)

the case of premature beats falling into the last 100 msec of the atrial cycle). Therefore, the shortening of the postextrasystolic cycle must be attributed completely to shortening of the duration of the premature action potential.

In literature a controversy exists between investigators about the effect of ectopic atrial premature beats on the automaticity of the sinus node (Klein et al., 1973 and Miller and Strauss, 1974). Since previous results were derived from analysis of single cells only, the reported differences (see Introduction) might be caused by the fact that not always the

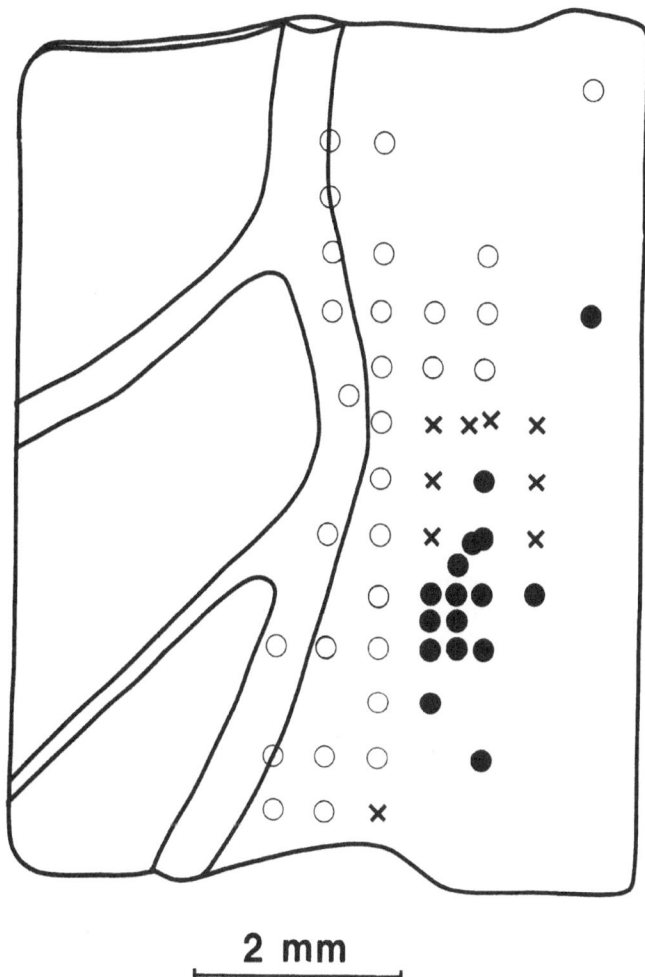

$\bigcirc$ **Lengthening of** $s_2 - s_3$

$\times$ **Constancy**   **of** $s_2 - s_3$

$\bullet$ **Shortening**   **of** $s_2 - s_3$

2 mm

Figure 4. Sketch of sinus node preparation indicating the spatial distribution of three different types of fiber responses to premature atrial stimulation. The fibers showing a lengthening of the postextrasystolic cycle of more than 5 msec compared to the basic cycle are indicated by open circles. The fibers in which the s_2-s_3 interval was more than 5 msec shorter than s_1-s_1 are indicated by filled circles. If the postextrasystolic cycle was not more than 5 msec shorter or longer than the basic cycle the fiber response was classified as constant (crosses).

(With permission of the American Heart Association.)

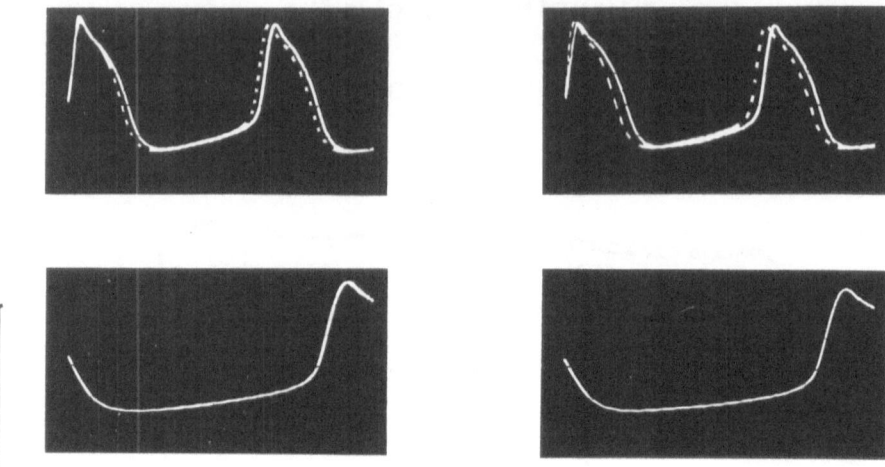

Figure 5. The course of the transmembrane potential of a dominant pacemaker fiber, during normal rhythm and after an atrial premature beat. The postextrasystolic cycle (s_2-s_3) is superimposed on the basic cycle (s_1-s_1). For the purpose of clarity the tracing during the postextrasystolic cycle is stippled. The left row gives the response of the fiber after an atrial premature impulse which penetrated over a certain distance into the sinus node, but did not capture the impaled fiber. The right row shows the response of the same fiber after an earlier atrial premature beat which captured the whole sinus node.

In the lower part the diastolic depolarization during normal rhythm and the postextrasystolic cycle are superimposed with a faster sweep of the oscilloscope. Calibration: vertical 100 mV, horizontal: 500 msec for upper panels and 250 msec for lower panels. See text for further discussion.

dominant pacemaker fiber was under investigation. With our results in mind, these differences are most probably not due to variation among preparations, but are caused by the fact that the behaviour of a single fiber, without sufficient justification, is taken as representative for the sinus node as a whole. As is demonstrated in Figure 5, shortening of the postextrasystolic cycle of the dominant pacemaker fibers is caused by a shortening of the premature action potential. As explanation one has to bear in mind that following a premature atrial beat the fibers along the sinoatrial border are depolarized earlier than the fibers in the pacemaker area. Concomitantly, also the process of repolarization starts earlier in the former group of fibers. This early repolarization of the fibers surrounding the dominant pacemaker fibers will accelerate the repolarization of these dominant fibers because of electrotonic interaction. It is further to be noted that shortening of the action potential and of postextrasystolic cycle of dominant pacemaker fibers are already apparent when the ectopic wave is approaching but still not yet capturing the pacemaker center (see Figure 5).

ANTEGRADE AND RETROGRADE CONDUCTION TIME

By making multiple microelectrode recordings in the sinus node, it was possible to get an accurate image of the spread of activation within the sinus node.

In Figure 6, maps of impulse propagation are shown during spontaneous rhythm (left map) and during a single premature atrial beat (right map). In the left hand sketch, earliest spontaneous discharge is taken as zero reference. For each impaled fiber the latency

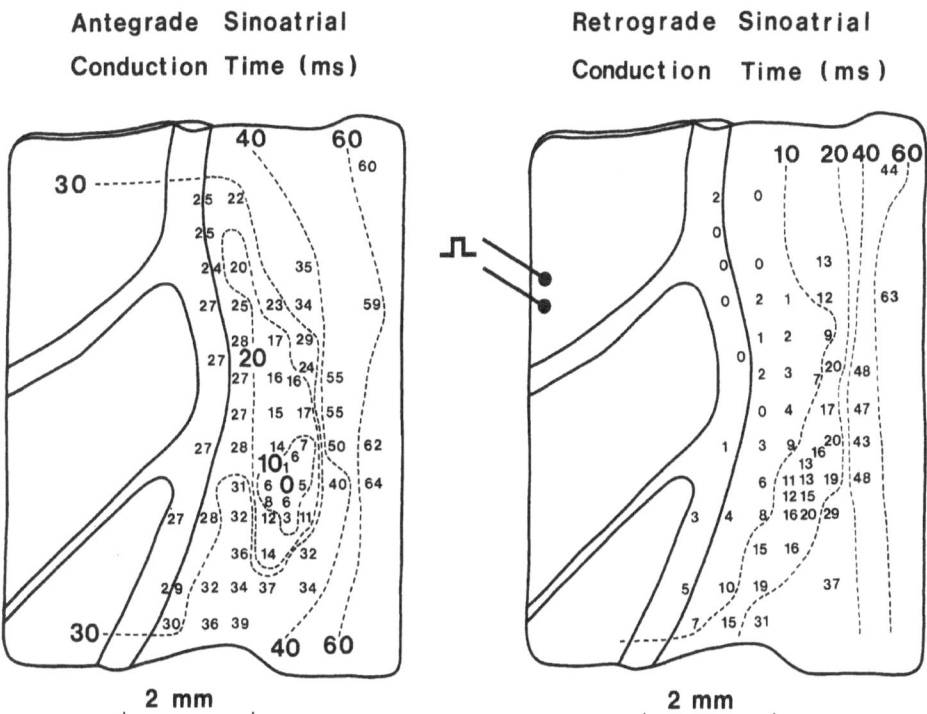

Figure 6. Maps of antegrade and retrograde sinoatrial conduction, as constructed from the time measurements of 54 fibers. During spontaneous rhythm (basic cycle length 440 msec) the earliest moment of spontaneous discharge is taken as zero reference (left map).

Following a single premature atrial beat (coupling interval 370 msec) capture of the crista terminalis is taken as zero reference (right map). Activation times of the fibers are given in msec and isochronic lines are drawn. (With permission of the American Heart Association.)

between this earliest activation and the discharge of the respective fiber is plotted in milliseconds. On the basis of these data, isochronic lines are drawn. The impulse arising in the center did not take the shortest route towards the atrium. Instead, there was preferential conduction towards the cranial end of crista terminalis. Activation of crista terminalis occurred about 25 msec after the spontaneous discharge of the dominant pacemaker cells. Impulse propagation towards the caval area was slow and apparently did not play any role in transmitting the impulse towards the atrium. Quite a similar pattern of the spread of spontaneous excitation from the sinus node of the rabbit has been reported by Sano and Yamagishi (1965). Retrograde sinoatrial conduction was studied after a premature beat which was initiated early enough to discharge the whole pacemaker area. In contrast to antegrade sinoatrial conduction, a preferential pathway through the sinus node during retrograde excitation cannot be distinguished. Instead, the impulse penetrates the sinus node as a broad wave front which decelerates gradually on its route through the sinus node towards the caval area.

If we combine the results given in Figure 4 and Figure 6 it is obvious that almost all the fibers demonstrating a shortening of the postextrasystolic cycle in reaction to an atrial premature beat (indicated with filled circels in Figure 4), belonged to the group of dominant pacemaker fibers (left map of Figure 6). In the six sinus node preparations in which a complete map could be made, retrograde sinoatrial conduction time (14.7 msec $\pm$ 2.2 [SD]) was shorter than antegrade sinoatrial conduction time (23.5 msec $\pm$ 2.3 [SD]) ($p < 0.001$); see also Table 1.

This finding is in accordance with the observation that dominant pacemaker fibers exhibit action potentials of higher amplitude and steeper rise of phase 0, when the impulse is coming from the atrium, than in case of spontaneous discharge. A possible explanation is that in case of spontaneous discharge of the sinus node, the impulse diverges from the group of dominant pacemaker fibers towards all directions. In such a situation, a relatively small number of fibers has to generate the excitatory current for a relatively large amount of surrounding fibers. Therefore, the depolarization of a dominant pacemaker fiber will be of smaller amplitude and lower rate of rise. If the impulse is coming from the atrium, the sinoatrial border is reached over a broad wave front. In the center of the sinus node, more fibers are discharged now simultaneously. Therefore, the action potentials of these fibers will in this case show higher amplitudes and increased rate of rise. Since the rate of rise of the upstroke of the action potential is an important factor for the conduction velocity, this might be the cause of the difference between antegrade and retrograde conduction within the sinus node. Differences in activation pattern during retrograde and antegrade conduction might also be of influence on the conduction time.

COLLISION BETWEEN AN ECTOPIC IMPULSE AND THE IMPULSE COMING FROM THE DOMINANT PACEMAKER

In case of premature beats elicited late in the atrial cycle and followed by a compensatory postextrasystolic cycle, two wave fronts are colliding somewhere in the sinus node. There is antegrade conduction of the impulse arising in the dominant pacemaker colliding against the ectopic impulse which is retrogradely conducted through the sinoatrial junction. Depending on the degree of prematurity of the ectopic impulse the collision between the antegrade and retrograde wave front can be expected to occur at a different region within the sinus node. Since the ectopic impulse is invading the sinus node more or less as a broad wave front (see Figure 6) the sites of collision will be determined almost exclusively by the pattern of antegrade conduction of the spontaneous discharge.

In Figure 7, the collision lines between nomotopic and ectopic activation were constructed for four premature beats with different prematurity. For that purpose, the degree of prematurity of stimulation that was necessary for capture, was determined for every fiber. This is expressed in the number of msec by which a_1-a_2 must be shorter than a_1-a_1. For simplicity, not all the values of the individual fibers are given, but only the collision lines. It should be emphasized that this map of collision lines does not represent the situation during one single beat. Instead, the numbers given with the lines indicate how much the atrial cycle has to be shortened for penetration of the ectopic wave front up to this border line. For example, if the curtailed atrial cycle a_1-a_2 is shorter than a_1-a_1 by 5 msec, the line indicated with "-5" represents the collision between the ectopic wave coming from the left, and the spontaneously emerging sinus impulse coming from the right. The earlier the ectopic beat occurs the more the line of collision is shifted towards the pacemaker center. If a_1-a_2 is more than 35–40 msec shorter than a_1-a_1, the pacemaker center is discharged prematurely by the ectopic impulse.

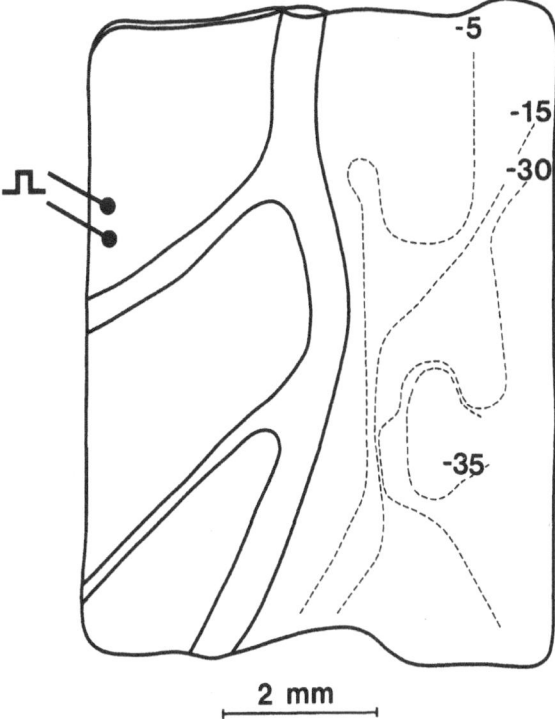

Figure 7. Sketch of sinus node preparation. The stippled lines are "collision lines". These indicate the site of collision between the impulse arising from the dominant pacemaker and conducting in an antegrade way, and the impulse elicited by premature stimulation of the atrium invading the sinus node retrogradely. The line indicated by "−5" represents the collision which occurs if the atrial cycle is curtailed 5 msec by the premature stimulus (thus a_1-a_2 is 5 msec shorter than a_1-a_1). At a prematurity of −35 msec the dominant pacemaker area is captured.
(With permission of the American Heart Association.)

ELECTROTONIC INTERACTION WITHIN THE SINUS NODE

In Figure 8 the effect of the penetrating ectopic wave front upon the dominant pacemaker fiber is shown. In the left part of this figure the course of the transmembrane potential of the dominant pacemaker fiber is shown during the induction of three ectopic beats of different prematurity (405, 385, and 370 msec respectively). In the right part of the figure the changes in curtailed and postextrasystolic cycle of this fiber are given together with a sketch of the preparation in which the site of recording is indicated as well as the lines of collision between the nomotopic wave front and the ectopic wave front for the different prematurities. In the left part of the figure, the curtailed cycle and the postextrasystolic cycle are superimposed on the recording during normal rhythm. In the upper panel a premature beat is elicited late in atrial diastole at a coupling interval of 405 msec. The curtailed atrial cycle is shortened by 10 msec. However, in the recorded fiber no change in cycle length or action potential configuration occurred under the influence of the atrial

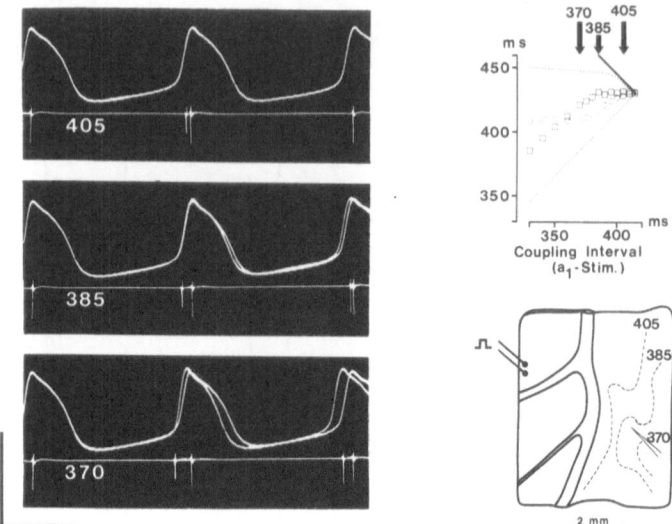

Figure 8. Left: transmembrane potential of a dominant pacemaker fiber and atrial electrogram during the induction of three atrial ectopic beats of different prematurity (405, 385, and 370 msec). Recordings during curtailed and postextrasystolic cycles are superimposed on recordings during spontaneous rhythm. Calibration: vertical: 100 mV, horizontal: 200 msec.

Right: curtailed cycle of the dominant pacemaker fiber (s_1-s_2: □) and postextrasystolic cycle (s_1-s_2: ○) as varied by the coupling interval of ectopic atrial beats. The stippled lines indicate the response of the atrium. The solid line represents the compensatory line. Below, a sketch of the preparation is given in which the sites of stimulation and intracellular recording are indicated. The atrial surface electrogram was taken from the crista terminalis. In this sketch the lines of collision between the impulse arising in the sinus node and the ectopic wave front elicited by premature atrial stimulation are given for the three different coupling intervals (405, 385, and 370 msec).

(With permission of the American Heart Association.)

premature beat. As can be seen in the sketch of the preparation the ectopic wave collided against the sinus impulse more than 1 mm away from the place where the microelectrode was impaled. In the middle panel a coupling interval of 385 msec produced a curtailed atrial cycle which is 30 msec shorter than a_1-a_1. Again, the pacemaker fiber is not captured by this premature beat, as can be concluded from the fact that s_1-s_2 is equal to s_1-s_1, and from the unchanged rate of rise and amplitude of the action potential upstroke. However, repolarization is accelerated, leading to shortening of the action potential duration. As phase 4 depolarization during the postextrasystolic cycle is unaffected (see Figure 5), this shortening of the action potential leads to shortening of the s_2-s_3 cycle although the fiber is not captured. Construction of the collision lines reveals that, following a coupling interval of 385 msec, the ectopic wave has approached the site of microelectrode recording up to about 0.5 mm. Thus, it must be concluded that the pacemaker center is influenced electrotonically over this distance. When the coupling interval is further shortened – as in the lower panel – the pacemaker fiber is prematurely discharged by the premature impulse as judged from the earlier onset and increased steepness of the upstroke of the action potential (phase 0). Following a premature beat curtailing the atrial cycle by 45 msec (coupling interval is 370 msec), the action potential is shortened more than in the case of the middle panel. This shortening is based on both a faster upstroke and a more rapid repolarization. Accordingly, the postextrasystolic cycle s_2-s_3 is shortened further. As to the electrotonic influence, our measurements allow some quantitative description of the distance across which this interaction can take place in the sinus node. The construction of the lines of collision between the ectopic and spontaneous wave front, and the resulting influence on the postextrasystolic cycle, revealed that the ectopic wave had to approach the pacemaker center up to 0.5 mm to exert an electrotonic effect. This is in accordance with the values for the space constant measured by use either of a large extracellular suction electrode ($\lambda = 465\ \mu$, Bonke, 1973) or the voltage clamp technique with a single sucrose gap ($\lambda = 828\ \mu$, Seyama, 1976).

RE-EVALUATION OF THE METHOD OF CALCULATING SINOATRIAL CONDUCTION TIME (SACT)

For the calculation of sinoatrial conduction time (SACT) in man, two modes have been used. Both are based on the relation between the atrial curtailed cycle and the postextrasystolic cycle as can be determined by the premature atrial stimulation technique. From this curve the SACT has been estimated either using the so-called plateau phase of the non-compensatory part of the curve (Strauss et al., 1973), or the point of transition from compensatory to non-compensatory values as reference point (Steinbeck et al., 1974). According to these criteria we have calculated the sinoatrial conduction time for our rabbit preparations. Since in our experiments the atrial curves did not show a plateau phase, we decided to use as reference the postextrasystolic cycle following a premature beat that curtailed the atrial cycle by 100 msec. By subtracting the normal interval (a_1-a_1) from the value of this postextrasystolic cycle (a_2-a_3) and dividing by two, the calculated unidirectional conduction time was derived ("non-compensatory phase" method). In the same way the calculation was done using the point of transition as reference ("transition" method).

Table 1 shows that both methods seriously underestimate true antegrade sinoatrial conduction time, since the calculated values are 14.2 msec $\pm$ 4.4 (SD) ("non-compensatory phase" method), and 10.2 msec $\pm$ 1.2 (SD) ("transition" method), compared with the true value for antegrade conduction of 23.5 msec $\pm$ 2.3 (SD). Underestimation is slightly less when the "non-compensatory phase" method is used. A satisfactory explana-

Table 1. Measured versus calculated sinoatrial conduction time.

	Measured values		Calculated values	
			Unidirectional conduction time	
Experiment	Antegrade conduction time	Retrograde conduction time	(non-compensatory phase)	(transition)
1	20 msec	16 msec	12 msec	10 msec
2	25 msec	15 msec	11 msec	9 msec
3	23 msec	14 msec	13 msec	10 msec
4	26 msec	18 msec	23 msec	12 msec
5	25 msec	13 msec	13 msec	9 msec
6	22 msec	12 msec	13 msec	11 msec
Mean $\pm$ SD	23.5 $\pm$ 2.3 msec (p < 0.001)	14.7 $\pm$ 2.2 msec	14.2 $\pm$ 4.4 msec (p < 0.025)	10.2 $\pm$ 1.2 msec

tion for this underestimation is given by our finding that

1. postextrasystolic cycle of the dominant pacemaker fibers is shortened,
2. antegrade and retrograde conduction in the sinus node are not equal, antegrade conduction being considerably slower than retrograde conduction.

REFERENCES

1. Bonke, F.I.M.: Electrotonic spread in the sinoatrial node of the rabbit heart. *Pflügers Arch* 339: 17, 1973
2. Bonke, F.I.M., Bouman, L.N., Van Rijn, H.E.: Change of cardiac rhythm in the rabbit after an atrial premature beat. Circ Res 24: 533, 1969
3. Bonke, F.I.M., Bouman, L.N., Schopman, F.J.G.: Effect of an early atrial premature beat on activity of the sinoatrial node and atrial rhythm in the rabbit. *Circ Res* 29: 704, 1971
4. Cushny, A.R., Matthews, S.A.: On the effects of electrical stimulation of the mammalian heart. *J Physiol* (*London*) 21: 213, 1897
5. Engelmann, T.W.: Über den Ursprung der Herzbewegung und die physiologischen Eigenschaften der grössen Herznerven des Frosches. *Arch f d ges Physiol* 65: 109, 1897
6. Klein, H.O., Singer, D.H., Hoffman, B.F.: Effects of atrial premature systoles on sinus rhythm in the rabbit. *Circ Res* 32: 480, 1973
7. Miller, H.C., Strauss, H.C.: Measurement of sinoatrial conduction time by premature atrial stimulation in the rabbit. *Circ Res* 35: 935, 1974
8. Sano, T., Yamagishi, S.: Spread of excitation from the sinus node. *Circ Res* 16: 423, 1965
9. Schreurs, A.W., Meijer, A.A., Bouman, L.N., Bonke, F.I.M.: Micromanipulator with an electrode driver used for microelectrode work. *Pflügers Arch* 346: 163, 1974
10. Seyama, I.: Characteristics of the rectifying properties of the sinoatrial node cell of the rabbit. *J Physiol* 255: 379, 1976
11. Steinbeck, G., Körber, H.J., Lüderitz, B.: Die Bestimmung der sinuatrialen Leitungszeit beim Menschen durch gekoppelte atriale Einzelstimulation. *Klin Wschr* 52: 1151, 1974
12. Strauss, H.C., Saroff, A.L., Bigger, J.T., Giardina, E.G.V.: Premature atrial stimulation as a key to the understanding of sinoatrial conduction in man. *Circulation* 47: 86, 1973
13. Wenckebach, K.F.: Über die Dauer der compensatorischen Pause nach Reizung der Vorkammer des Säugethierherzens. *Arch Anat Physiol*, 57–64, 1903

9

REVIEW OF THE SIGNIFICANCE OF DRUGS IN THE SICK SINUS NODE SYNDROME*

HAROLD C. STRAUSS, MELVIN M. SCHEINMAN, AN LaBARRE, DAVID J. BROWNING, THOMAS L. WENGER, AND ANDREW G. WALLACE

Although a review article such as this could summarize studies evaluating the effects of a variety of different drugs on sinus node function, we feel that this information is accessible in other articles and ask the interested reader to consult Breithardt et al. (1975, 1976, 1976a, and 1976b), Dhingra et al. (1975, 1976 and 1976a), Dighton (1974, 1975), Engel and Schaal (1973), Goodman et al. (1975), Jose and Taylor (1969), Reiffel et al. (1975), Schamroth (1966), Seides et al. (1974), Steinbeck and Lüderitz (1977), Stern and Eisenberg (1969). Instead, we will review the mechanisms underlying drug depression of sinus node function and discuss two variables that may influence the results obtained in any electro-pharmacologic study, namely, the population studied, the experimental protocol and a limitation of the testing procedures.

Since drugs are frequently used in patients with sick sinus syndrome to treat coexisting arrhythmias or other medical problems, it is well to consider those agents that may adversely affect sinus node function. By now it is established that antiarrhythmic drugs such as quinidine, procainamide, propranolol, verapamil and cardiac glycosides can adversely affect sinus node function (Short, 1954; Ferrer, 1974; Strauss et al., 1976; Breithardt et al., 1976c; Hewlett, 1907; Greenwood and Finkelstein, 1964; Margolis et al., 1975). Recent evidence would suggest that lithium and antihypertensive agents such as alpha-methyldopa, guanethidine and clonidine may also depress sinus node function in patients with sick sinus syndrome (Wellens et al., 1975; Scheinman et al.).

The adverse effects of these agents on sinus node automaticity and/or sinoatrial conduction may be directly or indirectly mediated. Indirect effects can result from vagomimetic properties (e.g., digitalis) (McLain et al., 1963; Chai et al., 1967) or from withdrawal of the supportive effects of catecholamines by beta-adrenergic receptor blockade (e.g., propranolol) or adrenergic neuron blockade (e.g. guanethidine, alpha-methyldopa) (Strauss et al., 1976; Scheinman et al.). Furthermore, drug combinations, such as reserpine and digoxin may be additive in eliciting adverse effects on sinus function (Bigger and Strauss, 1972).

The adverse effects of a drug on sinus node function may be manifest by an appearance of or an exacerbation of sinus bradycardia, sinus pauses, or sinoatrial exit block. The degree of depression is a complex outcome depending on the patient's sensitivity to the drug, the plasma drug concentration, vagal tone, and the presence or absence of congestive heart failure and/or ischemia of the sinus node. Patients without sinus node dysfunction may manifest depressed function when drug concentrations far exceed the therapeutic

* Supported in part by the U.S. Public Health Service Grants HL 19216, 05736, 15190, 07101, 01613 and RR 30 from the General Clinical Research Centers Program of the Division of Research Resources, National Institutes of Health, and by a Research Career Development Award (1-K04-HL-00268) to Dr. Strauss, by an American Heart Association Teaching Scholar Award to Dr. Scheinman.

range, as occurs in cases of overdosage with digitalis (Smith and Willerson, 1971). On the other hand, other patients having an increased sensitivity to a drug will demonstrate depressed sinus node function even at therapeutic concentrations (Margolis et al., 1975; Scheinman et al.). In addition, our observations of this latter group of patients lead us to believe that increased sensitivity to a drug is associated more often with the subgroup of patients with sinus pauses and/or sinoatrial exit block than with the subgroup with sinus bradycardia alone. Whether this reflects differences in the extent of the disease process or an actual difference in pathophysiology is unknown at present.

Although the clinician has several indicators of adverse drug reactions, each has its drawbacks. The most general indicators of adverse drug reactions are often symptoms. However, the severity of the symptoms does not always correlate with the degree of depression of sinus node function, for the former is also determined by the degree of depression of the pacemaker function elsewhere in the heart, cardiac contractility, blood pressure and cerebrovascular perfusion. Another indicator is heart rate, but since drugs can depress sinoatrial conduction as well as automaticity and therefore interfere with sinus node function without necessarily changing heart rate, its sensitivity as an indicator is limited too. Worse yet, drug induced disturbances may be intermittent and one may have to stress the patient to unmask the dysfunction. Patients are therefore referred for electropharmacologic study to document, if possible, the dysfunction and to elucidate the pathophysiology of the adverse drug reaction.

In the electrophysiology laboratory, spontaneous cycle length, responses to premature atrial stimulation and rapid atrial pacing are determined under control conditions and following intravenous administration of the appropriate drug (Strauss et al., 1976 and 1976a). In some instances, where acute administration of the drug may cause changes in autonomic nervous system tone the electropharmacologic effects are determined the following day, after oral administration of the drug (Margolis et al., 1975). In addition to the invasive procedure, ambulatory electrocardiograms are recorded when possible, both before and after the drug has been excreted to determine whether the rhythm disorder is present under control conditions as well as during drug therapy. Although often helpful, in many instances the results of such a pharmacologic study may be entirely negative. Furthermore, in comparing pharmacologic studies of a drug by different investigators, quite different results may be observed. It therefore seems appropriate to discuss the problems that may confound the interpretation of data.

The first problem concerns the variability in patient populations chosen for study, which is understandable since the diagnostic criteria for sick sinus syndrome are necessarily broad. These criteria have been outlined by Ferrer (1968), but do not quantitate the degree of sinus node dysfunction, a shortcoming made apparent in trying to compare two pharmacologic studies of the same drug in which the groups of patients differ in their degrees of sinus node dysfunction. For example, such differences may well explain why Steinbeck and Lüderitz (1977) observed a 47% decrease in sinoatrial conduction time whereas Dhingra et al. (1976b) saw only a 7% decrease following intravenous administration of atropine. In addition, quite apart from patient grouping on the basis of disease severity, some subdivision of patients by age should be made, since drug effects may depend on this variable. As an illustration, Dauchot and Gravenstein (1971) demonstrated that the tachycardic response to atropine diminishes with age.

A second problem concerns the manner and route of drug administration, which may influence experimental results in unexpected ways. For instance, rapid administration of a drug can change autonomic tone in either direction. On one hand, giving cardiac glycosides rapidly intravenously can cause vasoconstriction and sympathetic stimulation (Smith and Haber, 1973 and 1973a). The increased sympathetic tone may oppose the drug's depressant effects on sinus node automaticity and/or sinoatrial conduction and hence complicate the evaluation of the drug's effects. On the other hand, rapid intravenous administration of propranolol can cause hypotension and vagal withdrawal, leading to a less pronounced effect of this drug on sinus node automaticity and/or sinoatrial conduction. More predictably, declining plasma drug concentration following an intravenous dose may cause a decreasing pharmacologic effect as the study proceeds. The magnitude of this effect depends on drug elimination half-life, volume of distribution and number of compartments. In addition, the same dose of a drug given intravenously and orally can yield different plasma levels due to the first-pass effect (Nies and Shand, 1975). Finally, drug metabolites may augment the action of the parent compound so that the observed effect exceeds that expected if the metabolites are not measured along with the parent drug.

We will now review our experimental data on propranolol and disopyramide to support our view that patients with sinus pauses and/or sinoatrial exit block show more marked changes to the drugs during functional testing than do patients with sinus bradycardia alone. We will also discuss a limitation of the rapid atrial pacing technique and how this limitation may cause paradoxic responses.

When we administered propranolol 0.1 mg/kg intravenously over a 3–5 minute period to 12 patients with sick sinus syndrome, the spontaneous cycle length increased by 14.9% from 963 ± 149 msec (m± SD) to 1106 ± 187 msec (p < 0.005) (Figure 1). We then divided the patients into two groups, those with sinus pauses and/or sinoatrial exit block (group A, n = 5) and those with sinus bradycardia (group B, n = 7). Large increases (38 and 48%) in spontaneous cycle length were recorded in two patients from group A (Figure 1).

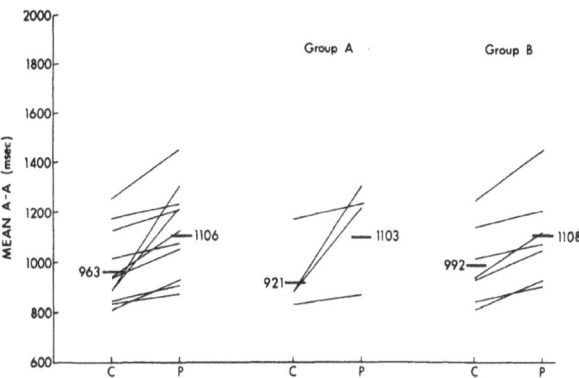

Figure 1. Effect of propranolol (0.1 mg/kg) on spontaneous cycle length.
Left: Twelve patients with sinus node dysfunction. Propranolol administration increased mean spontaneous cycle length (mean A-A) 14.9% from 963 ± 149 msec to 1106 ± 187 msec (p < 0.005).
Middle: Group A = 5 patients with sinoatrial block and/or sinus pauses. (Note: two patients had identical values for mean A-A before and after propranolol.) Two patients showed marked increases of 38% and 48%.
Right: Group B = 7 patients with sinus bradycardia. Mean A-A increased 12% from 992 ± 158 to 1108 ± 186 (p < 0.005).

The effect of intravenous propranolol on the maximum value of the first post pacing cycle length (normalized by the mean value of the spontaneous cycle length) in these patients is illustrated in Figure 2. The mean value of the maximum first post-pacing cycle increased from 1371 (1015–2222) msec to 2208 (1086–7014) msec (61%). The mean value of the normalized maximum first post-pacing cycle changed from 1.45 to 1.94 which was not statistically significant. Dramatic increases in the normalized maximum value of first post-pacing cycle of 81 and 145% were seen in two of the group A patients and a 43% increase in one of the group B patients. Intravenous atropine (0.02 mg/kg) administration failed to appreciably decrease the values of the first post-pacing cycle in the two group A patients (Figure 3) but did so in the group B patient.

$SACT_{A+R}$ was measured in nine of the twelve patients who received propranolol and was not significantly lengthened in these patients.

Disopyramide, an antiarrhythmic drug with quinidine-like effects, might be tolerated in patients with sick sinus syndrome because of its atropine-like effects. Intravenous administration of disopyramide (2 mg/kg) to 15 patients with sick sinus syndrome (group A = 6, group B = 9) caused the mean spontaneous cycle length to change from 938 ± 237 to 976 ± 282 msec (Figure 4). Although these changes were not significant, a large increase (91%) in spontaneous cycle length was seen in one group A patient. Disopyramide caused a decrease in spontaneous cycle length in 6/9 group B patients, consistent with its atropine-like effects.

Disopyramide phosphate changed the average value of maximum first post-pacing cycle from 2147 (988–6315) to 4830 (996–40680) msec and the average value of the normalized maximum first post-pacing cycle from 2.39 to 3.88 (Figure 5). Neither of these changes was significant. Large changes in the normalized maximum first post-pacing cycle occurred in 4 group A patients (Figure 5). In three group A patients large increases (93%,

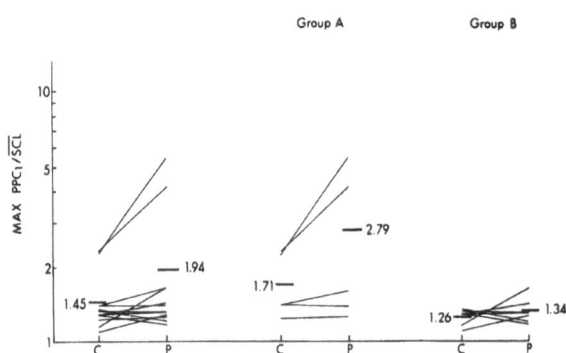

Figure 2. Effect of propranolol (0.1 mg/kg) on maximum first post-pacing cycle length.

Left: Twelve patients with sinus node dysfunction. Following propranolol administration the length of the maximum first post pacing cycle (max PPC_1) normalized by the spontaneous cycle length ($\overline{SCL}$) increased 34% from 1.45 (1.11–2.29) to 1.94 (1.17–5.48).

Middle: Group A = 5 patients with sinoatrial block and/or sinus pauses. Two of those patients showed marked increases in max $PPC_1/\overline{SCL}$ of 81% and 145%.

Right: Group B = 7 patients with sinus bradycardia. One patient increased max $PPC_1/\overline{SCL}$ by 43%.

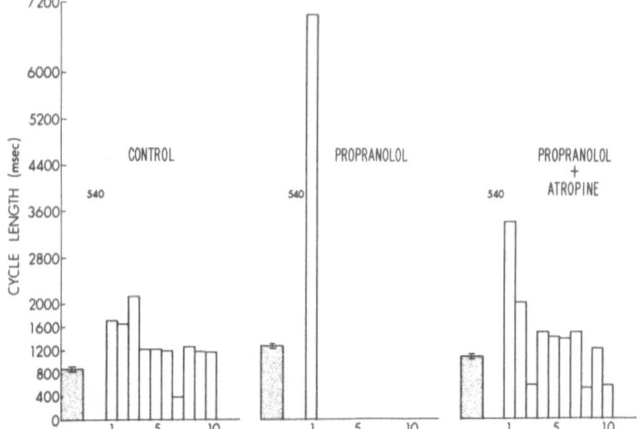

Figure 3. Effect of propranolol and propranolol plus atropine on post-pacing cycle lengths.

Mean spontaneous cycle lengths and SD prior to pacing is shown by the height of the stippled and error bars, respectively. Length of the post-pacing cycles is indicated by the clear bars. The post-pacing cycle number is plotted on the abscissa. A pacing cycle length of 540 msec was employed. Responses under control conditions are shown on left. Response following propranolol administration is shown in middle. Note only one post-pacing cycle is recorded as atrial pacing (CL 1000 msec) was started following the first post-pacing cycle. Responses following propranolol and atropine administration are shown on right. Note that atropine fails to decrease the value of first post-pacing cycle to that recorded under control conditions.

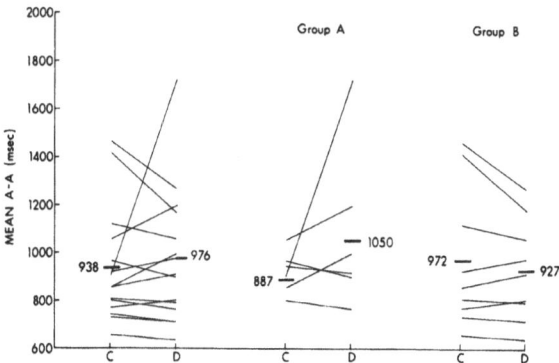

Figure 4. Effect of disopyramide phosphate 2 mg/kg on spontaneous cycle length.

Left: Fifteen patients with sinus node dysfunction. Following disopyramide administration mean spontaneous cycle length (mean A-A) increased 4% from 938 ± 237 to 967 ± 282.

Middle: Group A = 6 patients with sinoatrial block and/or sinus pauses. The only patient that merits comment is one who showed an increase in mean A-A of 91%.

Right: Group B = 9 patients with sinus bradycardia. Six showed a decrease in mean A-A consistent with its atropine like effect.

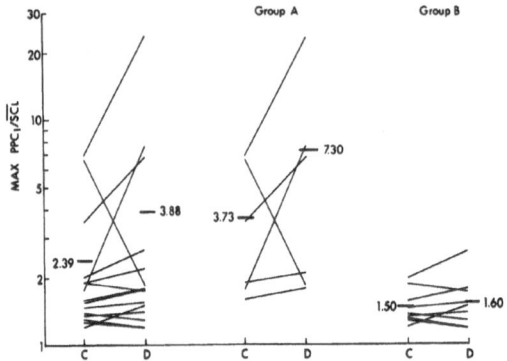

Figure 5. Effect of disopyramide phosphate (2mg/kg) on maximum first post-pacing cycle.
  Left: Fifteen patients with sinus node dysfunction. Following disopyramide administration the maximum post-pacing cycle (max PPC_1) normalized by the spontaneous cycle length ($\overline{SCL}$) changed from 2.39 to 3.88.
  Middle: Group A = 6 patients with sinoatrial block and/or sinus pauses. Four patients showed marked changes, 3 increased (93%, 242%, 337%), 1 showed a paradoxical decrease. (see text for explanation).
  Right: Group B = 9 patients with sinus bradycardia.

242%, and 337%) were seen. In the fourth patient a paradoxic response to rapid atrial pacing was recorded. In this patient the value of normalized maximum first post-pacing cycle decreased by 72% from 6.7 to 1.86. One might assume this to be due to the vagolytic effects of the drug. However, examination of the responses to premature atrial stimulation following disopyramide administration revealed a pattern consistent with first degree sino-atrial block with interference and second-degree sinoatrial block. Therefore, it is likely that in this patient, following disopyramide administration, sinus node entrance block occurred during rapid atrial pacing, causing the first post-pacing cycle length to decrease in value. This explanation of the paradoxic decrease in maximum value of the first post-pacing cycle has also been used to explain the decrease in maximum first post-pacing cycle following administration of cardiac glycosides (Engel et al., 1973; Dhingra et al., 1975).

Disopyramide caused a change in $SACT_{A+R}$ from 195 ± 62 to 171 ± 84 msec which was not significant (Figure 6). The only patient that merits comment is one group A patient with a marked decrease in $SACT_{A+R}$ from 278 msec to 138 msec (Figure 7). This change was associated with a change in A_1A_1 from 926 ± 16 to 1720 ± 102 msec. The decrease in $SACT_{A+R}$ in this one patient is likely to be due to the development of 2:1 sinoatrial exit block and is probably similar to the changes in atrioventricular conduction time that occur following transition from first degree to second degree atrioventricular block.

In summary, five patients demonstrated large increases in maximum value of the first post-pacing cycle following administration of propranolol (n = 2) or disopyramide (n = 3) (Figures 2, 3 and 5). All five patients belonged to group A (demonstrating sinus pauses and/or sinoatrial exit block prior to study). It should also be noted that secondary pauses following termination of rapid atrial pacing (Strauss et al., 1978) were observed under control conditions in all five patients, suggesting that secondary pauses may identify patients who are at high risk for developing prolonged post-pacing cycles and presumably

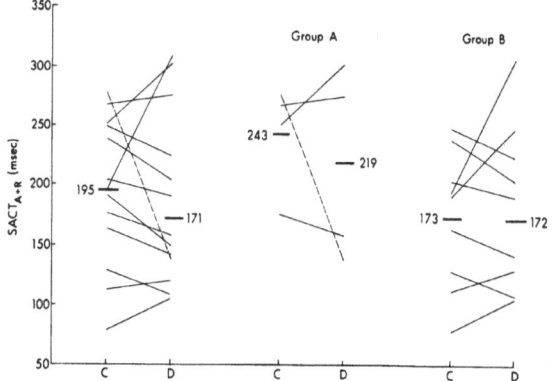

Figure 6. Effect of disopyramide phosphate (2 mg/kg) on SACT$_{A+R}$.
SACT$_{A+R}$ decreased following disopyramide phosphate administration from 195 ± 62 msec to 171 ± 84 msec. Note patient in group A (interrupted line) whose SACT$_{A+R}$ fell from 278 msec to 138. This was associated with a change in mean A$_1$A$_1$ from 926 ± 16 to 1770 ± 102 msec.

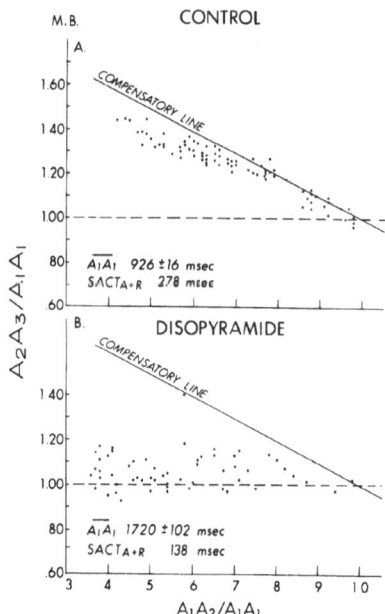

Figure 7. Change in SACT$_{A+R}$ following disopyramide administration in a patient whose mean A$_1$A$_1$ changed from 926 to 1720 msec. This change in mean A$_1$A$_1$ is consistent with the development of 2:1 sinoatrial exit block.

prolonged spontaneous sinus pauses following drug administration. Although a decrease in maximum value of the first post-pacing cycle after disopyramide occurred in one patient, this should not be equated with a beneficial effect of the drug since sinotrial conduction was further depressed. Rather, the decrease points up a limitation of the testing procedure. Also the decrease in value of the maximum first post-pacing cycle does not mean that the bradyarrhythmias occurring during chronic therapy with disopyramide will be less severe.

Although we demonstrated that drugs may increase spontaneous cycle length, $SACT_{A+R}$ or the maximum value of the first post-pacing cycle, the relationship of these acute effects to the effects that the drugs cause during chronic oral administration is unclear, since only a few of these patients received chronically administered propranolol or disopyramide. Preliminary insights into the possible relationship of acute and chronic effects has been provided in a study of Scheinman et al., in which 8 hypertensive patients presented with depression of sinus node function while being treated with antihypertensive agents (guanethidine (1), clonidine (2), alpha-methyldopa (3) and propranolol (2)). Following discontinuation of drug therapy, electrophysiologic studies were performed in four patients and propranolol challenge was performed in three of the four patients. All of the four patients demonstrated secondary pauses following termination of rapid atrial pacing during the control period. Intravenous propranolol administration increased the maximum normalized post-pacing cycle by 11%, 40%, and 300% in the three patients. While no firm conclusions can be drawn it is of interest that secondary pauses following rapid atrial pacing occurred in 4/4 patients tested. In a separate case report (Margolis et al., 1975) a similar association was seen, in which one patient who experienced marked depression of sinus node function during chronic digoxin therapy also had secondary pauses during the control post-pacing period. Our observations on the acute and chronic effects of the different drugs would suggest that the detection of secondary pauses during the post-pacing period under control conditions may identify patients at high risk for adverse drug reactions.

ACKNOWLEDGEMENT

We would like to express our thanks to Laura Cook and Don Kopp for their help in the electrophysiology laboratory during the studies. Our thanks also goes to Don Powell for the art work and to Dave Hugett for the photography. We would also like to express our appreciation to Marilyn McIntosh for typing the manuscript.

REFERENCES

1. Bigger, J.T. Jr., Strauss, H.C.: Digitalis toxicity: Drug interactions promoting toxicity and the management of toxicity. *Sem Drug Treat* 2: 147, 1972
2. Breithardt, G., Seipel, L., Höhfeld, E., Both, A., Loogan, F.: Pharmakologische Beeinflussung der "sinuatrialen Leithungszeit" und der Sinusknotenautomatie beim Menschen. *Z Kardiol* 64: 895, 1975
3. Breithardt, G., Seipel, L.: The influence of drugs on sinoatrial conduction time in man. In Cardiac Pacing. Diagnostic and Therapeutic Tools, edited by Lüderitz, B., Springer-Verlag, Berlin, 1976, p 58
4. Breithardt, G., Seipel, L., Both, A., Loogen, F.: The effect of atropine on sino-atrial conduction time in man. *Eur J Cardiol* 4: 49, 1976a
5. Breithardt, G., Seipel, L., Wiebringhaus, E., Loogan, F.: Effect of verapamil on sinus node in patients with normal and abnormal sinus node function. *Circulation* 54 (Suppl II): II–19, 1976b

6. Chai, C.Y., Wang, H.H., Hoffman, B.F., Wang, S.C.: Mechanisms of bradycardia induced by digitalis substances. *Am J Physiol* 212: 26, 1967
7. Dauchot, P., Gravenstein, J.S.: Effects of atropine on the electrocardiogram in different age groups. *Clin Pharmacol Ther* 12:274, 1971
8. Dhingra, R.C., Amat-Y-Leon, F., Wyndham, C., Wu, D., Denes, P., Rosen, K.M.: The electrophysiological effects of ouabain on sinus node and atrium in man. *J Clin Invest* 56: 555, 1975
9. Dhingra, R.C., Amat-y-Leon, F., Wyndham, C., Denes, P., Wu, D., Pouget, J.M., Rosen, K.M.: Electrophysiologic effects of atropine on human sinus node and atrium. *Am J Cardiol* 38: 429, 1976
10. Dhingra, R.C., Amat-y-Leon, F., Wyndham, C., Denes, P., Wu, D., Miller, R.H., Rosen, K.M.: Electrophysiologic effects of atropine on sinus node and atrium in patients with sinus nodal dysfunction. *Am J Cardiol* 38: 848, 1976a
11. Dighton, D.H.: Sinus bradycardia. Autonomic influences and clinical assessment. *Br Heart J* 36: 791, 1974
12. Dighton, D.H.: Sinoatrial block, autonomic influences and clinical assessment. *Br Heart J* 37: 312, 1975
13. Engel, T.R., Schaal, S.F.: Digitalis in the sick sinus syndrome. The effects of digitalis on sinoatrial automaticity and atrioventricular conduction. *Circulation* 48: 1201, 1973
14. Ferrer, M.I.: The sick sinus syndrome in atrial disease. *JAMA* 206: 645, 1968
15. Ferrer, M.I.: The Sick Sinus Syndrome. Futura, Mount Kisco, New York, 1974
16. Greenwood, R.S., Finkelstein, D.: Sinoatrial Heart Block. Charles C. Thomas, Springfield Illinois, 1964
17. Goodman, D.J., Rossen, R.M., Ingham, R., Rider, A.K., Harrison, D.C.: Sinus node function in the denervated human heart. Effect of digitalis *Br Heart J* 37: 612, 1975
18. Hewlett, A.W.: Digitalis heart block. *JAMA* 48: 47, 1907
19. Jose, A.D., Taylor R.R.: Autonomic blockade by propranolol and atropine to study intrinsic myocardial function in man. *J Clin Invest* 48: 2019, 1969
20. Margolis, J.R., Strauss, H.C., Miller, H.C., Gilbert, M., Wallace, A.G.: Digitalis and the sick sinus syndrome. Clinical and electrophysiologic documentation of a severe toxic effect on sinus node function. *Circulation* 52: 162, 1975
21. McLain, P.L., Kruse, T.K., Redick, T.F.: The effect of atropine on digitoxin bradycardia in cats. *J Pharmacol Exp Ther* 139: 42, 1963
22. Nies, A.S., Shand, D.G.: Clinical pharmacology of propranolol. *Circulation* 52: 6, 1975
23. Reiffel, J.A., Bigger, J.T. Jr., Giardina, E.G.V.: "Paradoxical" prolongation of sinus nodal recovery time after atropine in the sick sinus syndrome. *Am J Cardiol* 36: 98, 1975
24. Schamroth, L.: Immediate effects of intravenous propranolol on various cardiac arrhythmias. *Am J Cardiol* 18: 438, 1966
25. Scheinman, M.M., Strauss, H.C., Evans, G.T., Ryan, C., Massie, B., Wallace, A.G.: Adverse effects of sympatholytic agents in patients with hypertension and sinus node dysfunction. (*Am J Med*, in press)
26. Seides, S.F., Josephson, M.E., Batsford, W.P., Weisfogel, G.M., Lau, S.H., Damato, A.N.: The electrophysiology of propranolol in man. *Am Heart J* 88: 733, 1974
27. Short, D.S.: The syndrome of alternating bradycardia and tachycardia. *Br Heart J* 16: 208, 1954
28. Smith, T.W., Willerson, J.T.: Suicidal and accidental digoxin ingestion. Report of five cases with serum digoxin level correlations. *Circulation* 44: 29, 1971
29. Smith, T.W., Haber, E.: Digitalis (First of four parts). *N Engl J Med* 289: 945, 1973
30. Smith, T.W., Haber, E.: Digitalis (Second of four parts). *N Engl J Med* 289: 1010, 1973a
31. Steinbeck, G., Lüderitz, B.: Störungen der Sinusknotenfunktion. Diagnostik und klinische Bedeutung. *Dtsch Med Wochenschr* 102: 35, 1977
32. Stern, S., Elnsenberg, S.: The effect of propranolol (inderal) on the electrocardiogram of normal subjects. *Am Heart J* 77: 192, 1969
33. Strauss, H.C., Gilbert, M., Svenson, R.H., Miller, H.C., Wallace, A.G.: Electrophysiologic effects of propranolol on sinus node function in patients with sinus node dysfunction. *Circulation* 54: 452, 1976
34. Strauss, H.C., Scheinman, M.M., Evans, G.T., Bashore, T., Wallace, A.G.: Electrophysiologic effects of disopyramide in patients with sinus node dysfunction. *Circulation* 54 (Suppl. II): II–17, 1976a
35. Strauss, H.C., Scheinman, M.M., LaBarre, A., Browning, D.J., Benditt, D.G., Wallace, A.G.: Programed atrial stimulation and rapid atrial pacing in patients with sinus pauses and sinoatrial exit block, in this book, 1978
36. Wellens, H.J., Cats, V.M., Düren, D.R.: Symptomatic sinus node abnormalities following lithium carbonate therapy. *Am J Med* 59: 285, 1975

10

EFFECT OF PROPRANOLOL ON NORMAL AND ABNORMAL SINUS NODE FUNCTION

ONKAR S. NARULA, MIGUEL VASQUEZ, NARASIMHAN SHANTHA
REUBEN CHUQUIMIA, WILLIAM D. TOWNE, AND JOSEPH W. LINHART

INTRODUCTION

During the last decade, propranolol has been used clinically in the management of patients with arrhythmias, angina pectoris and hypertension (1–8). However, in man little data are available pertaining to the electrophysiological effects of propranolol on the normal sinus node function. In most of the previous studies the effect of propranolol has been analyzed regarding only one parameter of sinus node function, i.e. the changes in spontaneous cycle length or rate. Despite isolated reports in man, published data on the effects of propranolol on other parameters of sinus node function are limited (9–15). In view of its extensive clinical use in patients with various types of arrhythmias, especially supraventricular tachycardias (SVT), i.e. atrial fibrillation, atrial flutter, or atrial tachycardia, which inherently produce overdrive suppression of the sinus node, it is of clinical importance to learn the effects of propranolol on various parameters of sinus node function, both in patients with normal and abnormal sinus node function. The purpose of this paper is to present our data on the effects of intravenous propranolol on 3 parameters of sinus node function: 1) spontaneous cycle length, 2) sinoatrial conduction time and 3) sinus node recovery time.

METHODS AND MATERIALS

The electrophysiological effect of propranolol on sinus node function was analyzed in thirty patients. In twenty patients sinus node function was considered to be normal on the basis of electrocardiographic and clinical evidence. In addition, none of these twenty patients exhibited sinus bradycardia or any evidence of sinus node dysfunction during electrophysiological studies. The other ten patients were symptomatic with dizziness or syncope and were suspected of having sinus node dysfunction. These patients either showed consistent sinus bradycardia or exhibited spontaneous periods of sinoatrial (SA) block or SA arrest.

All patients were studied in the post absorptive state after premedication with 100 mg Nembutal administered intramuscularly, one half hour prior to study. A bipolar electrode catheter was placed in the His bundle region as described previously (16). A second quadripolar pacing catheter, with electrodes 10 mm apart was also introduced into the right atrium and positioned so that the proximal electrode pair was located in the region of the sinus node for recording of the high right atrial electrogram and the distal pair was used for atrial stimulation. Atrial stimulation studies were performed at double the diastolic threshold with stimuli 2 msec in duration. Multiple ECG leads representing the three planes of the ECG were recorded simultaneous with the intracardiac recordings. After catheter placement, for purposes of control, observations of the spontaneous sinus rhythm were made for a period of 10 minutes. During the last minute of the control period, ten consecutive spontaneous cycles were measured to calculate the mean sinus cycle length (mean A_1A_1). Sinoatrial conduction time (SACT) was measured by the method of Strauss et al. (17). Following this, spontaneous sinus rhythm was observed for another period of two minutes prior to analysis of sinus node recovery time (SNRT).* SNRT was measured by atrial pacing (AP) at two different cycle lengths (500 and 430 msec, sometimes 370 and 330 msec were used) for a period of two minutes at each level (18). A rest period of 2–3 minutes was provided between each pacing period to permit sinus rhythm to return to control levels.

After control determinations were completed, propranolol was administered intravenously in dosage of 0.1 mg/kg body weight over a period of 5–7 min. Ten minutes after the infusion of the last drop of propranolol, the studies were repeated to measure SACT and SNRT. Following propranolol some of the patients who were suspected to have sinus node dysfunction were given an intravenous bolus of 2.5 mg of Atropine. The studies for the measurement of SACT and SNRT were again repeated.

The estimated SACT was calculated by the most recently described method of Strauss et al., based on a mean of A_2A_3 intervals falling in the latter portion of zone 2 (reset zone). SACT $= A_2A_3-A_1A_1$. The value thus obtained represents the total of conduction time into and out of the sinus node (19). Sinus node recovery time was measured as described previously (Narula et al., 1972). The longest interval after a period of atrial pacing was taken as sinus node recovery time. It does not matter whether this is the first interval after the pacing period or one of the subsequent intervals. The corrected SNRT (CSNRT) was obtained by deducting the mean of 10 consecutive spontaneous sinus cycles recorded immediately preceding each atrial pacing cycle length.

RESULTS

Results are discussed separately for those patients with normal sinus node function and those suspected to have sinus node dysfunction.

1. PATIENTS WITH NORMAL SINUS NODE FUNCTION

In these patients, the spontaneous cycle length ranged from 680–955 msec. Following propranolol a statistically significant (P < 0.005) increase of 12% in mean cycle length (range 705–1020 msec) was noted which increased from 776 msec to 853 msec (Figure 1). The SACT changed in a random fashion after propranolol. Although the mean SACT for the entire group lengthened slightly with propranolol from 167 to 185 msec, this increase was not statistically significant (Figure 1).

With atrial pacing at a cycle length of 500 msec, the mean CSNRT lengthened slightly with propranolol from a control of 258 ± 120 msec to 287 ± 124 msec (Figure 1). The CSNRT with propranolol was unchanged in two, prolonged in twelve, and shortened in six patients. Similarly with atrial pacing at a cycle length of 430 msec the mean CSNRT lengthened slightly after propranolol from a control of 216 ± 114 msec to 236 ± 116 msec (Figure 1). In both cases of atrial pacing the slight increase in mean CSNRT was not statistically significant. Following propranolol fifty percent of the patients (10 out of 20) showed a shortening in CSNRT at either of the atrial pacing cycle lengths. Although during

---

*The author introduced in 1972 the abbreviation SRT for sinus node recovery time; the editor has chosen SNRT for reasons of uniformity of the different chapters.

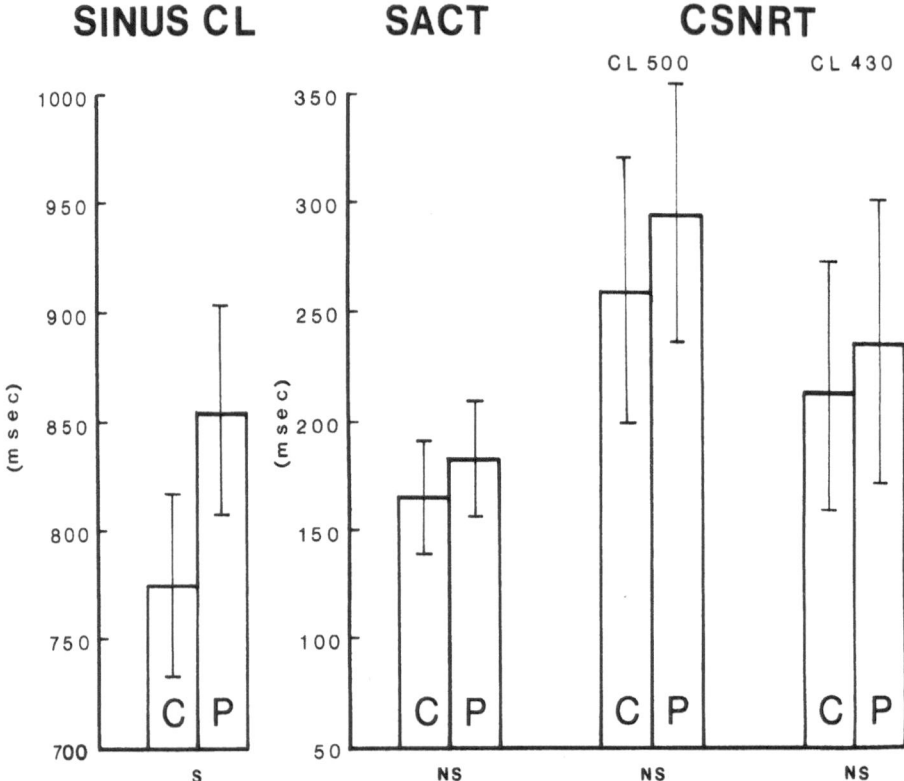

Figure 1. In patients with normal sinus node function the effect of propranolol is shown on cycle length (CL), sinoatrial conduction time (SACT) and corrected sinus node recovery time (CSNRT) at two atrial pacing CLs of 500 and 430 msec. The mean values during control (C) and following propranolol (P) are depicted by vertical bars and also show the standard deviation. S = statistically significant, NS = statistically nonsignificant.

control most of these patients had exhibited a shortening in CSNRT at high atrial pacing rates, after propranolol a shortened CSNRT was seen at a comparably slower atrial pacing rate. This shortening in CSNRT following propranolol was probably due to an enhancement or occurrence of entrance block into the sinus node at a comparable slower atrial pacing interval. An analysis of data on the longest or the maximum CSNRT observed, at either of the atrial pacing intervals, showed an average increase of 7% following propranolol (from 290 to 310 msec).

2. PATIENTS SUSPECTED OF SINUS NODE DYSFUNCTION

In these ten patients control electrophysiological studies showed that in five despite a consistent sinus bradycardia the sinus node function was normal. In the other five patients both the SACT and CSNRT were prolonged during control. In these 10 patients during control the spontaneous cycle length ranged from 800 to 1235 msec. Following propranolol the cycle length remained unchanged in two, and lengthened in 8 patients. Patients with normal and abnormal electrophysiological studies of sinus node function could not be

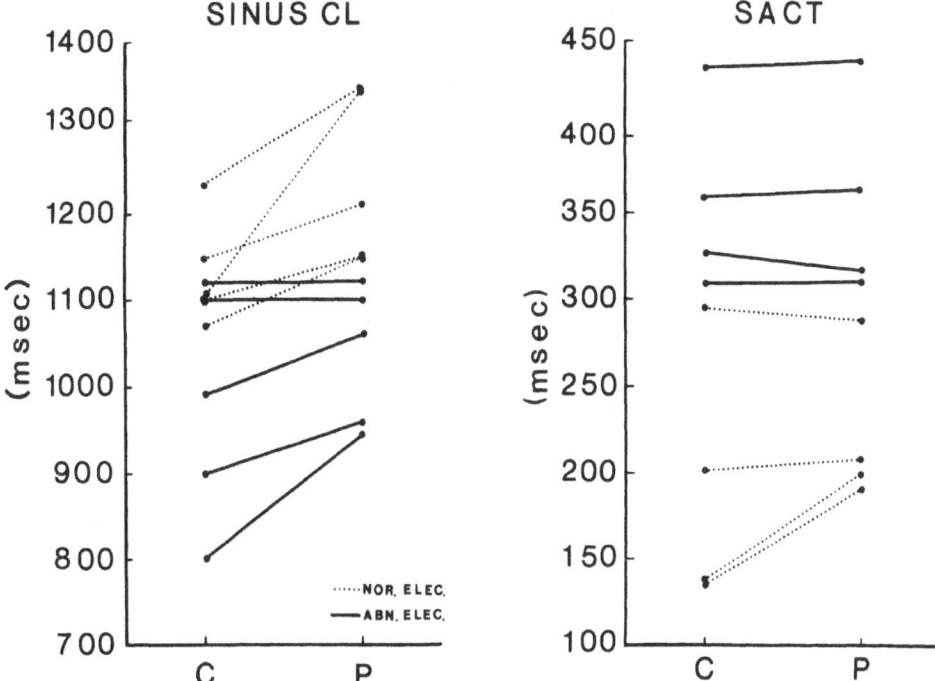

Figure 2. The effect of propranolol on cycle length and SACT is shown in 10 patients suspected to have sinus node dysfunction. Left panel shows changes in cycle length (CL) and the right panel shows changes in SACT. Patients with sinus bradycardia and a normal sinus node function based on electrophysiological studies are depicted by the dotted lines. Patients with sinus node dysfunction based on electrophysiological studies are depicted by a solid line. In one patient, the SACT could not be defined either during control of following propranolol.

differentiated on the basis of changes in cycle length with propranolol (Figure 2). In 9 of the ten patients the SACT was not altered significantly with propranolol (Figure 2). In the tenth patient the SACT could not be calculated as zone 2 responses could not be defined either during control or following propranolol.

In the five patients with sinus bradycardia and a normal sinus node function during control electrophysiological studies the CSNRT lengthened slightly at atrial pacing with 500 msec interval and was essentially unchanged after atrial pacing with 430 msec interval (Figure 3). In these five patients the CSNRT remained normal (< 525 msec) during control, with propranolol, and with atropine which was administered following propranolol. A typical response is illustrated in Figures 4, 5 and 6. In this patient the longest CSNRT during control (Figure 4, panel D) and with propranolol (Figure 5, panel C) was 220 and 140 msec, respectively. With atropine the spontaneous cycle length was shortened from 1220 to 900 msec and the longest CSNRT was 460 msec (Figure 6). Although the CSNRT after atropine was longer than that during control or with propranolol, it was still within the normal range (Figure 6).

The other five patients with abnormal sinus node function during control electrophysiological studies, exhibited a pronounced prolongation of CSNRT following propranolol (Figure 3). A marked prolongation of CSNRT with propranolol is illustrated by

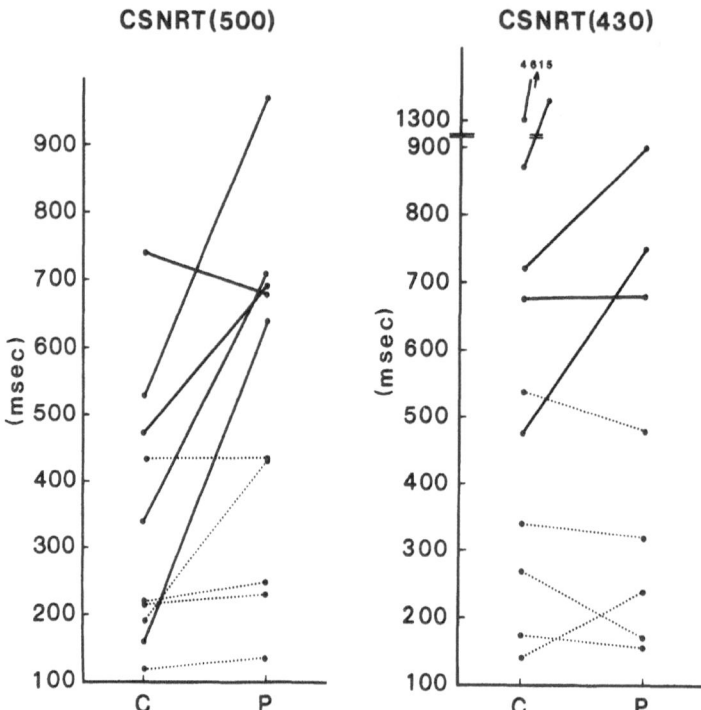

Figure 3. Shows the effect of propranolol on CSNRT at two different atrial pacing cycle lengths in 10 patients with sinus bradycardia who were suspected to have sinus node dysfunction. Similar to Figure 2, the dotted lines represent patients with sinus bradycardia but with normal function and the solid lines represent patients with sinus bradycardia and sinus node dysfunction. In one of the patients the CSNRT after propranolol at a CL of 430 msec was markedly prolonged to 4615 msec. This prolongation could not be depicted on the scale in the right hand panel and therefore, is indicated by an arrow next to the solid bar representing this patient.

recordings in a patient who during control showed a mean cycle length of 800 msec and occasional periods of 2:1 SA block (Figures 7 and 8). In this patient the prolongation of CSNRT was directly related to the rate of atrial pacing both during control and following propranolol. However, such a direct relationship between the atrial pacing rate and the prolongation of CSNRT could not always be correlated in each patient. This is illustrated by recordings in another patient with sinus bradycardia (Figure 9 and 10). In this patient the mean control spontaneous cycle length was 1100 msec. During control this patient exhibited a direct relationship between the duration of CSNRT and atrial pacing rate. The CSNRT increased from 465 to 2375 msec with a shortening in atrial pacing interval from 500 to 375 msec (Figure 9). After propranolol the CSNRT showed a prolongation at atrial pacing intervals of 500 and 440 msec. However, at faster atrial pacing rate (interval 375 msec) the CSNRT was markedly shorter as compared to the control (825 vs. 2375 msec) (Figure 10). The observations in this patient suggest that propranolol enhanced entrance block into the sinus node and prevented rapid atrial impulses from penetrating the sinus node. This resulted in a comparatively shorter CSNRT following propranolol despite an atrial pacing rate similar to the control as lesser number of impulses

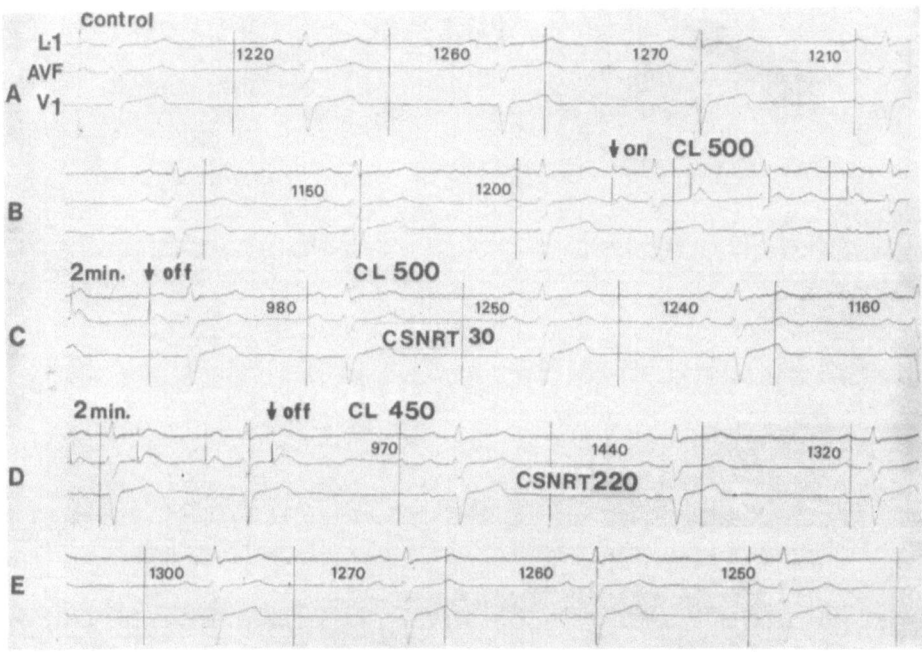

Figure 4. Recordings of CSNRT during control in a symptomatic patient with sinus bradycardia suspected to have sinus node dysfunction.

A: During control, spontaneous cycle length varied between 1210 and 1270 msec.

B and C: Show the onset and termination of atrial pacing (CL = 500 msec) after two minutes and the CSNRT is 30 msec.

D and E: Shows that after atrial pacing at a CL of 450 msec the CSNRT is 220 msec. Panels D and E show continuous recordings. All the numbers depicted in this figure and subsequent figures represent measurements in milliseconds, whereas the time lines are at 1 second intervals.

reached the sinus node. In these five patients with sinus node dysfunction the CSNRT with several atrial pacing rates both during control and following propranolol is detailed in Figure 11. This figure shows that in three patients, at comparable atrial pacing rates, the CSNRT was shortened following propranolol.

DISCUSSION

The mechanism of overdrive suppression of the sinus node is probably based on the release of acetylcholine and perhaps on accumulation of potassium outside the cell (20–22). Electrical stimulation of the heart releases acetyl-choline and catecholamines from storage sites or nerve terminals. However, overdrive suppression is not solely dependent upon the release of acetylcholine as it may be noted even after parasympathetic blockade with atropine (18, 22, 23). Similarly infusion of norepinephrine reduces but does not abolish overdrive suppression (21). These findings are further supported by electrophysiological studies in man with denervated hearts, after cardiac transplantation (23). Overdrive suppression of the sinus node was also demonstrated in these hearts and

PROPRANOLOL

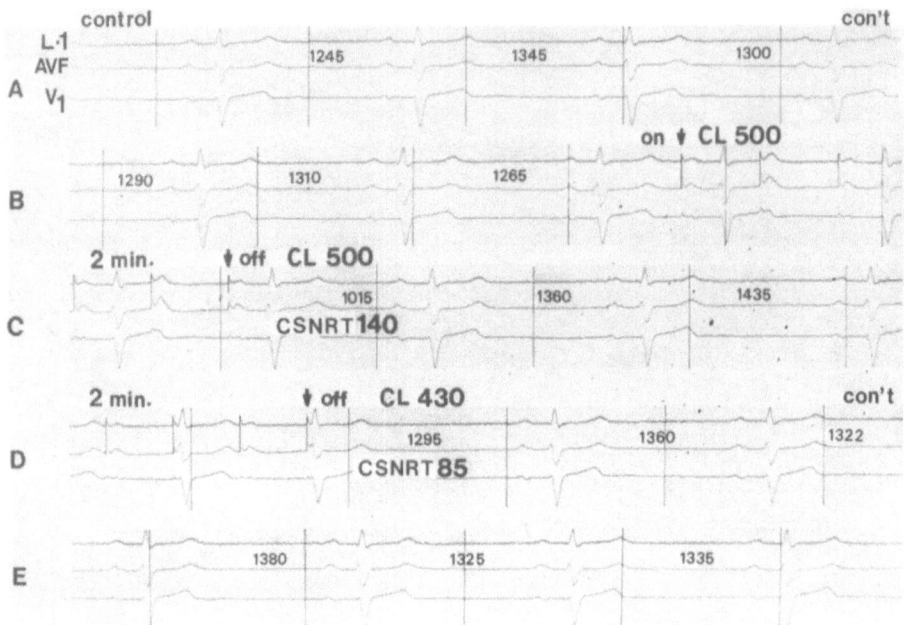

Figure 5. Shows the effect of propranolol on SNRT in the same patient as in Figure 4.

A: Shows that the sinus cycle length is slightly prolonged as compared to the control (Figure 4, panel A).

B and C: Show a CSNRT of 140 msec with propranolol after atrial pacing with a CL of 500 msec.

D and E: Show a CSNRT of 85 msec following atrial pacing at a CL of 430 msec. The CSNRT is essentially unchanged with propranolol as compared to that of control (Figure 4).

the range of CSNRT was similar to that reported in normal cases with intact cardiac innervation (23).

Previous experimental studies have demonstrated that changes in autonomic influences effect the response to overdrive suppression to a significant degree. The post drive suppression is augmented or greatly prolonged a) by stimulation of the vagi, b) by sectioning of the sympathetic cardiac accelerator nerves with removal of the thoracic ganglia and c) after pretreatment with guanethidine or reserpine (21). Atrial pacing during control results in a release of both the acetylcholine and the catecholamines. The administration of propranolol, by blocking the neutralizing effect of the released catecholamines results in an unopposed effect of acetylcholine on the SN and hence a comparatively greater degree of overdrive suppression or prolongation of SNRT.

Studies in isolated cardiac tissues have shown that propranolol results in a change of various parameters of action potential, i.e. a decrease of membrane responsiveness, a lowering of the overshoot and of the maximal velocity of the upstroke, and a slowing of spontaneous phase four depolarization and conduction velocity (24–27). Propranolol in the concentrations used clinically has little direct effect and only the levo or racemic propranolol can block the changes in the action potential induced by epinephrine (Howitt et al., 1968). The results of the present study may be explained on the basis of changes in the action potential described above.

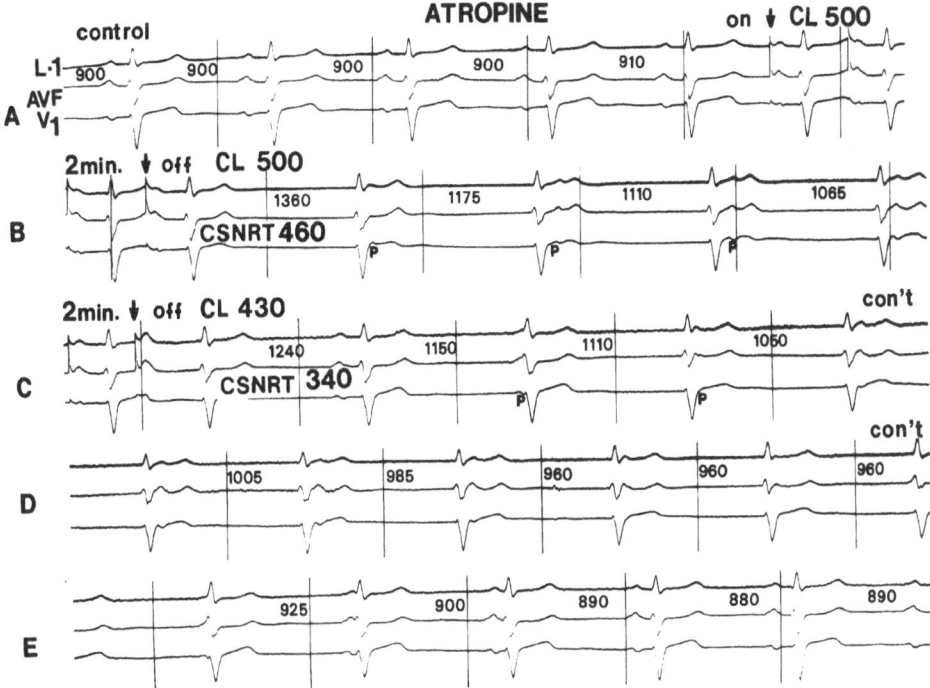

Figure 6. Shows measurements of CSNRT after atropine in the same patient as in Figures 4 and 5. In this patient 2.5 mg of atropine was administered intravenously immediately following measurements with propranolol.

A: Sinus cycle length is shortened significantly.

B: Shows the CSNRT (460 msec) after atrial pacing at a CL of 500 msec.

C – E: Shows the CSNRT (340 msec) after atrial pacing at a CL of 430 msec.

On cessation of atrial pacing the first escape beat originates from the sinus node. However, subsequent beats show an iso-rhythmic dissociation between the sinus P waves and the junctional QRS complexes, until the ventricles are completely captured by the sinus P waves (panel E). Panel C to E show continuous recordings.

The dosage of propranolol used in this study is similar to that used by others during electrophysiological studies in man (12, 13). With this dosage regimen mean serum levels of 13.6 ng/ml have been reported 45 to 60 minutes after propranolol administration and it has been demonstrated that this will have a significant β-adrenergic blocking effect (12). Our studies were generally completed in ≦30 minutes after the last dose of propranolol. In addition, this dosage regimen was selected to ward off unnecessary side effects or complications, i.e. hypotension which in turn may artificially alter the sympathetic or parasympathetic influences and thereby confuse interpretation of the results. In clinical practice, propranolol is generally not used in intravenous doses larger than that utilized in the present study. Therefore, it is believed that the results obtained from our studies should be applicable during clinical management of patients with arrhythmias.

Our data in patients with normal sinus node function show that with propranolol the sinus cycle length increased by an average of 12%. This is slightly less than that reported previously by others (15% and 22%) (12, 29). This difference may be explained by the fact that our patients were premedicated by Nembutal whereas others obtained their data in nonsedated patients, possibly with higher levels of released catecholamines. Although

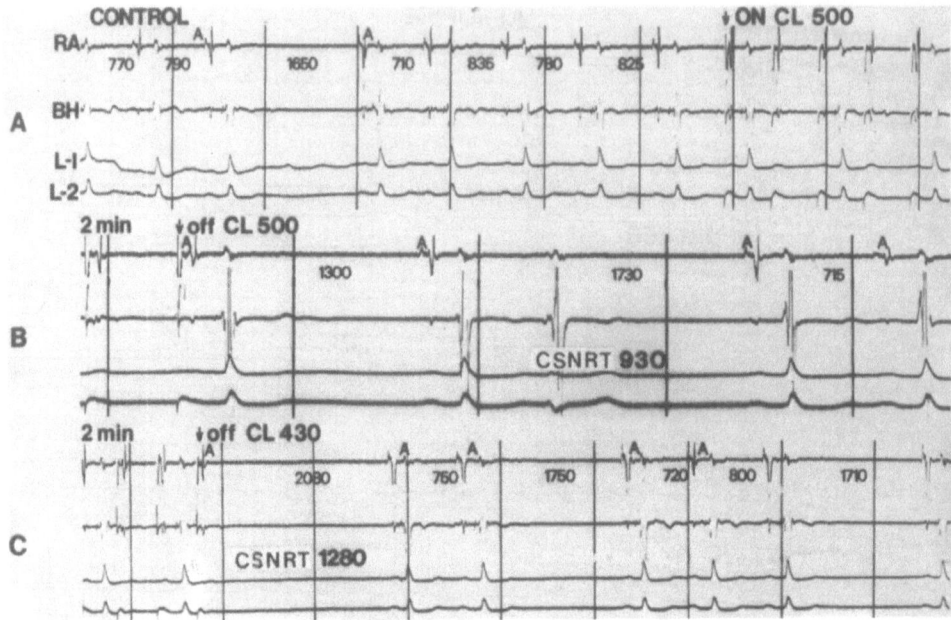

Figure 7. Shows control measurements of CSNRT after atrial pacing at CLs of 500 and 430 msec in a patient with sinus node dysfunction and 2:1 SA block. On cessation of atrial pacing at CL of 430 msec the frequency of 2:1 SA block was markedly increased as is shown in panel C.

there was a slight increase in the mean SACT, in the patients with normal sinus node function, it was not statistically significant. It is difficult to properly evaluate the effect of propranolol on SACT due to limitations inherent in the present technique for estimation of SACT. The problems with the technique for measurement of SACT have been reviewed recently (Narula, 1975: Strauss and Wallace, 1976).

Our data show that in patients with normal heart rate and normal sinus node function the CSNRT slightly lengthened with propranolol, this lengthening was neither statistically nor clinically significant. Our data in symptomatic patients with sinus bradycardia, who were suspected to have sinus node dysfunction, is of special clinical interest. Those patients who had a normal sinus node function, based on electrophysiological studies, despite a sinus bradycardia exhibited a response similar to those with normal heart rates and normal sinus node function. In these patients with propranolol the CSNRT was prolonged only slightly. None exhibited an exacerbation of sinus bradycardia when the sinus rate was decreased by an average of 5 beats/minute. These patients usually exhibited A-V conduction abnormalities or bundle branch block patterns with a prolonged H-V interval. This might be the explanation of their symptoms of dizziness and syncope.

The patients with sinus bradycardia and sinus node dysfunction, documented during electrophysiological studies, exhibited a pronounced prolongation of CSNRT following propranolol. The patients with sinus bradycardia and a normal or abnormal prolongation of CSNRT with propranolol could not be differentiated on the basis of changes in the spontaneous cycle length. These studies suggest that it may be possible to clinically differentiate patients in whom sinus node function with propranolol may not be further

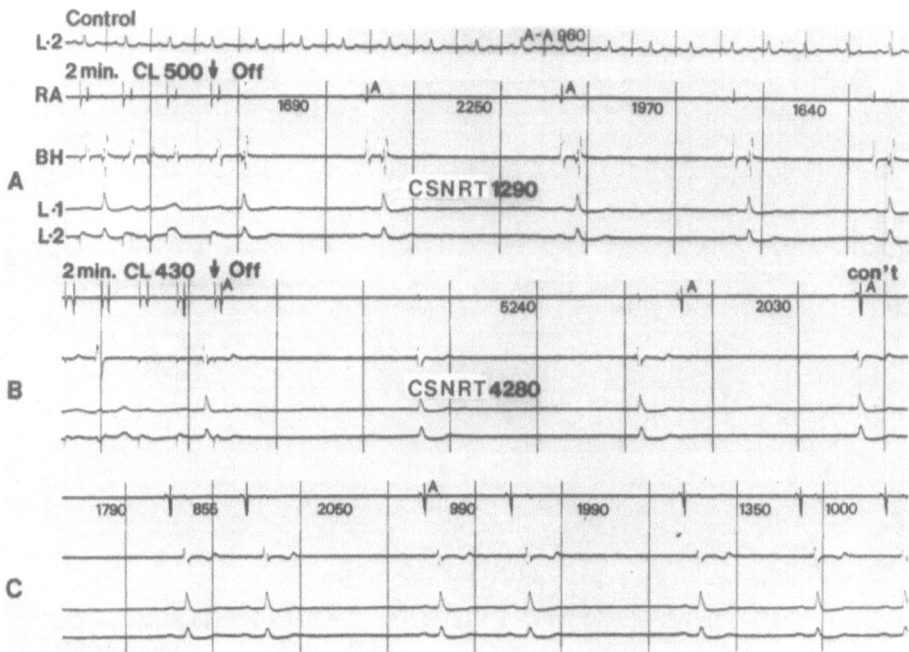

Figure 8. Shows the effect of propranolol in the same patient as shown in Figure 7. On top the control rhythm strip (L-2) shows a slight lengthening of mean spontaneous cycle length from 800 to 960 msec with propranolol

A: Shows a CSNRT of 1290 msec after atrial pacing at a CL of 500 msec.

B and C: Show a CSNRT of 4280 msec after atrial pacing at a CL of 430 msec. On cessation of the pacing the frequency of 2:1 SA block in increased. The recordings in panels B and C are continuous.

adversely affected as opposed to those in whom it may deteriorate significantly. Such a differentiation may permit preselection of patients being considered for therapy with propranolol in whom it may be administered safely, with caution, or may be contraindicated without the support of an artificial pacemaker to prevent serious sinus bradycardia or periods of asystole.

These conclusions are also supported by a critical review of the data reported by others which shows that in patients with clinically diagnosed sinus node dysfunction but with a normal result of an electrophysiological study, the response to overdrive suppression after propranolol was not pronounced (Strauss et al., 1976). They also could not differentiate between patients with sinus node dysfunction and those with normal sinus node function, on the basis of response to propranolol (13). However, a critical review of their data suggests that such a conclusion may not be valid. The ten patients included in their study were ascribed to have "symptomatic sinus node dysfunction." The criteria utilized for determining sinus node dysfunction and how the latter was correlated with the patient's symptoms were not described. Only five of the ten patients had either symptoms of syncope or dizziness. In the other five patients the symptoms of fatigue, dyspnea or palpitations were attributed to sinus node dysfunction. Two patients exhibited a hypersensitive

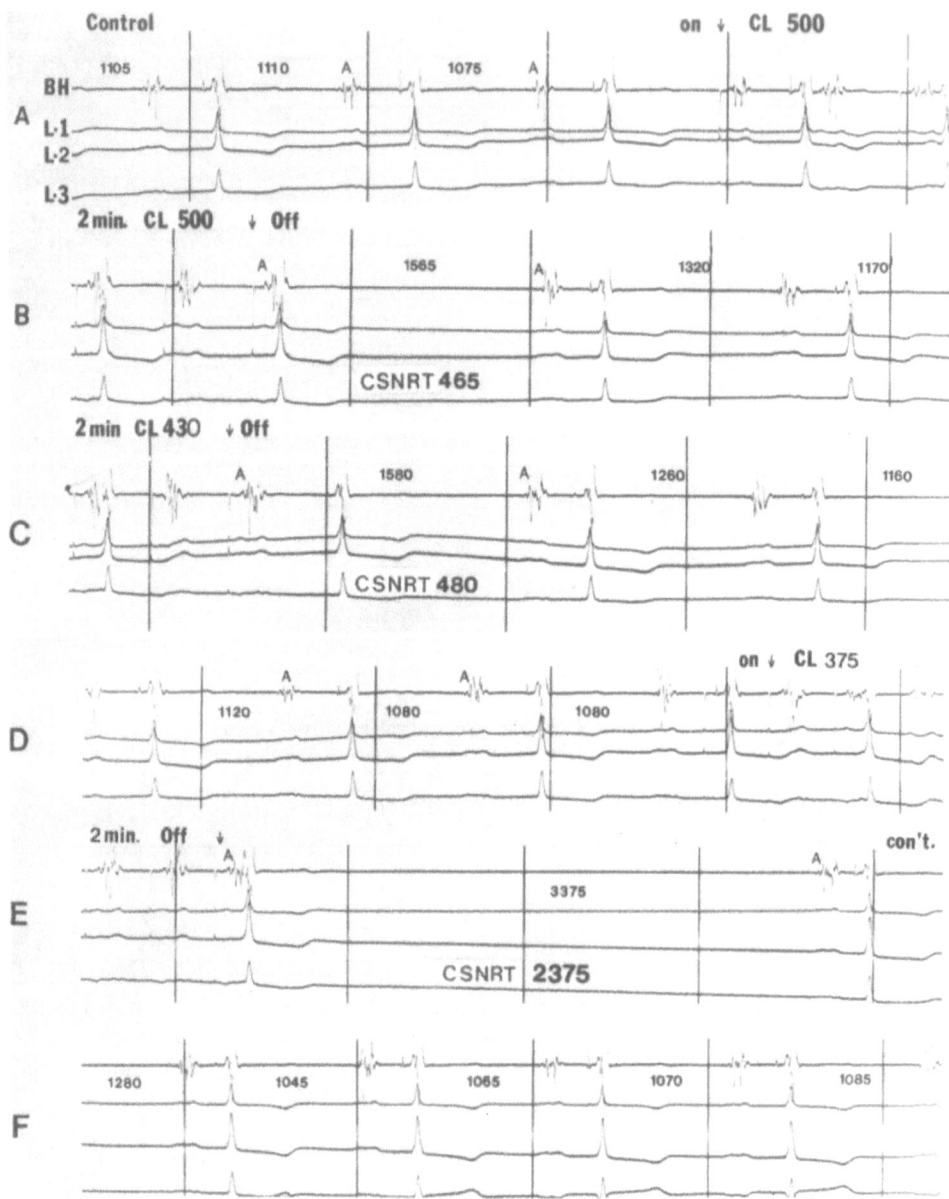

Figure 9. Shows control measurements of CSNRT in a patient with sinus node dysfunction. CSNRT ranges between 465 msec to 2375 msec after atrial pacing at CLs of 500 and 375 msec.

carotid sinus reflex. In their series at the time of study heart rates were ≧56 beats/ minute in all except two patients. It appears that a heart rate of 60 beats/min was used for defining sinus bradycardia. However, others have defined sinus bradycardia as heart rates less than 50 or 55 beats/minute. During control, the CSNRT was abnormal in

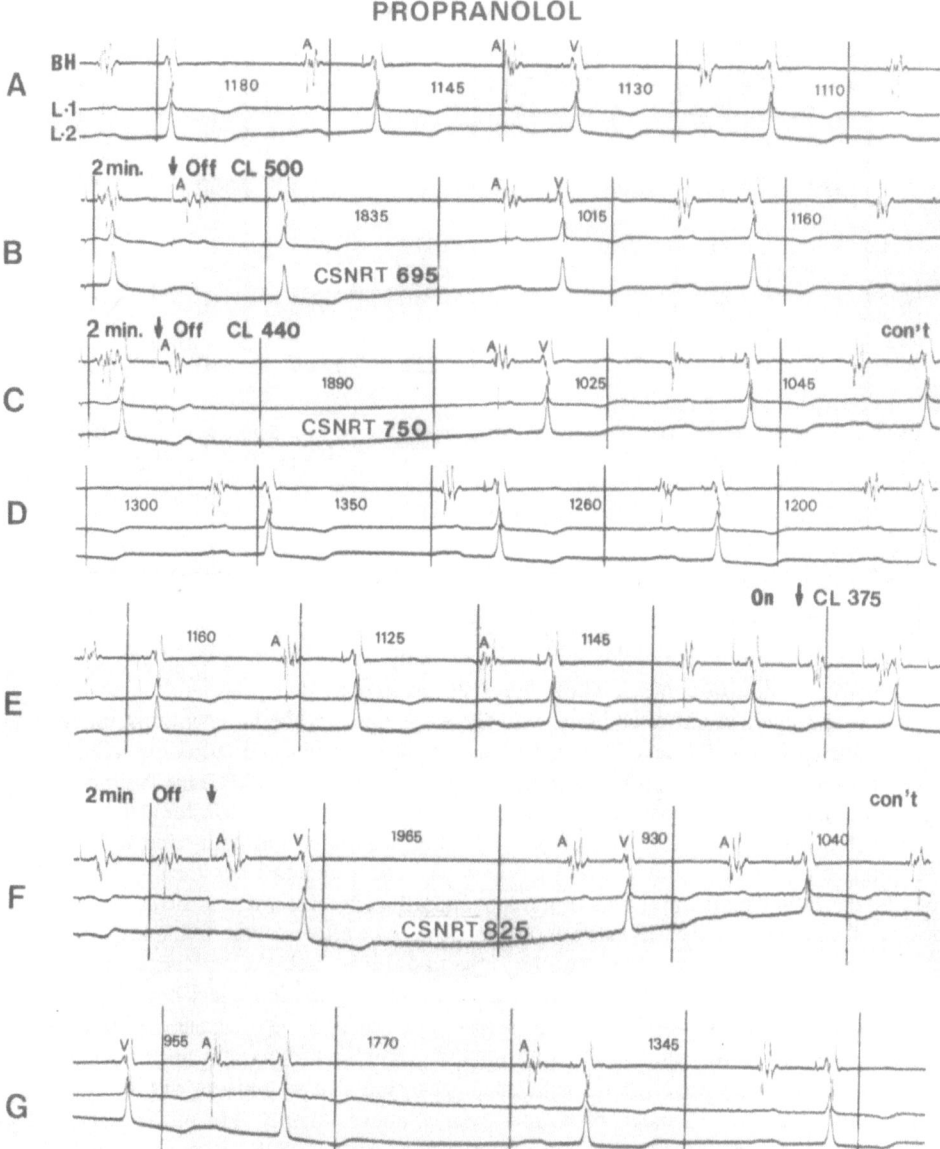

Figure 10. Shows the effect of propranolol on the CSNRT in the same patient as shown in Figure 9. The mean sinus cycle length is only slightly prolonged with propranolol as compared to the control (Figure 9, panel A). The CSNRT ranges between 695 to 825 msec with atrial pacing CLs between 500 and 375 msec.

only two of the ten patients and both exhibited a severe prolongation of CSNRT following propranolol. In five other patients, the CSNRT changed to ≦58 msec with propranolol. This suggests that the results of the latter study or not discordant with those of ours. It is obvious from both of these studies that a marked prolongation of CSNRT

Effect of Propranolol on CSNRT

No.	CL 500		CL 430		CL 370		CL 330	
	C	P	C	P	C	P	C	P
1	160	640	720	900	1600	2340	4500	4900
2	530	966	1300	4615	900	2712	1860	9155
3	475	690	475	750	2375	+855	520	490
4	740	680	675	680	690	820	1780	+740
5	340	710	870	1340	1310	+1140	390	340

Figure 11. Tabulates CSNRT at various atrial pacing cycle lengths both during control and following propranolol in 5 patients with sinus node dysfunction documented with electrophysiological studies.

with propranolol was noted only in those patients who exhibited an abnormal CSNRT even during control.

In our study 50% of the patients with normal sinus node function exhibited a shortening of CSNRT following propranolol. This was generally noted at slower atrial pacing rates as compared to that of control. These observations suggest that propranolol may result in an enhancement of entrance block into the sinus node. If the latter interpretation is correct, then it is possible that patients with sick sinus syndrome and a prolonged CSNRT may be protected from overdrive suppression following propranolol. This is supported by the observations in a patient with sinus node dysfunction who, at faster atrial pacing rates, exhibited a shortening in CSNRT following propranolol as compared to control measurements. Although in this patient at lower atrial pacing rates the CSNRT was lengthened following propranolol (Figures 9 and 10). Therefore, it is possible that sinus node dysfunction in such cases may not be unmasked even after propranolol, due to further enhancement of entrance block into the sinus node. If in fact, the patients included in the series by Strauss et al. (1976), did have a sinus node dysfunction, a lack of marked prolongation of CSNRT in most of their patients may be explained on this basis, i.e. enhanced entrance block into the sinus node and thus the protection of the sinus node from overdrive suppression. However, these data do suggest that a) if in patients with sinus node dysfunction, a protective mechanism does exist, it does not apply to all of the cases with sich sinus node as is illustrated by a marked prolongation of CSNRT with propranolol in a patient with documented SA block during control (Figures 7 and 8); b) depending upon the response to propranolol it may be possible to differentiate the various underlying mechanisms or the dominant mechanism responsible for sick sinus syndrome, i.e. abnormalities of sinoatrial conduction and of the generator function of the sinus node.

In isolated tissues, it was demonstrated that in order to produce lower sinus rates or asystole, it was necessary to affect all sinus node pacemaker fibers by acetylcholine, whereas only a few pacemaker fibres need be accelerated by norepinephrine to produce an increment in the heart rate (32). Therefore, it may be reasoned that in patients with a sick sinus node, only a few pacemaker fibers may be functioning under the influence of available catecholamines which are sufficient enough to sustain sinus rhythm. In such patients, a withdrawal of catecholamine influences and β-adrenergic blockade with propranolol may not only result in slower rate but also show a pronounced suppression to overdrive pacing or a marked prolongation of SNRT. It is suggested that the duration of SNRT or the response to overdrive suppression is dependent upon: 1) the amount of acetylcholine during basal levels and that resulting from overdrive pacing; 2) the degree to which pacemaker fibers in a diseased sinus node are dependent upon available catecholamines to sustain a stable sinus rhythm; and 3) the capability of the atrial paced beats to enter the sinus node and thereby produce its suppression. It may be argued that patients with sinus node dysfunction, who exhibit a lesser degree of suppression to overdrive pacing after propranolol have a relatively greater number of functional pacemaker fibers which are also dependent to a lesser degree on the release of catecholamines to sustain a stable sinus rhythm. However, studies in additional patients with sinus node dysfunction are required to further elucidate this hypothesis.

During our studies it was noted that with propranolol in some patients with sinus node dysfunction, although the CSNRT lengthened at slower atrial pacing rates, it was shortened at faster atrial pacing rates as compared to the control CSNRT. In another patient with sinus node dysfunction, the CSNRT during control was minimally prolonged (685 msec) and was essentially unchanged with propranolol (Figure 12, panels A and B). As atropine was administered immediately after propranolol, the CSNRT was markedly lengthened to 2445 msec (Figure 12, panel C). Based on the observations in this patient, it is suggested that in patients suspected to have sinus node dysfunction, during electrophysiological studies both propranolol and atropine should be administered either simultaneously or one after the other. Such a procedure would permit abolition of sinus node entrance block and/or a reduction in sino-atrial conduction time and thus enable the effect of overdrive suppression to become fully manifested following propranolol. If propranolol alone is administered, it may lead to an increase in SN entrance block and thereby protection of SN from overdrive suppression. On the other hand if atropine alone is administered, although sinoatrial conduction is enhanced, the effect of normal or increased amounts of circulating catecholamines cannot be negated and may thus prevent overdrive suppression of an abnormal sinus node. The advantage of the combined administration of propranolol and atropine, in patients during electrophysiological evaluation of sinus node function, is obvious from this reasoning.

In summary, our results show that intravenous propranolol in the dosages commonly used in clinical practice has little effect on the response to overdrive suppression in patients with normal sinus node function. However, the sinus cycle is lengthened with propranolol both in normal and in abnormal patients on the average of 12 to 16%. Although the number of patients analyzed in this study is small, it does suggest that in symptomatic patients with sinus bradycardia or those suspected to have sinus node dysfunction, following propranolol: a) the SACT is not appreciably lengthened; b) despite sinus bradycardia the SNRT is not significantly prolonged in those with normal sinus node function during electrophysiological testing; c) in patients with electrophysiologically documented ab-

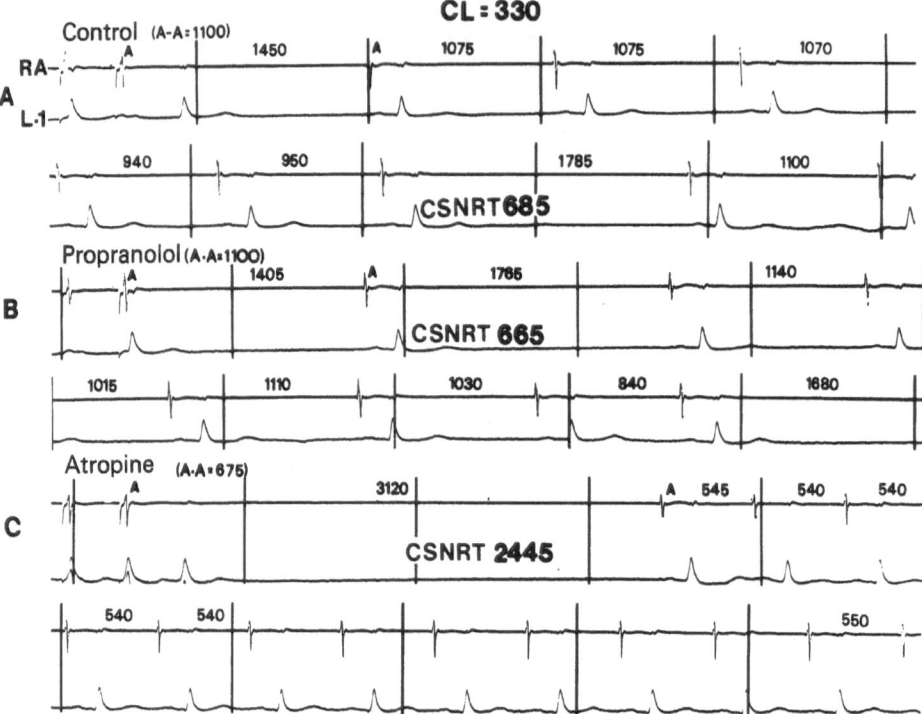

Figure 12. Shows measurements of CSNRT (atrial pacing with 330 msec interval) in a patient with sinus node dysfunction during control, with propranolol and following atropine. Atropine was administered immediately after measurements with propranolol were obtained. Shows simultaneous recordings of RA and LI. Each panel consists of two rows of continuous recordings.

normal sinus node function, the SNRT is significantly prolonged. Propranolol appears to enhance sinus node entrance block and this affect appears to be negated by atropine. Our data suggest that propranolol may be administered safely in patients with normal sinus node function without the fear of producing a severe sinus bradycardia, SA block, SA pauses and a prolonged period of sinus asystole during spontaneous or stimulation induced conversion of an arrhythmia. These data indirectly also suggest that patients exhibiting marked sinus bradycardia or asystole following conversion of a supraventricular arrhythmia with propranolol administration probably have an underlying sinus node dysfunction. Such patients should not be neglected and in these patients sinus node function should be further investigated in the absence of propranolol.

ACKNOWLEDGEMENTS

The authors are extremely indebted to Mrs. Jackie Porter for her superb secreterial assistance in the preparation of this manuscript. We also express our thanks to Ms. Erna Braun, Mr. Jack deBruin and the Photography Section of the Chicago Medical School for the preparation of illustrations.

REFERENCES

1. Bath, J.C.L.: Treatment of cardiac arrhythmias in unanesthetized patients. Role of adrenergic beta-receptor blockade. *Am J Cardiol* 18: 415, 1966
2. Szekely, P., Jackson, F., Wynne, N.A., Vohra, J.K., Batson, G.A., Dow, W.I.M.: Clinical observations on the use of propranolol in disorders of cardiac rhythm. *Am J Cardiol* 18: 426, 1966
3. Stock, J.P.P.: Beta-adrenergic blocking drugs in the clinical management of cardiac arrhythmias. *Am J Cardiol* 18: 44, 1966
4. Schamroth, L.: Immediate effect of intravenous propranolol on various cardiac arrhythmias. *Am J Cardiol* 18: 438, 1966
5. Lemberg, L., Castellanos, A., Arcebal, A.G.: The use of propranolol in arrhythmias complicating acute myocardial infarction. *Am Heart J* 80: 479, 1970
6. Turner, J.R.B.: Propranolol in the treatment of digitalis-induced and digitalis-resistant tachycardias. *Am J Cardiol* 18: 450, 1966
7. Howitt, G., Husaim, M., Rowlands, D.J., Logan, W.F.W.E., Shanks, R.G., Evans, M.G.: The effect of the dextro isomer of propranolol in sinus rate and cardiac arrhythmias. *Am Heart J* 76: 736, 1968
8. Dimich, I., Steinfeld, L., Richman, R., Lasser, R.: Treatment of recurrent paroxymal ventricular tachycardia. *Am Heart J* 79: 811, 1970
9. Berkowitz, W.D., Wit, A.L., Lau, S.H., Steiner, C., Damato, A.N.: The effects of propranolol in cardiac conduction. *Circulation* 40: 855, 1969
10. Rosen, K.M., Barwolf, G., Ehasaui, A., Rahimtoola, S.H.: Effects of lidocaine and propranolol in the normal and anomalous pathways in patients with pre-excitation. *Am J Cardiol* 30: 801, 1972
11. Smithen, C.S., Balcon, R., Sowton, E.: Use of bundle of His potentials to assess changes in atrioventricular conduction produced by a series of beta-adrenergic blocking agents. *Br Heart J* 33: 955, 1971
12. Seides, S.F., Josephson, M.E., Batsford, W.P., Weisfogel, G.M., Lau, S.H., Damato, A.N.: The electrophysiology of propranolol in man. *Am Heart J* 88: 733, 1974
13. Strauss, H.C., Gilbert, M., Svenson, R.H., Miller, H.C., Wallace, A.G.: Electrophysiologic effects of propranolol on sinus node function in patients with sinus node dysfunction. *Circulation* 54: 452, 1976b
14. Grendahl, H., Miller, M., Sivertssen, E.: Registration of sinus node recovery time in patients with sinus rhythm and in patients with dysrhythmias. *Acta med Scand* 197: 403, 1975
15. Chiquimia, R., Vasquez, M., Qureshi, T., Khan, M., Towne, W.D., Narula, O.S.: Effects of propranolol on sinus node recovery time and sinoatrial conduction time. *Clin Res* 25: 212A, 1977
16. Narula, O.S., Cohen, L.S., Scherlag, B.J., Samet, P., Lister, J.W., Hildner, F.J.: Localization of AV conduction defects in man by recordings of the His bundle electrogram. *Am J Cardiol* 25: 228, 1970
17. Strauss, H.C., Saroff, A.L., Bigger, J.T., Giardina, E.G.V.: Premature atrial stimulation as a key to the understanding of sinoatrial conduction in man. *Circulation* 47: 88, 1973
18. Narula, O.S., Samet, P., Javier, R.P.: Significance of the sinus node recovery time. *Circulation* 45: 140, 1972
19. Strauss, H.C., Bigger, J.T., Saroff, A.L., Giardina, E.G.V.: Electrophysiologic evaluation of sinus node function in patients with sinus node dysfunction. *Circulation* 53: 763, 1976a
20. West, T.C.: Effects of chronotropic influences on subthreshold oscillations in the sinoatrial node. In specialized tissues of the heart. Editors: Paes de Carvalho, A., De Mello, W.C., Hoffman, B.F., Elsevier Publishing Co., Amsterdam-London-New York-Princeton, 1961, p 81
21. Lange, G.: Action of driving stimuli from intrinsic and extrinsic sources on in situ pacemaker tissues. *Circ Res* 17: 449, 1965
22. Lu, H.H., Lange, G., McC. Brooks, C.: Factors controlling pacemaker action in cells of the sinoatrial node. *Circ Res* 17: 460, 1965
23. Goodman, D.J., Rossen, R.M., Ingham, R., Rider, A.K., Harrison, D.C.: Sinus node function in the denervated human heart. Effect of digitalis. *Br Heart J* 37: 612, 1975
24. Davis, L.D., Temte, J.V.: Effects of propranolol in the transmembrane potentials of ventricular muscle and Purkinje fibers of the dog. *Circ Res* 22: 661, 1968
25. Pollen, D.W., Scott, A.C., Wallace, W.F.M.: A comparison of the direct effects of d/l and d-propranolol in the electrical and mechanical behaviour of isolated frog ventricle. *Cardiovasc Res* 3: 7, 1969
26. Shinebourne, E., White, R., Hamer, J.: A qualitative distinction between the beta-receptor-blocking and local anesthetic actions of anti-arrhythmic agents. *Circ Res* 24: 853, 1969
27. Vaughan-Williams, E.M.: Mode of action of beta-receptor antagonists on cardiac muscle. *Am J Cardiol* 18: 399, 1966
28. Abrams, W.B., Davies, R.O.: The antiarrhythmic mechanisms of beta-adrenergic blocking agents, in "Cardiac arrhythmias", edited by Driefus, L.S., Likofew, Likoff, W. Grune & Stratton, New York, 1973, p 517
29. Scherlag, B.J., Lau, S.H., Helfant, R.H., Berkowitz, W.D., Stein, E., Damato, A.N.: Catheter technique for recording His-bundle activity in man. *Circulation* 39: 13, 1969

30. Strauss, H.C., Wallace, A.G.: Direct and indirect techniques in the evaluation of sinus node function. In: The conduction system of the Heart. Editors: Wellens, H.J.J., Lie, K.I., Janse, M.J., Stenfert Kroese, Leiden, 1976, p 227
31. Narula, O.S.: Disorders of sinus node function: electrophysiologic evaluation. In: His bundle electrocardiography and clinical electrophysiology. Editor: Narula, O.S., Publ.: FA Davis, Philadelphia, 1975, p. 275
32. Rosenbleuth, A.: Transmission of nerve impulses at neuroeffector junctions and peripheral synapses. New York, The Technology Press of Massachusetts Institute of Technology and John Wiley and Sons, 1950, p 96

11

DUAL EFFECT OF VERAPAMIL ON SINUS NODE FUNCTION IN MAN*

GÜNTER BREITHARDT, LUDGER SEIPEL, AND EBERHARD WIEBRINGHAUS

Verapamil is the prototype of slow-channel inhibiting drugs which exert their effect mainly on the sinus and atrioventricular node (Bayer et al., 1975; Kohlhardt et al., 1976; Wit and Cranefield, 1974; Zipes and Fischer, 1974). Experimental studies in the isolated sinoatrial preparation have shown that it has a marked depressant effect on sinus node activity (Bayer et al., 1975; Chiba, 1975; Obayashi et al., 1975; Wit and Cranefield, 1974). Verapamil causes a decrease in the amplitude of the action potential and a small decline in the maximal diastolic potential (Wit and Cranefield, 1974). Sinus node discharge is decreased and may be followed by subthreshold oscillations leading to irregular failure of impulse initiation (Bayer et al., 1975; Kohlhardt et al., 1976; Wit and Cranefield, 1974). Selective injections of verapamil into the right coronary artery of the dog also caused a decrease in heart rate with appearance of nodal rhythms which was not the case if it was administered intravenously (Garvey, 1969). In contrast to the experiments in isolated preparations, studies in the intact animal have failed to demonstrate a depressant effect of verapamil on the sinus node at therapeutic doses (Garvey, 1969; Obayashi et al., 1975). Heart rate increases after iv injection of verapamil (Garvey, 1969). However, after high doses not used in the clinical setting, marked sinus suppression also ensued in the conscious dog (Obayashi et al., 1975).

Studies in man have shown that verapamil may increase heart rate after acute injection (Belz and Bender, 1974; Disertori et al., 1976; Husaini et al., 1973). This is in contrast to the markedly depressant effect of verapamil on sinus node function in some patients with sick sinus syndrome which we recently reported (Breithardt et al., 1976). In order to elucidate these apparent discrepancies, we studied its effect on the sinus node in man both with and without autonomic blockade.

METHODS

Patients were studied in the non-sedated, postabsorptive state after having given written informed consent. All cardioactive drugs had been withdrawn during at least 48 hours, in case of digoxin during at least 5 to 7 days. All patients were free of any signs of heart failure. For the identification of the underlying arrhythmias, in all patients routine 12 lead ECG's and ten hours' ambulatory tape-recordings were performed. Additionally, some patients were kept on bed-side monitors for 24 hours or more. Except for two cases only patients were studied in whom the clinical evaluation did not show any signs of sinus node dysfunction. One patient (case no. 16) had previous digoxin intoxication. On the day of study, the digoxin level had decreased to 0.3 ng/ml.

* Supported in part by Landesamt für Forschung, NRW.

For the study of sinus node function spontaneous cycle length, sinus node recovery time (SNRT), corrected SNRT (CSNRT), and sinoatrial conduction time (SACT) were evaluated using previously described methodology and equipment (Breithardt and Seipel, 1976; Seipel et al., 1978). After a control recording over a period of at least ten minutes, high rate atrial pacing was performed for estimation of SNRT. Pacing was started just above the spontaneous rate. After 30 seconds of pacing, it was stopped abruptly and started again after restoration of a regular sinus rhythm not before an interval of 15 seconds. The rate of pacing was increased in increments of 20 beats per minute up to 180 or 200 beats per minute. The longest pause irrespective of the rate of pacing at which it was achieved, was considered as maximal SNRT. Then, single premature atrial stimuli with increasing prematurity were introduced after each eighth spontaneous atrial beat. Single SACT was calculated from return cycles during reset responses (Strauss et al., 1973). The mean spontaneous cycle length was calculated from all $A_1 A_1$ intervals measured during premature atrial stimulation or, in case premature atrial stimulation had not been performed, it was calculated from at least ten spontaneous cycles before and 10 to 15 minutes after administering verapamil.

The following patients were studied:

Group I: 18 patients received 0.1 mg/kg verapamil intravenously after the control study via an indwelling catheter line into the left antecubital vein within two or three minutes.

Group II: Eight patients in whom autonomic blockade was performed after the control study. First, 0.1 mg/kg propranolol was injected at a rate of 1 mg per minute. Then, atropine was given rapidly at a dose of 0.02 mg/kg iv within half a minute. Finally, verapamil was injected using the dosage and kind of administration as described for group I. After each of these injection, spontaneous cycle length, SNRT and SACT were estimated as described.

In addition, two patients with sinus node dysfunction were studied in the same way.

In four of the eight patients with normal sinus node function of group II and in the latter two patients with sinus node dysfunction, verapamil was injected without prior autonomic blockade on a different day. On that occasion, only the spontaneous cycle length was measured 10 to 15 minutes after injection of verapamil and compared to the response after autonomic blockade in the same patients. In these six patients who received verapamil both with and without autonomic blockade, blood pressure was measured with a sphygmomanometer. Mean blood pressure was calculated from systolic and diastolic values.

STATISTICAL ANALYSIS

Statistical analysis was performed by use of the Wilcoxon rank test for paired or unpaired data using a program implemented on a Dietz Mincal 621 computer.

RESULTS

The clinical data and the electrophysiological findings during the control study are presented in Table 1 and 2. Mean age did not differ significantly between both groups. Similarly, there was no significant difference between the various electrophysiological findings during the control study with exclusion of patients no. 27 and 28 who presented sinus node dysfunction.

Table 1. Group 1. Clinical data and electrophysiological findings before (control) and after verapamil in patients with normal sinus node function. The changes of spontaneous cycle length (A₁A₁), sinus node recovery time (SNRT), corrected SNRT (CSNRT), and sino-atrial conduction time (SACT) are listed for each patient. All intervals in milliseconds (msec) (mean ± S.D.). Abbreviations: AVB = atrioventricular block, RBBB = right bundle branch block, LBBB = left bundle branch block, SB = sinus bradycardia, LAH = left axis deviation, SVT = supraventricular tachycardia, AF = atrial fibrillation, LGL = Lown-Ganong-Levine syndrome, WPW = Wolff-Parkinson-White syndrome, VEB = ventricular ectopic beats.

Case no.	Age	Sex	ECG	Mean A_1A_1 control	verapamil	SNRT control	verapamil	CSNRT control	verapamil	SACT control	verapamil
1	36	m	normal	714	625	–	–	–	–	–	–
2	24	f	1° AVB	667	535	–	–	–	–	–	–
3	14	m	VEB	600	600	790	830	190	230	–	–
4	38	m	LGL	750	706	780	640	30	66	–	–
5	42	m	LAH	833	800	–	–	–	–	–	–
6	45	m	LGL	896	800	700	900	196	160	–	–
7	23	f	VEB	600	600	1190	1030	590	430	–	–
8	22	f	LGL	750	750	820	880	70	130	–	–
9	68	f	LGL	769	759	1150	1300	381	540	–	–
10	32	f	SVT	943	849	1180	950	373	100	52	59
11	30	m	WPW Type A, SVT	899	853	1200	1300	300	447	63	73
12	27	m	Ventr. rhythm	1029	842	1300	1520	270	678	88	173
13	21	f	LGL	750	750	1000	950	250	200	–	–
14	42	f	LGL	664	594	1050	700	386	106	93	62
15	45	m	SVT, RBBB	624	792	990	2600	366	1808	131	186
16	17	f	previous digoxin intoxication	896	857	1170	1230	274	373	66	84
17	46	m	VEB, intermitt. AF	722	766	1200	1020	478	254	112	130
18	39	f	LGL	550	450	750	680	200	230	–	–
	34 ± 13.3			759 ± 133.5	718 ± 121.8	1018 ± 206.9	1102 ± 484.7	264 ± 192.4	371 ± 442.0	86 ± 28	110 ± 53.4
				P < 0.01		n.s.		n.s.		n.s.	

GROUP I: RESPONSE TO VERAPAMIL WITHOUT AUTONOMIC BLOCKADE

Mean spontaneous cycle length decreased significantly from 759 ± 133.5 msec (mean ±
S.D.) to 718 ± 121.8 msec (P < 0.01, n = 18) ten to fifteen minutes after injection of
verapamil. Sinus node recovery time (SNRT) (n = 15), corrected SNRT (CSNRT) and
calculated sinoatrial conduction time (SACT) (n = 7) increased slightly (Figure 1). However, these changes were not significant.

GROUP II: RESPONSE TO VERAPAMIL AFTER AUTONOMIC BLOCKADE

Mean spontaneous cycle length increased in all patients after injection of propranolol,
whereas it decreased again below the control level after additional administration of
atropine (Table 2, Figure 2). Subsequent administration of verapamil caused a significant
increase in spontaneous cycle length from 641 ± 98.3 msec (atropine) to 704 ± 125.3 msec
(verapamil) (P < 0.025).

After administering propranolol and atropine, SNRT (CSNRT) increased from 846 ±
160.1 msec (221 ± 93.2 msec) to 1045 ± 240.0 msec (380 ± 131.6 msec) (P < 0.025, resp.).
SACT showed also a significant increase from 63 ± 22.3 msec (atropine) to 80 ± 24.0 msec
(verapamil) (P < 0.001).

For the individual responses to the various drugs, we refer to the data in Table 2.

COMPARISON OF RESULTS WITH AND WITHOUT AUTONOMIC BLOCKADE

The changes of the mean values of group I (without blockade) and group II (with blockade)
are illustrated in Figure 1. Without blockade verapamil caused a significant decrease in
spontaneous cycle length which, on the contrary, increased after prior autonomic blockade.
SNRT, CSNRT and SACT increased significantly after autonomic blockade whereas these
parameters did not show any significant change without blockade though there was a
tendency to an increase of these parameters.

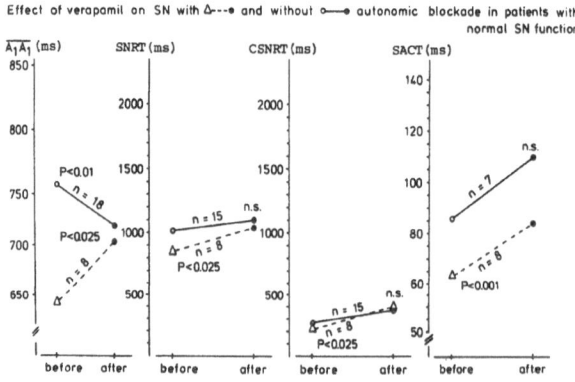

Figure 1. Effect of verapamil on sinus node in patients with normal sinus node function without(o—•) (group 1)
and with (△----•) (group II) autonomic blockade. The values before verapamil represent either the control
value (0) or in case of autonomic blockade the value after atropine (△).

Table 2. Group II. Clinical data and electrophysiological findings in patients with normal sinus node function in whom autonomic blockade (propranolol and atropine) was performed prior to injection of verapamil. Abbreviations: see Table 1.

Case no.	Age	Sex	ECG	Mean A_1A_1 control	prop	atro	vera	SNRT control	prop	atro	vera	CSNRT Control	prop	atro	vera	SACT Control	prop	atro	vera
19	62	f	LBBB	781	898	801	821	1060	1140	1040	1240	279	242	239	419	137	135	100	103
20	25	f	1° and 2° AVB	940	1096	723	830	1470	1480	990	1160	530	384	267	330	122	124	87	112
21	32	f	1° AVB	495	555	545	560	640	820	740	780	330	343	353	343	85	122	75	103
22	40	f	1° AVB	773	898	644	848	1167	1202	793	1443	393	335	142	648	93	66	55	76
23	44	f	LGL	790	950	720	750	1010	1320	1060	1100	220	370	340	350	59	83	50	76
24	36	m	LBBB	937	987	591	679	1272	1449	780	1028	395	462	159	438	144	125	41	63
25	38	f	SVT	550	780	524	546	937	1505	634	860	387	725	110	314	89	98	54	69
26	36	f	LBBB	793	845	580	598	1155	1180	752	752	336	313	155	192	109	104	38	41
	39			757	876	641	704	1089	1262	846	1045	359	397	221	380	105	107.1	63	80
	10.8			160.6	160.5	98.3	125.3	245.2	228.5	160.1	240.0	92.2	146.7	93.2	131.6	28.7	23.8	22.3	24.0
p<				} 0.0025	} 0.0025	} 0.025		} 0.025	} 0.0025	} 0.025		} n.s.	} 0.025	} 0.025		} n.s.	} 0.0005	} 0.0025	
27	57	f	SB	1246	1361	1107	1262	1744	2037	–	7300	592	741	–	6055	193	217	–	90
28	33	f	SB	1250	1540	880	970	2000	2680	1120	1600	750	1140	240	630	104	94	39	47

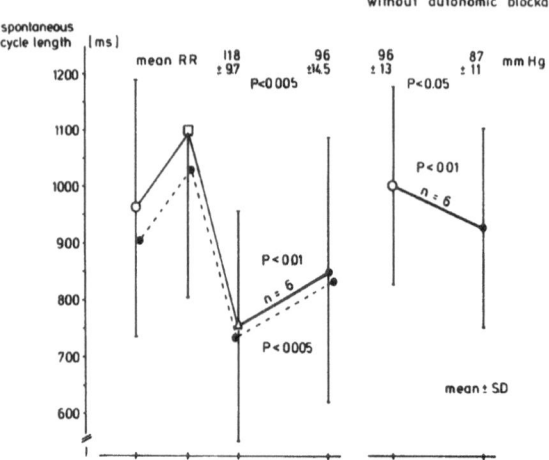

Figure 2. Changes of spontaneous cycle length in response to verapamil in 6 patients in whom the effect of verapamil was tested both with (left) and without (right) autonomic blockade. Additionally, the change of spontaneous cycle length in all ten patients in whom autonomic blockade was performed is indicated by interrupted lines. The response of blood pressure (mean RR) is indicated above.

In six patients (cases 22–24, 26–28), who had received verapamil after autonomic blockade, verapamil was administered without prior blockade on a different day. Only spontaneous cycle length was monitored. Furthermore, in these patients blood pressure response to the injection of verapamil was documented both with and without prior autonomic blockade. The results are shown in Figure 2.

Spontaneous cycle length decreased from 1005 ± 176.9 msec (control) to 928 ± 175.9 msec (verapamil) (P < 0.01). This response was opposite to the response with autonomic blockade (increase of cycle length from 754 ± 205.2 msec to 851 ± 239.5 msec (P < 0.0125)). The fall in blood pressure in response to verapamil was more pronounced after prior autonomic blockade than without blockade (Figure 2). It fell from an average of 118 ± 9.7 mm Hg (calculated mean blood pressure) to 96 ± 14.5 mm Hg (P < 0.005) with prior autonomic blockade and from 96 ± 13.1 mm Hg to 89 ± 11.2 mm Hg (P < 0.05) without prior autonomic blockade.

DISCUSSION

Verapamil is a potent antiarrhythmic drug that exerts its predominant action on the A-V node (Belz and Bender, 1974; Gleichmann et al., 1973; Husaini et al., 1973; Krikler, 1974; Neuss and Schlepper, 1971; Rosen et al., 1975; Schamroth et al., 1972; Seipel et al., 1974). Therefore it has mainly been used in the treatment of A-V nodal reentrant tachycardias or in order to slow ventricular response in atrial fibrillation (Bender, 1967; Rosen et al., 1975; Schamroth et al., 1972). The effect of verapamil on the sinus node in man has been less well documented.

Though available data suggest that verapamil has no pronounced effects on the normal sinus node in man (Belz and Bender, 1974; Gleichmann et al., 1973; Husaini et al., 1973; Grendahl et al., 1975; Seipel et al., 1974), we recently observed a severely depressant effect of the drug in some patients with sick sinus syndrome (Breithardt et al., 1976). In most of these patients with sinus node dysfunction, spontaneous cycle length increased which is in contrast to the lack of response or even a decrease in patients with normal sinus node function (Breithardt et al., 1976; Belz and Bender, 1974; Husaini et al., 1973). In 3 out of 11 patients with sinus node dysfunction (control SNRT > 525 msec), SNRT increased markedly (from 2480 msec to 8050 msec, from 2380 msec to 10.4 sec, and from 3860 msec to 49 sec) after injection of verapamil. In the latter case, an atrial standstill occurred during 49 sec. The ventricles were activated by a His bundle escape rhythm that was retrogradely blocked. This response of SNRT in patients with abnormal sinus node function is clearly different to the slight changes to SNRT seen in patients with normal sinus node function (Breithardt et al., 1976; Grendahl et al., 1975; Husaini et al., 1973).

As previous experimental studies suggested that autonomic effects might be involved in the response of the sinus node to verapamil (Angus et al., 1976; Garvey, 1969; Ross and Jorgensen, 1967), we studied the effect of verapamil on the sinus node in man both with and without prior autonomic blockade. Three parameters of sinus node function (spontaneous cycle length, sinus node recovery time, sinoatrial conduction time) were evaluated in 28 patients. The methodological aspects and limitations of the estimation of sinus node recovery time and sinoatrial conduction time have previously been discussed (Breithardt and Seipel, 1976; Breithardt et al., 1977; Mandel et al., 1971; Miller and Strauss, 1974; Narula et al., 1972; Seipel et al., 1974; Seipel and Breithardt, 1975; Steinbeck and Lüderitz 1976; Strauss et al., 1973; Strauss and Wallace, 1976; Ticzon et al. 1975).

In our study, the dosage of autonomically blocking drugs (propranolol and atropine) was lower than in previous studies (Jordan et al., 1976; Jose, 1966); it nevertheless proved sufficient to produce different effects of verapamil. As the invasive study could not be repeated in the same patient, two groups of patients with normal sinus node function were studied who did not differ significantly as to their electrophysiological findings during the control study. Furthermore, to ascertain that verapamil caused a different effect on spontaneous cycle length without blockade, it was injected in six patients who had received autonomic blockade on a different day.

The opposite effects of verapamil on sinus node function, especially spontaneous cycle length, with and without autonomic blockade provide evidence that the autonomic nervous system is involved in the action of verapamil. An increase in spontaneous cycle length as in our study was also found after autonomic blockade in the experimental animal (Angus et al., 1976; Ross and Jorgensen, 1967; Zipes and Fischer, 1974). Moreover, recently Wagner et al. (1977) noted that the acute toxic effect of verapamil in mice was nearly doubled by a partial depletion of catecholamines by reserpine.

The different effects of verapamil may be explained in the following way. Verapamil has a relaxing effect on smooth vascular tone leading to a decrease in peripheral resistance and a fall in blood pressure (Angus et al., 1976; Belz and Bender, 1974; Ross and Jorgensen, 1967; Rydén and Saetre, 1971; Schmahl and Betz, 1964; Brittinger et al., 1970). This causes a reflex cardioacceleration that may either be due to an increase in beta-adrenergic stimulation or a withdrawal of parasympathetic tone or both (Glick and Braunwald, 1965; Higgins et al., 1973; Thames and Kontos, 1970; Vatner et al., 1972). Epinephrine or isoproterenol are able to reverse the effect of slow channel inhibiting drugs (Chiba, 1975; Iijima and Taira, 1976; Wit and Cranefield, 1974; Zipes and Fischer, 1974). Similarly cholinergic blockade with atropine is still effective after pretreatment with verapamil (unpublished data). Whatever the mechanisms, they will counteract the depressing effect of verapamil on sinus node function which is known from studies in the isolated sinoatrial preparation (Bayer et al., 1975; Kohlhardt et al., 1976; Okada and Konishi, 1975; Wit and Cranefield, 1974; Zipes and Fischer, 1974). The net effect of verapamil on the sinus node depends on the balance between the direct (depressant) and indirect (stimulating) effects.

Another mechanism that might be responsible for the increase in heart rate has been demonstrated by Garvey (1969) who found that pretreatment with verapamil effectively antagonized the effect of acetylcholine or vagal stimulation on the sinus node. However, this antagonism to vagal effects could not be shown by injection of verapamil into the right coronary artery (Garvey, 1969). This suggests that the vagolytic effect of verapamil in this study must have been exerted at a level in the nervous system that is above the sinus node itself.

The opposite effects of verapamil on spontaneous cycle length which could be shown in our study, resemble the effects of verapamil in patients with sick sinus syndrome. However, we were not able to demonstrate similar marked effects on sinus node recovery time after autonomic blockade as in the sick sinus syndrome. SACT consistently increased after autonomic blockade whereas the response without blockade was insignificant. These differences in the action of verapamil in the sick sinus syndrome and after autonomic blockade suggest that either the degree of autonomic blockade, which was achieved in our patients, was too weak or that some other mechanisms might be involved in the deleterious effect of verapamil in some patients with sick sinus syndrome. It might well be that in the sick sinus syndrome, besides a reduced responsiveness to autonomic stimuli (Dighton, 1975), there is an increased sensitivity to the directly depressant effect of verapamil. A similar increase in sensitivity has been found in response to propranolol (Narula, 1978; Seipel et al., 1978; Strauss et al., 1976), to quinidine (Damato, 1978) and to disopyramide (Seipel and Breithardt, 1976). To date no comparable data exist whether the effect of verapamil in the sick sinus syndrome may be aggravated by autonimic blockade.

The role of the autonomic nervous system in modulating the effect to antiarrhythmic drugs on the sinus node needs further studies. Recently, Birkhead and Vaughan Williams (1977) showed that the depressant effect of disopyramide to which a vagolytic action is attributed, was only apparent after cholinergic blockade with atropine.

Concluding, verapamil has significant effects on sinus node function which are modulated by the autonomic nervous system. With respect to the different response of patients with normal and abnormal sinus node function, verapamil should be used with caution if sinus node dysfunction is suspected. However, these data are only relevant to the acute administration of verapamil. It is not possible to accurately predict the response to verapamil on a chronic oral therapy, though the indirect (stimulating) effect might be less pronounced.

REFERENCES

Angus, J.A., Richmond, D.R., Dhumma-Upakorn, P., Cobbin, L.B., Goodman, A.H.: Cardiovascular action of verapamil in the dog with particular reference to myocardial contractility and atrioventricular conduction. *Cardiovasc Res* 10: 623, 1976

Bayer, R., Kalusche, D., Kaufmann, R. Mannhold, R.: Inotropic and electrophysiological actions of verapamil and D 600 in mammalian myocardium. III. Effects of the optical isomers on transmembrane action potentials. Naunyn-Schmiedeberg's *Arch Pharmacol* 290: 81, 1975

Belz, G.G., Bender F.: Therapie der Herzrhythmusstörungen mit Verapamil. Gustav Fischer Verlag, Stuttgart, 1974

Bender, F.: Isoptin zur Behandlung der tachykarden Form des Vorhofflatterns. *Med Klinik* 62: 634, 1967

Birkhead, J.S., Vaughan Williams, E.M.: Dual effects of disopyramide on atrial and atrioventricular conduction and refractory periods. *Brit Heart J* 39:657, 1977

Breithardt, G., Seipel, L.: The effect of premature atrial depolarization on sinus node automaticity in man. *Circulation* 53: 920, 1976

Breithardt, G., Seipel, L., Wiebringhaus, E., Loogen, F.: Effect of verapamil on sinus node in patients with normal and abnormal sinus node function. *Circulation* 54: suppl. II–19, 1976

Breithardt, G., Seipel, L., Loogen, F.: Sinus node recovery time and calculated sinoatrial conduction time in normal subjects and patients with sinus node dysfunction. *Circulation* 56: 43, 1977

Brittinger, D.W., Schwarzbeck, A., Wittenmeier, K.W., Twittenhoff, W.D., Stegaru, B., Huber, W., Ewald, R.W., v. Henning, G.E. Fabricius, M., Strauch, M.: Klinisch-experimentelle Untersuchungen über die blutdrucksenkende Wirkung von Verapamil. *Dtsch med Wschr* 95: 1871, 1970

Chiba, S.: Effects of verapamil on the blood-perfused, isolated atrium preparation of the dog heart. *Jap Heart J* 16: 709, 1975

Damato, A.N.: Quinidine and the sick sinus syndrome. In: F.I.M. Bonke, ed., The sinus node: Structure, function, and clinical relevance. 1978

Dighton, D.H.: Sinoatrial block. Autonomic influences and assessment. *Brit Heart J* 37: 321, 1975

Disertori, M., Molinis, G., Lanzetta, T., Antonini, L., Furlanello, F.: Effetti del verapamil sulla funzione sinusale e sulla conduzione atrio-ventricolare, lungo le vie normali ed anomale, in pazienti con preesistenti alterazioni della eccito-conduzione. *G Ital Cardiol* 6: 300, 1976

Garvey, H.L.: The mechanism of action of verapamil on the sinus and av nodes. *Europ J Pharmacol* 8: 159, 1969

Gleichmann, U., Seipel, L., Loogen, F.: Der Einflusz von Antiarrhythmika auf die intrakardiale Erregungsleitung (His-Bündel-Elektrographie) und Sinusknotenautomatie beim Menschen. *Dtsch med Wschr* 98: 1487, 1973

Glick, G., Braunwald, E.: Relative roles of the sympathetic and parasympathetic nervous system in the reflex control of the heart. *Circ Res* 16: 363, 1965

Grendahl, H., Miller, M., Sivertssen, E.: Registration of sinus node recovery time in patients with sinus rhythm and in patients with dysrhythmias. *Acta med scand* 197: 43, 1975

Higgins, C.B., Vatner, S.F., Braunwald, E.: Parasympathetic control of the heart. *Pharmacol Rev* 25: 119, 1973

Husaini, M.H., Kvasnicka, J., Rydén, L., Holmberg, S.: Action of verapamil on sinus node, atrioventricular and intraventricular conduction. *Brit Heart J* 35: 734, 1973

Iijima, T., Taira, N.: Modification by manganese ions and verapamil of the response of the atrioventricular node to norepinephrine. *European J Pharmacol* 37: 55, 1976

Jordan, J., Yamaguchi, I, Mandel, W.J.: Studies on the mechanism of sinus node dysfunction in the sick sinus syndrome. *Circulation* 54: suppl. II–230, 1976

Jose, A.D.: Effect of combined sympathetic and parasympathetic blockade on heart rate and cardiac function in man. *Amer J Cardiol* 18: 476, 1966

Kohlhardt, M., Figulla, H.-R., Tripathi, O.: The slow membrane channel as the predominant meadiator of the excitation process of the sinoatrial pacemaker cell. *Basic Res Cardiol* 71: 17, 1976

Krikler, D.: Verapamil in cardiology, *Europ J Cardiol* 2: 3, 1974

Mandel, W.J., Hayakawa, H., Danzig, R., Marcus, H.S.: Evaluation of sino-atrial node function in man by overdrive suppression. *Circulation* 44: 59, 1971

Miller, H.C., Strauss, H.C.: Measurement of sinoatrial conduction time by premature atrial stimulation in the rabbit. *Circ Res* 35: 935, 1974

Narula, O.S., Samet, P., Javier, R.P.: Significance of the sinus node recovery time. *Circulation* 45: 140, 1972

Narula, O.S.: Effect of intravenous propranolol on sinus node recovery time and sinoatrial conduction time in patients with sinus node dysfunction. In: F.I.M. Bonke, ed.: The sinus node: Structure, function, and clinical relevance. 1978

Neuss, H., Schlepper, M.: Der Einflusz von Verapamil auf die atrioventrikuläre Überleitung. *Verh Dtsch Ges Kreisl Forschg* 37: 433, 1971

Okada, T., Konishi, T.: Effects of verapamil on SA and AV nodal action potentials in the isolated rabbit heart. *Jap Circulation J* 39: 913, 1975

Obayashi, K., Nagasawa, K., Mandel, W.J., Vyden, J.K.,: Cardiovascular effects of the new antiarrhythmic agent, verapamil. *Amer J Cardiol* 35: 161, 1975

Rosen, M.R., Wit, A.L., Hoffman, B.F.: Electrophysiology and pharmacology of cardiac arrhythmias. VI. Cardiac effects of verapamil. *Amer Heart J* 89: 665, 1975

Ross, G, Jorgensen, C.R.: Cardiovascular action of ipoveratril. *J Pharmacol Exper Therapeut* 158: 504, 1967

Rydén, L., Saetre, H.: The haemodynamic effects of verapamil. *Eurp J Clinical Pharmacol* 3: 153, 1971

Schamroth, L., Krikler, D.M., Garrett, C.: Immediate effects of intravenous verapamil in cardiac arrhythmias. *Brit Med J* 1: 660, 1972

Schmahl, F.W., Betz, E.: Die Wirkung von α-Isopropyl-α-(N-methyl-N- homoveratryl) -γ-amino-propyl-3,4-dimethoxyphenylacetonnitrile auf die Durchblutung von Myokard, Leber, Niere, Skeletmuskulatur und Gehirn der Katze. *Arzneimittel-Forsch* 14: 1159, 1964

Seipel, L., Breithardt, G., Both, A., Loogen, F.: Messung der "sinu-atrialen Leitungszeit" mittels vorzeitiger Vorhofstimulation beim Menschen. *Dtsch med Wschr* 99: 1895, 1974

Seipel, L., Both, A., Breithardt, G., Gleichmann, U., Loogen, F.: Action of antiarrhythmic drugs on His bundle electrogram and sinus node function. *Acta Cardiol (Brux.)* suppl. 18, 251, 1974

Seipel, L., Breithardt, G.: Sinusknotenautomatie und sinu-atriale Leitung. *Z Kardiol* 64: 1014, 1975

Seipel, L., Breithardt, G.: Sinus recovery time after disopyramide phosphate *Amer J Cardiol* 37: 1118, 1976

Seipel, L., Breithardt, G., Leuner, Ch.: Programmed atrial stimulation used for the measurement of sino-atrial conduction time. In: F.I.M. Bonke, ed.: The sinus node: Structure, function, and clinical relevance. 1978

Seipel, L., Breithardt, G., Döhring, H.P.: Die Wirkung von Atenolol auf Sinusknoten und intrakardiale Erregungsleitung beim Menschen im Vergleich zu Propranolol. Z. Kardiol 66: 719, 1977

Steinbeck, G., Lüderitz, B.: Sinus node recovery time and sinoatrial conduction time. In: Cardiac Pacing. Diagnostic and therapeutic tools, edited by B. Lüderitz, Springer Verlag, Berlin-New York, 1976, p. 45–57

Strauss, H.C., Saroff, A.L., Bigger, J.T., Jr., Giardina, E.G.V.: Premature atrial stimulation as a key to the understanding of sinoatrial conduction in man. Presentation of data and critical review of the literature. *Circulation* 47: 86, 1973

Strauss, H.C., Wallace, A.G.: Direct and indirect techniques in the evaluation of sinus node function. In: The conduction system of the heart, edited by H.J.J. Wellens, K.I. Lie, M.J. Janse. 1976, p. 227–237

Strauss, H.C., Gilbert, M., Svenson, R.H., Miller, H.C., Wallace, A.G.: Electrophsiologic effects of propranolol on sinus node function in patients with sinus node dysfunction. *Circulation* 54: 452, 1976

Thames, M.D., Kontos, H.A.: Mechanisms of baroreceptor-induced changes in heart rate. *Amer J Physiol* 218: 251, 1970

Ticzon, A.R., Strauss, H.C., Gallagher, J.J., Wallace, A.G.: Sinus nodal function in the intact dog heart evaluated by premature atrial stimulation and atrial pacing. *Am J Cardiol* 35: 492, 1975

Vatner, S.F., Higgins, C.B., Franklin, D., Braunwald, E.: Autonomic components of reflex tachycardia induced by hypotension. *Physiologist* 15: 294, 1972

Wagner, J., Schümann, H.J., Görlitz, B.D.: Änderung der Toxität des Calciumantagonisten Verapamil durch Brenzkatechinaminverarmung. *Arzneim-Forsch/Drug Res* 27: 558, 1977

Wit, A.L., Cranefield, P.F.: Effect of verapamil on the sinoatrial and atriventricular nodes of the rabbit and the mechanism by which it arrests reentrant atrioventricular nodal tachycardia. *Circ Res* 35: 413, 1974

Zipes, D.P., Fischer, J.C.: Effects of agents which inhibit the slow channel on sinus node automaticity and atriventricular conduction in the dog. *Circulation Res* 34: 184, 1974

12

GENERAL CONCLUSIONS:
LIMITATIONS OF SINUS NODE FUNCTION TESTING IN PATIENTS WITH KNOWN OR SUSPECTED SINUS NODE DISEASE

KENNETH M. ROSEN, RAMESH C. DHINGRA, PABLO DENES, DELON WU, CHRISTOPHER WYNDHAM, AND FERNANDO AMAT-Y-LEON

The electrophysiological evaluation of sinus node function is extensively reviewed in this symposium on the sinus node. In addition, several excellent studies review the effects of pharmacologic agents on sinus node function. In this presentation, we will not attempt to duplicate that which has been said already in this symposium. This manuscript instead will be somewhat philosophic in its tone, and deal with trying to evaluate the current place of electrophysiological evaluation of sinus node function.

NORMAL SINUS NODE FUNCTION

The clinical indications for analysis of sinus node function, relate to delineation of patients who have, or will develop sinus node dysfunction. This task cannot be accomplished, until the behavior of the normal human sinus node is well characterized. Since the most important function of the sinus node, is the regular generation of impulses, it is this particular function that needs specific attention in terms of definition of normality. Before defining which patients have sinus node disease, it is absolutely necessary to define the normal behavior of heart rates in a healthy population.

We have recently attempted to do this by continuous 24-hour electrocardiographic monitoring in people without apparent heart disease (1). The study group consisted of 50 male medical students who met the following criteria: 1) Absence of history of cardiovascular disease and absence of systemic disease. 2) Normal cardiovascular examination. 3) Normal electrocardiogram. 4) Normal chest x-ray. 5) Normal echocardiogram (patients with mitral valve prolapse and asymmetric septal hypertrophy were excluded). Medical students who met the above criteria were felt to be free of apparent heart disease.

The following definitions were utilized in our study: 1) Normal sinus rhythm was defined by the presence of the antegrade P wave morphology, and heart rates of 60–100 beats/min, with less than 10% change in adjacent cycle lengths. Sinus tachycardia was defined when sinus rates were faster than 100 beats/min, and sinus bradycardia when sinus rates were less than 60 beats/min. Sinus arrhythmia was defined by the presence of an irregular sinus rhythm with adjacent cycle lengths varying by 10% or more. Mild sinus arrhythmia was defined by irregular sinus rhythm with variation in adjacent cycle length by 10% to less than 50%. Moderate sinus arrhythmia was defined when adjacent cycle lengths varied by 50% to less than 100%. Marked sinus arrhythmia was defined as sinus arrhythmia with changes in adjacent cycle lengths greater than 100% or more.

Heart rate data is summarized in Table 1. Twenty-four hour average heart rates in our 50 subjects ranged from a high of 87 to a low of 60 beats/min with a mean ± SD of 73 ± 7 beats/min. Waking periods average rates ranged from 95 to 67 beats/min (mean 80 ± 7). Waking

Table 1. Heart rates and sinus pauses in 50 normal subjects.

	Mean ± Standard Deviation	Range
24 hour period		
Total recording time (minutes)	1434 ± 90	1260–1957
Average heart rate (beats/min)	73 ± 7	59–87
Waking periods		
Average rate (beats/min)	80 ± 7	67–90
Maximal rate (beats/min)	141 ± 17	107–180
Minimal rate (beats/min)	54 ± 6	37–65
Longest pause (seconds)	1.36 ± 0.16	1.00–1.68
Sleeping periods		
Average rate (beats/min)	56 ± 6	45–70
Maximal rate (beats/min)	86 ± 9	70–115
Minimal rate (beats/min)	43 ± 5	33–55
Longest pause (seconds)	1.62 ± 0.20	1.20–2.06

period maximum heart rates ranges from a high of 180 to a low of 107 beats/min (mean 141 ± 17), and usually corresponded to periods of physical activity. Waking period minimal rates ranged from a high of 65 to a low of 37 beats/min (mean 53 ± 6). In each subject, the longest sinus pause was also averaged during the waking period, and ranged from 1.68 seconds to 1.00 seconds (mean 1.36 ± .16 secs). All subjects had a waking rate of more than 100 beats/min at least one time during the day and thirteen subjects had a waking rate of less than 50 beats/min at least one time during a day.

Sleeping heart rates were considerably slower, as expected. Average sleeping average rates ranged from a high of 70 to a low of 45 beats/min (mean 56 ± 6). Sleeping period maximal rates ranged from a high of 115 to a low of 70 beats/min (mean 86 ± 9). Sleeping period minimum rates ranged from a high of 55 to a low of 33 beats/min (mean 43 ± 5). Longest pauses observed during sleeping periods ranged from a high of 2.06 to a low of 1.20 seconds (mean 1.62 ± 0.20).

All subjects had sleeping rates of less than 60 beats/min at least one time during the night. Twelve subjects (24%) had sleeping rates of less than 40 beats/min at least one time during the night. In thirty-four subjects (68%), the longest pause of the sleeping periods was greater than 1.5 seconds; in 26 subjects, ranged from 1.5 to 1.75 seconds and 12 subjects from 1.75 to 2.00 seconds; in two subjects, it was greater than 2.00 seconds. In regard to sinus arrhythmias, all subjects had episodes of mild sinus arrhythmia. Eighty-six percent of our patients had at least one episode of moderate sinus arrhythmia, and 50% of our patients had at least one episode of marked sinus arrhythmia.

These observations in male medical students without apparent heart disease, are relevant to the understanding of sinus node function. The demonstration of sinus rates as slow as 33 beats/min, the demonstration of sinus pauses of up to 2 seconds in normal subjects, and the pauses slightly greater than 2 seconds in two of our subjects, suggest that this range of bradyarrhythmia, may be encountered in a normal population. These rates and pauses are frequently in the range at which patients may be considered for pacemaker implantation because of sinus node dysfunction. It is obvious that therapy predicted upon results of continuous electrocardiographic monitoring, must take into account the arrhythmias and variations in heart rates encountered in a normal population.

The difficulty of defining normality is further extended by recognizing that our own study dealt with a relatively limited population of young healthy males. There are no normal values established for normal healthy females, which could be different than the male population reported by us. In addition, since heart rates slow with aging, it is very likely that normally encountered rates in middle aged and aged population would be significantly slower than the above described ranges of normality. These difficulties in establishing normality, compound the difficulty in attempting to define what constitutes abnormal sinus node function.

PROSPECTIVE ELECTROPHYSIOLOGICAL EVALUATION OF SINUS NODE FUNCTION

It is quite obvious that electrophysiological evaluation of sinus node function has been extremely helpful in understanding the physiology of the sinus node as well as the pathophysiology of the sinus node (2–15). Electrophysiological studies have also yielded important insights concerning the effects of pharmacologic agents upon the sinus node (16–22). However, a major question before us has yet to be answered, and that is the place of testing sinus node function in the delineation of patients who either need pacemakers for control of symptomatic bradyarrhythmias, or prophylactic pacemakers for control of arrhythmias yet to develop in the future.

In regard to sinus node function, there are a number of problems inherent in the prospective evaluation of sinus function studies. This is in marked contrast to the evaluation of patients with bifascicular block. We have been concerned for the past six years with a prospective study of patients with intact conduction and bifascicular block (23–26). In our study, the group at risk is relatively well defined, consisting of a group of patients with a specific electrocardiographic abnormality that is quite definitely abnormal (bifascicular block with intact A-V conduction). Electrophysiological techniques for evaluating these patients are relatively straight forward and consist of His bundle recordings, measurement of pacing responses, and measurements of refractory periods of the specialized conduction system with atrial extra-stimulus technique. The normal range of intervals and stimulatory responses are relatively well defined in terms of normality. The end point which the study is attempting to predict is relatively well defined, and consists of A-V block distal to the His bundle and/or the development of sudden death (which could reflect either ventricular fibrillation or lethal bradyarrhythmia).

In attempting to set up a similar study of patients with sinus node of dysfunction, there are several obvious immediate problems. What is to be considered the group at risk? The group or groups at risk could consist on one or more of the following: 1) Patients with electrocardiographically documented severely symptomatic sinus node dysfunction. However, this group obviously needs pacemakers, so that the results of electrophysiologic testing, although interesting, cannot be used to delineate therapy. 2) Patients with electrocardiographically documented sinus node dysfunction (note that this group is difficult to define since the range of normality of electrocardiographic behavior is quite large), in whom symptoms are suspected of being due to sinus bradyarrhythmia. In regard to this group, at least at the present, there does not appear that any test that will replace the documentation in real time of a cause and effect relationship between bradyarrhythmia and symptoms. 3) Asymptomatic patients with electrocardiographically documented sinus node dysfunction (this group could have sinus bradycardia, or sinus pauses). 4) Elderly patients without electrocardiographically documented sinus node dysfunction, who are considered at risk because elderly patients are prone to sinus node disease. 5) Patients with no electrocardiographic evidence of sinus node dysfunction, in whom symptoms are possibly consistant with symptomatic sinus node disease.

The above paragraph delineates possible groups in whom sinus node function testing could conceivably be of value. It is not at all clear which of these groups would be most satisfactory, in terms of delineating clinically useful information from sinus node function testing. It should also be pointed out, that if sinus node function testing were of value, it might be of value in only some of the above groups.

If one were to attempt a prospective study in attempt to delineate those patients needing pacemakers, or those who would need pacemakers in the future, one would also have to define which tests of sinus node function were worth performing. Sinus node recovery times could be measured, but it is not clear specifically which rates would provide the most useful data. In patients with peri-sinus nodal disease, the problem would be compounded by unidirectional sinus entrance block at faster heart rates, precluding meaningful measurement of recovery times. It is also not clear whether sinus node recovery time should be corrected for sinus cycle length. There is no prospective data concerning sinus node recovery times (uncorrected or corrected) in the evaluation of sinus node dysfunction.

Sino-atrial conduction times could be measured with extra-stimulus techniques. However, with the latter type of testing, the confounding effect of cycle length upon this measurement cannot be solved at the moment. All interventions which might change cycle length would probably also effect sino-atrial conduction time (27). There is no reason at the moment to believe that these electrophysiological tests of sinus node function, which utilize pacing catheters, are any better than other varieties of sinus node function testing. For example, sinus node responses to atropine, propranolol, and isoproterenol, might yield useful insights into normal and abnormally functioning sinus node. Treadmill testing, with noting of sinus node response to graded exercise, could also provide important information concerning normal and abnormal sinus node. Perhaps the best test of all, would be the 24-hour recording over one or more days of sinus rates utilizing the holter recorder.

Assuming that appropriate test of sinus node function were chosen, one would then be faced with the delineation of suitable end points for the study. The development of asymptomatic bradyarrhythmias doesn't seem suitable, because asymptomatic bradyarrhythmias probably do not usually need therapy with permanent pacing. The development of symptomatic bradyarrhythmias would be a suitable end point, but one would be faced with proving a cause and effect of relationship between the bradyarrhthmia and symptoms. Sudden death is another conceivable end point in the prospective study of sinus node function. However, sudden death in a patient with sinus bradyarrhythmia could be tachyarrhythmic.

The difficulties inherent in prospective evaluation of sinus node function utilizing electrophysiological techniques are highlighted by a recent study reported by our laboratory. We attempted to prospectively evaluate the significance of prolonged sino-atrial conduction time (15). In our study, 152 msec was considered the upper limit of normal, so that patients with sino-atrial conduction times greater than 152 msec were considered to have prolonged SACT. Between January 1974 and January 1976, 470 patients underwent diagnostic electrophysiological studies in our laboratory utilizing atrial extra-stimulus technique. Indications for study in this group included AV and intra-ventricular conduction defects, atrial or ventricular tachyarrhythmia, and suspected sinus node disease. The latter category accounted for 52 of the 470 patients studied.

Of the 470 patients, 24 patients had a prolonged (greater than 152 msec) calculated sino-atrial conduction time. These 24 included 15 with suspected sinus node disease (29% of 52 patients with suspected sinus node disease) and 9 without previous suspected sinus node disease (2% of the 418 patients without suspected sinus node disease).

The group of 24 patients with prolonged SACT consisted of 18 males and 6 females with a mean age of 65 years. Electrocardiographic monitoring in this group of patients revealed significant sinus or atrial dysrhythmia in 19 (79%). Of these 19, 15 had persistent sinus bradycardia and/or sino-atrial block, three had sinus bradyarrhythmia with paroxysmal atrial tachyarrhythmia, and one had isolated tachyarrhythmia. However, there was not a suitable age matched control group to compare in terms of incidence of dysrhythmia with this detected group. Four of the patients with prolonged SACT needed permanent pace-makers during a mean follow-up period of 427 days, because of development of sympto-matic bradyarrhythmia. Three of our patients died non-suddenly.

We concluded from this study that prolonged calculated sino-atrial conduction time was associated with a high incidence of electrocardiographic abnormalities of sinus node and atrium. Despite this, bradyarrhythmic morbidity was relatively low, suggesting that prolonged sino-atrial conduction time in the absence of initial symptoms, was not an indication for prophylactic pacing.

Similar and more extensive studies are necessary regarding all the currently available tests of sinus node function. It is very likely, that no one test of sinus node function will be ideal in achieving delineation of which group of patients needs permanent pacing. It is very likely that a combination of tests, possibly including a catheter evaluation, exercise testing, and pharmacologic manipulation, will eventually allow us to delineate a group that needs pacing for prevention of significant morbidity and mortality.

CURRENT STATUS OF ELECTROPHYSIOLOGICAL SINUS NODE FUNCTION TESTING

Before attempting to delineate groups of patients in whom sinus node function testing is currently useful, it is helpful to try to summarize what is currently known regarding the value of these tests. If one performs electrophysiological studies in patients with obviously symptomatic sinus node disease, a significant percentage will have detectable abnormal-ities of sinus node function (2, 4–7, 10, 15). These abnormalities may include prolongation of sinus node recovery time, prolongation of corrected sinus node recovery time and pro-longation of sino-atrial conduction time. There will be patients detected who have paroxys-mal severe bradyarrhythmia in whom electrophysiological study during intervals when sinus rates are normal or near normal, will have totally normal electrophysiological studies (8, 11, 12, 14).

Patients with questionably symptomatic sinus node disease (intermittent periods of dizziness without a demonstrated cause and effect relationship to bradyarrhythmia), may or may not have abnormalities of sinus node function detectable with electrophysio-logical study. However, in this group, the question of whether bradyarrhythmia produces symptoms, may frequently not be clarified by the finding of either normal or abnormal sinus function studies. In an occasional patient, the abnormalities of sinus node function detected with electrophysiological studies, will be so severe as to strongly implicate the sinus node in a genesis of symptoms. An example (I would consider this a rather rare example), would be a patient in whom sinus rates are normal, but sinus node recovery times are markedly prolonged to the extent of several seconds, with accompanying symptoms. In our experience, this type of patient is a rare exception.

If one studies patients who are asymptomatic but who have electrocardiographic evidence of sinus node dysfunction, electrophysiological studies again may be normal or abnormal. There is little prospective data regarding the significance of either normal or abnormal function as detected electrophysiologically in this group of patients. One would be hard pressed to make a decision for a pacemaker based upon the results of electro-physiologic studies in this group of patients. Again, it is possible that on rare occasions such severe abnormalities might be encountered, that pacemaker would be advisable.

If one studies asymptomatic patients without electrocardiographic abnormalities of sinus node function, then electrophysiological studies will be normal in most (normal recovery times, corrected recovery times, and sino-atrial conduction times) (6, 9). An occa-sional patient may be encountered who has abnormalities of sinus node function, but who has no electrocardiographic evidence of sinus node disease. If one were to study trained athletes with sinus bradycardia, then the number of patients demonstrating abnormal findings would be significantly increased.

INDICATIONS FOR ELECTROPHYSIOLOGICAL TESTING OF SINUS NODE FUNCTION

With all the above limitations, there is still a role for electrophysiological testing of sinus node function. Patients in whom these studies are indicated would include: 1) *Patients with obviously symptomatic sinus node disease*: In this group, the need for permanent pacing is obvious. Electrophysiological findings however are of interest, and could relate to sub-sequent clinical course. Demonstration of conduction defects, would preclude the use of permanent atrial pacing (2). Demonstration of tachyarrhythmias replicable with cardiac stimulation, would provide a clue to additional problems not yet encountered (28).

2) *Questionably symptomatic patients with sinus node disease*: The electrophysiological studies are of interest in this group of patients, and can sometimes provide a clue as to the significance of previously recorded bradyarrhythmias. Marked abnormalities of sinus node function, such as major prolongation of sinus node recovery time, are supportive findings in regard to necessity of permanent pacing. It should be pointed out, that decision making regarding the need for permanent pacing, will seldom be made from the results of sinus node function testing alone.

3) *Patients with no electrocardiographic evidence of sinus node dysfunction, but with symp-toms suggestive of bradyarrhythmia*: In this group, if electrophysiological studies are per-formed, they should be aimed at delineating A-V and I-V conduction disease, sinus node dysfunction, and supraventricular and ventricular tachyarrhythmia. Again, it would be rare for electrophysiological studies to determine the absolute necessity for or against pacemaker implantation.

4) *Asymptomatic patients with sinus node abnormalities*: In this group of patients there is no particular set of electrophysiological abnormalities which should necessitate perman-ent pacing. We do not believe that electrophysiological testing is ordinarily indicated in this group except under unusual circumstances.

It should be emphasized that decision making regarding therapy, will rarely depend upon electrophysiological testing alone. History, physical examination, other indicated laboratory investigation (for example, CNS work-up if symptoms relate to the central nervous system), 24-hour electrocardiographic recordings, treadmill testing, will all play a role in clinical decision making. It should be recognized that the natural history of sinus node disease, is frequently dependent upon the state of the underlying myocardium. It is crucial to delineate the presence and significance of underlying myocardial disease in these patients.

REFERENCES

1. Brodsky, M, Wu, D., Denes, P., Kanakis, C., Rosen, K.M.: Arrhythmias documented by 24-hour continuous electrocardiographic monitoring in 50 male medical students without apparent heart disease. *Amer J Card* 39: 390, 1977
2. Rosen, K.M., Loeb, H.S., Sinno, M.Z., Rahimtoola, S.H., Gunnar, R.M.: Cardiac conduction in patients with symptomatic sinus node disease. *Circulation* 43: 836, 1971
3. Mandel, W., Hayakawa, H., Danzig, R., Marcus, H.S.: Evaluation of sino-atrial function in many by overdrive suppression. *Circulation* 44: 59, 1971
4. Narula, O.S., Samet, P., Janvier, R.P.: Significance of the sinus node recovery time. *Circulation* 45: 140, 1972
5. Mandel, W.J., Hayakawa, H., Allen, H.N., Danzig, R., Kermaier, A.I.: Assessment of sinus node function in patients with the sick sinus syndrome. *Circulation* 46: 761, 1972
6. Dhingra, R.C., Rosen, K.M., Rahimtoola, S.H.: Normal conduction intervals and responses in sixty-one patients using His bundle recording and atrial pacing. *Chest* 64: 55, 1973
7. Strauss, H.C., Saroff, A.L., Bigger, J.T., Giardina, E.G.V.: Premature atrial stimulation as a key to the understanding of sino-atrial conduction in man. *Circulation* 47: 86, 1973
8. Gupta, P.K., Lichstein, E., Chadda, K.D., Badui, E.: Appraisal of sinus nodal recovery time in patients with sick sinus syndrome. *Amer J card* 34: 265, 1974
9. Dhingra, R.C., Wyndham, C., Amat-y-Leon, F., Denes, P., Wu, D., Rosen, K.M.: Sinus nodal responses to atrial extra-stimuli in patients without apparent sinus node disease. *Amer J Card* 36: 445, 1975
10. Masini, G., Dianda, R., Graziina, W.: Analysis of sino-atrial conduction in man using premature atrial stimulation. *Cardiovasc Res* 9: 498, 1975
11. Steinbeck, G., Luderitz, B.: Comparative study of sino-atrial conduction time and sinus node recovery time. *Brit Heart J* 37: 956, 1975
12. Strauss, H.C., Bigger, J.T., Saroff, A.L., Giardina, E.G.V.: Electrophysiologic evaluation of sinus node function in patients with sinus node dysfunction. *Circulation* 53: 763, 1976
13. Breithardt, G., Seipel, L.: The effect of premature atrial depolarization on sinus node automaticity in man. *Circulation* 53: 920, 1976
14. Scheinman, M.M., Kunkel, F.W., Peters, R.W., Hirschfeld, G., Schoenfeld, P.L., Abbott, J.A., Modin, G.: Atrial pacing in patients with sinus node dysfunction. *Amer J Med* 61: 641, 1976
15. Dhingra, R.C., Amat-y-Leon, F., Wyndham, C., Deedwania, P.C., Wu D., Denes, P., Rosen, K.M.: Clinical significance of prolonged sino-atrial conduction time. *Circulation* 55: 8, 1976
16. Dhingra, R.C., Amat-y-Leon, F., Wyndham, C., Wu, D., Denes, P., Rosen, K.M.: The electrophysiological effects of ouabain on sinus node and atrium in man. *J Clin Invest* 56: 555, 1975
17. Dhingra, R.C., Amat-y-Leon, F., Wyndham, C., Denes, P., Wu, D., Pouget, J.M., Rosen, K.M.: Electrophysiologic effects of atropine on human sinus node and atrium. *Amer J Card* 38: 429, 1976
18. Dhingra, R.C., Amat-y-Leon, F., Wyndham, C., Denes, P., Wu, D., Miller, R.H., Rosen, K.M.: Electrophysiologic effects of atropine on sinus node and atrium in patients with sinus node dysfunction. *Amer J Card* 38: 848, 1976
19. Goodman, D.J., Rosen, R.M., Ingham, R., Rider, A.K., Harrison, D.C.: Sinus node function in the denervated human heart. Effect of digitalis. *Brit Heart J* 37: 612, 1975
20. Strauss, H.C., Gilbert, M., Svenson, R.H., Miller, H.C., Wallace, A.G.: Electrophysiologic effects of propranolol on sinus node function in patients with sinus node dysfunction. *Circulation* 54: 452, 1976
21. Reiffel, J.A., Bigger, J.T., Giardina, E.G.V.: "Paradoxical" prolongation of sinus nodal recovery time after atropine in the sick sinus syndrome. *Amer J Card* 36: 98, 1975
22. Dhingra, R.C., Deedwania, P.C., Cummings, J.M., Amat-y-Leon, F., Wu, D., Denes, P., Rosen, K.M.: Electrophysiologic effects of lidocaine on sinus node and atrium in patients with and without sinoatrial dysfunction. *Circulation*, in press.
23. Dhingra, R.C., Denes, P., Wu, D., Chuquimia, R., Amat-y-Leon, F., Wyndham, C., Rosen, K.M.: Syncope in patients with chronic bifascicular block. Significance, causative mechanisms, and clinical implication. *Ann Intern Med* 81: 302, 1974
24. Denes, P., Dhingra, R.C., Wu, D., Chuquimia, R., Amat-y-Leon, F., Wyndham, C., Rosen, K.M.: Chronic H-V interval in patients with bifascicular block, right bundle branch block and left anterior hemiblock. Clinical, electrocardiographic, and electrophysiologic correlations. *Amer J Card* 35: 23, 1975

25. Dhingra, R.C., Denes, P., Wu, D., Wyndham, C., Amat-y-Leon, F., Towne, W.D., Rosen, K.M.: Prospective observations in patients with chronic bundle branch block and marked H-V prolongation. *Circulation* 53: 600, 1976

26. Dhingra, R.C., Denes, P., Wu, D., Chuquimia, R., Amat-y-Leon, F., Wyndham, C., Rosen, K.M.: Chronic right bundle branch block and left posterior hemiblock. Clinical, electrophysiologic and prognostic observations. *Amer J Card* 35: 23, 1975

27. Reiffel, J.A., Bigger, J.T., Konstam, M.A.: The relationship between sinoatrial conduction time and sinus cycle length during spontaneous sinus arrhythmia in adults. *Circulation* 50: 924, 1974

28. Amat-y-Leon, F., Wu, D., Dhingra, R., Denes, P., Wyndham, R., Simpson, R., Rosen, K.M.: Electrophysiological mechanisms of supraventricular tachyarrhythmia in patients with sinus node disease. *Circulation* 56 (suppl. III): 106, 1977

SECTION TWO

RELATION BETWEEN STRUCTURE AND FUNCTION OF THE SINUS NODE

13

THE FINE STRUCTURE OF THE SINUS NODE: A SURVEY

J. TRANUM-JENSEN

In this survey it is attempted to summarize the present knowledge about the fine structure of the sinus node with a main emphasis on structures of possible physiological interest, and to illustrate the points with material from dog, pig, and rabbit hearts*. In view of several recent reviews, some of which are very comprehensive, on both light- and electron-microscopial aspects of the sinus node structure (Challice, 1971; Virágh and Challice, 1973b; Truex, 1974, 1976; Tranum-Jensen, 1976), it will not be attempted to review the literature in great detail. The survey is confined to adult mammalian hearts.

The sinus node has been studied with the light microscope in a large number of species (for review see e.g. Robb and Petri, 1961; Truex, 1974, 1976) and with the electron microscope in several: *mouse* (Maekawa et al., 1967), *rat* (Virágh and Porte, 1961; Cheng, 1971), *rabbit* (Torii, 1961; Trautwein and Uchizono, 1963; Challice, 1966; Tranum-Jensen and Bojsen-Møller, 1973), *dog* (Kawamura, 1961; James et al., 1966; Hayashi, 1971), *mole* (Kikuchi, 1976), *cow* (Hayashi, 1962), *monkey* (Colborn and Carsey, 1972; Virágh and Porte, 1973), *human embryos* (Yamauchi, 1965), and *adult man* (James et al., 1966).

When the literature on the fine structure of the sinus node is considered it should be recalled that nearly all ultrastructural studies are performed on morphological nodal tissue, not preceeded by electrophysiological identification, – the only exceptions being studies on the rabbit node (Trautwein and Uchizono, 1963; and by Janse et al. and Masson-Pévet et al., both published in this book). This poses a problem because the boundaries of the morphological node are not sharply defined in several species.

Several types of muscle cells have been described in the sinus node. Though termed differently in different studies, they can be grouped into: a) "typical nodal cells" which is the predominant or exclusive cell type in the central nodal area, b) "transitional cells" which prevail in the peripheral nodal areas, particularly noticed where the nodal tissue joins working atrial myocardium, and c) "intercalated clear cells" which are usually found singly, scattered in the node, though occasionally in small groups. There seems at present no basis for a more detailed morphological classification, and as yet, there is not sufficient direct evidence to specify the precise functional differences between these cell types. It seems therefore advisable to employ functionally neutral terms as those mentioned above.

---

* The material used for illustrations in this contribution is derived from young dogs, pigs and rabbits, fixed in vivo during Nembutal – N₂O anaestesia, while artificially ventilated by vascular perfusion at controlled physiological pressures retrogradely through the aorta, with phosphate or cacodylate buffered glutaraldehyde-formaldehyde mixtures. Tonicity of fixative vehicles kept at 280–300 mOsm, – of total fixatives 700–750 mOsm, pH 7.2–7.3. Postfixation in OsO₄ and embedding in Epon 812. Sections for light microscopy stained with toluidine blue, – for EM with uranyl and lead stains. Labelling of adrenergic fibers was obtained according to Tranzer and Thoenen (1967) by slow intravenous injection of 5-OH-dopamine (80 mg/kg body weight) in dilute aquous solution, 1/2 hour prior to fixation. Staining with ruthenium red was performed on tiny biopsies according to Luft (1971).

THE "TYPICAL NODAL CELLS"

These cells form the bulk of the central part of the node. They are recognized in the light microscope as small, pale staining cells, clustered in irregular strands spaced by connective tissue, vessels and nerves (Figures 1a, b, 2a, b). The cells have diameters at the level of the nucleus of 3–9 μ, mostly around 5 μ. Three dimensional reconstructions of single cells have not been made on the sinus node, but comparison of profiles seen in cross- and longitudinal sections suggests a roughly spindle shaped cell, furnished with irregular extensions (Kawamura, 1961), probably very similar to the reconstructions obtained on atrio-ventricular nodal cells (Thaemert, 1970).

Ultrastructural studies on sinus nodes of mammalia are, with some reservations due to technical limitations in early studies, in good accordance with their descriptions of these main cells of the node, and what is stated below can be taken as a general description of the typical nodal cells in the adult sinus node. For the embryonic sinus node (Yamauchi, 1965) the descriptions will not apply on several points.

THE SARCOLEMMA

The sarcolemma comprises the cell membrane (plasmalemma) and the cell coat (glycocalyx). Several pertinent questions on cell membrane structure in nodal cells cannot be answered since freeze fracture studies are not yet complete. So far, it can only be said that the membrane has the usual thickness of cell membranes, i.e. 8–9 nm, and has a distribution of particles apparently similar to working atrial cardiocytes (see contribution of Masson-Pévet et al. in this book).

The specialized system for inward spread of excitation, the T-tubule system, occurs irregularly in atrial working cardiocytes (Forssmann and Girardier, 1970; Berger and Rona, 1971); it has never been demonstrated in nodal cells.

Small invaginations of the cell membrane, caveolae, having the shape of a small vesicle, 60–80 nm in diameter, connected to the surface by a short neck about 30 nm in diameter, are very frequent along the surface of nodal cells (Figures 4,5,6). It appears that a majority, if not all, of these vesicles seen in the cytoplasm immediately adjacent to the cell membrane, are connected to the surface. Occasionally a vesicle may be seen budding from another vesicle producing a short beaded tube (Figure 6) which is reminiscent of the early stages in the formation of T-tubules (Ezerman and Ishikawa, 1967). Caveolae occur in all cardiocytes, but in greatly varying numbers (Simpson et al., 1973). Their frequency in nodal cells is high and it seems likely that they have an electrophysiological significance. At least on some areas of the cell surface, like in Figure 6, their presence will more than double the membrane area per unit area of the cell surface and herewith probably also the membrane capacitance as suggested for T-tubules in working cardiocytes (Sommer and Johnson, 1968). The membranes of T-tubules and caveolae are morphologically similar in skeletal muscle in that they have no or few intercalated membrane particles, suggesting

Figure 1a. Low power light micrograph of a 1 μ Epon section cut perpendicularly to the sulcus terminalis (st) of a dog heart. The palely stained tissue of the cross sectioned sinus node (N) partly surrounds the nodal artery (A). Cr – working myocardium of crista terminalis. e – endocardium.

b. The area marked by frame in Figure 1a at the border between the nodal tissue (N) and the working myocardium. Transitional cells of small diameter, but well stained, are mixed with palely stained nodal cells in the middle third of the picture.

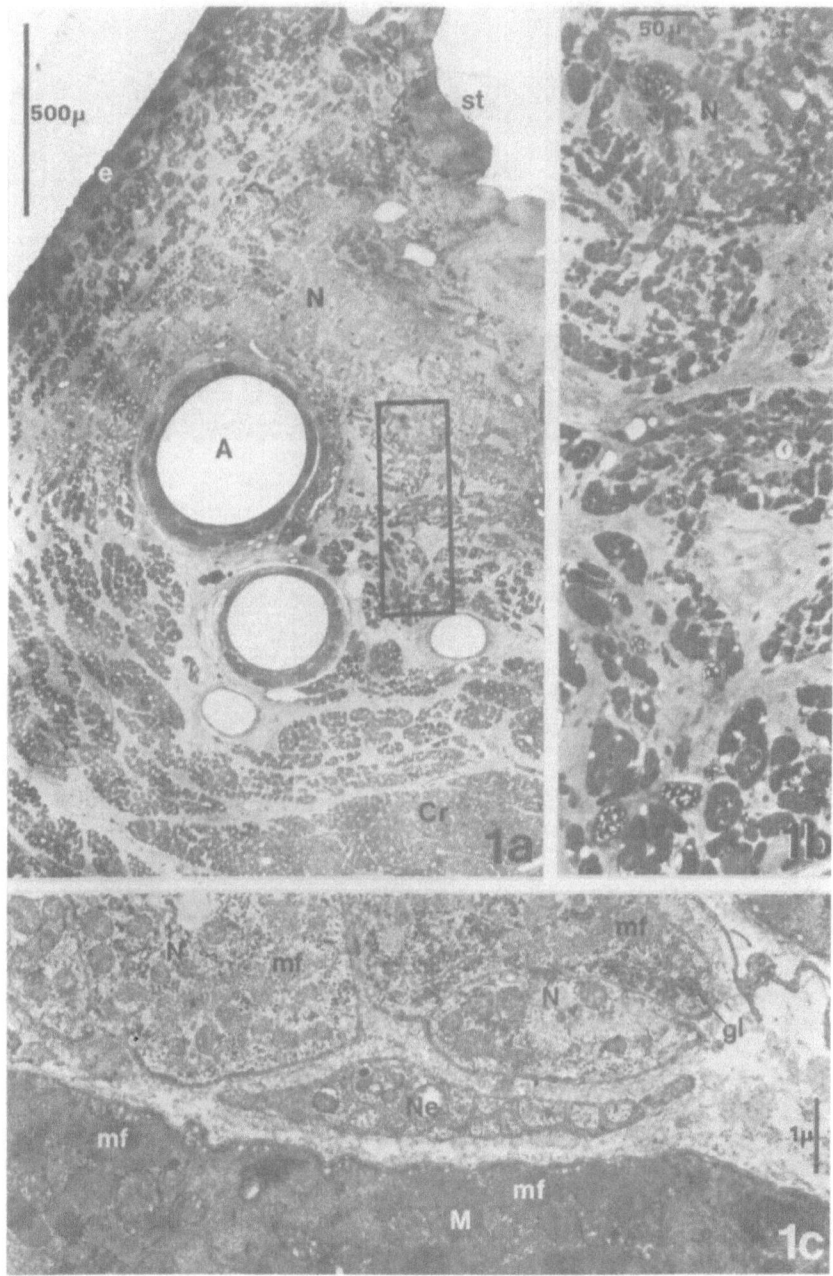

c. Low power electron micrograph from the border zone corresponding to Figure 1b. Part of a transitional cell (M), packed with myofibrils (mf) is seen together with nodal cells (N), poor in myofibrils, but rich in glycogen (gl). Ne – nerve.

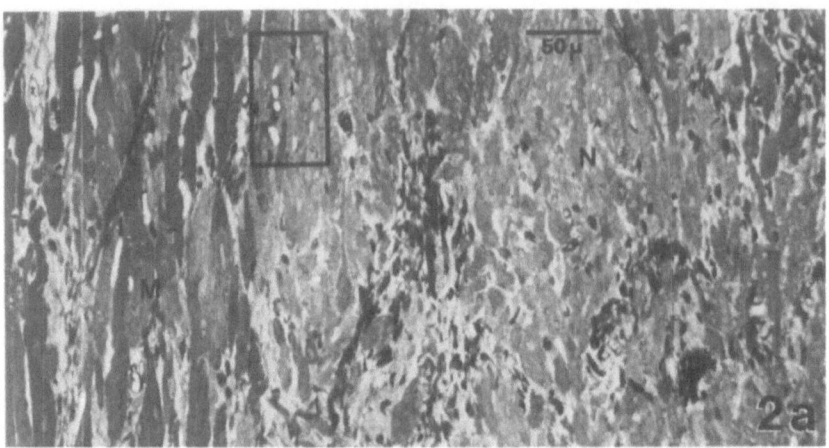

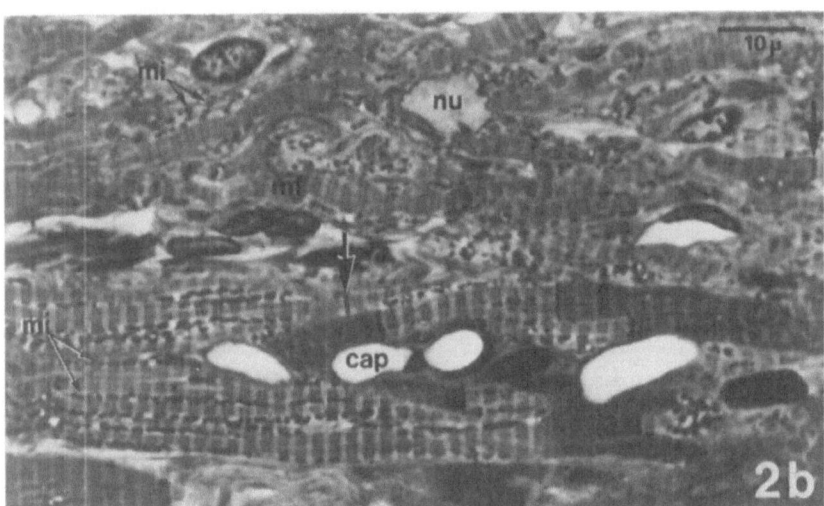

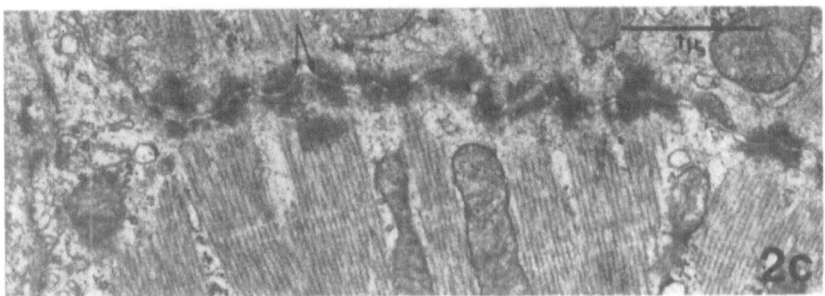

Figure 2a. Light micrograph of a longitudinal section through the sinus node (N) at the border to the working myocardium (M) in a dog heart.

that they, compared to the surrounding cell membrane, are more passive in phenomena involving hydrophilic conductance channels (Dulhunty and Franzini-Armstrong, 1974; Franzini-Armstrong, 1975).

The cell coat covers the exterior of the cell membrane and is seen in ordinary electron micrographs as a 20–40 nm thick fuzzy layer along membranes facing wider intercellular spaces. The outermost layer of the coat has a higher density and is separated from the cell membrane by a lighter stratum; it is often referred to as the external lamina (Figures 5,9, 10a). A cell coat is present on all cardiocytes and its main components are believed to be glycoproteins and acidic mucosubstances (Howse et al., 1970). Ruthenium red which is a positively charged electron dense marker (Luft, 1971; Blanquet, 1976) stains the coat intensely (Figure 7). It has recently been reported that a sarcolemmal preparation obtained by cell fractionation did have an appreciable capacity for binding of calcium ions, and that this binding decreased in the presence of lanthanum ions or ruthenium red (Limas, 1977). It seems reasonable to view the cell coat as a polyanionic, immobile layer which may act as a buffering layer for cations and perhaps as a barrier for some substances. Because components of the cell coat are synthetized in the cell to which the coat belongs (Bennett et al., 1974), it should probably be considered a cell specific, functionally integrated component of the sarcolemma.

FILAMENTOUS AND FIBRILLAR STRUCTURES

One of the most conspicuous features of the typical nodal cells is their poorly developed contractile apparatus, which together with their small size, is one of the main characteristics for their light microscopical identification. Organized sarcomeric fibrils occupy less than half the cell volume and the fibrils are less axially aligned in the cells compared to working cardiocytes. The fibrils are often seen to branch and split off unorganized filaments. The characteristic banding of sarcomeres is less distinct. Particularly H-bands and M-lines are often slurrish and Z-discs are often irregular and show interruptions and thickenings.

Unorganized thin filaments are widely distributed in the cytoplasm. Many of these have a thickness comparable to actin, while others are somewhat thicker (Figure 9) and are likely to be so-called "10 nm filaments" (Small and Sobieszek, 1977). Such filaments have been identified in bovine Purkinje fibres where, as elsewhere, they are supposed to have the function of a cytoskeleton (Eriksson et al., 1976).

Leptomeric fibrils, which are small bundles of thin filaments with a 16 nm transverse banding pattern, occur scattered in various types of cardiocytes (Virágh and Challice, 1969; Bogusch, 1976) and are also found in sinus nodal cells (Figure 9). Their composition and significance are unknown. They are often found in a subsarcolemmal position, but may be found in the cell interior as well, and in the latter case, frequently associated with Z-discs.

---

b. High power light micrograph corresponding to the frame in Figure 2a. Nodal cells with few and wavy myofibrils (mf) occupy the upper half of the picture, while transitional cells containing more and parallel aligned myofibrils are seen in the lower half. Mitochondria (mi) are seen as small dark bodies irregularly distributed in the nodal cells, while they are aligned in regular rows between the myofibrils of the transitional cells. Small transverse stretches of intercalated discs are marked by larger arrows. nu – nucleus of nodal cell. cap – capillary.

c. An intercalated disc similar to those marked in Figure 2b at the border zone of the sinus node towards working myocardium. The disc has a straight, primitive form. Only fasciae adherentes (arrows) are clearly seen.

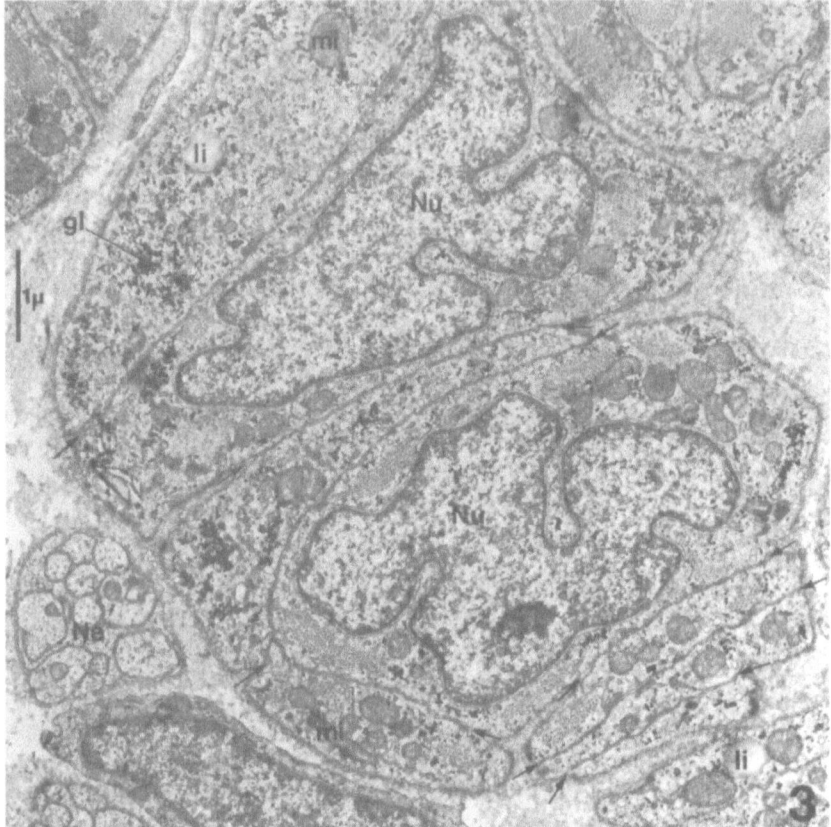

Figure 3. Low power electron micrograph of cross sectioned typical nodal cells of a dog sinus node. Two cells are sectioned at level with the nucleus (Nu) and are in close apposition with several processes of other cells. The narrow (20 nm) clefts between the cells are marked by small arrows. gl – glycogen granules. li – lipid droplets. mi – mitochondria. Ne – small nerve.

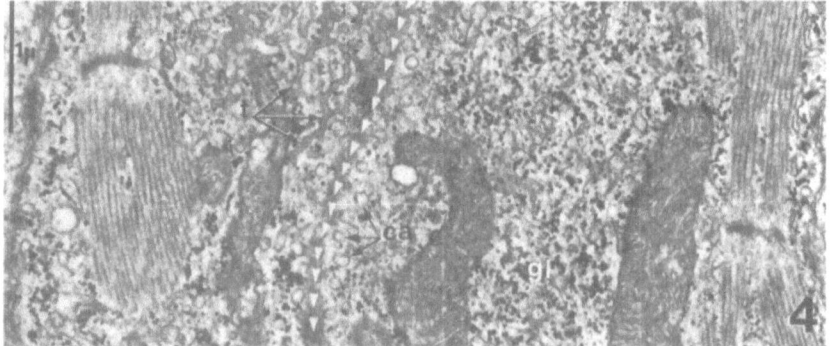

Figure 4. Longitudinal section of two closely apposed processes of typical nodal cells in a dog sinus node. Two cell membranes in close apposition are obliquely sectioned along the line marked by arrowheads. The small vesicles (ca) beneath the cell membranes are likely to be caveolae. Irregular and branching tubular profiles (t) of sarcoplasmic reticulum are seen without relation to myofibrils. A branching myofibril is seen to the right, and numerous glycogen granules (gl) are present in the cytoplasm.

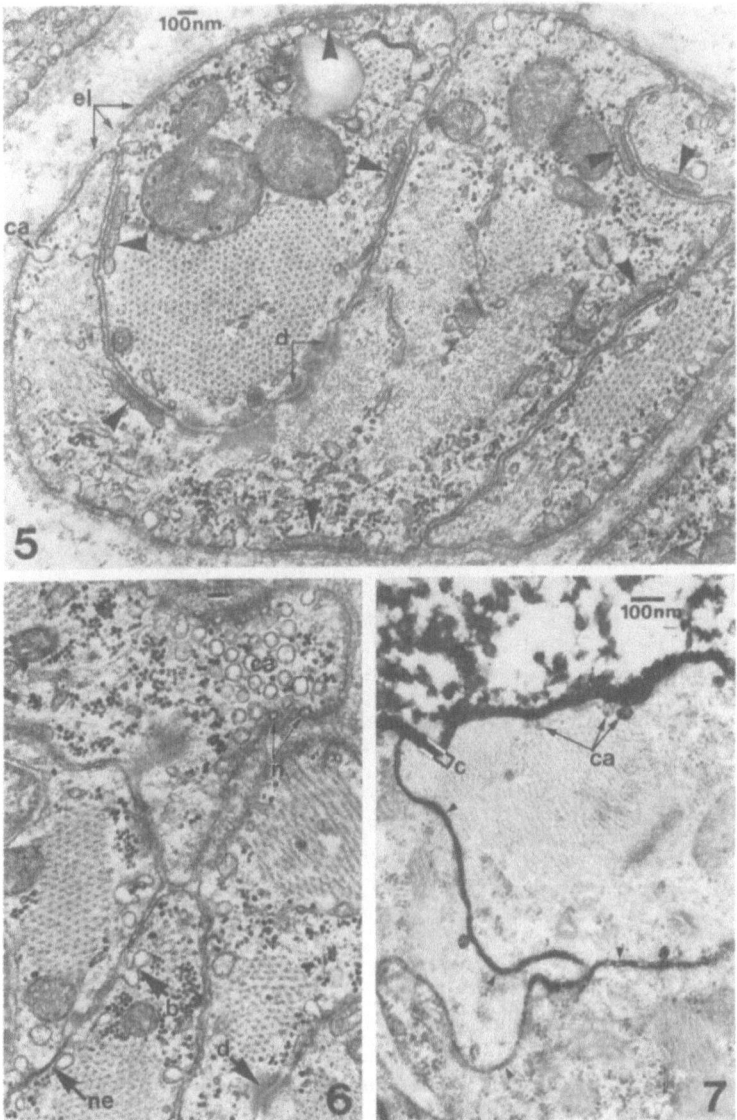

Figure 5. Cross section of a small bundle formed by closely apposed processes of typical nodal cells in a dog sinus node. The external lamina (el) of the cell coat does not enter into the narrow clefts between the cells. Numerous caveolae (ca) and several subsurface cisterns (arrowheads) of the sarcoplasmic reticulum are seen along the cell membranes. d – desmosomes.

Figure 6. Section through processes of nodal cells in a dog showing a small nexus (ne). At upper right a process has been cut tangentially to its surface revealing numerous caveolae, the narrow necks of which (n) are seen in the obliquely sectioned cell membrane. A branching caveola is seen at arrow (b). d – desmosome. Bar indicates 100 nm.

Figure 7. Electron micrograph of typical nodal cells from a rabbit sinus node stained *en bloc* with ruthenium red which binds strongly to the cell coat (c). The marker is present also in the narrow clefts between the cells (small arrowheads). Caveolae (ca) are filled to varying degrees. The structures in the extracellular space in the upper fourth of the picture are transversely sectioned collagen fibrils.

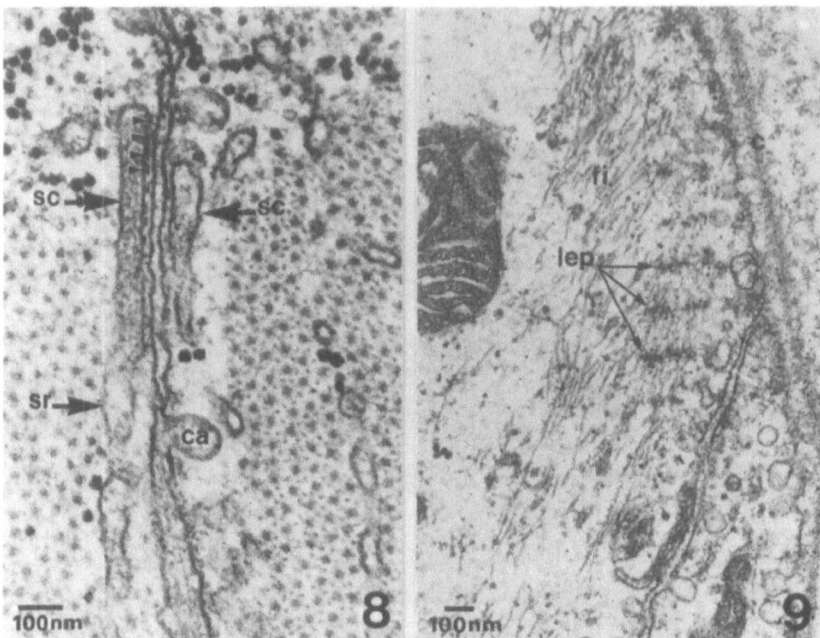

Figure 8. Electron micrograph of parts of two typical nodal cells in a dog sinus node. Subsurface cisterns (sc) containing granular material are seen on each side of the narrow cleft between the cells. Small and regularly spaced densities can be seen in the gap between the cisterns and the cell membrane, most clearly in the cistern to the left (small arrowheads), which is also seen in luminal continuity with a profile of sarcoplasmic reticulum (sr). ca – caveola.

Figure 9. Electron micrograph from the periphery of two nodal cells in a rabbit sinus node. The external lamina of the cell coat (c) is clearly seen. A leptomere fibril with the characteristic transverse banding (lep) is seen in a subsarcolemmal position together with filaments (fi) measuring about 10 nm across. The empty spaces in the cell to the left in the picture did contain glycogen which has been eluated during the preparation.

The myofibrils of nodal cells are structurally reminiscent of myofibrils in embryonic (Virágh and Challice, 1973a) and cultured cardiocytes (Legato, 1972). It has been suggested that the similarly poor development of the contractile apparatus in Purkinje fibres of some species is caused by an imbalance in the synthesis and degradation of myofibrillar proteins (Thornell, 1973), reflecting a decreased selection for contractile properties (Oliphant and Loewen, 1976).

THE SARCOPLASMIC RETICULUM (SR)

Subsarcolemmal cisterns (junctional SR) of the SR are observed in ordinary electron micrographs of nodal cells as elongated membrane bound profiles separated from the inside of the cell membrane by a gap of about 20 nm bridged by small, regularly spaced densities ("feet"). The cisterns contain stained material, usually of a granular appearance (Figures 5, 8). Thus the structure of the cisterns appears similar to those of working cardiocytes (Sommer and Johnson, 1970; Sommer and Waugh, 1976) and skeletal muscle cells (Franzini-Armstrong, 1975). The subsarcolemmal cisterns have been identified as accumulation sites for calcium (Winegrad, 1965; Legato and Langer, 1969; Saetersdal et al., 1974). ATP-ase activity has been demonstrated cytochemically at these sites (Rostgaard and Behnke, 1965) and they are considered a principal site of calcium release in the excitation-contraction coupling (Bassingthwaighte and Reuter, 1972), though their roles in skeletal versus cardiac muscle may be somewhat different (Langer, 1971).

The subsarcolemmal cisterns are in luminal continuity with tubules of SR extending deep into the cell. The nodel cells are obviously not specialized for a contractile function. The SR likewise does not have the degree of organization seen in working cardiocytes (Sommer and Waugh, 1976), and the irregular and branching profiles of SR in nodal cells are often observed without apparant relation to myofibrils (Figure 4).

STRUCTURES ENGAGED IN INTRACELLULAR SYNTHESIS

Nodal cells contains free ribosomes, but because of overlap in size with small glycogen particles, their number is difficult to estimate without special measures taken (Thornell, 1974). Small profiles of rough endoplasmic reticulum are occasionally seen, and small Golgi complexes are usually seen in sections near the nucleus. The atrial specific granules (Jamieson and Palade, 1964; Bencosme and Berger, 1971) which occur regularly in atrial working cardiocytes, and which are often numerous close to the Golgi, have been reported to occur in nodal cells of the monkey (Colborn and Carsey, 1972). However, they are not reported in most studies on the sinus node and it may safely be stated that they do not occur in typical nodal cells with a frequency comparable to that observed in atrial working cardiocytes. These granules were once thought to be storage sites for catecholamines. There is now accumulating evidence that this is not the case (Bencosme and Berger, 1971; De Bold and Bencosme, 1973) and cytochemical analysis indicates a content of complex carbohydrates (Huet et al., 1974). Their significance remains obscure.

STRUCTURES INVOLVED IN CELL METABOLISM

Mitochondria occur in sinus nodal cells with an apparently random distribution and occupy a cell volume fraction, estimated to be lower than in working cardiocytes. They are of very variable shapes and sizes, and their matrix density in well preserved specimen is roughly equal to that of mitochondria in working cardiocytes.

A high content of glycogen is a widely recognized characteristic of the conducting system. Sinus node cells sometimes contain appreciable amounts of glycogen granules, usually in the form of 25–30 nm β-particles (Figures 3, 4); larger aggregate α-particles may also be seen. However the cell volume fraction of glycogen varies considerably between the nodal cells. Some cells contain an amount approaching half the cell volume while others contain amounts comparable to those of working cardiocytes (Virágh and Challice, 1973b; Virágh and Porte, 1973). Conversely, the frequency of lipid droplets seen in thin sections of sinus node cells seems lower compared to working cardiocytes (Figure 3). These features may seem in rough accordance with histochemical studies on the conducting system (Schiebler et al., 1956; Isaacson and Boucek, 1968; Gossrau, 1971) demonstrating enzyme activities indicative for a preponderance of glycolytic over oxidative metabolism.

A NOTE PERTINENT TO THE NATURE OF "CLEAR CELLS"

The glucose residues bound in the osmotically inactive macromolecular glycogen particles represent, when metabolized to low molecular metabolites, as lactate, an osmotic potential for an increase in cell volume. A constant declining number of glycogen granules until complete disappearance has been observed under conditions of ischemic hypoxia in working myocardium, followed by explosive cell swelling upon reperfusion (Jennings and Ganote, 1974), suggesting that such osmotic mechanisms may be operating. Glycogen in the cells of the atrioventricular bundle is rapidly mobilized by isoproterenol, epinephrine, hypoxia, and somewhat less by norepinephrine (Gossrau, 1971), indicating that the stores are labile. The capillary density in conducting tissues seems generally to be lower than in working myocardium (Gallo, 1956; Schiebler and Doer, 1963; Pape et al., 1969) and, therefore, distances of diffusion are longer. This, together with a relatively low coefficient of diffusion for lactate (Eggleton et al., 1928) might cause an accumulation of lactate under certain conditions of enhanced glycogen metabolism and reduced or abolished vascular flow, which are likely to occur in many experimental situations. Cells in a block of tissue, which has been ischemic for some time before removal from the animal and transferred to an approximately normotonic solution, could be expected to swell, particularly those cells with a high glycogen content. In an animal which was frightened before anaestesia and insufficiently ventilated so that circulating catecholamines reach a high level, and in which fixation by perfusion was not completely successful, glycogen-rich cells could be expected to accumulate water by the same mechanism.

The "intercalated clear cells" described in several studies on the sinus- and atrioventricular node and found in various positions in the atria as well (Kawamura, 1961; James et al., 1966; Truex, 1974, 1976; Virágh and Challice, 1973b) do often exhibit a structure which, according to descriptions and published micrographs, could formally be explained by osmotic swelling together with some internal disorganization of a cell of the particular type among which the aberrant cell is found. Furthermore these cells have many similarities to damaged cells, produced by ischemic hypoxia followed by reperfusion (Jennings and Ganote, 1974). The above considerations make it tempting to assume that many of the "intercalated clear cells" described in literature have an artifactual origin, or at least do not represent a normal cell type. It is tentatively suggested that they arise as a product of unphysiological metabolism where glycogen is mobilized more rapidly than low molecular metabolites, particularly lactate, can be removed. In the atrioventricular node it was observed that the frequency of "intercalated clear cells" can vary considerably between preparations from different animals of the same species (Tranum-Jensen, 1976). Individual differences between cells in their capacity for glycolytic metabolism might explain their uneven distribution in the tissue.

INTERCELLULAR CONTACTS

A paucity in specialized intercellular junctions is one of the characteristic features of nodal cells (Kawamura and James, 1971). The typical nodal cells approximate each other quite close for large areas of their surface, being separated by a rather uniform gap of about 20 nm. The nodal cells are not observed in a similar close apposition with other cell types except for axons. The external lamina of the cell coat, covering the cell membrane on surfaces exposed to wider intercellular spaces, does not enter into these narrow clefts (Figure 5). However, some cell coat material is present in the clefts and after staining with ruthenium red the marker is present in these clefts too (Fig. 7), which may indicate the presence of anionic binding sites, though it must be emphasized that the marker is not proven absolutely specific.

The only specialized intercellular contacts regularly found along the 20 nm clefts are fasciae adherentes and small desmosomes. The fasciae adherentes are the sites where myofibrils insert and transfer pull to myofibrils in neighbouring cells and are generally believed to serve·this mechanical purpose only (Dewey, 1969; McNutt, 1970). Mechanical adhesion is likewise the only function so far ascribed to the desmosomes. They have the shape of small rounded discs between apposed cell membranes, – in sections seen as a dense filling with an intermediate line between the cell membranes which at these sites exhibit a distinct layer of dense material on the cytoplasmic side (Rayns et al., 1969). In various epithelia these junctions serve very clearly as attachment sites for numerous 10 nm tonofilaments (Farquhar & Palade, 1963). Such filament attachments may be seen on cardiac desmosomes as well (Muir, 1965). The structural integrity and mechanical stability of fasciae adherentes and desmosomes are dependent of the presence of calcium ions in the extracellular fluid (Dreifuss et al., 1966; Muir, 1967).

Nexuses are widely accepted as the principal low resistance junction between working cardiocytes (Berger, 1972). They appear in electron micrographs with conventional techniques as a stretch of very close (2–3 nm) apposition of distinct and strict parallel membranes. Utilizing small size extracellular tracers and freeze fracture replicas, hexagonally arranged particles are observed which spand the narrow gap. These particles are generally believed to contain the hydrophilic channels responsible for the low electrical resistance across these junctions (Revel and Karnovsky, 1967; McNutt and Weinstein, 1970; Loewenstein, 1976).

The low speed of conduction in the central nodal region (Paes de Carvalho, 1961) and the low margin of safety have often been ascribed to the relative sparsity of nexuses in this tissue, and have lead to proposals for alternative mechanisms of conduction in nodal tissues (Pollack, 1974, 1976, 1977). Recent freeze fracture studies on frog atrial fibers, where the occurrence of nexuses has been questioned, revealed the presence of what was considered a less orderly structured variant of the nexus (Mazet and Cartaud, 1976). It cannot be excluded that similar aberrant types of junctions, difficult to observe in sectioned material, might appear in freeze fracture replicas of nodal tissues.

THE "TRANSITIONAL CELLS"

The boundaries of the typical sinus node tissue towards the surrounding atrial working myocardium are not sharply defined, and the term "transitional cells" is used by many investigators to designate cells, particularly at the border zone, which do not fall into either category. The "transitional cells" are thus separated as a class of small cells with diameters comparable to those of typical nodal cells, but with a higher estimated cell volume fraction of myofibrils which moreover are better organized and more axially aligned than in the typical nodal cells. These cells also form nexuses more frequently than the typical nodal cells. This zone of transition is very broad in the rabbit heart. In the pig and dog heart, the zone of transition is narrower and the various cell types are well illustrated because they can all be seen in the same field at higher magnification (Figures 1a–c, 2a–c).

INNERVATION OF THE SINUS NODE

The sinus node receives an abundant supply of nerve fibers in all mammalian hearts studied (Yamauchi, 1973). Using techniques of catecholamine fluorescence a proportion of the fibers is identified as adrenergic in several species (Angelakos et al., 1963; Dahlström et al., 1965; Nielsen and Owman, 1968; Ehinger et al., 1968; Ellison, 1974). Enzyme histochemical staining for cholinesterase equally reveals an abundant nerve supply (Ehinger et al., 1968; Bojsen-Møller and Tranum-Jensen, 1971, 1972), but the reaction for cholinesterase is not sufficient for the identification of cholinergic fibers (Koelle, 1955). With the electron microscope it is possible to distinguish different types of terminals based on the morphology of synaptic vesicles (Burnstock and Iwayama, 1971), but the preservation of granular cores in vesicles of adrenergic terminals is fortuitous with conventional techniques (Richardson, 1966). The introduction of false transmitter precursors, producing stable precipitates in adrenergic terminals (Tranzer and Thoenen, 1967; Chiba, 1973) now has greatly facilitated the ultrastructural identification of adrenergic fibres. The cholinergic fibers still being identified mostly *per exclusionem* as non-adrenergic (Figure 10c).

By far, most of the axon profiles seen in the sinus node are located in small nerves comprising 5–15 axons, and are located in wider intercellular spaces. Coming down to smaller nerves, the Schwann cell investment becomes incomplete, and finally naked axons travel in the clefts between the nodal cells. Clusters of synaptic vesicles occur regularly in varicosities of naked axons or where the Schwann cell covering is incomplete on small nerves. By far, most varicosities are separated from the nodal cells by more than 100 nm (Figure 10b) and an external lamina is present on both the opposed membranes. Close contacts of 20 nm membrane apposition without investment of external laminae are also found, not frequently, in some species. In the dog they are rarely found (Hayashi, 1970). However in the pig and rabbit heart they are easily found (Figure 10a, c). Close contacts have been pictured clearly in other species also (Cheng, 1971), and they are extremely numerous in the mole heart (Kikuchi, 1976), which is unique also because of the numerous myelinated fibers present among the nodal cells of this species, otherwise being an unusual finding.

Pairs of adrenergic and non-adrenergic varicosities (Figure 10c) are a common finding at least in the rabbit, and a morphological specialization of the apposed axonal membranes has been described, indicative for an interaction between the terminals (Nilsson and Sporrong, 1970).

Besides the efferent nerve terminals, which contain synaptic vesicles, a different type of nerve terminal is found, characterized by its large size and a high content of mitochondria, vacuoles of autophagic activity and residual bodies (Figure 10d). Based on a close structural similarity with known mechanoreceptor endings (Burnstock and Iwayama, 1971, Tranum-Jensen, 1975) such endings are considered to be solitary afferent endings.

Parasympathetic ganglia are located close to and occasionally also within the sinus node. Besides the cholinergic ganglion cells these ganglia contain a population of small granule-containing cells, which form reciprocal synapses with cholinergic terminals. The

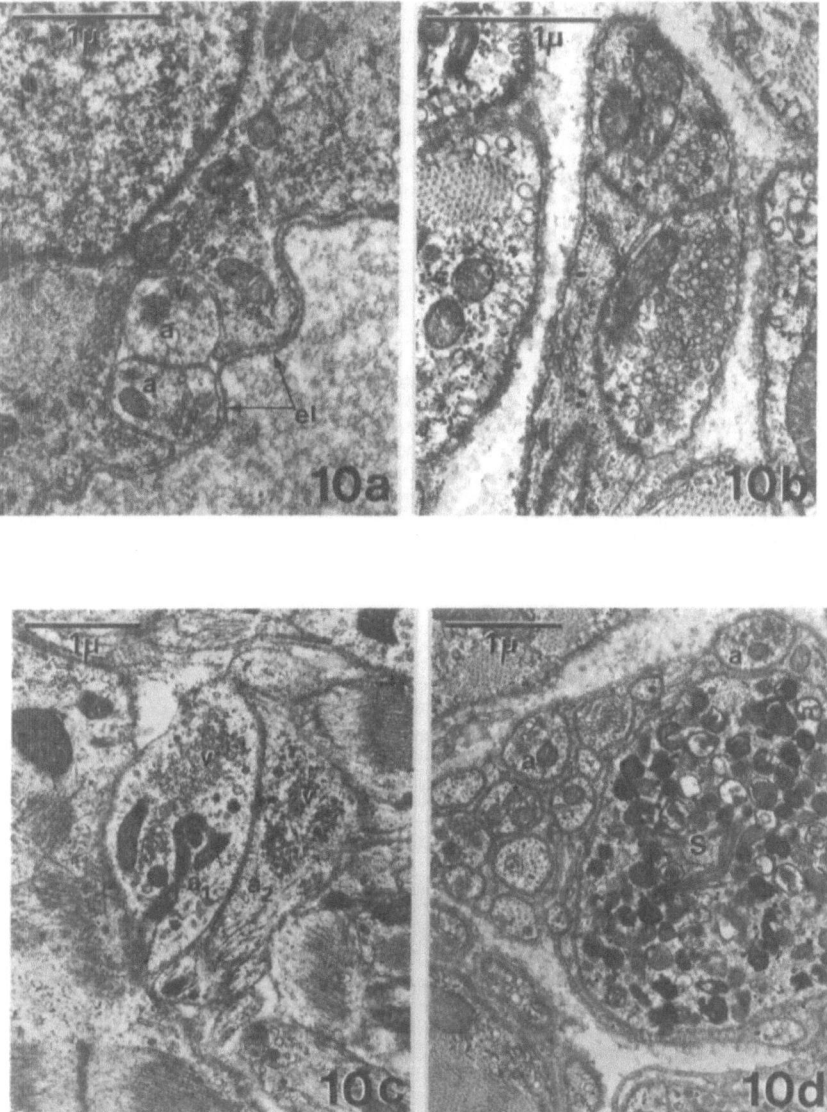

Figure 10a. Electron micrograph of a typical nodal cell from a pig sinus node. The nucleus is seen at upper left. Two adjacent axon profiles (a) containing clusters of synaptic vesicles (v) form close contact with the nodal cell. The external lamina of the cell coat (el) does not enter the 20 nm gap of the close contacts.

b. Electron micrograph from the sinus node of a dog heart. A small nerve enters from below and an axon varicosity containing synaptic vesicles (v) is exposed to the extracellular space to the right, separated from the nearest nodal cell by a gap of 100–200 nm. An external lamina is present on both opposing cell membranes.

c. Electron micrograph of a pair of axon varicosities (a$_1$ and a$_2$) in close contact with surrounding typical nodal cells in a rabbit heart. The animal received 5-OH-dopamine, and the varicosity (a$_2$) is identified as adrenergic because its synaptic vesicles (v) possess distinct dense cores. The neighbouring varicosity (a$_1$) is identified as non-adrenergic because its synaptic vesicles (v) possess no cores.

d. Cross section of a small nerve in a dog sinus node. The nerve contains several small axon profiles with clusters of synaptic vesicles (a), and one large varicosity (S) which contains many mitochondria, autophagic vacuoles, and dense residual bodies, suggestive for it being a sensory terminal.

granule-containing cells are believed to store dopamine and to function in an inhibitory system of the parasympathetic ganglionic transmission. (Jacobowitz, 1967; Yamauchi, 1975; Papka, 1976). Biochemical analysis has indicated dopamine to occur in the sinus node region in a markedly higher concentration than in any other region of the heart analyzed (Angelakos et al., 1963; Angelakos, 1965) and at least part of this dopamine is likely to originate from the granule containing cells of the many parasympathetic ganglia of the region.

REFERENCES

Angelakos, E.T.: Regional Distribution of Catecholamines in the Dog Heart. *Circ Res* 16: 39, 1965
Angelakos, E.T., Fuxe, K., Torchiana, M.L.: Chemical and Histochemical Evaluation of the Distribution of Catecholamines in the Rabbit and Guinea Pig Hearts. *Acta physiol scand* 59: 184, 1963
Bassingthwaighte, J.B., Reuter, H.: Calcium Movements and Excitation-Contraction Coupling in Cardiac Cells. *In*: Electrical Phenomena in the Heart, W.C. De Mello (ed.), p. 353. Academic Press, 1972
Bencosme, S.A., Berger, J.M.: Specific Granules in Mammalian and Non-Mammalian Vertebrate Cardiocytes. *Meth Achievm exp Path* 5: 173, 1971
Bennett, G., Leblond, C.P., Haddad, A.: Migration of Glycoprotein from the Golgi Apparatus to the Surface of Various Cell Types as Shown by Radioautography after Labelled Fucose Injection into Rats. *J Cell Biol* 60: 258, 1974
Berger, J.M., Rona, G.: Functional and Fine Structural Heterogeneity of Atrial Cardiocytes. *Meth Achievm exp Path* 5: 540, 1971
Berger, W.K.: Correlation between the Ultrastructure and Function of Intercellular Contacts. *In*: Electrical Phenomena in the Heart, W.C. De Mello (ed.), p. 63. Academic Press, 1972
Blanquet, P.R.: Ultrahistochemical Study on the Ruthenium Red Surface Staining. II. Nature and Affinity of the Electron Dense Marker. *Histochemistry* 47: 175, 1976
Bogusch, G.: Enzymatic Digestion and Urea Extraction on Leptomeric Structures and Normomeric Myofibrils in Heart Muscle Cells. *J Ultrastructure Res* 55: 245, 1976
Bojsen-Møller, F., Tranum-Jensen, J.: Rabbit heart nodal tissue, sinuatrial ring bundle and atrioventricular connexions identified as a neuromuscular system. *J Anat* 112: 367, 1972
Bojsen-Møller, F., Tranum-Jensen, J.: Whole-mount demonstration of cholinesterase-containing nerves in the right atrial wall, nodal tissue, and atrioventricular bundle of the pig heart. *J Anat* 108: 375, 1971
Burnstock, G., Iwayama, T.: Fine-Structural Identification of Autonomic Nerves and their Relation to Smooth Muscle. *Prog Brain Res* 34: 389, 1971
Challice, C.E.: Studies on the Microstructure of the Heart. I. The sinu-atrial node and sinu-atrial ring bundle. *J Roy Micr Soc* 85: 1, 1966
Challice, C.E.: Functional Morphology of the Specialized Tissues of the Heart. *Meth Achievm exp Path* 5: 121, 1971
Cheng, Y.-P.: The Ultrastructure of the Rat Sino-Atrial Node. *Acta anat Nipponica* 46: 339, 1971
Chiba, T.: Electron Microscopic and Histochemical Studies on the Synaptic Vesicles in Mouse Vas Deferens and Atrium after 5-Hydroxydopamine Administration. *Anat Rec* 176: 35, 1973
Colborn, G.L., Carsey, E. Jr.: Electron Microscopy of the Sino-Atrial Node of the Squirrel Monkey (Saimiri sciureus). *J Mol Cell Cardiol* 4: 525, 1972
Dahlström, A., Fuxe, K., Mya-Tu, M., Zetterström, B.E.M.: Observations on adrenergic innervation of dog heart. *Amer J Physiol* 209: 689, 1965
De Bold, A.J., Bencosme, S.A.: Studies on the Relationship between the Catecholamine Distribution in the Atrium and the Specific Granules Present in Atrial Muscle Cells. 2. Studies on the Sedimentation Pattern of Atrial Noradrenaline and Adrenaline. *Cardiovasc Res* 7: 364, 1973
Dewey, M.M.: The Structure and Function of the Intercalated Disc in Vertebrate Cardiac Muscle. *In*: Comparative Physiology of the Heart, McCann, F.V. (ed.), *Experientia*, suppl. 15: 10, 1969
Dreifuss, J.J., Girardier, L., Forssmann, W.G.: Etude de la propagation de l'excitation dans le ventricule de rat au moyen de solution hypertonique. *Pflügers Arch* 292: 13, 1966
Dulhunty, A.F., Franzini-Armstrong, C.: Caveolae as specialized structural components of the surface membrane of skeletal muscle. *Fed Proc* 33: 401, 1974
Eggleton, G.P., Eggleton, P., Hill, A.V.: The Coefficient of Diffusion of Lactic Acid through Muscle. *Proc Roy Soc, ser B*, 103: 620, 1928
Ehinger, B., Falck, B., Persson, H., Sporrong, B.: Adrenergic and Cholinesterase-Containing Neurons of the Heart. *Histochemie* 16: 197, 1968

Ellison, J.P.: The Adrenergic Cardiac Nerves of the Cat. *Am J Anat* 139: 209, 1974

Eriksson, A., Thornell, L.E., Stigbrand, T.: Ultrastructural and biochemical observations on cytoplasmic filaments of heart Purkinje fibers. *J Ultrastructure Res* 54: 481, 1976

Ezerman, E.B., Ishikawa, H.: Differentiation of the Sarcoplasmic Reticulum and T System in Developing Chick Skeletal Muscle In Vitro. *J Cell Biol* 35: 405, 1967

Farquhar, M.G., Palade, G.E.: Junctional Complexes in Various Epithelia. *J Cell Biol* 17: 375, 1963

Forssmann, W.G., Girardier, L.: A Study of the T System in Rat Heart. *J Cell Biol* 44: 1, 1970

Franzini-Armstrong, C.: Membrane particles and transmission at the triad. *Fed Proc* 34: 1382, 1975

Gallo, P.: A study on the topographical and quantitative relations between capillaries and fibres of the conduction system of the heart and on their functional significance. *Cardiologia (Basel)* 29: 241, 1956

Gossrau, R.: Histochemische, fluoreszenzmikroskopische und experimentelle Untersuchungen am Reizleitungssystem von Goldhamster, Maus und Ratte. *Histochemie* 26: 44, 1971

Hayashi, K.: An Electron Microscope Study on the Conduction System of the Cow Heart. *Jap Circ J* 26: 765, 1962

Hayashi, S.: Electron Microscopy of the Heart Conduction System of the Dog. *Arch histol jap* 33: 67, 1971

Hayashi, S., Oga, K., Otsuka, N.: The Fine Structure of Nerve Endings in the Sinus Node of the Canine Heart. *J Electron Micr* 19: 176, 1970

Howse, H.D., Ferrans, V.J., Hibbs, R.G.: A Comparative Histochemical and Electron Microscopic Study of the Surface Coatings of Cardiac Muscle Cells. *J Mol Cell Cardiol* 1: 157, 1970

Huet, M., Benchimol, S., Castonguay, Y., Cantin M.: Ultrastructural Cytochemistry of Atrial Muscle Cells, III. Reactivity of Specific Granules in Man. *Histochemistry* 41: 87, 1974

Isaacson, R., Boucek, R.J.: The atrioventricular conduction tissue of the dog. Histochemical properties; influence of electric shock. *Am Heart J* 75: 206, 1968

Jacobowitz, D.: Histochemical studies on the relationship of chromaffin cells and adrenergic nerve fibers to the cardiac ganglia of several species. *J Pharmacol exp Ther* 158: 227, 1967

James, T.N., Sherf, L., Fine, G., Morales, A.R.: Comparative Ultrastructure of the Sinus Node in Man and Dog. *Circulation* 34: 139, 1966

Jamieson, J.D., Palade, G.E.: Specific Granules in Atrial Muscle Cells. *J Cell Biol* 23: 151, 1964

Jennings, R.B., Ganote, C.E.: Structural Changes in Myocardium During Acute Ischemia. *Circ Res* 34–35, suppl. III: 156, 1974

Kawamura, K.: Electron Microscope Studies on the Cardiac Conduction System of the Dog. II. The Sino-atrial and Atrioventricular Nodes. *Jap Circ J* 25: 973, 1961

Kawamura, K., James, T.N.: Comparative Ultrastructure of Cellular Junctions in Working Myocardium and the Conduction System under Normal and Pathologic Conditions. *J Mol Cell Cardiol* 3: 31, 1971

Kikuchi, S.: The Structure and Innervation of the Sinu-Atrial Node of the Mole Heart. *Cell Tiss Res* 172: 345, 1976

Koelle, G.B.: The Histochemical Identification of Acetyl-Cholinesterase in Cholinergic, Adrenergic and Sensory Neurons. *J Pharm exp Ther* 114: 167, 1955

Langer, G.A.: Coupling calcium in mammalian ventricle: its source and factors regulating its quantity. *Cardiovascular Res* suppl. I: 71, 1971

Legato, M.J.: Ultrastructural Characteristics of the Rat Ventricular Cell Grown in Tissue Culture, with Special Reference to Sarcomerogenesis. *J Mol Cell Cardiol* 4: 299, 1972

Legato, M.J., Langer, G.A.: The Subcellular Localization of Calcium Ion in Mammalian Myocardium. *J Cell Biol* 41: 401, 1969

Limas, C.J.: Calcium-Binding Sites in Rat Myocardial Sarcolemma. *Arch Biochem Biophys* 179: 302, 1977

Loewenstein, W.R.: Permeable Junctions. *Cold Spring Harbor Symp Quant Biol* 40: 49, 1976

Luft, J.H.: Ruthenium Red and Violet. II. Fine Structural Localization in Animal Tissues. *Anat Rec* 171: 369, 1971

Maekawa, M., Nohara, Y., Kawamura, K., Hayashi, K.: Electron Microscope Study of the Conduction System in Mammalian Hearts. *In*: Electrophysiology and Ultrastructure of the Heart, T. Sano, V. Mizuhira, K. Matsuda (eds.), p. 41. Bunkodo, Tokyo, 1967

Mazet, F., Cartaud, J.: Freeze-Fracture Studies of Frog Atrial Fibres. *J Cell Sci* 22: 427, 1976

McNutt, N.S.: Ultrastructure of Intercellular Junctions in Adult and Developing Cardiac Muscle. *Amer J Cardiol* 25: 169, 1970

McNutt, N.S., Weinstein, R.S.: The Ultrastructure of the Nexus. *J Cell Biol* 47: 666, 1970

Muir, A.R.: Further observations on the cellular structure of cardiac muscle. *J Anat* 99: 27, 1965

Muir, A.R.: The effects of divalent cations on the ultrastructure of the perfused rat heart. *J Anat* 101: 239, 1967

Nielsen, K.C., Owman, Ch.: Difference in cardiac adrenergic innervation between hibernators and non-hibernating mammals. *Acta physiol scand*, suppl. 316: 1, 1968

Nilsson, E., Sporrong, B.: Electron Microscopic Investigation of Adrenergic and Non-Adrenergic Axons in the Rabbit SA-Node. *Z Zellforsch* 111: 404, 1970

Oliphant, L.W., Loewen, R.D.: Filament Systems in Purkinje Cells of the Sheep Heart: Possible Alterations of Myofibrillogenesis. *J Mol Cell Cardiol* 8: 679, 1976

Paes de Carvalho, A.: Cellular Electrophysiology of the Atrial Specialized Tissues. *In*: The Specialized Tissues of the Heart, A. Paes de Carvalho, W.C. De Mello, B.F. Hoffman (eds.), p. 115. Elsevier, Amsterdam, 1961.

Pape, C., Kübler, W., v. Smekal, P.: Morphometrie am Reizleitungssystem und Arbeitsmyokard des Kalbherzens. *Beitr path Anat* 140: 23, 1969

Papka, R.E.: Studies of Cardiac Ganglia in Pre- and Postnatal Rabbits. *Cell Tiss Res* 175: 17, 1976

Pollack, G.H.: AV nodal transmission: A proposed electromechanical mechanism. *J Electrocardiol* 7: 245, 1974

Pollack, G.H.: Intercellular Coupling in the Atrioventricular Node and Other Tissues of the Rabbit Heart. *J Physiol* 255: 275, 1976

Pollack, G.H.: Cardiac Pacemaking: An Obligatory Role of Catecholamines? *Science* 196: 731, 1977

Rayns, D.G., Simpson, F.O., Ledingham, J.M.: Ultrastructure of desmosomes in mammalian intercalated disc; appearances after lanthanum treatment. *J Cell Biol* 42: 322, 1969

Revel, J.P., Karnovsky, M.J.: Hexagonal Array of Subunits in Intercellular Junctions of the Mouse Heart and Liver. *J Cell Biol* 33: C7, 1967

Richardson, K.C.: Electron Microscopic Identification of Autonomic Nerve Endings. *Nature* 210: 756, 1966

Robb, J.S., Petri, R.: Expansions of the Atrio-Ventricular System in the Atria. *In*: The Specialized Tissues of the Heart, A. Paes de Carvalho, W.C. De Mello, B.F. Hoffman (eds.), p. 1. Elsevier, Amsterdam, 1961

Rostgaard, J., Behnke, O.: Fine Structural Localization of Adenine Nucleoside Phosphatase Activity in the Sarcoplasmic Reticulum of Striated Muscle. *In*: Intracellular Transport, p. 103, Academic Press, 1966

Saetersdal, T.S., Myklebust, R., Berg Justesen, N.-P.: Ultrastructural Localization of Calcium in the Pigeon Papillary Muscle as Demonstrated by Cytochemical Studies and X-Ray Microanalysis. *Cell Tiss Res* 155: 57, 1974

Schiebler, T.H., Starck, M., Caesar, R.: Die Stoffwechsel-situation des Reizleitungssystems. *Klin Wschr* 34: 181, 1956

Schiebler, T.H., Doer, W.: Ortholigie des Reizleitungssystems. *In*: Das Herz des Menschen, W. Bargman, W. Doer, eds., Thieme, Stuttgart, 1963

Simpson, F.O., Rayns, D.G., Ledingham, J.M.: The Ultrastructure of Ventricular and Atrial Myocardium. *In*: Ultrastructure of the Mammalian Heart, C.E. Challice, S. Virágh, eds., p. 1. Academic Press, 1973

Small, J.V., Sobieszek, A.: Studies on the Function and Composition of the 10 nm (100 A) Filaments of Vertebrate Smooth Muscle. *J Cell Sci* 23: 243, 1977

Sommer, J.R., Johnson, E.A.: Cardiac Muscle, – A Comparative Study of Purkinje Fibers and Ventricular Fibers. *J Cell Biol* 36: 497, 1968

Sommer, J.R., Johnson, E.A.: Comparative Ultrastructure of Cardiac Cell Membrane Specializations. A Review. *Amer J Cardiol* 25: 184, 1970

Sommer, J.R., Waugh, R.A.: The Ultrastructure of the Mammalian Cardiac Muscle Cell – with Special Emphasis on the Tubular Membrane Systems. *Amer J Pathol* 82: 192, 1976

Thaemert, J.C.: Atrioventricular Node Innervation in Ultrastructural Three Dimensions. *Am J Anat* 128: 239, 1970

Thornell, L.E.: Evidence of an Imbalance in Synthesis and Degradation of Myofibrillar Proteins in Rabbit Purkinje Fibres. *J Ultrastructural Res* 44: 85, 1973

Thornell, L.E.: Distinction of Glycogen and Ribosome Particles in Cow Purkinje Fibers by Enzymatic Digestion *En bloc* and in Sections. *J Ultrastructure Res* 47: 153, 1974

Torii, H.: Electron Microscope Observations of the S-A and A-V Nodes and Purkinje Fibers of the Rabbit. *Jap Circ J* 26: 39, 1962

Tranum-Jensen, J.: The ultrastructure of the sensory end-organs (baroreceptors) in the atrial endocardium of young mini-pigs. *J Anat* 119: 255, 1975

Tranum-Jensen, J.: The fine structure of the atrial and atrioventricular (AV) junctional specialized tissues of the rabbit heart. *In*: The Conduction System of the Heart, H.J.J. Wellens, K.I. Lie, M.J. Janse (eds.), p. 55. H.E. Stenfert Kroese, Leiden, 1976

Tranum-Jensen, J., Bojsen-Möller, F.: The ultrastructure of the Sinuatrial Ring Bundle and of the Caudal Extension of the Sinus Node in the Right Atrium of the Rabbit Heart. *Z Zellforsch* 138: 97, 1973

Tranzer, J.P., Thoenen, H.: Electronmicroscopic Localization of 5-hydroxydopamine (3,4,5-trihydroxy-phenyl-ethylamine), a New "False" Sympathetic Transmitter. *Experientia* 23: 743, 1967

Trautwein, W., Uchizono, K.: Electron Microscopic and Electrophysiologic Study of the Pacemaker in the Sino-Atrial Node of the Rabbit Heart. *Z Zellforsch* 61: 96, 1963

Truex, R.C.: Structural Basis of Atrial and Ventricular Conduction. *Cardiovasc Clin* 6: 1, 1974

Truex, R.C.: The sinoatrial node and its connections with the atrial tissues. *In*: The Conduction System of the Heart, H.J.J. Wellens, K.I. Lie, M.J. Janse (eds.), p. 209. H.E. Stenfert Kroesé, Leiden, 1976

Virágh, S., Challice, C.E.: Variations in filamentous and fibrillar organization, and associated sarcolemmal structures, in cells of the normal mammalian heart. *J Ultrastructure Res* 28: 321, 1969

Virágh, S., Challice, C.E.: Origin and Differentiation of Cardiac Muscle Cells in the Mouse. *J Ultrastructure Res* 42: 1, 1973a.

Virágh, S., Challice, C.E.: The Impulse Generation and Conduction System of the Heart. *In*: Ultrastructure of the Mammalian Heart, C.E. Challice, S. Virágh (eds.), p. 43. Academic Press, 1973b

Virágh, S., Porte, A.: Structure Fine du Tissu Vecteur dans le Coeur de Rat. *Z Zellforsch* 55: 263, 1961

Virágh, S., Porte, A.: The Fine Structure of the Conducting System of the Monkey Heart (Macaca mulatta). I. The Sino-atrial Node and the Internodal Connections. *Z Zellforsch* 145: 191, 1973

Winegrad, S.: Autoradiographic studies of intracellular calcium in frog skeletal muscle. *J Gen Physiol* 48: 455, 1965

Yamauchi, A.: Electron Microscopic Observations on the Development of S-A and A-V Nodal Tissues in the Human Embryonic Heart. *Z Anat Entw Gesch* 124: 562, 1965

Yamauchi, A.: Ultrastructure of the Innervation of the Mammalian Heart. *In*: Ultrastructure of the Mammalian Heart, C.E. Challice, S. Virágh (eds.), p. 127. Academic Press, 1973

Yamauchi, A., Yokota, R., Fujimaki, Y.: Reciprocal Synapses between Cholinergic Axons and Small Granule-containing Cells in the Rat Cardiac Ganglion. *Anat Rec* 181: 195, 1975

14

THE DEVELOPMENT OF THE SINOATRIAL NODE*

ROBERT H. ANDERSON, HO SIEW YEN, ANTON E. BECKER, AND
JOHN A. GOSLING

INTRODUCTION

In contrast to the many investigations devoted to the morphological development of the atrioventricular specialized tissues (see James, 1970; Anderson and Taylor, 1972 for review) few researchers have studied the development of the sinoatrial node. Amongst the reports existing on this subject, descriptions of the initial histological differentiation of the node differ markedly. Some investigations have failed to distinguish nodal tissue until relatively late in development. Thus, Shaner (1929) first observed structurally distinct nodal cells in a 100 mm calf fetus while Robb, Kaylor and Turman (1948) first noted this tissue in a 160 mm human fetus. In contrast, Sanabria (1936), Walls (1947), Muir (1951), Van Mierop and Gessner (1970) and Yamauchi (1965) have all recognized specialized tissue at much earlier stages prior to completion of septation of the developing heart. Further disagreement concerns the origin of the node as either a paired (Patten, 1956) or as a unilateral structure (Van Mierop and Gessner, 1970). An entirely different area of controversy surrounds the presence or absence of specialized connexions extending from the sionatrial node through the atrial myocardium (James, 1970; Janse and Anderson, 1974).

In an effort to resolve some of these discrepancies, we have examined the histological and histochemical features of the sinoatrial node in a series of human fetuses from stages prior to completion of septation to the mid-term stage. In addition, we have studied a series of neonatal hearts to assess the structure, disposition and connexions of the sinoatrial node at the time of birth.

MATERIALS AND METHODS

The material (see Anderson and Taylor, 1972; Anderson et al., 1976, 1977 for details) comprises a graded series of human fetuses prepared either by routine paraffin wax embedding techniques or by fresh frozen cryostat sectioning methods. The latter procedures permitted the application of histochemical techniques for the demonstration of tissue cholinesterase activity (Anderson and Taylor, 1972). In demonstrating the latter enzymes, specific inhibitors (Gosling, 1969) were used in eight newly prepared fetuses between the ages of $6\frac{1}{2}$ and 14 weeks to distinguish between acetyl- and non-specific cholinesterase activity. In addition we have examined four fetuses of crown-rump length 12, 16, 28, and 40 mm, respectively, provided by Dr. L.M. Gerlis.

* Supported by a grant from the British Heart Foundation.
* The editor preferred "sinoatrial" instead of "sinuatrial,"

Finally, a series of eight neonatal hearts was studied in which the junctional regions of the superior and inferior venae cavae together with the right atrium were removed as a single block of tissues. Prior to processing the blocks were graphically drawn to scale, embedded in paraffin wax and serially sectioned at 10 micron thickness. One section in each twenty-fifth cut was mounted and stained using a trichrome technique. Following study of these sections, the position of the sinoatrial node together with its principal blood supply were superimposed on the graphic representations of the original blocks.

RESULTS

(a) EARLY DEVELOPMENT

The youngest fetuses studied were of crown-rump length 12 mm, 15 mm and 16 mm, respectively, and in all three the venous valves (particularly the right) were prominent structures located at the junction of the sinus venosus and the primitive atrium (Figure 1). When traced inferiorly, the inferior commissure of the valves was related to the atrioventricular endocardial cushion tissues, which together with atrioventricular sulcus tissue separated it from the primordium of the compact atrioventricular node derived from atrioventricular ring tissue (Figure 1). Superiorly, the venous valve tissue was aggregated into a second commissure, the septum spurium. The junction of venous valves, primitive atrium and wall of the superior vena cava was thickened as a semi-circular cushion which encircled the anterior margin of the superior vena cava (Figure 2a). Close examination of this cushion revealed that it had several specific tissue components. On its endocardial aspect the wall of the superior vena cava and the wall of the primitive atrium extended down in bilaminar fashion to form the substance of the venous valves. However, in the region in which these two layers joined to form the valve, a discrete cylinder of cells was identified in the epicardial aspect of the stem of the junction (Figure 2b). This cylinder was arranged so as to encircle the anterior quadrants of the superior vena caval – right atrial junction, and also extended laterally and downwards towards the opening of the inferior vena cava (Figure 2a).

Histologically the cells of the superior vena cava, right atrium and venous valves were of similar size, shape, arrangement and staining affinity. However, the cells of the epicardial cylinder were smaller and more loosely arranged in reticulated interweaving fashion (Figure 3a and b).

(b) CONTINUING FETAL DEVELOPMENT

In the present study, data on fetal development of the node from the 28 mm to mid-term stages were obtained from freshly prepared material in which histological and histochemical techniques were employed on serial sections. Four fetuses were studied ranging between 28 mm and 40 mm crown rump length (approximately 7 weeks age). In all these specimens, the sinoatrial node was clearly identified histologically as an epicardial collection of cells in the sulcus terminalis. The cell mass was concentrated at the lateral quadrant of the junction of the superior vena cava and the right atrium and was composed of tightly packed cells set in a collagen matrix (Figure 4). The cells formed interconnecting fasciculi which were separated by connective tissue elements. Nodal cells and developing atrial

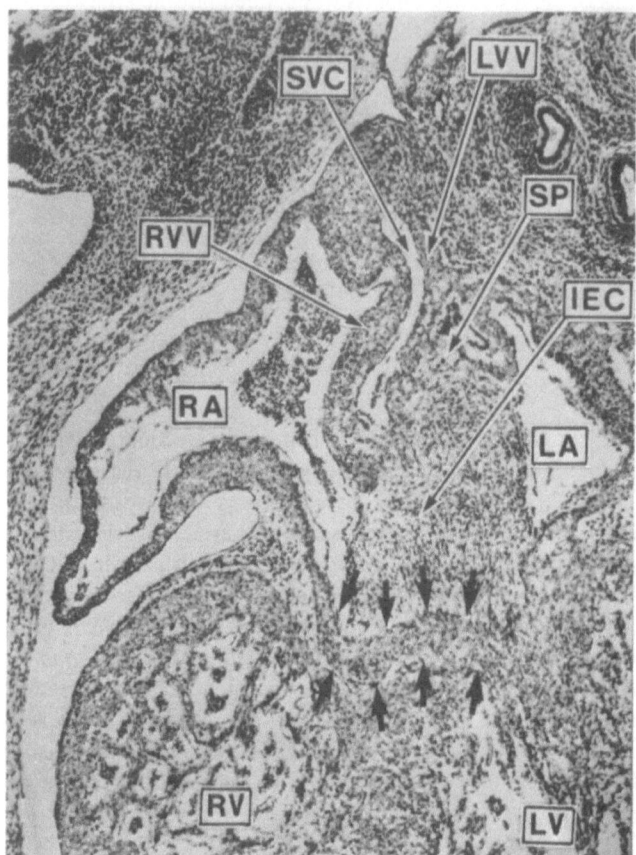

Figure 1. Section through the developing right atrium (RA) of a 15 mm human fetus. The section passes through the lower part of the junction of the superior vena cava (SVC) with the atrium. Note the prominent right venous valve (RVV) and the left venous valve (LVV) fused with the septum primum (SP). Note also that although the venous valve extends towards the atrioventricular junction, it is separated from the atrioventricular ring specialized tissue (between arrows) by the inferior endocardial cushion (IEC). LA – left atrium; RV – right ventricle; LV – left ventricle.

myocardium were histologically distinct and were separated by a very narrow zone of intermediate transitional cells (Figure 5). The node extended epicardially and medially in front of the superior vena cava for a short distance, but a distinct prolongation, the cauda, extended downwards alongside the orifice of the inferior vena cava (Figure 5). In all hearts studied, the cells of the node were cholinesterase positive when compared with the cells of the atrial myocardium (Figures 4–6). Numerous cholinesterase positive autonomic ganglion cells were identified epicardially in relation to the nodal cells. In addition large cholinesterase-positive nerve bundles extended into the node. The enzyme activity in these specimens was predominantly due to non-specific tissue cholinesterases.

Other than for the cauda of the node, distinct projections or discrete tracts of nodal tissue extending into the surrounding atrial myocardium were not observed. In a single specimen of 60 mm length a strand of larger cells was observed on the endocardial

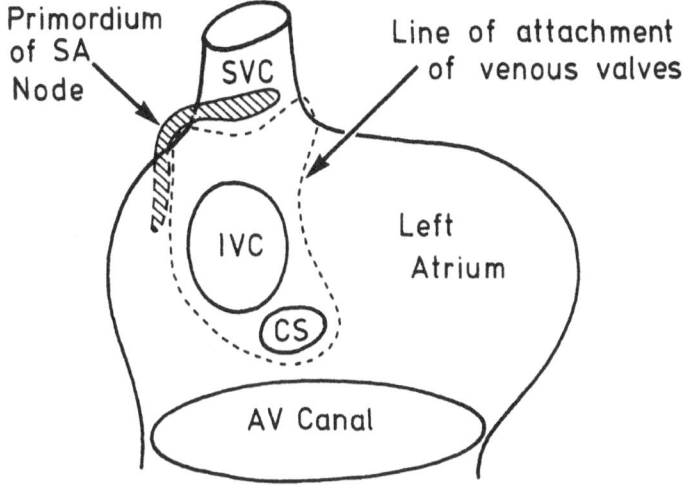

Figure 2a. Diagram representing the location of the cylinder of cells forming the primordium of the sinoatrial (SA) node and its relationship to the attachment of the venous valves. (SVC – superior vena cava; IVC – inferior vena cava; CS – coronary sinus; AV – atrioventricular). Figure 2b shows a cross-section through the sinoatrial junction, illustrating the relationship of the nodal primordium to the atrial wall and the venous valves.

aspect of the right side of the atrial septum (Figure 7a). The cells were cholinesterase positive (Figure 7b). However, when traced in serial sections, the strand made no contact with either node, fading out in the substance of the septum. Such strands were not identified in any other specimen.

    In specimens in excess of 28 mm in length it was considerably easier to identify nodal tissue in the freshly prepared material than in the paraffin embedded material. The reasons for this were threefold. Firstly, intercellular relationships were better preserved in fresh material, secondly the collagen matrix of the node was more readily stained and thirdly it

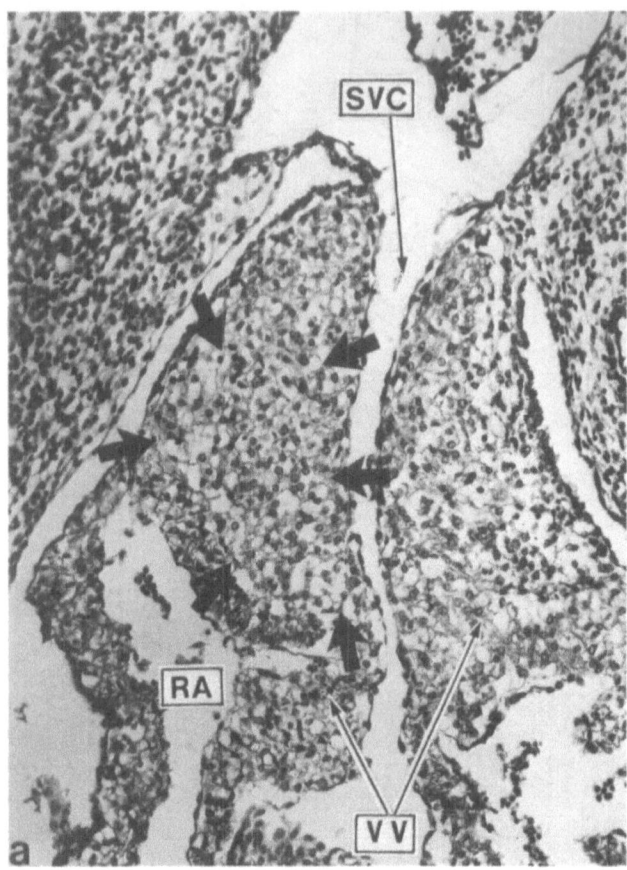

was possible to examine the cholinesterase differentiation of the node in cryostat sections (Figures 4–6).

At mid-term, as in earlier material, the node consisted histologically of densely packed and interconnecting fasciculi of small cells (Figure 6a) frequently arranged around a prominent nodal artery. At the margins of the node, the transitional zone was evident between the nodal fasciculi lying in their fibrous matrix and the dispersed and individually separated atrial myocardial cells of the crista terminalis and the superior caval wall (Figure 6). This short transitional zone surrounded the nodal cells and separated them from adjacent myocardium. Histologically distinct tracts of nodal tissue (other then for the extensive epicardial cauda and the shorter medial extension across the crista terminalis) were absent. In terms of size, the node itself was decreased relative to the remainder of the right atrial structures. In essence, during development the atrial myocardium outstrips the growth of nodal cells resulting in a relative increase in size of the atrium compared with that of the node (compare Figures 3, 5 and 6). In addition the left venous valve was virtually absent. The right valve, whilst still appearing to form a valve for the inferior vena cava, was considerably attenuated.

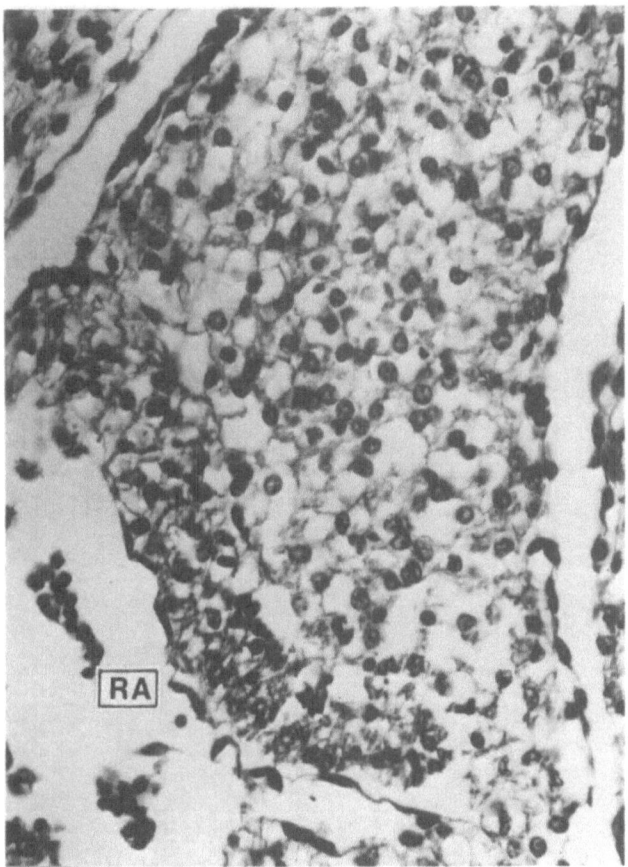

Figure 3. Histological sections of the junction of the superior vena cava (SVC) with the right atrium (RA) in a 15 mm human fetus. Note how the atrial cells are continued into the venous valves (VV), and how a cylinder of slightly different cells is located in the epicardial fold of the lateral junction (between arrows). This cylinder is shown in higher magnification in Figure 3b.

As in earlier material, the sinoatrial node and atrioventricular node together with nervous tissue were clearly cholinesterase positive (Figure 6).

NEONATAL MATERIAL

In all eight hearts studied the sinoatrial node was clearly identified in epicardial position in the sulcus terminalis. Whilst there was marked individual variation in size, shape and vascular supply of the nodes examined in this study (Figure 8), all had the principal mass of nodal cells lying lateral to the junction of the superior vena cava and the right atrium. In only one heart did a medial extension of the node pass over the crest of the junction

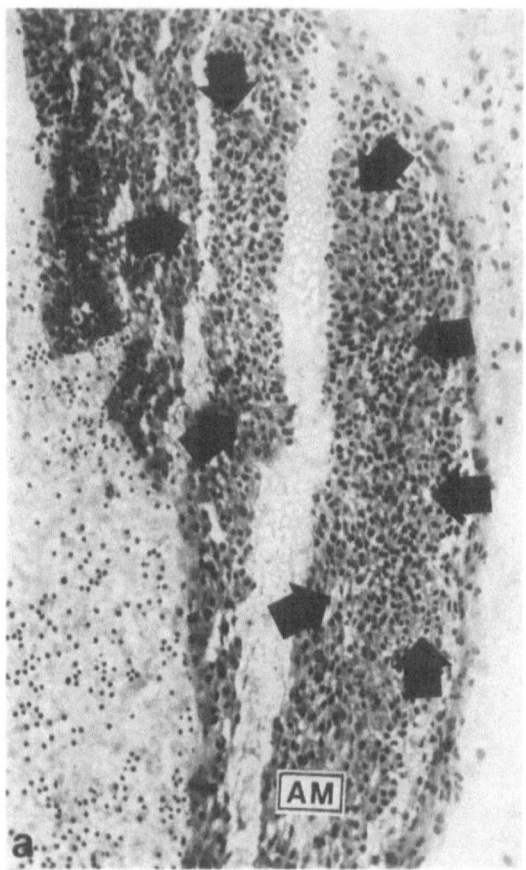

between the atrial appendage and the superior vena cava. A cauda was present in all hearts, varying considerably in size and extent. In those hearts in which the caudae were particularly extensive, nodal tissue passed amongst atrial myocardium as a small column of tightly packed sinoatrial nodal cells (Figure 9). However, the transition between node and atrial myocardial tissue was distinct in all preparations, and as in the fetal hearts, intraatrial tracts were not identified. Concerning the arrangement of vessels, only in 4 specimen was a single large artery found to extend throughout the length of the node. In the remaining 4 hearts a large artery entered either at one or both ends of the node and subsequently divided to ramify within the nodal substance (Figure 8). The course of the main artery was inconstant, usually running along the anterior atrial wall and then passing either in front (2 cases), behind (4 cases) or encircling (2 cases) the superior vena cava to enter the node (Figure 8).

In the neonatal series, nodal size was relatively small when compared to the bulk of the atrial tissues. It is also noteworthy that the nodal cells were interspaced between a fibrous tissue matrix in these specimens. Indeed, this collagen was useful as a guide to the position of the sinoatrial node in trichrome stained sections (Figure 9).

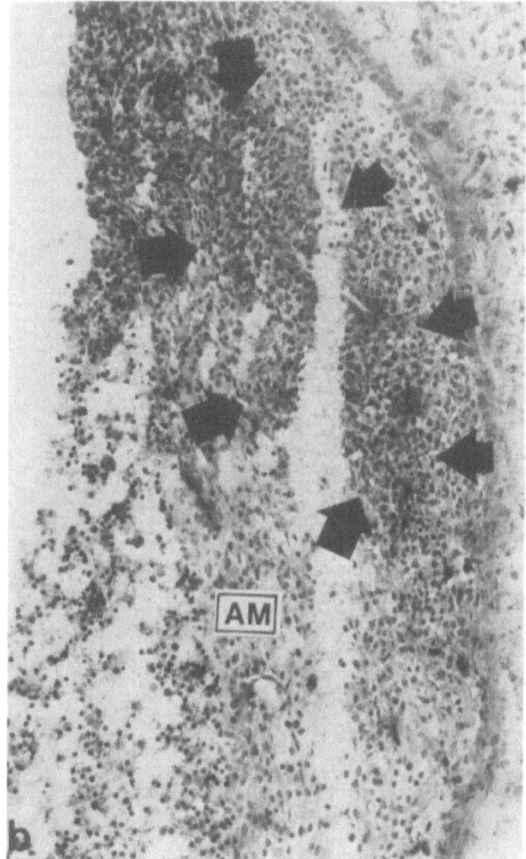

Figure 4. Sections of the sinoatrial node from a 28 mm human fetus processed to demonstrate histology (Figure 4a) and non-specific cholinesterase activity (Figure 4b). Note that the nodal cells (between arrows) are more densely packed than the atrial myocardium (AM) and are cholinesterase positive. The crack in the node is an artefact due to the cryostat method of tissue preparation.

DISCUSSION

(a) EARLY DEVELOPMENT AND ORIGIN OF THE SINOATRIAL NODE

There has been disagreement concerning the time at which the sinoatrial node is first recognizable as a histologically discrete structure. Shaner (1929) and Robb et al. (1948) argued that differentiation is a relatively late event while Sanabria (1936), Walls (1947), Muir (1951), Yamauchi (1965) and Van Mierop and Gessner (1970) all found the node in very early fetuses. Electrophysiological evidence has been obtained to show activity in very early stages (Van Mierop, 1967) and our findings support the evidence for early existence of an anatomically discrete pacemaker. Cellular differentiation has been

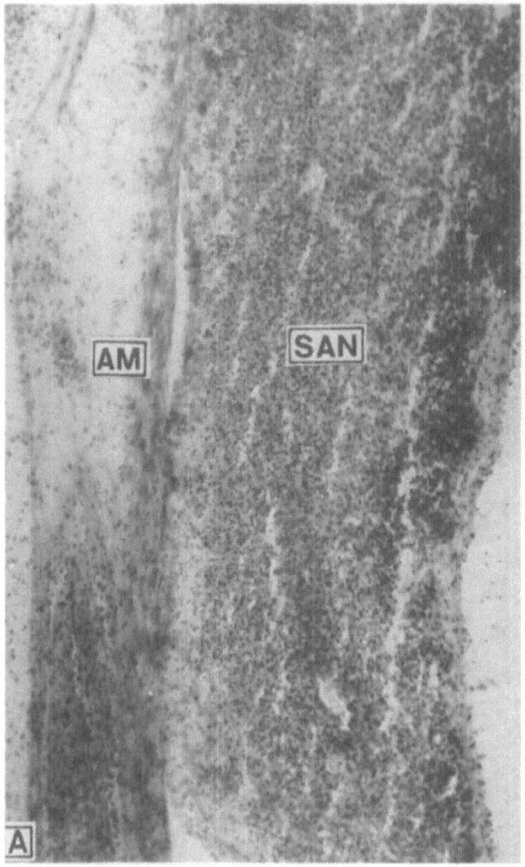

recognized at the anticipated site of the node in the youngest fetuses in the present
investigation. In our previous studies (Anderson et al., 1976) considerably thickening of
the sinoatrial junction was noted but at that time we had not successfully identified the
epicardial cylinder of cells presently described and considered to represent the nodal
primordium. This cylindrical cell mass is epicardially situated and is located in the
sulcus terminalis; the precise position of the definitive node. Furthermore, the cholinesterase technique has demonstrated histochemically positive cells in this exact location – an
enzyme known to be associated with conducting tissue. Thus, although cytological differences are subtle, we believe that the sinoatrial node forms a single, histologically
distinct structure in these early stages and is situated in a position directly comparable
with that seen in the neonate. Whether the node is differentiated from the more extensive
ring of sinoatrial junctional tissue (Anderson et al., 1976) or is differentiated in situ from
atrial myocardium cannot be determined from the material presently at our disposal. However, we are unable to provide evidence to support the concept of Patten (1956) that the
sinoatrial and atrioventricular nodes are paired structures derived from right and left
sinus horn, respectively. At the earliest stage studied, both sinoatrial and atrioventricular
nodal primordia were identified, the latter being derived from the atrioventricular ring

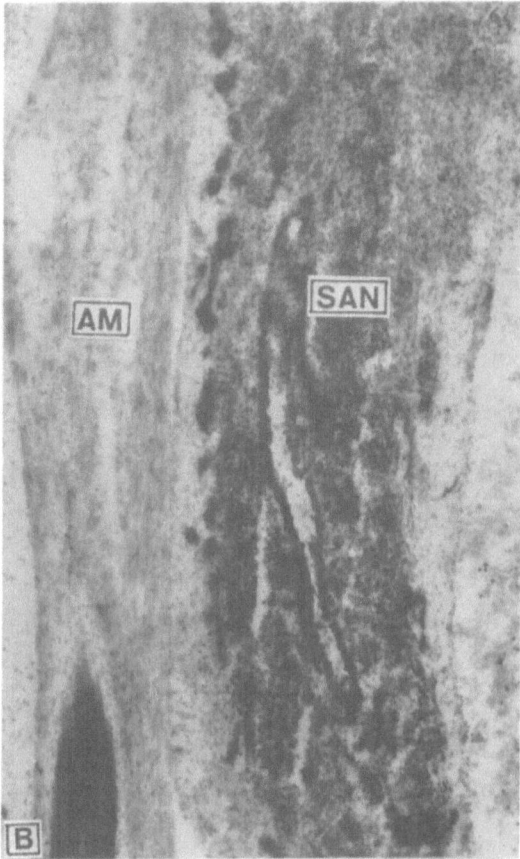

Figure 5. Sections of a sinoatrial node from a 60 mm human fetus processed to demonstrate histology (Figure 5a) and non-specific cholinesterase activity (Figure 5b). Note that the node is an extensive structure surrounding a prominent artery with a cauda extending towards the inferior vena cava.

specialized tissue (Figure 1). Our findings therefore endorse the observations of Van Mierop and Gessner (1970) that the sinoatrial node is a unilateral structure. One important feature emerged from our study regarding subsequent development of the sinoatrial node. Initially the node forms a large structure when compared with the size of the right atrium. At birth, however, the node is relatively small despite individual variations in size, shape and vascular supply. This trend of relative diminution of nodal size occurs throughout the experimental series and indicates that growth of atrial myocardium outstrips the growth of sinoatrial nodal tissue. A similar relative decrease in size is noted in the venous valves. Initially these structures are comparable in thickness to the atrial walls and septum and extend from sinoatrial to atrioventricular junctions, a fact previously doubted by one of us (Janse and Anderson, 1974). However, at birth the valves are markedly reduced and are composed predominantly of fibrous tissue.

It is on considerable significance to note that throughout its development, the sinoatrial

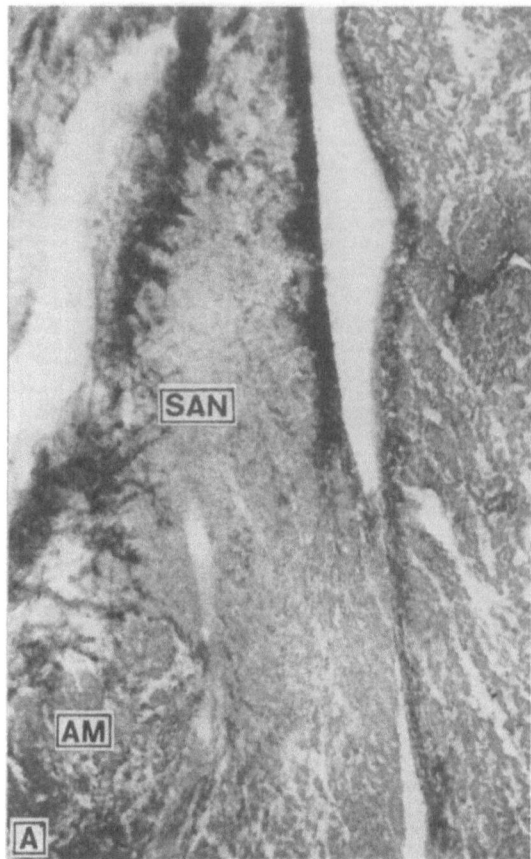

node contains a high proportion of collagen. The collagen forms a matrix which separates the fasciculi of tightly packed cells constituting the node. The presence of fibrous tissue is particularly well seen in the freshly prepared material, in which the collagen is more readily stained than in the paraffin embedded material. However, even in paraffin sections collagen is easily identified at birth. It may be that subsequent "fibrosis" of the node with increasing age is due to a decrease in nodal cells per unit area rather than an increase in fibrous tissue.

(b) THE ANATOMICAL LOCATION OF THE NODE

Throughout its development the sinoatrial node has been identified as a laterally placed structure relative to the junction of the superior vena cava and the right atrium. This lateral position was originally reported by Keith and Flack (1907) and endorsed by Lev and Watne (1954) and James (1961). In contrast, Hudson (1960) described the node as a horseshoe shaped structure encircling the anterior caval junction and suggested that the auricular crest was a guide to the node. Whilst our study shows considerable individual

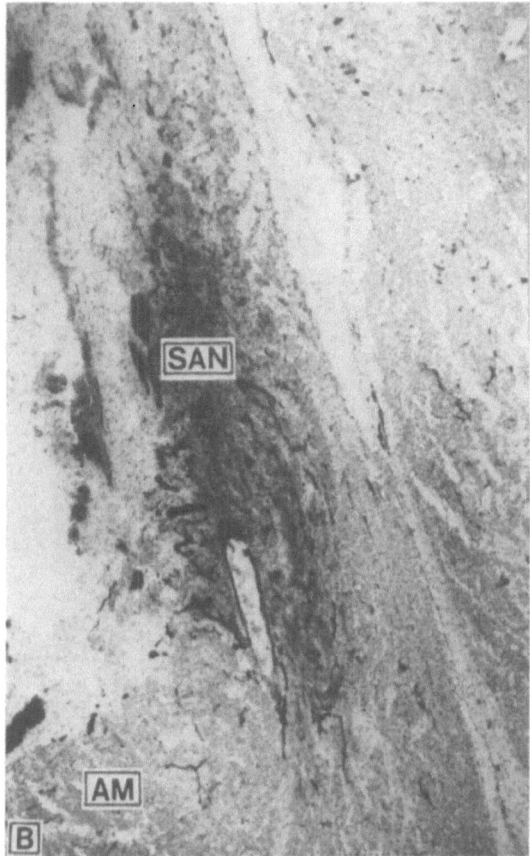

Figure 6. Sections of a sinoatrial node from a mid-term human fetus (220 mm). Note that the node is now relatively smaller. In the cholinesterase preparation (Figure 6b) it can be seen that the nodal cells themselves are cholinesterase positive but are additionally supplied with cholinesterase positive nerves. Note the short transitional zone between node (SAN) and atrial myocardium (AM).

variation in nodal position, in only one of our eight cases was nodal tissue present at the auricular crest. Precise knowledge of the position of the node is essential in order that specialized tissue may be avoided during atrial surgery. Our findings suggest that the lateral part of the caval-atrial junction is the area most "at risk", particularly since the node is an eipcardial structure, lying superficially in the sulcus terminalis. In this context two further points warrant consideration. Firstly, the node frequently has an extensive cauda which passes downwards alongside the orifice of the inferior vena cava. Secondly, the vascular supply is particularly variable. In our small series, the major artery supplying the node usually approached from the anterior atrial wall but could pass either clockwise or anticlockwise around the superior vena cava. Such variations suggest that the entirety of the sulcus terminalis and the junctional region of the right atrium and superior vena cava should be treated with extreme caution during atrial surgery.

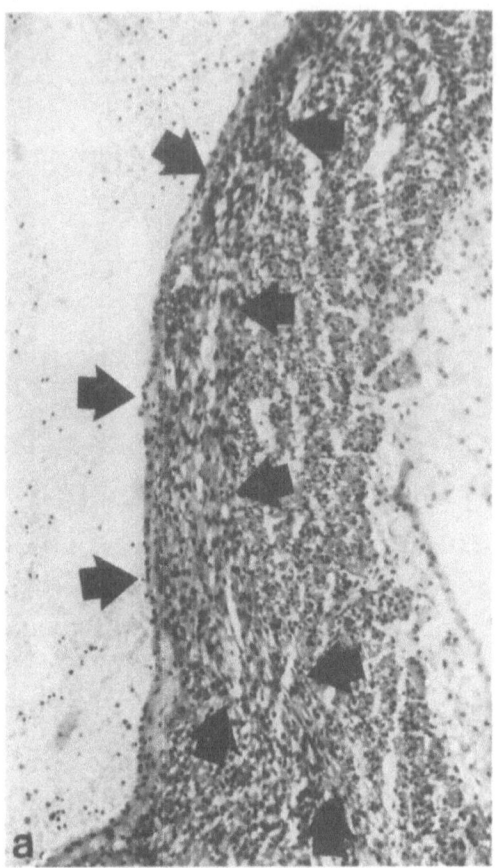

(c) THE PERIPHERAL CONNEXIONS OF THE SINOATRIAL NODE

Our present studies have shown that the sinoatrial node merges imperceptibly and rapidly into atrial myocardium around its margins. We have failed to obtain either histological or histochemical evidence to support the concept that tracts of specialized tissue extend between the sinoatrial and atrioventricular nodes (James, 1963) and it is difficult from our findings to suggest an anatomical substrate for the perinodal fibers which are detected electrophysiologically (Strauss and Bigger, 1972). The transition from sinoatrial nodal cells to atrial myocardial cells is such that there is no extensive zone of transitional cells similar to that which occurs in the atrioventricular junctional area (Becker and Anderson, 1976).

Concerning the nature of the internodal myocardium, electrophysiological studies (Spach et al., 1969, 1971) have demonstrated unequivocally that the impulse spreads preferentially from the sinus node along broad bands of atrial tissue which extend between the orifices of the right atrium. Our findings show that such bands are composed of cells indistinguishable either histologically or histochemically from the myocardium of the right atrial appendage or the left atrium.

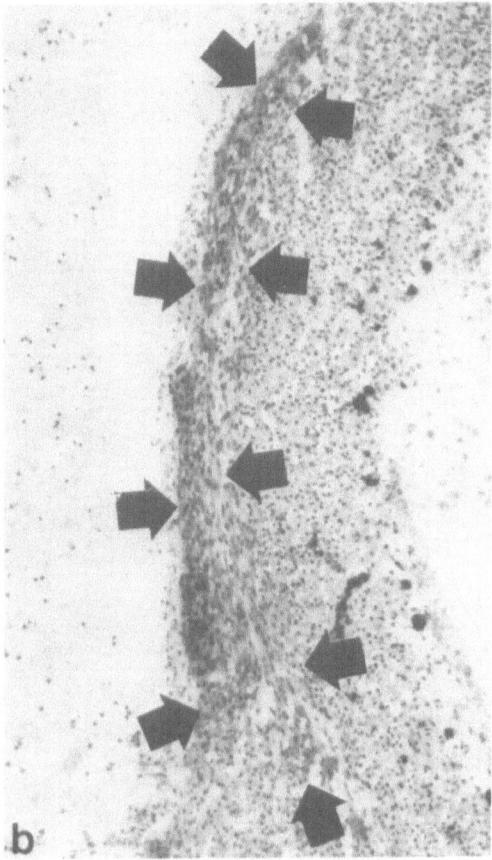

Figure 7. Sections of a strand of cells (between arrows) from the anterior atrial wall of a 65 mm fetus. Histology (Figure 7a) shows that the cells are larger than the surrounding myocardial cells and they are also cholinesterase positive (Figure 7b).

Recently, Isa and his associates (1976) found extensions of "Purkinje-like" cells emanating from the sinoatrial node in adult material, and suggested that these may have significance in preferential conduction. A group of cells possessing "Purkinje-like" histological characteristics has also been observed in one of the specimen examined in the present series. However, although cholinesterase positive, these cells were separate from both the sinoatrial and atrioventricular nodes. They formed an isolated cell group confined to the right atrial wall adjacent to the anterior atrioventricular junction. Since these cells were not in continuity with nodal tissue it seems unlikely that they served as a preferential pathway for impulse conduction. Until more data is available, the developmental origin and functional significance of these cells must remain enigmatic. Therefore the findings of the present investigation add support to the view that conduction between the sinoatrial and atrioventricular nodes occurs in the absence of morphologically specialized atrial tracts.

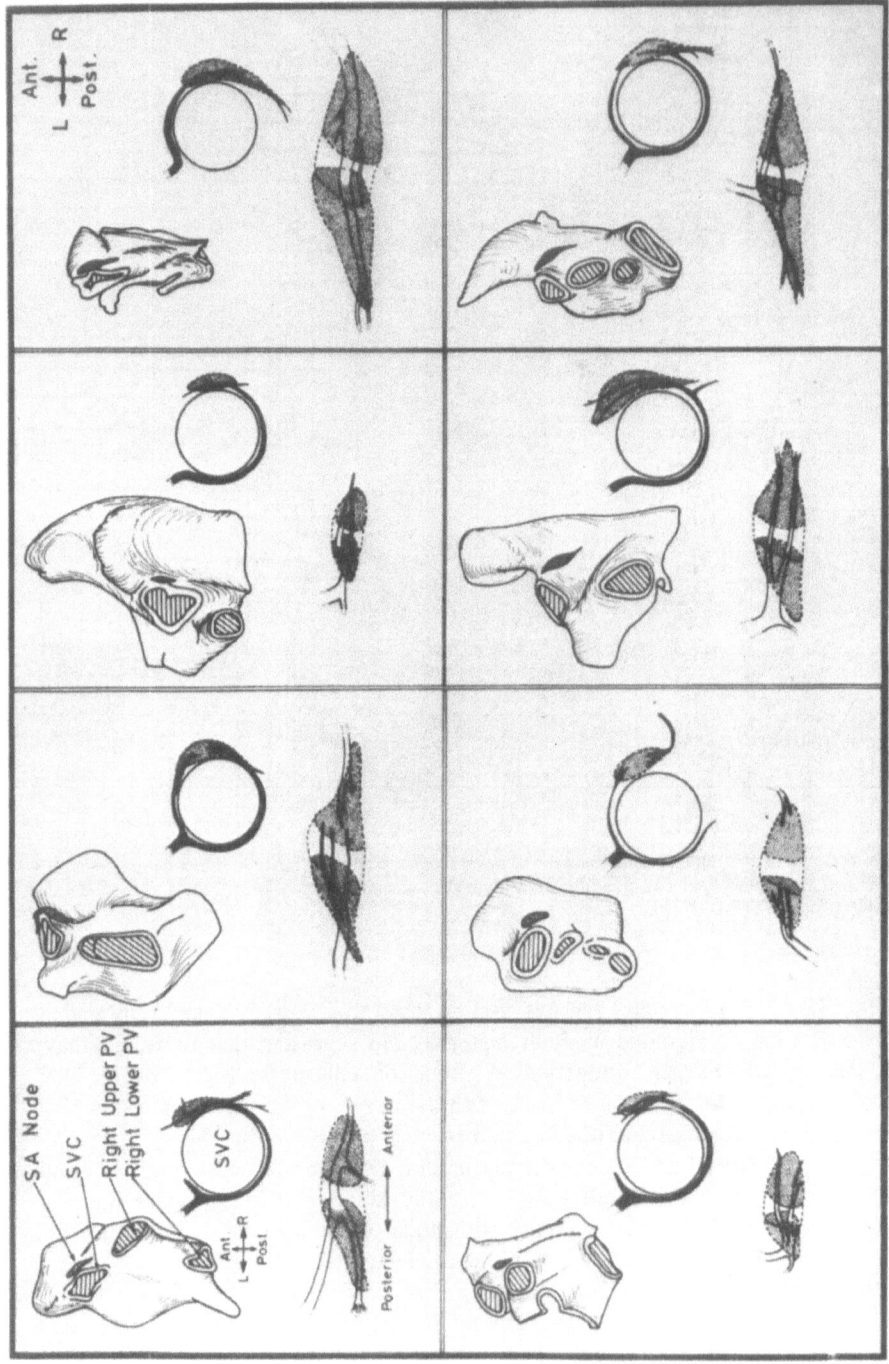

Figure 8. Diagrammatic representation of the position and vascular supply of the sinoatrial node in eight neonatal hearts.

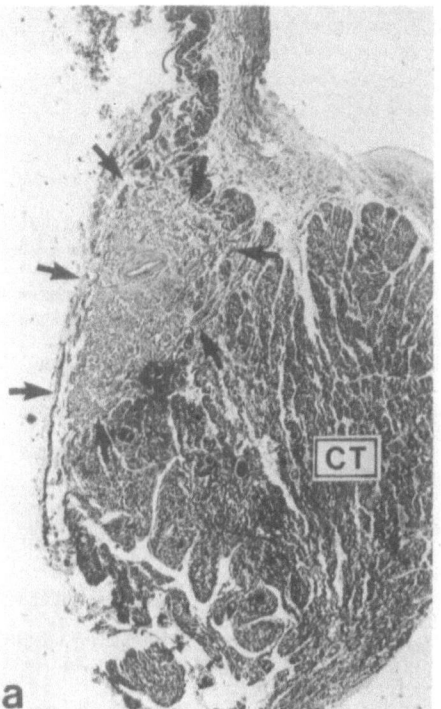 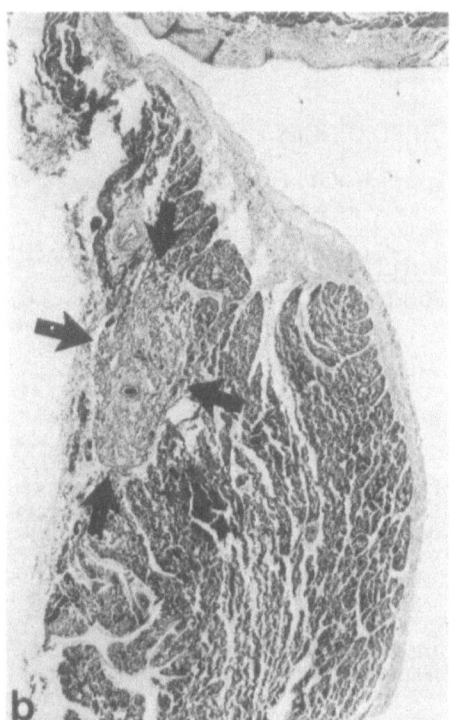

Figure 9. Sections of the sinoatrial node from a neonatal heart. Note the discrete junction between the node (between arrows) and the crista terminalis (CT). Note also its epicardial position. Figure 9b shows the extensive cauda of the node which burrows amongst the atrial myocardium (between arrows).

CONCLUSIONS

The primordium of the sinoatrial node was distinguished histologically in all specimens including a fetus of approximately six weeks gestational age. Nodal tissue was identified sub-epicardially in the sulcus terminalis at the lateral junction of the superior vena cava and the right atrium and was cholinesterase positive in all specimens which were processed histochemically. Throughout fetal development the nodal cells were associated with numerous connective tissue elements. In older fetal material, the node retained its morphological position but decreased in size relative to the atrial myocardium while an extension of nodal cells ran towards the inferior vena cava in all cases. Histologically or histochemically distinct internodal tracts amongst the atrial cells were not observed. At birth, although constant in location, considerable variation was noted in the size, shape, and vascular supply of individual sinoatrial nodes.

ACKNOWLEDGEMENTS

We are indebted to our colleagues who placed embryonic material at our disposal, particularly Prof. F. Harris and Mrs. A. Smith of the Institute of Child Health, Alder Hey Children's Hospital, Liverpool, United Kingdom and Dr. Leon M. Gerlis, Grimsby General Hospital. We thank Miss Sally A. Thompson for technical assistance. The photography was performed by Mr. K. Moreman. Finally, we are indebted to Miss Noelle de Freitas for secretarial assistance.

REFERENCES

Anderson, R.H., Taylor, I.M.: Development of atrioventricular specialized tissue in human heart. *Brit Heart J* 34: 1205, 1972

Anderson, R.H., Janse, M.J., Van Capelle, F.J.L., Billette, J., Becker, A.E., Durrer, C.: A combined morphological and electrophysiological study of the atrioventricular node of the rabbit heart. *Circulation Res* 35: 909, 1974

Anderson, R.H., Wenink, A.C.G., Becker, A.E., Janse, M.J.: Development of the Specialized Tissues. in Conduction System of the Heart: Structure, function and clinical implications, edited by Wellens, H.J.J., Lie, K.I., Janse, M.J. Stenfert Kroese, Leiden, p 1–28, 1976

Anderson, R.H., Wenink, A.C.G., Losekoot, R.G., Becker, A.E.: Congenitally Complete Heart Block – Developmental Aspects. *Circulation*, 56:90, 1977

Becker, A.E., Anderson, R.H.: Morphology of the Human Atrioventricular Junctional Area. in Conduction System of the Heart: Structure, function and clinical implications, edited by Wellens, H.J.J., Lie, K.I., Janse, M.J. Stenfert Kroese, Leiden, p. 263–286, 1976

Gosling, J.A.: Observations on the distribution of intrarenal nervous tissue. *Anat Rec* 163: 81, 1969

Hudson, R.E.B.: The human pacemaker and its pathology. *Br Heart J* 22: 153, 1960

Isa, L., Matturi, L., Rossi, L.: Contributo isto-citologico al riconoscimento delle connessioni internodali atriali. *G Ital Cardiol* 6: 1024, 1976

James, T.N.: Anatomy of the human sinus node. *Anat Rec* 141: 109, 1961

James, T.N.: The connecting pathways between the sinus node and the A-V node and between the right and left atrium in the human heart. *Am Heart J* 66: 498, 1963

James, T.N.: Cardiac conduction system: fetal and post-natal development. *Am J Cardiol* 25: 321, 1970

Janse, M.J., Anderson, R.H.: Specialized Internodal Atrial Pathways: Fact or Fiction? *Eur J Cardiol* 2: 117, 1974

Keith, A., Flack, M.W.: The form and nature of the muscular connections between the primary divisions of the vertebrate heart. *J Anat Physiol* 41: 171, 1907

Lev, M., Watne, A.L.: Method for routine histopathologic study of human sinoatrial node. *AMA Arch Path* 57: 168, 1954

Muir, A.R.: The development of the sino-atrial node in the heart of the sheep. *J Anat* 85: 430, 1951

Patten, B.M.: Development of the sinoventricular conduction system. *Univ Mich Med Bull* 22: 1, 1956

Robb, J.S., Kaylor, C.T., Turman, W.G.: A study of specialized heart tissue at various stages of development of the human fetal heart. *Am J Med* 5: 324, 1948

Sanabria, T.: Recherches sur la differenciation du tissu nodal et connecteur du coeur des mammiferes. *Arch Biol* 47: 1, 1936

Shaner, R.F.: The development of the atrioventricular node, bundle of His and sinoatrial node in the calf; with a description of a third embryonic nodelike structure. *Anat Rec* 44: 85, 1929

Spach, M.S., King, T.D., Barr, R.C., Boaz, D.C., Morrow, M.N., Herman-Giddens, S.: Electrical potential distribution surrounding the atria during depolarization and repolarization in the dog. *Circulation Res* 24: 857, 1969

Spach, M.S., Lieberman, M., Scott, J.C., Barr, R.C., Johnson, E.A., Kootsey, J.M.: Excitation sequences of the atrial septum and AV node in isolated hearts of the dog and rabbit. *Circulation Res* 29: 156, 1971

Strauss, H.C., Bigger, J.T. Jr.: The electrophysiological properties of the rabbit sinoatrial perinodal fibers. *Circulation Res* 31: 490, 1972

Van Mierop, L.H.S.: Location of pacemaker in chick embryo heart at the time of initiation of heartbeat. *Am J Physiol* 212: 407, 1967

Van Mierop, L.H.S., Gessner, I.H.: The morphologic development of the sinoatrial node in the mouse. *Am J Cardiol* 25: 204, 1970

Walls, E.W.: The development of the specialized conducting tissue of the human heart. *J Anat* 81: 93, 1947

Yamauchi, A.: Electron microscopic observations on the development of S-A and A-V nodal tissues in the human embryonic heart. *A Anat Entwickl Gesch* 124: 562, 1965

15

TECHNIQUES AND PROBLEMS IN CORRELATING CELLULAR ELECTROPHYSIOLOGY AND MORPHOLOGY IN CARDIAC NODAL TISSUES

MICHIEL J. JANSE, JORGEN TRANUM-JENSEN, ANDRÉ G. KLÉBER, AND
FRANS J.L. VAN CAPELLE

It is evident that it is very difficult to predict the functional behaviour of a cell, or a group of cells, on the basis of morphological data alone. It is equally clear that one cannot be informed of the cellular morphology of a particular part of the heart when only electrophysiological information is available. However, these two different kinds of information are combined when models are created, and to do this one has to ensure identity between structures studied by the different methods. Because the cardiac nodes are complex both with respect to structure and function, and the topographical landmarks for the small volumes of tissue are few and variable, combined studies in the same preparation are necessary. Yet there are very few studies in which electrophysiological and morphological investigations were carried out in the same preparation. A notable exception is the study of Trautwein and Uchizono (1963) in which the ultrastructure was determined of cells which were at least close (i.e. < 1 mm) to cells of which typical pacemaker action potentials had been recorded in the sinoatrial node of rabbits.

Previously we have attempted to correlate the electrophysiology and morphology of different parts of the atrioventricular node using iontophoretical ejection of cobalt ions from the microelectrode after recording of intracellular action potentials. The preparations were subsequently cut into serial 20 μ (thick) frozen sections. This allowed a three-dimensional reconstruction of the AV node to be made showing its architecture, but details of cellular morphology could not be observed in the frozen sections. (Anderson et al., 1974).

Another problem we faced was that in only 50% of the experiments we were able to find a single cobalt deposit at the expected site; in the remaining experiments we either found no deposits, or even more surprising, multiple diffuse cobalt deposits were found, suggesting leakage of cobalt all along the shaft of the microelectrode. In conclusion, this method was found satisfactory for marking a region of the AV node, but inappropiate for precise marking at the cellular level and for the study of cellular details. The present paper describes an attempt to arrive at a more reliable way of identifying the cell from which the microelectrode recording was made. As will be shown, it is not at all necessary to mark the cell recorded from with an injected dye.

NOTES ABOUT THE USE OF ISOLATED, SUPERFUSED PREPARATIONS

It is well known that for isolated preparation of cardiac muscle placed in a tissue bath and superfused with an oxygenated Tyrode solution, the rate of diffusion of oxygen and of small molecules like glucose into the preparation becomes restrictive, when a cylindrical preparation (e.g. a papillary muscle) is more than about 600 microns in diameter, and physiological studies will reflect partially hypoxic conditions (Cranefield and Greenspan, 1960). In a plane sheet of tissue this critical thickness is even less, because for a thickness of the sheet equal to the diameter of the cylinder, the surface area per unit volume across the sheet is half of that of a unit volume along the cylinder.

Figure 1A shows a photomicrograph of a piece of interventricular septum from a preparation which had been superfused with oxygenated Tyrode solution for a period of 5 hours at 36°C. As can be seen, the layer of cells exhibiting a normal morphology extends only 150 microns below the endocardium. Beyond this depth there is a stratum of swollen cells and extracellular spaces are indistinguishable. At a depth of about 300 microns from the endocardial surface, the cells are necrotic. Figure 1B shows a section from the anterior part of the atrioventricular node from the same preparation. the layer of well preserved cells is here only about 100 microns thick, and consists almost exclusively of atrial overlay cells. Nearly the full thickness of the atrioventricular node itself is morphologically abnormal. From an electrophysiological point of view these superfused preparations remained functionally constant for a period of 3 hours, using as parameters conduction time through the node, the ability to conduct and block premature atrial impulses, and the atrial pacing rate at which a Wenckebach phenomenon would be elicited in the AV node. Yet it was found that even within three hours, cells in the deeper layers of the AV node showed a highly abnormal morphology. It may be that conduction through the atrioventricular node remains unimpaired even though large parts of the node are destroyed, or perhaps that morphologically abnormal cells can function normally for some time, as far as conduction

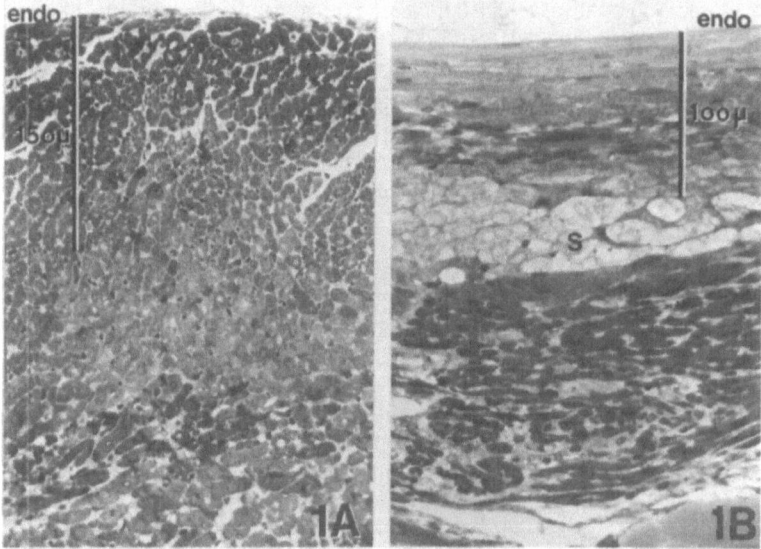

Figure 1A. Right side of rabbit interventricular septum, superfused with oxygenated Tyrode solution for 5 hours. The tissue was then uniformly exposed to the fixative through a cut made perpendicularly to the endocardium at the onset of fixation. The Epon section shown was located immediately below this previously cut surface. Morphologically normal cells extend about 150 μ below the endocardial surface (endo). Deeper to this, the cells are slightly swollen and intercellular spaces are narrowed. At a depth of about 250 μ the tissue is necrotic.

Figure 1B. Section cut perpendicularly to the endocardium across the atrioventricular node, treated and fixed as in Figure 1A. Morphologically well preserved cells extend here only about 100 μ below the endocardial surface (endo), and comprise in this case almost only atrial overlay tissue. Nearly the full thickness of the node is morphologically abnormal. Superficial cells of the node are markedly swollen (S) and still deeper the cells are pyknotic. Toluidine blue stain.

of the electrical impulse is concerned. At any rate it is evident that the layer of cells which remains morphologically normal after prolonged periods of superfusion is not thicker than 150 microns. A sheet-like preparation over which oxygenated Tyrode solution is flowing on both sides should therefore not be thicker than 300 microns, which is about half the critical diameter from a cylindrical preparation calculated by Cranefield and Greenspan (1960). Additionally, from a morphological point of view optimal fixation can best be achieved by vascular perfusion. In our experiments, which were primarily devised for studies of the atrioventricular node, we therefore developed a perfused preparation.

THE ISOLATED, PERFUSED AND OPENED PREPARATION OF THE RABBIT HEART

Rabbits were anaesthetized by intravenous injection of nembutal. After intravenous injection of heparin, the heart was rapidly removed and placed in a large volume of oxygenated Tyrode solution at 37°C. Both the right and the left coronary artery were then cannulated using the largest possible catheter diameter and perfused at 100 mmHg hydrostatic pressure with an oxygenated standard Tyrode solution to which 4% dextran (T 70 pharmacia, m.w. 70.000) was added. Because of the individual variations in the distribution of the coronary arteries, dual cannulation was necessary to ensure homogeneous and reproducible perfusion of the preparation. This was particularly important for the lower part of the interatrial septum, containing the atrioventricular node. The time interval between removal of the heart and beginning of dual coronary perfusion was on the average about 3 minutes. The right atrium was then opened according to Paes de Carvalho et al. (1959) by cutting through the crista supraventricularis and superior vena cava. Additionally, the aorta was divided between the right an left coronary artery (see Figure 2). Opened in this way, the crista terminalis is cut and atrial activation is not completely normal. However, both the SA node and the AV node are well exposed. Arteries in the cut surfaces of the interventricular septum and ventricular walls, were clamped by small agraffes. The preparation was pinned on a disc of cork and transferred to a tissue bath, where, in addition to being perfused, it was also superfused with oxygenated normal Tyrode solution.

THE MARKING TECHNIQUE

Microelectrodes were filled with filtered 0.2 M KCl containing 2% procion yellow M4RS or 2% pontamine sky blue 6 BX, (G.T. Gurr), which have been used successfully by others to mark nerve cell bodies (Stratton and Kravitz, 1973; Boakes et al., 1974). The microelectrodes had a resistance of about 60 megOhm, the equivalent resistance of the electrodes when filled with 3 M KCl being around 20 megOhm. Because of the vigorous contractions of the perfused preparation, floating microelectrodes had to be used for intracellular recording (Woodbury and Brady, 1956). After recording, hyperpolarizing current pulses of 400–800 Nano Ampere were applied to the microelectrode with the purpose of expelling the dye into the cell. The preparation was then immediately fixed by perfusion through the coronary arteries with a fixative (2.5% glutaraldehyde + 1% formaldehyde in 0.11 M phosphate buffer, pH 7.2), while the microelectrode remained in the tissue. The preparation was fixed within seconds. A second microelectrode filled with india ink, and of which the very

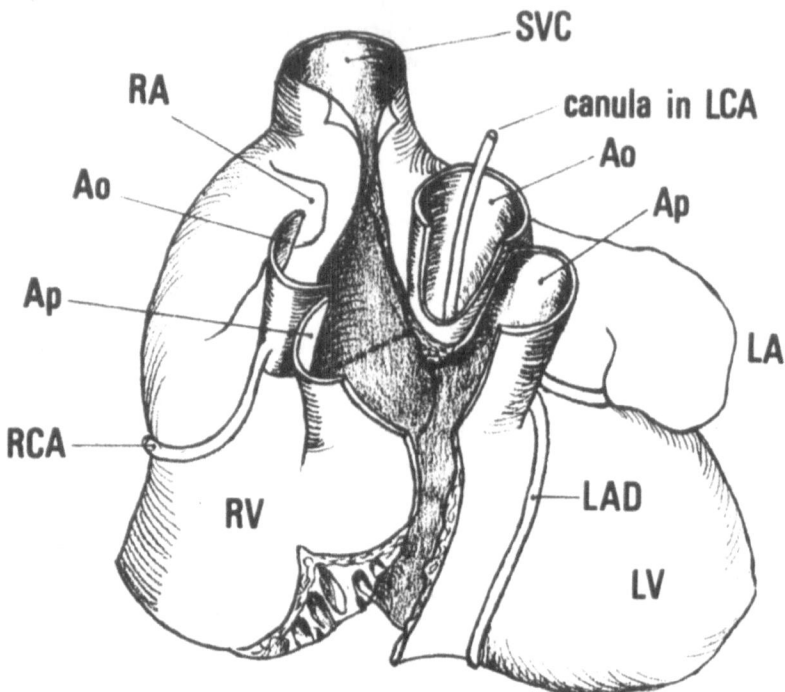

Figure 2. Schematic drawing indicating how the isolated perfused rabbit heart preparation was opened. SVC = superior vena cava; LA: left auricle; RA: right auricle; Ao: aorta; Ap: arteria pulmonalis; RCA: right coronary artery; LCA: left coronary artery; LAD: left anterior descending artery; LV: left ventricle; RV: right ventricle. The dotted line indicates the attachment of the tricuspid valve.

tip was broken, was then positioned very close to the recording microelectrode and by hydraulic pressure small deposits of india ink were placed subendocardially to mark the position of the recording microelectrode, and a photograph of the preparation was taken through a dissecting microscope. The perfusion with fixative was maintained for 20 minutes before the recording microelectrode was withdrawn. The entire preparation was then kept at 4°C in a fixative for three hours. A tiny block of 1–2 mm³ of precisely known orientation was then cut at the position marked by the india ink dots. The block was washed for one hour in the buffer of the fixative, and positioned in 2% OsO_4 in the same buffer for 15–30 minutes. Following a 15 minutes wash in the buffer, the block was dehydrated in ethanol and embedded in Epon 812 (Luft, 1961) or Spurr's resin (Spurr, 1969). Block marked with procion yellow were not postfixed in OsO_4. Pontamine sky blue 6 BX bleaches slowly in OsO_4 and postfixation should therefore not be extended beyond 30 minutes, and the period of dehydration should be as short as possible because the dye slowly elutes from cells in the lower ethanol concentrations. The blocks were cut with glass knives into a complete series of 4 micron sections which were mounted unstained in Epon. The section containing the microelectrode tip position was identified with phase contrast optics, and this section, together with its adjacent sections could then be remounted on pre-cast epon blocks (Woodcock and Bell, 1967) and resectioned for electron microscopy. Usually a series of 30 to 50 ultrathin sections could be obtained.

RESULTS

The use of the perfused preparations markedly improved the cellular preservation; after perfusion periods up to 3 hours, the cellular morphology was almost indistinguishable from that of optimally in vivo fixed tissue. The recovery of the dye marks was very unsatisfactory. No marks of procion yellow were found in 9 experiments, and in only 2 out of 16 experiments could distinct pontamine sky blue marks be found. However, in nearly all blocks (19 out of 22) in which the microelectrode was left in the tissue during fixation, the track of the microelectode could be found, allowing identification of the tip position to within a volume of 2 to 4 cells. In some cases even the very cell impaled could be identified. We believe that the main reason for the lack of success in retrieving the dye marks was due to an insufficient concentration of the dye in the cells. In its turn, this was probably caused by the fact that due to the vigorous contractions of the perfused preparation, the microelectrode could not be maintained in an intracellular position for long, so that the period of intracellular dye injection may have been too short.

MORPHOLOGICAL IDENTIFICATION OF CELLS IN THE SINOATRIAL NODE FROM WHICH INTRACELLULAR ACTION POTENTIALS HAD BEEN RECORDED – LIGHT MICROSCOPY AND ULTRASTRUCTURE

Figure 3A shows a preparation drawn from a colour photograph made through a dissecting microscope. The microelectrode is situated just medially to the crista terminalis, about halfway between the superior and inferior caval veins. Atrial surface electrodes are positioned on both sides of the microelectrode. The preparation was spontaneously active. The action potentials shown have the configuration of a true pacemaker, with a smooth transition between phase 4 and phase 0, yet the cell is clearly activated later than the tissue under both atrial surface electrodes. The cell is a potential pacemaker which does not contribute to the pacing of this preparation. Yet it does not seem to be activated by the atrial wavefront since the configuration of the action potential is unlike that of a latent pacemaker: there is no sharp transition between phase 4 and phase 0. Figure 3 B-E shows low and high power photomicrographs of 4 micron sections at the site of impalement in the cauda of the sinus node. Although dye was injected, it was not found. Nevertheless, the microelectrode track is clearly visible, even though it is not exactly in the plane of sectioning. The tip position could, in this preparation, be determined to the very cell that had been impaled. This cell belongs to a group of cells located just medially to the crista terminalis which have the structure of typical nodal cells (see contribution by Tranum-Jensen in this book) and which form the cauda of the sinus node (Tranum-Jensen and Bojsen-Møller, 1973). It is to be noted that the cells along the microelectrode track are stretched, but that the cell at the tip position is not distorted in this case.

Figure 4A shows the position of the recording microelectrode and the atrial surface electrode in another spontaneously active preparation. The former is located in the thin tissue of the superior caval vein, the latter is on the crista terminalis. The action potentials have the configuration of a true pacemaker potential and occur earlier than the atrial electrogram. Again dye was injected, and the microelectrode remained in the tissue during fixation. In serial section of 4 micron thickness no dye was found. However, the microelectrode track, which was exactly in the plane of sectioning, could easily be identified, as

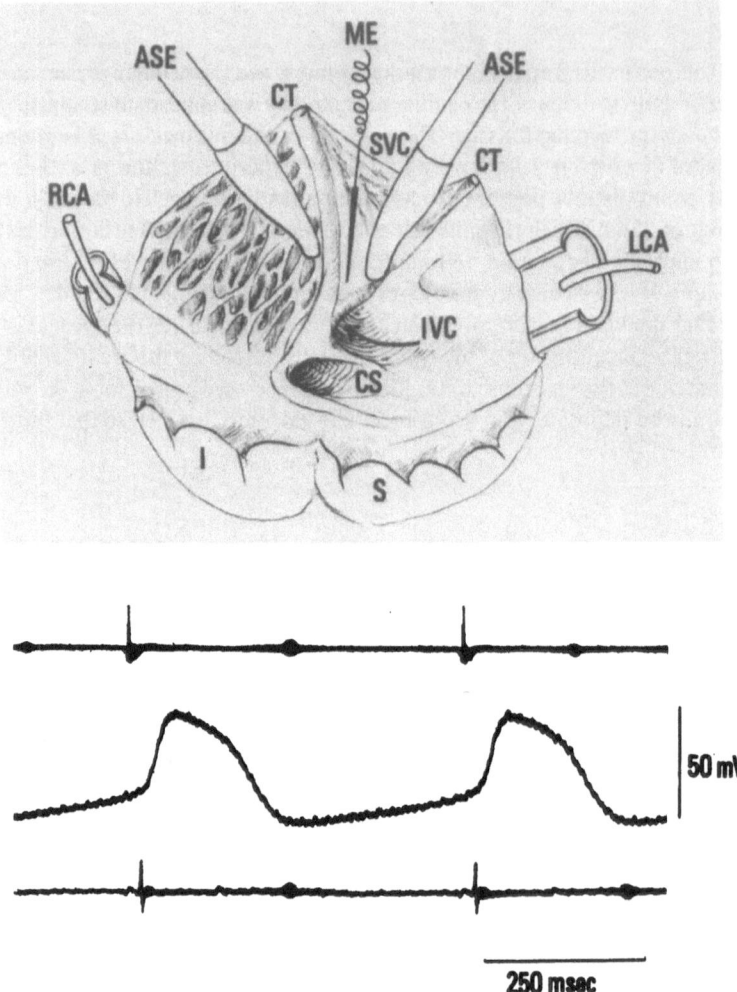

Figure 3A. Upper panel: endocardial surface of the opened right atrium. Abbreviation as in Figure 1; CT; crista terminalis; ASE: atrial surface electrode; ME: microelectrode; IVC: inferior vena cava; CS: coronary sinus; I: infundibulum of right ventricle; S: interventricular septum.
Lower panel: upper and lower trace: surface electrograms recorded by surface electrodes shown above. Middle trace: intracellular action potentials recorded with microelectrode shown above. Note true pacemaker configuration of action potential which occurs later than atrial activations.

shown in Figure 4B and C. Upon withdrawal from the tissue, the last 25 μ of the micro-electrode broke and remained in the tissue. As shown, the tip has a diameter of about 0.8 micron, and has several holes along its shaft. It is tempting to suggest that these holes are caused by the high current density during dye injection. It offers an additional possible explanation for the infrequent finding of dye deposits, because a large part of the dye may have escaped through these holes. Such holes close to the tip may in larger cells, such as nerve cell bodies, still be located intracellularly. The porous crystalline structure of the microelectrode seen in electron micrographs (Figure 4D) may also be a result of the high current density during dye injection but might also result from the preparative procedure

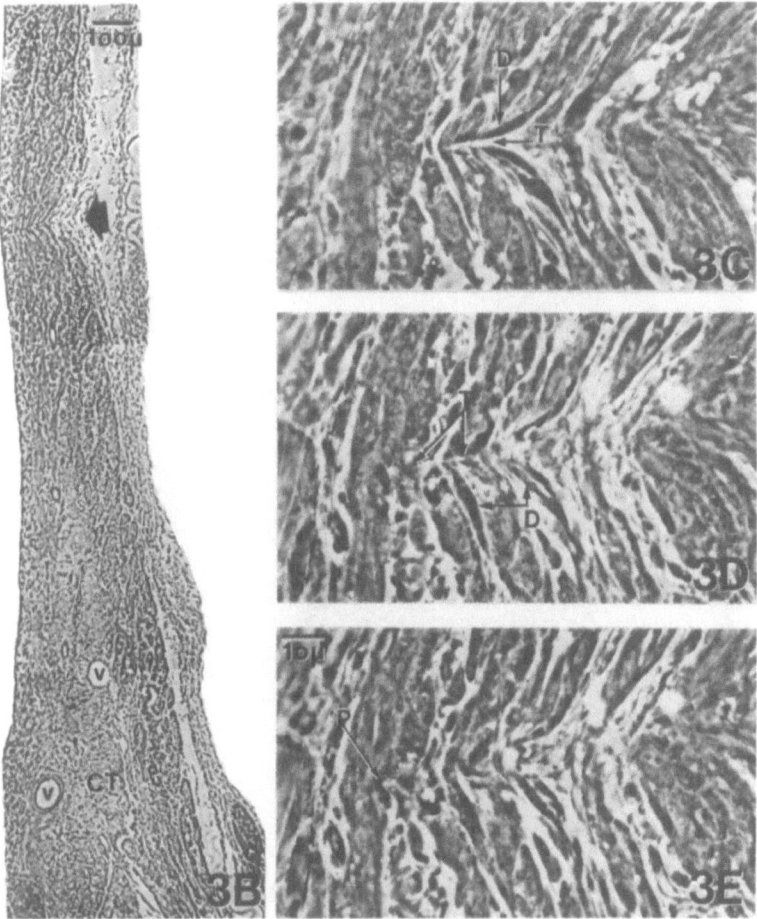

Figure 3B. 4 μ Epon section viewed with phase contrast optics, showing the track of the microelectrode corresponding to Figure 3A, situated in the cauda of the sinus node. CT – crista terminalis; v – vessels fixed in an opened state due to perfusion.

C. The microelectrode track (T) of Figure 3B seen at higher magnification. Cells along the track are markedly stretched and dark (D). In the neighbouring section (Figure 3D) the track is followed still deeper to the site of impalement (P), best seen in another plane of focus in Figure 3E.

and the passage of time, since the sections were cut several months after the experiment. The cellular distortion along the microelectrode track is substantial. The damage caused by the microelectrode consists of a funnel shaped depression at the site of entrance in the tissue, and of a cone of stretched cells along the shaft. This distortion was seen in all experiments, and the deeper the impalement, the more pronounced the distortion. In our perfused preparations, in which contractions are vigorous, stable recordings from surface cells are usually not possible. The mechanical distortion of cells around the microelectrode track may be a consequence of the fact that the floating microelectrode remained in a stable position only when the tip was relatively deeply embedded in the tissue. As can be seen in Figure 4G, some of the stretched cells are more dense than others. Remounting and sec-

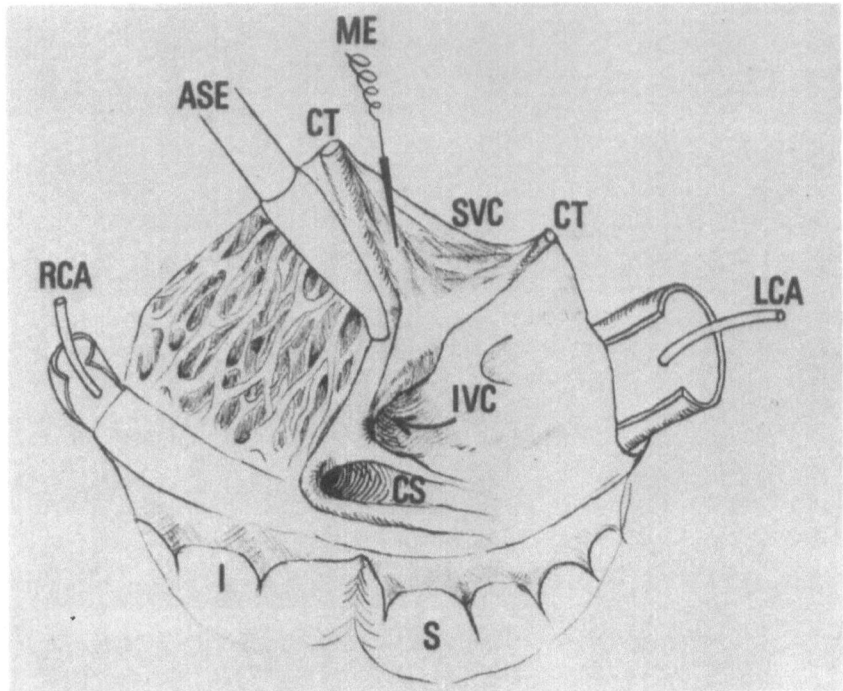

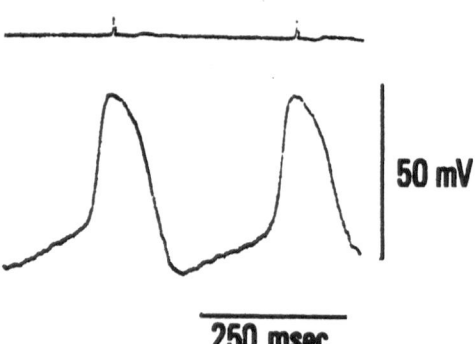

Figure 4A. Diagram indicating microelectrode position and position of atrial surface electrode. In lower panel atrial electrogram and intracellular action potentials. Cell recorded from is true pacemaker; upstroke occurs earlier than atrial activity.

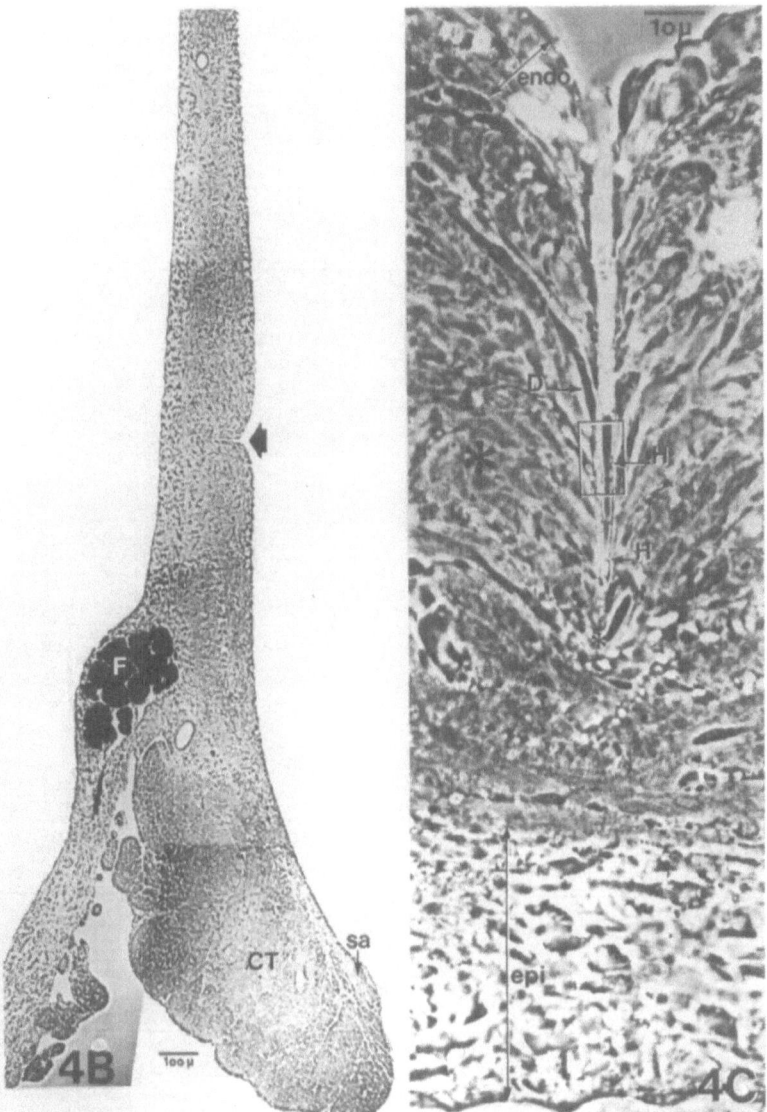

Figure 4B. 4 μ Epon section viewed with phase contrast optics, showing the track of the microelectrode corresponding to Figure 4A, positioned centrally in the sinus node about 0.5 mm medial to the crista terminalis (CT). The tissue of the node can be followed onto the medial aspect of the CT where it reaches to the sinu-atrial ring bundle (sa). F – fat cells in the sulcus terminalis.

C. The microelectrode track of Figure 4B seen at higher magnification. The track coincides precisely with the plane of sectioning. The outer 25 μ of the microelectrode tip has remained in the tissue. Several small holes (H) are seen in the microelectrode. The electrode has been retracted slightly before breaking and the empty track can be followed to the position marked by small asterisk. The oblong dark structure to the right of the asterick is an optical artefact caused by a grain of dirt on the section. The microelectrode has produced a funnelshaped depression of the endocardium (endo), and several stretched and darkened cells (D) are seen along the track. epi – epicardium.

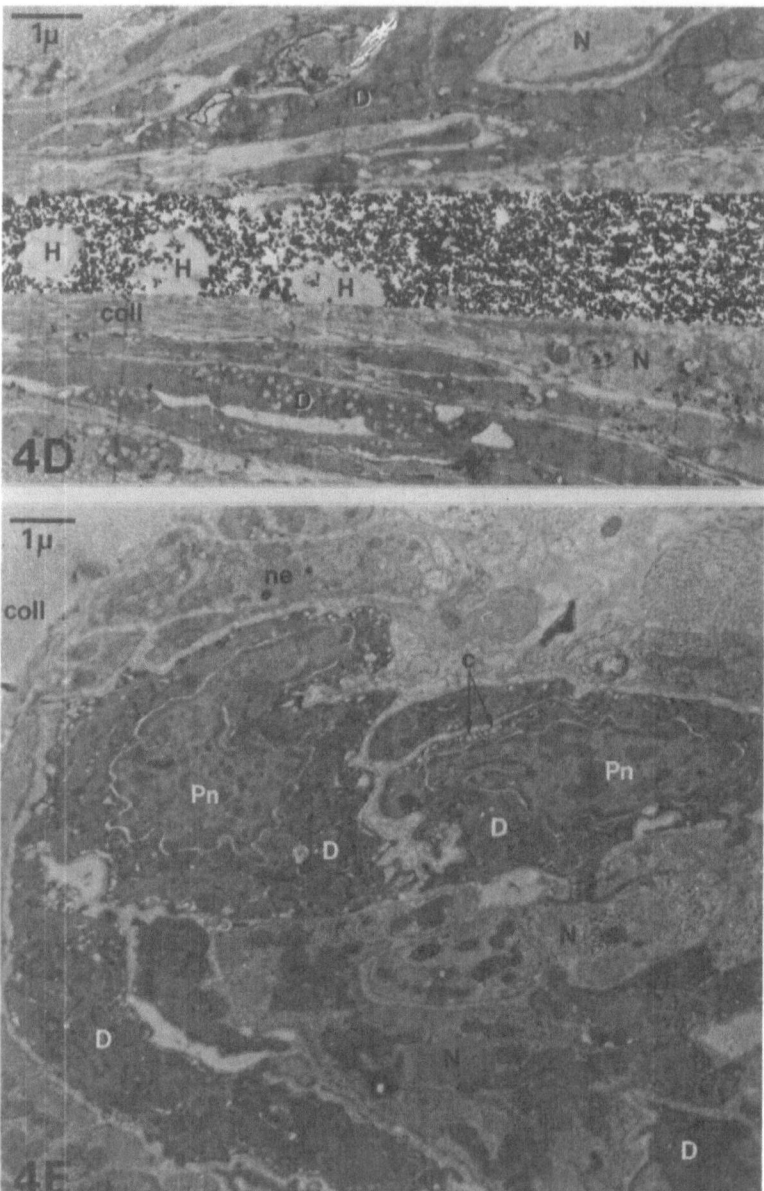

Figure 4D. Lower power electron micrograph corresponding to the frame in Figure 4C, obtained by re-mounting and ultrathin sectioning of the 4 μ Epon section of Figure 4B. The glass of the microelectrode has a porous crystalline structure and the holes (H) seen in phase contrast are verified. The cells surrounding the electrode are extremely stretched and many of these may appear abnormally dark (D), while extensions of others appear normal (N). coll – collagen.

E Ultrathin section obtained after remounting a neighbouring 4 μ section to that of Figure 4B. The section is cut parallel to the track of the microelectrode in a distance of about 3 μ and the picture is taken at the site overlying the tip position. Several of the cells (D) are markedly shrunken and have pyknotic nuclei. The cytoplasma is homogeneously dark and only mitochondria are discerned. Caveolae (c) stand out in increased contrast along the cell membrane. Processes of the dark cells are mingled with processes of normal cells (N). ne – small nerve; coll – collagen.

tioning this 4 micron section for electron microscopy revealed that these cells were severely damaged (see Figures 4D and E). We do not know whether this damage is due to mechanical distortion or to the passage of current through the microelectrode or to both. However, the distortion itself must be a mechanical phenomenon. Therefore, intracellular action potentials with "normal" amplitudes may be recorded from cells that are either damaged themselves, or have damaged neighbours. Outside the cone of distortion caused by the microelectrode but still within 50 μ of the tip position, the cells had the structure of typical nodal cells (Figure 5). (Described more detailed in contributions by Masson-Pévet et al. and by Tranum-Jensen in this book).

CONCLUSIONS

In conclusion, we believe that correlation between cellular electrophysiology and fine structural morphology in the cardiac nodes is possible by using preparations perfused and fixed through their coronary artery system. Electrophoretic injection of dyes is not neces-

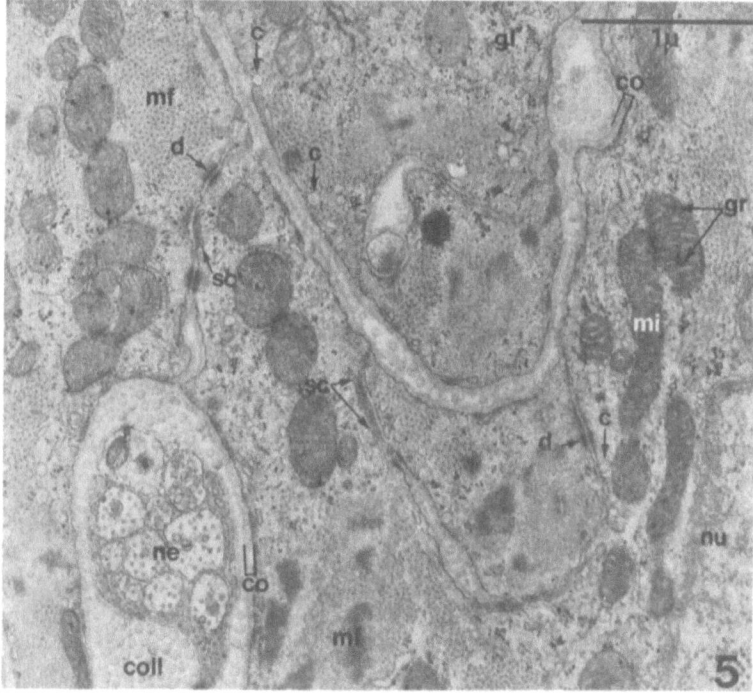

Figure 5. Electron micrograph of section obtained at the approximate position marked by larger asterisk in Figure 4C outside the cone of distortion around the microelectrode. Intermingled processes of several well-preserved typical nodal cells with a low content of myofibrils (mf) are seen. Mitochondria (mi) are of normal structure and density, and contain normal mitochondrial granules (gr). Small desmosomes (d) are seen between cell membranes in close (200A) apposition, and the cell coat (co) with its external lamina can be distinguished in several places. sc – subsurface cisterns of sarcoplasmic reticulum; c – caveolae; gl – glycogen granules; nu – nucleus; ne – small nerve; coll – collagen.

sary since the microelectrode track consistently can be identified when the microelectrode remains in the tissue during fixation. The mechanical distortion of cells along the microelectrode track may be considerable. The possibility should be considered that action potentials recorded with microelectrodes from nodal cardiac tissue are in fact recorded from damaged cells, or from cells whose neighbours are damaged.

REFERENCES

Anderson, R.H., Janse, M.J., van Capelle, F.J.L., Billette, J., Becker A.E., Durrer, D.: A combined morphologic and electrophysiologic study of the atrioventricular node of the rabbit heart. *Circulation Res* 35: 909, 1974

Boakes, R.J., Bramwell, G.J., Briggs, I., Candy, J.M., Tempesta E.: Localization with pontamine skye blue of neurones in the brainstem responding the micro iontophoretically applied compounds. *Neuropharmacology* 13: 475, 1974

Cranefield, P.F., Greenspan, K.: The role of oxygen uptake of quiescent cardiac muscle. *J Gen Physiol* 44: 235, 1960

Luft, J.H.: Improvement in epoxy resin embedding methods. *J Biophys Biochem Cytol* 9: 409, 1961

Paes de Carvalho, A., de Mello, C.W., Hoffman, B.F.: Electrophysiological evidence for specialized fiber types in rabbit atrium. *Am J Physiol* 196: 483, 1959

Spurr, A.R.: A low viscosity epoxy resin embedding medium for electron microscopy. *J Ultrastructure Res* 26: 31, 1969

Stretton, A.O.W., and Kravits, E.A.: Intracellular dye injection: the selection of procion yellow and its application in preliminary studies of neuronal geometry in the lobster nervous system. In: Intracellular staining in neurobiology, edited by S.B. Kater, C. Nicholson. Springer Verlag, Berlin, Heidelberg, New York, 1973, p. 21

Tranum-Jensen, J., Bojsen-Møller, F.: The ultrastructure of the sinoatrial ring bundle and of the caudal extension of the sinus node in the right atrium of the rabbit heart. *Z Zellforsch* 138: 97, 1973

Trautwein, W, Uchizono, K.: Electron microscopic and electrophysiologic study of the pacemaker in the sinoatrial node of the rabbit heart. *Z Zellforsch* 61: 96, 1963

Woodbury, J.W., Brady, A.J.: Intracellular recording from moving tissue with a flexibly mounted ultra microelectrode. *Science* 123: 100, 1956

Woodcock, C.L.F., Bell, P.R.: A method for mounting 4 μ resin sections routinely for ultra thin sectioning. *J Roy Micr Soc.* 3/4; 485, 1967

From:
The department of Cardiology and Clinical Physiology, Wilhelmina Gasthuis, Amsterdam
The Interuniversity Institute of Cardiology, The Netherlands,
and the Anatomy dept. C, University of Copenhagen, Denmark.

16

ULTRASTRUCTURAL AND FUNCTIONAL ASPECTS OF THE RABBIT SINOATRIAL NODE

MIREILLE MASSON-PÉVET, W.K. BLEEKER, A.J.C. MACKAAY,
D. GROS, AND L.N. BOUMAN

INTRODUCTION

The heart beat originates within a certain group of cells of the sinoatrial node (SA node), and from this location, the excitation is propagated through the entire node, the right atrium and the other parts of the heart. Using intracellular recordings of electrical activity, West showed already in 1955 that within small areas of the SA node large differences in the shape of the recorded action potentials could be found. In addition it is known that the leading pacemaker site is small (for review see Brooks and Lu, 1972) and that its location within the node is variable even in animals from the same species (Sano and Yamagishi, 1965; Bleeker et al., 1978). Also morphologically the SA node is not homogeneous while a gradual transition between different territories is observed within the node. So it is difficult to localize precisely the leading pacemaker center. Nevertheless, among the numerous studies dealing with the ultrastructure of the SA node of several mammalian species: mole (Kikuchi, 1976), rat (Bompiani et al., 1959; Virágh and Porte, 1960; Cheng, 1971), rabbit (Torii, 1962; Trautwein and Uchizono, 1963; Challice, 1966; Tranum-Jensen, 1976), dog (Kawamura, 1961; James et al., 1966; Hayashi, 1971), cow (Rhodin et al., 1961; Hayashi, 1962), monkey (Colborn and Carsey, 1972; Viragh and Porte, 1973) and man (James et al., 1966), only that of Trautwein and Uchizono (1963) has been made after electrophysiological identification, but they selected rather large pieces (1 mm²) for morphological examination.

The study we present here was undertaken to investigate the ultrastructural features of the electrophysiologically identified group of leading pacemaker fibers. Therefore, we had to study, in ultrathin sections and freeze-cleaved replicas, pieces of nodal tissue small enough to ensure electrophysiological homogeneity. To this aim, we used the microelectrode technique in order to localize and to delimit the leading pacemaker center as exactly as possible in combination with electron-microscopical techniques to study its ultrastructure. We had to map the SA node more or less extensively to be able to localize precisely the leading center of the node, and that is why we combined the ultrastructural study of the pacemaker site with a mapping of the propagation of the excitation within the node.

MATERIAL AND METHODS

PREPARATION

Rabbits of both sexes weighing 2.5–3 kg, were anesthetized with either Na-pentobarbital (Nembutal) 20 mg/kg i.v., followed by Ether inhalation or 10 mg Fluanison + 0.2 mg Fentanyl. base (Hypnorm)/kg i.m.. The heart was rapidly excised and immersed in an oxygenated salt solution (Mc Ewen 1956; NaCl 130.6 mM, NaHCO₃ 24.2 mM, KCl 5.6 mM,

CaCl$_2$ 2.2 mM, MgCl$_2$ 0.5 mM, glucose 11.1 mM, saccharose 13.2 mM, saturated with a mixture of 95% O$_2$ and 5% CO$_2$, pH 7.35). The preparation which included the sinoatrial node (SA node), the intercaval region and the roof of the right atrial appendage was pinned up on a perforated silicon rubber block in a tissue bath so as to expose the endocardial surface. Oxygenated salt solution was continuously circulated through the 5 ml tissue bath, entering at the bottom at a rate of 20 ml/min and being sucked off from the surface. Temperature was kept constant within 0.1°C at 38°C.

LOCALIZATION OF LEADING PACEMAKER CELLS

The procedure of the localization of the leading pacemaker cells is discussed in detail elsewhere (Bleeker et al., 1978). In summary the exact localization is achieved in two steps. First, the excitation of the nodal area was mapped by recording of the electrical activity from a great number of cells according to Sano and Yamagishi (1965). The group of the earliest discharging cells was delimited by timing the moment of maximal rate of rise of the action potential to an atrial reference electrogram. Secondly, the leading fibers within this group were identified by comparing the slopes of the pacemaker potential. Action potentials were recorded by means of conventional microelectrode technique. The exploring microelectrode was mounted on a micromanipulator on a mechanical stage, the lateral movements of which were read with vernier scales accurate to 0.01 mm (Schreurs et al., 1974). Each impaled cell was marked with two coordinates. In the pacemaker center, the distance between two impalements was 0.1–0.2 mm.

ELECTRON MICROSCOPY

At the end of the electrophysiological mapping, which took 1 to 3 hours, the site of the leading pacemaker group was iontophoretically marked. For that purpose, the microelectrode was filled with a 1% solution of Alcian Blue (Lee et al., 1969) and two dots were made 200 micrometers (μm) apart, one on each side. Then the preparation, still mounted to the silicon rubber block, was immersed in cold 2% paraformaldehyde and 2.5% glutaraldehyde in 0.1 M cacodylate buffer pH 7.4 (Karnovsky, 1967). The fixation was performed during one night for the preparations intended for ultrathin sectioning and half an hour for the preparations destined for freeze fracturing. Afterwards, the preparations were washed in cacodylate buffer 0.2 M pH 7.4 and the small selected pieces were cut in blocks of 50–80/200 μm, parallel to the crista terminalis (CT), using two razor blades glued together.

For thin sectioning, the small fixed fragments were subsequently postfixed in OsO$_4$ 1% in cacodylate buffer 0.1 M one hour at 4°C, washed again in cacodylate buffer 0.2 M pH 7.4, immersed in magnesium uranyl acetate 0.5% in NaCl 0.9% at room temperature during 20 min, dehydrated in acetone and embedded in Araldite (Glauert and Glauert, 1958). The sections were cut on a Reichert ultramicrotome with glass or diamond knife and stained with lead citrate (Reynolds, 1963).

For freeze fracturing, the briefly fixed specimen were washed quickly in cacodylate buffer 0.2 M pH 7.4 and infiltrated successively with 10, 20 and 30% glycerol in the same buffer. The pieces were then mounted on gold discs and frozen in Freon 22 cooled with liquid nitrogen. Freeze fracturing at −100°C, and platinum-carbon shadowing were carried out using a Balzers freeze-etch apparatus according to Moor and Mühlethaler (1963). Replicas and ultrathin sections were examined with a Philips EM 301 electron microscope.

QUANTIFICATION

The point counting method (Weibel et al., 1966) was applied. This procedure is based on superimposing a regular point lattice on a micrograph and counting the points which fall on transections of the structures to be analysed quantitatively. A square lattice of 1 cm side-length was used over micrographs at a final magnification × 25,000. Magnifications were calibrated using a germanium shadowed carbon replica (54,864 lines per inch). Three hearts were used for quantitative determination of the volume density of the following structures: nucleus, myofilaments, mitochondria, caveolae, tubules of the sarcoplasmic reticulum, subsarcolemmal cisterns. For each of these three hearts, sections from 2 sites were used for measurements: – leading pacemaker cells and – atrium cells from the CT. For each group of cells, the structures mentioned were counted in 20 micrographs 18/18 cm. All the measured cellular components were expressed as percentages of the volume of the entire cellular mass in the section.

RESULTS

MAPPING OF THE PROPAGATION OF EXCITATION

In 25 spontaneously beating right atria, the origin and spread of excitation was mapped by multiple impalements (Bleeker et al., 1978). The preparations beated regularly; beat to beat intervals were between 320 and 420 msec at the beginning of the recording and gradually increased during the experiment (10–15 msec/hour); differences between consecutive intervals were less than 2 msec. Preparations beating irregularly were excluded because shape of action potentials and arrival time were not constant during impalation.

In 11 preparations an area of about 4 × 6 mm was explored in detail (Figure 1); this took 3 to 5 hours. The site of earliest discharge was found in the intercaval region, 0.5–2 mm away from the macroscopically visible border of the crista terminalis. From this leading pacemaker center, the excitation wave was propagated preferentially in an oblique, cranial direction towards to crista terminalis. This is in accordance with the results of Sano and Yamagishi (1965). In 14 preparations intended for electron microscopy (10 for ultrathin sectioning and 4 for freeze fracturing) we mapped extensively the leading pacemaker center and in addition but less precisely the rest of the node to be sure that the spread of excitation showed in these preparations essentially the same pattern as described previously.

QUANTITATIVE DESCRIPTION OF LEADING PACEMAKER CELLS

1. Fine structure
The cells observed within the pacemaker center will always be compared with atrial cells (Figure 2) which are so much better known from description in the literature (Mc Nutt and Fawcett, 1969). Table 1 presents a quantitative description of their composition. The cells observed in the pacemaker center (Figure 3) are of one type only: roughly spindle-shaped cells with a maximum length of 20–30 μm and a diameter of less than 8 μm, showing often an extremely irregular profile in cross section. The long axis of the cells is roughly parallel to the crista terminalis (CT). The nucleus is large and lobulated and is situated near the

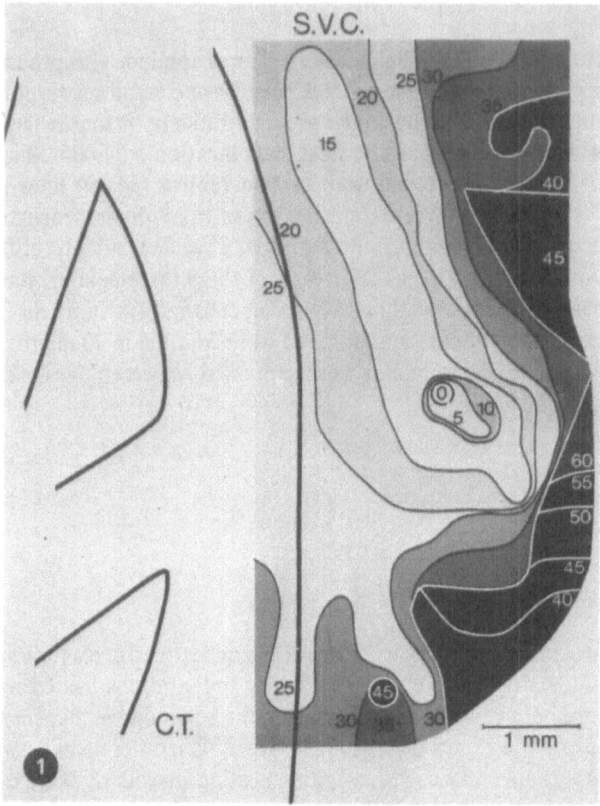

Figure 1. Propagation of excitation in the SA node. The site of earliest discharge is marked O. From here the excitation is propagated preferentially (velocity 50 cm/sec) in an oblique cranial direction towards the crista terminalis (CT); propagation is slower in other directions (5 cm/sec) and extremely slow towards the interatrial septum (less than 0.5 cm/sec). SVC: superior vena cava.

center of the cell. Chromatin is mainly concentrated in a zone adjoining the nuclear envelope, but some chromocentra are also present in the nucleoplasma. Nuclei occupy about 13% of the entire cellular volume (Table 1). The contractile system of pacemaker cells is extremely poorly developed in two respects 1) quantitatively it is much less abundant than that of the working myocardium, occupying 15% of the cellular volume instead of 53% in the CT, 2) qualitatively, its degree of organization is very low. Isolated thin and thick myofilaments are dispersed through the sarcoplasm or are bundled into myofibrils which are loosely organized with thick irregular Z lines. A and I bands are not distinctly marked, and H bands are nearly always absent (Figure 4). Myofibrils often branch or follow a zigzag course. The contractile system is also often inequally distributed; it is possible to find in the same cell a large zone where no myofilaments are present and another one where the density of contractile material is much higher. When the SA node has been cut perpendicularly to the CT, fibrils are seen running in every direction and no preferential orientation can be found (Figure 3). Nevertheless, when cut parallelly to the CT, myofibrils are observed in a great number parallel to the long axis of the cell (Figure 4). Thus it seems that the contractile system has a preferential orientation, although it is definitely less axially

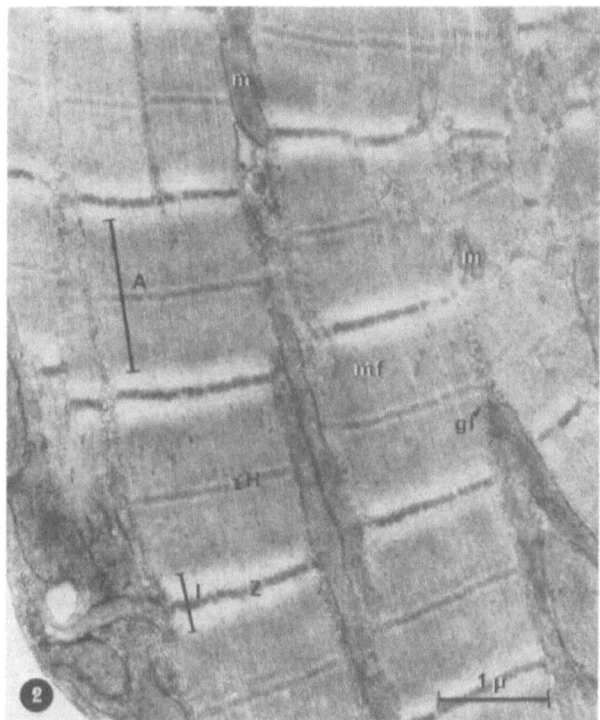

Figure 2. Some myofibrils (mf) from the crista terminalis are cut more or less longitudinally showing the pattern of the sarcomeres. Between myofibrils, mitochondria (m) and glycogen granules (gl) are present. × 25,000.

organized than that in atrial cells. Accumulations of electron dense material which presumably contains Z line material are often found in the sarcoplasm just beneath the sarcolemma (Figure 3).

Mitochondria with well developed cristae (Figures 3–4) seem to be distributed randomly in the sarcoplasm. They occupy about 15% of the cellular volume (Table 1). The sarcoplasmic reticulum (SR) is poorly developed in pacemaker cells. It represents only 1% of the volume of the sarcoplasm (Table 1). In all three preparations quantified SR tubules are more numerous in atrial cells than in nodal cells, but this does not apply to the subsarcolemmal cisterns (couplings). No relation has been found between tubules of the SR and myofibrils. They are found at random in the sarcoplasm (Figure 3). Golgi apparatus is present in the vicinity of the nucleus. Short tubules of poorly developed endoplasmic reticulum are observed in the sarcoplasm (Figure 3). The specific atrial dense granules (Bencosme and Berger, 1971) which are found in great number in atrium cells have only been observed very occasionally. Dense particles having a diameter ranging between 15–30 nm are present in the cytoplasm (Figure 9). Some of them, associated with the membranes of the reticulum, can be recognized as ribosomes. We have not performed any specific staining enabling a more definite identification, and as they overlap the size ranges of glycogen particles and ribosomes around 20 nm, we are not able to identify them pre-

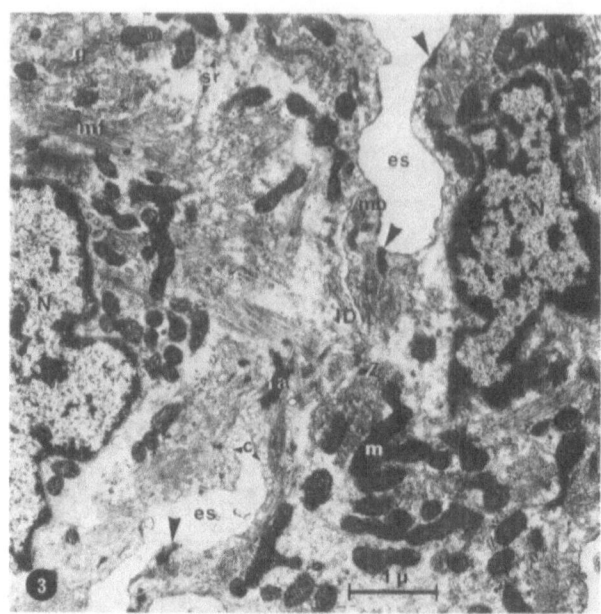

Figure 3. General view of 2 cross-sectioned cells from the SA node centre. The contractile system (mf) is extremely poorly developed and randomly distributed. At higher left, myofilaments in longitudinal and in cross section are seen side by side. Z lines (z) are thick, and z line material is found under the sarcolemma (large arrow heads). The extracellular space is often large (es) after 3 hours superfusion, and the cells are in close apposition, where they form rather straight intercalated discs (ID). A fascia adherens (fa) is present. N: nucleus SR: sarcoplasmic reticulum; g: golgi apparatus; c: caveolar invaginations; m: mitochondria; mb: multivesicular body. × 21,000.

Table 1. Composition of myocardial cells from

	Rabbit SA node	*Rabbit crista terminalis*
	Per cent of total cellular volume	Per cent of total cellular volume
Organelle	± SD. (n = 3)	± SD. (n = 3)
Myofibrils	14.7 ± 5.3	53.6 ± 3.6
Mitochondria	14.7 ± 1.5	23.0 ± 4.4
Nuclei	13.1 ± 2.7	4.3 ± 1.0
Caveolae	1.8 ± 0.1	0.8 ± 0.4
Subsarcolemmal cisternae	0.24 ± 0.07	0.38 ± 0.14
SR tubules	0.8 ± 0.7	2.6 ± 0.5
SR total	1.0 ± 0.8	3.0 ± 0.4

cisely. Nevertheless, it is clear that these granules are much less numerous in cells from the SA node than in cells from the CT. Two organelles are more abundant in the sarcoplasm of SA node cells than in that of atrium cells: multivesicular bodies (Figure 3) and leptomere fibrils (Figure 5).

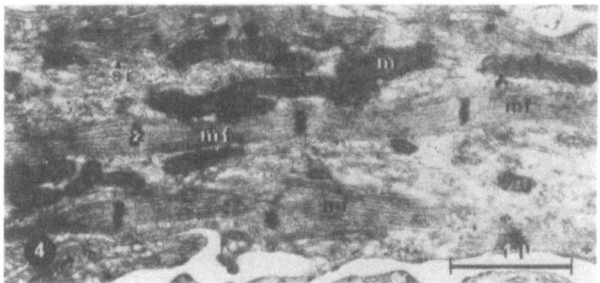

Figure 4. Longitudinal section of a SA nodal cell. The myofibrils (mf) are poorly developed and exhibit thick Z lines (z). Some tubules of sarcoplasmic reticulum (sr) are present. mit: Mitochondria. × 28,000.

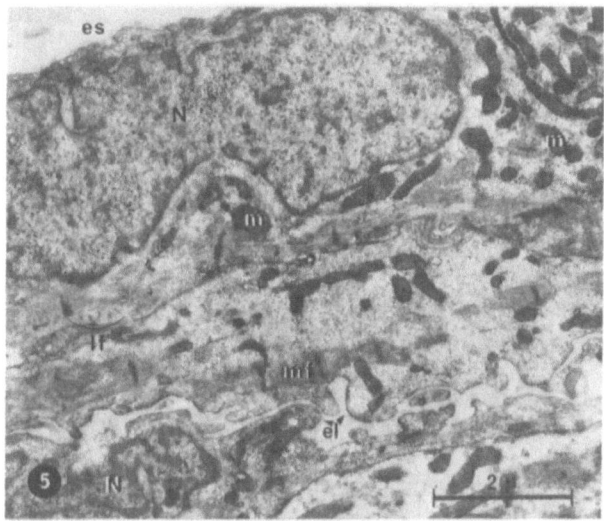

Figure 5. Longitudinal section of 4 SA nodal cells. This preparation has been fixed without prior electrophysiological study, and the cells are in close apposition. They have an elongated shape. The external lamina (el) is observed. A leptomeric fibril (lf) is located in the sarcoplasm under the sarcolemma. N: nucleus; m: mitochondria; mf: myofibrils; es: extracellular space. × 15,600.

2. Cell membranes and associated structures. Extracellular space.

The freeze cleave technique has been used parallelly with the ultrathin sections technique to demonstrate more clearly the structure of the membranes and especially the junctions present between the cells. The freeze cleave process splits plasma membranes along their hydrophobic interior, producing 2 fracture faces (Branton, 1966): PF face associated with cytoplasmic matrix and directed toward the exterior of the cell, and EF face associated with the extracellular space and directed toward the cytoplasm (for nomenclature see Branton et al., 1975) (Figure 6). The fracture faces PF and EF of the SA node cells, as all membranes examined so far, are studded with intramembranous particles of about 9 nm of diameter distributed at random (Figure 6). PF faces show 4 to 6 times more particles than EF faces (Figure 6). Figure 7 gives a general view of freeze cleaved SA nodal cells. Caveolar

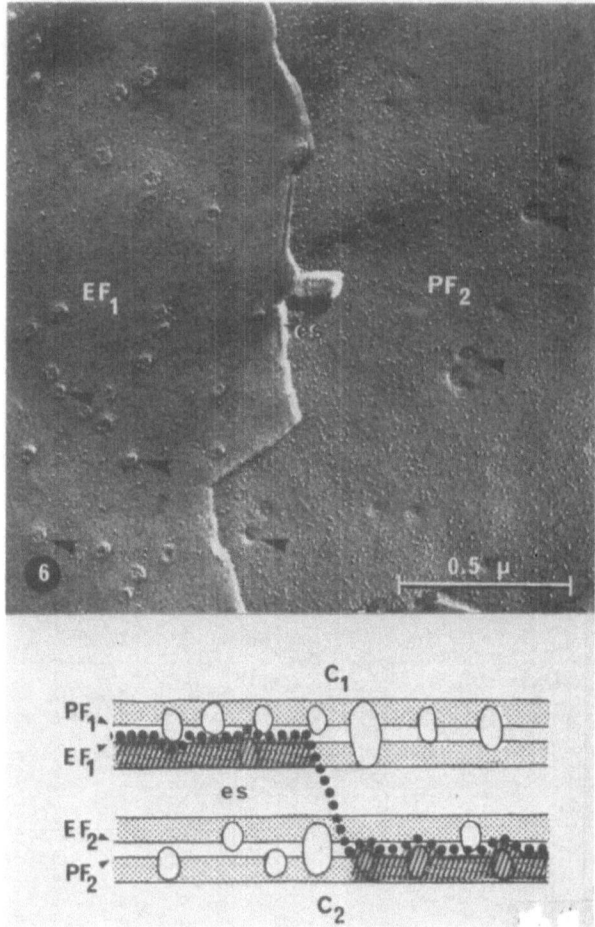

Figure 6. The cleavage plane has broken through two myocardial cells (C_1 and C_2) revealing the plasma membrane fracture faces EF_1 and EF_2. The PF faces are studded with numerous intramembranous particles whereas the EF faces show few particles. Arrows indicate openings of caveolar invaginations. es: extracellular space. × 68,800
Interpretation: Each membrane is composed of two lamellae. The fracture plane (dotted line) passes through the middle of the membrane revealing either the external face of the protoplasmic lamella (PF) or the internal face of the external lamella (EF).

invaginations are very abundant along the sarcolemma (Figure 8b) and represent about 2% of the cellular volume (Table 1). With the freeze cleave technique, caveolar invaginations can be observed in the cytoplasm, abutting to the sarcolemma (Figure 8a) and they clearly demonstrate the presence of a short neck. On the PF faces, the openings of the caveolae are found as circular depressions of 20–40 nm diameter (Figures 6 and 8a). On the EF faces, they take an other appearance. In this case, the observer is to be situated in the cell, looking at the outer leaflet of the plasma membrane. The caveolae have been broken away during fracturing and they appear as small walled craters (Figure 6). A T system has never been observed in SA node cells in ultrathin sections and no openings of the cleaved membranes have been found which could correspond to invaginations of the sarcolemma into the cells other than caveolar invaginations.

The three types of specialized junctions found between atrial cells – fascia adherens, desmosome or macula adherens and gap junction or nexus – are also present between nodal cells. However, here these junctions are not incorporated in well developed intercalated discs as they are in the CT (Figure 9). Desmosomes are recognized on PF and EF faces as patches of more or less packed and irregular particles which are larger than the usual intramembraneous particles of the undifferentiated membrane (Figure 11). Gap junctions are identified without ambiguity in freeze cleaved specimen. They appear on PF faces as arrays of particles with a 9 nm center-to-center distance (Figures 10a and 10c) which may be organized hexagonally (Figure 10c), on the EF faces as similar arrays of depressions (Figure 10b). In cells from the leading pacemaker, gap junctions are not found at preferential sites as they are in atrial cells. In ultrathin sections, punctate junctions are often observed (Figure 12); however, we have not been able to find back, in replicas, any membraneous structure which could correspond to these.

The extracellular space present between the individual leading nodal cells was quite large (Figure 3), and most of the time no external lamina was observed lining the sarcolemma. In control experiments, however, in which the preparation was fixed without prior electrophysiological study, most of the cells were in close apposition (not further than about 20 nm apart) on a great part of their surface (Figure 5). Then, when the extracellular space was larger, an external lamina was present (Figure 5). Collagenous fibers are abundant and can easily be identified in ultrathin sections as well as in freeze fractured specimen (Figures 13a and 13b). The same holds true for the extremely numerous axon profiles which are observed (Figures 14a and 14b).

DISCUSSION

Under our experimental conditions, the preparation beated regularly for longer than six hours, and reproducible action potentials could be registrated, even after this long period of time. We suppose that these results were obtained because of the fact that the preparation is very thin at the level of the SA node (maximal thickness: 0.3 mm), so that all the cells were well oxygenated. At the level of the CT which is much thicker (more than 1 mm) the oxygenation seemed to be not so good: the cells in the center were often necrotic. Nevertheless, the superfusion during the electrophysiological study gave some problems also at the SA node level. We saw that when SA node cells were observed without prior electrophysiological study, they were associated in small groups in which they were tightly packed to each other. However, when fixed after a mapping experiment, the extracellular space appeared large without an external lamina lining the sarcolemma. In both cases, (with and without prior electrophysiological study) the fixation conditions were exactly the same. Thus the superfusion with the salt solution seems to be responsible of this partial loosening of the cells. However it does not seem that the long superfusion causes other damages at the ultrastructural level, and more particularly, in most cases, the fine structure of the cells seemed to be perfectly preserved.

The method of mapping was based on the following assumptions: 1) the site of pacemaking and the route and velocity of the excitation propagation are constant during the experiment. 2) two dimensions suffice to describe the spread of excitation in the SA node.

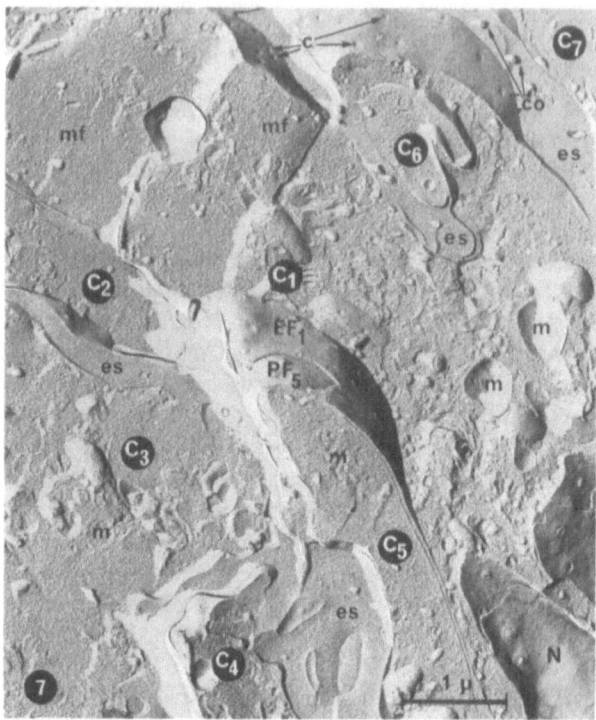

Figure 7. General view of fractured cells from the SA node. The interpretation is shown on the apposed page. The fracture reveals seven cells ($C_1 \ldots C_7$). g: golgi apparatus; mf: myofibrils; es: extracellular space; c: openings of caveolar invaginations; co: collagen fibers; N: nucleus; EF_1: external lamella of the sarcolemma of C_1; PF_5: protoplasmic lamella of the sarcolemma of C_5. × 23,400.

These assumptions were justified by the following observations: – during long impalement of a single cell ($\frac{1}{2}$ hour) the arrival time remained constant within 2 msec; – repeated impalements at the same site resulted in reproducible shape of the action potential and arrival time within 2 msec, even after some hours; – action potentials recorded at the same site but at different depths were identical.

The accuracy of determination of the impalement site was limited mainly by the movements of the contracting preparation which never exceeded 50 micrometers. Because the transition from diastolic depolarization to fast depolarization is very smooth in leading pacemaker cells, it is not possible to indicate a threshold. So as arrival time we chose the moment of steepest rise of the action potential as did Sano and Yamagishi (1965). Other criteria have been chosen by other authors, but this point is discussed elsewhere (Bleeker et al., 1978).

The electrophysiologically identified group of leading pacemaker cells of the SA node has been found to cover an area of maximally 0.2 × 0.4 mm. Taking into account the dimensions of the cells it can be estimated that the leading pacemaker center will contain only a few thousands cells. According to our criteria, it seems that all these cells have the same electrophysiological and morphological properties. In other words, the leading pacemaker function has been found to be confined to a group of cells of one type only as also

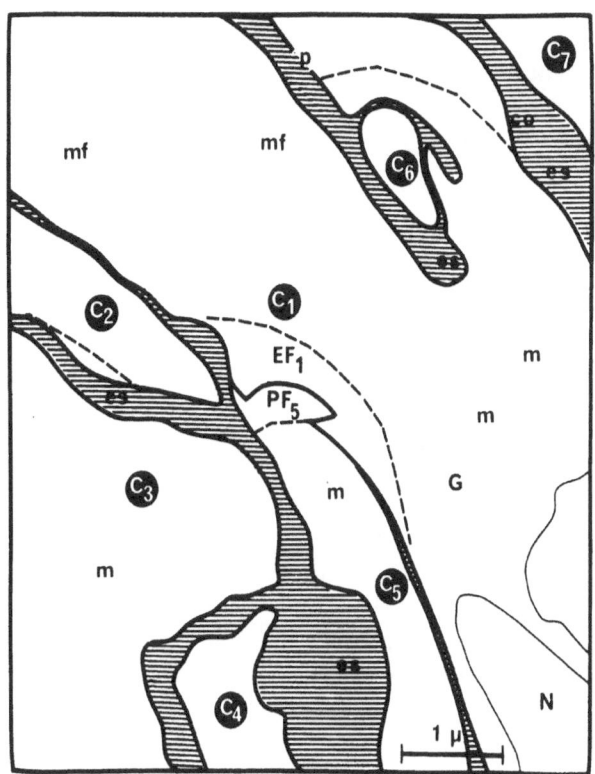

stated by Trautwein and Uchizono (1963). But we get the impression that this cell group is larger than the electrophysiologically leading pacemaker group (Bleeker et al., 1978). This cell type is named in literature P cells (James et al., 1966) or typical nodal cells (Virágh and Porte, 1973; Hayashi, 1971); they are characterized by the fact that they are the "palest" or "clearest" cells of the SA node in E.M. micrographs and probably from the entire heart. From the results shown in Table 1, we can see that only 46% of the volume of the SA nodal cells is occupied by the quantified structures compared to 86% of the volume of the atrium cells. Thus their content in organelles is low. With 15% of the cellular volume occupied by the myofilaments, these cells are clearly not very well adapted for contraction. Sometimes they are so devoid of organized myofilaments that one may wonder if they are able to contract at all.

We found that the total SR was three times less abundant in leading nodal cells than in atrium cells. There are less SR tubules in the pacemaker cells than in the CT. In the nodal cells the couplings are relatively more numerous than the SR tubules. It is not known whether in the nodal cells, where the contractile system is so rudimentarily developed, the function of the SR couplings is the same as in working myocardium. In ultrathin sections as well as with freeze cleaved replicas of SA node cells, the presence of a very great number of vesicles 20–40 nm in diameter under the sarcolemma has clearly been shown. We called these vesicles caveolae or caveolar invaginations, but in literature they are also often named micropinocytotic vesicles (e.g. Virágh and Porte, 1973). As we saw, their number in atrial cells was smaller than in leading nodal cells. A lot of questions arise as far as their function is concerned:

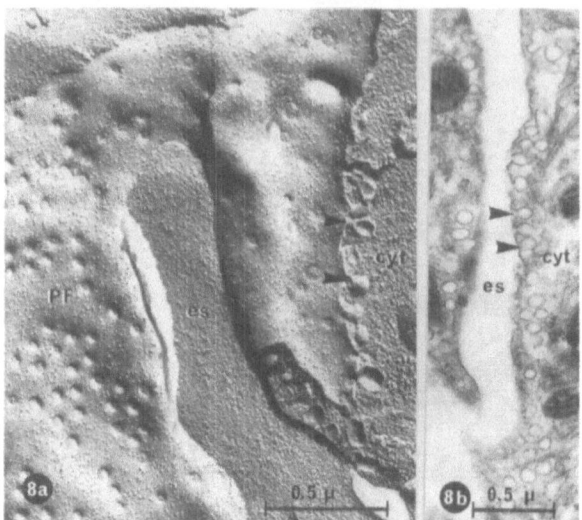

Figure 8a. On the left side of the micrograph see the PF face of a myocardial cell of the SA node. Note the numerous openings of the caveolar invaginations. The fracture revealed on the right side a part of the cytoplasm (cyt) in which caveolar invaginations are observed. Arrows indicate connections between the vesicles and the membranes. es: extracellular space. × 60,000.

b. Ultrathin section of a SA nodal cell demonstrating the presence of a great number of caveolar invaginations under the sarcolemma. Note the openings of these vesicles in the extracellular space (arrows). At the top, some vescicles seem to have fused. × 40,600.

1. to what extent do they alter the total surface of the sarcolemma?,
2. are they involved in a transport process? and if they are,
3. on which scale?,
4. which type of transport, and
5. in which direction?

Mobley and Page (1971) gave an answer to the first question; they found that in sheep cardiac Purkinje bundles the surface area of the individual fibers increased 260% with the vesicles included. We did not measure it, but from what we can see on the electronmicrographs, we think that the caveolae are even more numerous in nodal cells than in Purkinje cells, and if this is the case, the surface area in SA node cells would be increased more than 2.6 times by the presence of the vesicles. This point is, of course, rather important when the membrane capacitance or resistance per unit area of cell surface has to be calculated from electrical measurements. The problem whether the caveolar invaginations are involved in a transport process is to date not yet solved. Nevertheless, it has been shown in secretory cells, that in freeze fracturing the process of exocytosis appears different from that of endocytosis (Orci et al., 1973; Smits et al., 1973). If the same criteria can also be applied to heart cells, the vesicles we are talking about could be endocytotic vesicles, but absolutely not exocytotic vesicles. This is in contradiction with the suggestion of Pollack (1977). But according to the results of Lorber and Bertaud (1971), it seems also rather improbable that these vesicles are endocytotic. These authors studied these vesicles in frog atrial muscle where they are numerous. They used lanthanum as an extracellular marker, but they did administer it after fixation of the muscle. Thus they could make sure that all the marked vesicles communicate with the extracellular space, even if it was not evident in a particular

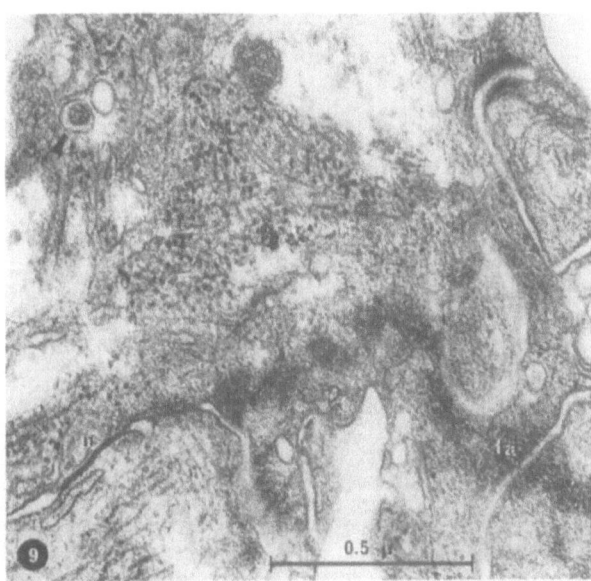

Figure 9. Desmosomes (d), fascia adherens (fa) and nexus (n) are present between cells from the SA node.
×96,000.

thin section. These authors were not able to find any vesicle without lanthanum; they consequently suggest that micropinocytosis does not occur in these cells, and if it does, pinching off of vesicles is a rare event, else the free vesicles formed will have a short life. Thus it would seem that these vesicles act as extension of the cell membrane and serve to enlarge its area, and therefore we called them caveolae or caveolar invaginations and not micropinocytotic vesicles. Ishikawa and Yamada (1975) presented evidence in mouse cardiac muscle that the sarcolemma of the T system arises by progressive addition of caveolae.

SA nodal cells are in contact with each other in all directions, and it is often stated that no intercalated discs are present (e.g. James et al., 1966). Nevertheless, it is obvious (see Figure 9) that often the membranes of two neighbouring cells are forming structures which arc like the rather straight intercalated discs observed between embryonic heart cells or young heart cells in culture (Masson-Pévet et al., 1976). In these intercalated discs, fasciae adherentes, desmosomes and gap junctions are observed. Gap junctions have been mentioned to be either absent (James et al., 1966) or exceedingly rare (Tranum-Jensen, 1976). We do not agree with these opinions because we found, using both ultrathin sectioning and freeze fracturing techniques, that although nexuses are less numerous than between atrial cells, they are not rare. Rather large nexuses have also been observed, although small nexuses are more numerous. It is believed that the nexuses are the low resistance junctions between heart cells (for review see Berger, 1972). The fact that we found an appreciable amount of gap junctions conforms with the finding of Bonke (1972) that the space constant in SA node of the rabbit is relatively large.

We can state that none of the observed cellular details seems to be the structural basis of the spontaneous discharge. This is not so surprising because it is known that every myocardial cell can become spontaneously beating if it is isolated (Harary and Farley, 1963); in addition, under certain circumstances a shift in dominant pacemaker site can occur within

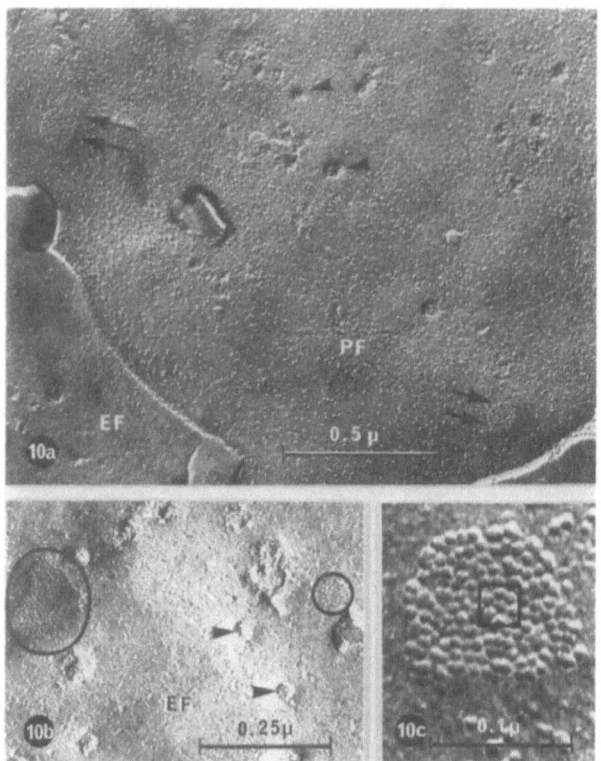

Figure 10a. The fracture plane, revealed PF and EF faces. Arrows indicate gap junctions on the PF face. Arrow heads show openings of caveolar invaginations. × 71,300.

b. EF fracture face. In the circles note the regular arrangement of small pits corresponding to nexal structures. × 120,000.

c. High magnification of one of the gap junctions seen in Figure 10a, where the hexagonal arrangement of the junctional particles is shown. × 320,000.

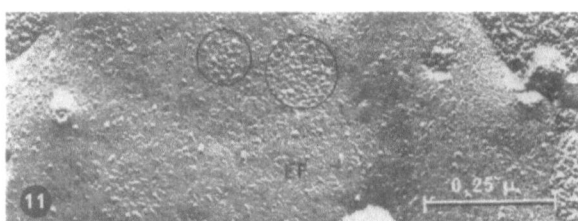

Figure 11. Aspect of desmosomes on a EF fracture face. × 120,000.

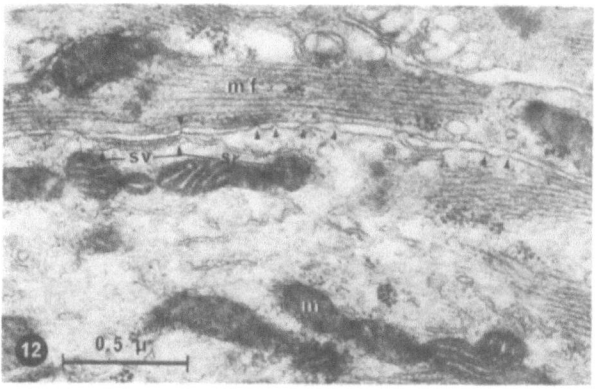

Figure 12. Aspect of the punctate junctions (arrows) observed between SA nodal cells. A continuity is seen between a subsarcolemmal vesicle (sv) and a tubule of the SR (sr). mf: myofilaments. × 60,000.

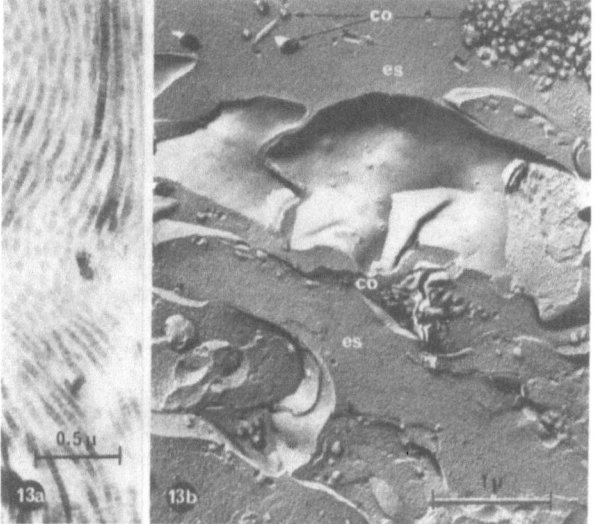

Figure 13a. Collagen fibers in ultrathin sections. × 40,800.

b. Collagen fibers (co) are present in great number in the extracellular space (es). × 28,400.

the node (Brooks and Lu, 1972). Probably pacemaking is a membrane bound process which cannot be detected with the electron microscopical techniques now available.

ACKNOWLEDGEMENTS

We wish to thank Dr. Elisabeth C.M. Hoefsmit, Electron microscopy Laboratory of the Free University, Amsterdam, for the generous offering of her facilities to us. We also wish to thank her and Prof. Dr. J. James for their helpful discussions, and C.E. Besselsen and J.O. Boorsma for technical assistance.

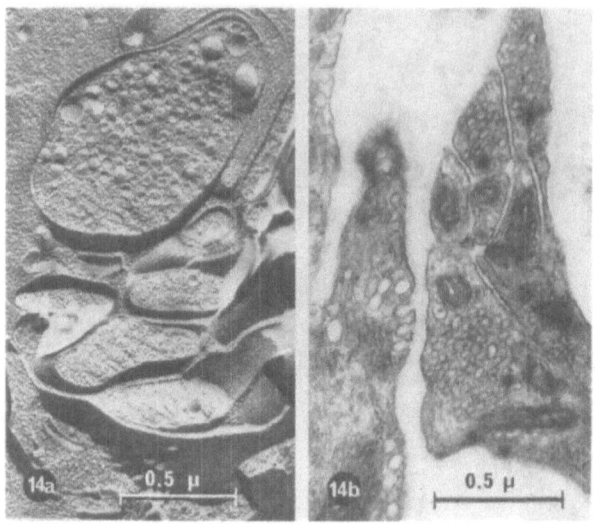

Figure 14a. The freeze fracture has broken through a bundle of axons. × 50,000.
  b. A bundle of axons is present between SA nodal cells. × 57,300.

REFERENCES

Benscosme, S.A., Berger, J.M.: Specific granules in mammalian and non-mammalian vertebrate cardiocytes. In: *Meth Achievm Exp Path* vol. 5. Bajusz, E., Jasmin, G. (eds.), Basel, 1971, p. 173

Berger, W.K.: Correlation between the ultrastructure and function of intercellular contacts. In: Electrical phenomena in the heart, edited by de Mello, W.C. Acad. Press, New York and London, 1972, p. 63

Bompiani, G.D., Rouiller, C., Hatt, P.Y.: Le tissu de conduction du cœur chez le rat. Etude au microscope électronique. I. Le tronc commun du faisceau de His et les cellules claires de l'oreillette droite. *Arch des maladies du cœur et des vaisseaux* 52: 1257, 1959

Bonke, F.I.M.: Electrotonic spread in the sinoatrial node of the rabbit heart. *Pflügers Arch* 339: 17, 1973

Branton, D.: Fracture faces of frozen membranes. *Proc Nat Acad Sci USA* 55: 1048, 1966

Branton, D., Bullivant, S., Gilula, N.B., Karnovsky, M.J., Moor, A., Mühlethaler, K., Northcote, D.H., Packer, L., Satir, B., Satir, P., Speth, V., Staehlin, L.A., Steer, R.L., Weinstein, R.S.: Freeze-etching nomenclature. *Science* 190: 54, 1975

Brooks, C.Mc.C., Lu, H.H.: The sinoatrial pacemaker of the heart. Springfield, Ill., 1972

Challice, C.E.: Studies on the microstructure of the heart. I. The sinoatrial node and the sinoatrial ring bundle. *J Roy Micr Soc* 85: 1, 1966

Cheng, Y.P.: The ultrastructure of the rat sinoatrial node. *Acta Anat Nipponica* 46: 339, 1971

Colborn, G.L., Carsey, E. Jr.: Electron microscopy of the sinoatrial node of the squirrel monkey (saimiri sciureus). *J Mol Cell Cardiol* 4: 525, 1972

Glauert, A.M., Glauert, R.H.: Araldite as an embedding medium for electron microscopy. *J Biophys Biochem Cytol* 4: 191, 1958

Harary, I., Farley, B.: In vitro studies on single beating heart cells. *Exptl Cell Res* 29: 451, 1963

Hayashi, K.: An electron microscopy study on the conduction system of the cow heart. *Jap Cir J* 26: 765, 1962

Hayashi, S.: Electron miscroscopy of the heart conduction system of the dog. *Arch Histol Jap* 33: 67, 1971

Ishikawa, H., Yamada, E.: Differentiation of the sarcoplasmic reticulum an T-system in developing mouse cardiac muscle. In: Developmental and physiological correlates of cardiac muscle, edited by Lieberman, M., Sano, T. Raven Press, 1975, p. 21

James, T.N., Sherf, L., Fine, G., Morales, A.R.: Comparative ultrastructure of the sinus node in man and dog. *Circulation* 34: 139, 1966

Karnovsky, M.J.: The ultrastructural basis of capillary permeability studied with peroxidase as tracer. *J Cell Biol* 35: 213, 1967

Kawamura, K.: Electron microscope studies on the cardiac conduction system of the dog. II. The sinoatrial and atrioventricular nodes. *Jap Cir J* 25: 973, 1961

Kikuchi, S.: The structure and innervation of the sinu-atrial node of the mole heart. *Cell Tiss Res* 172: 345, 1976

Lee, B.B., Mandl, G., Stean, J.P.B.: Microelectrode tip position marking in nervous tissue: a new dye method. *Electroenceph Clin Neurophysiol* 27: 610, 1969

Lorber, V., Bertaud, W.S.: Cellular surfaces of amphibian atrial muscle. *J Cell Sci* 9: 427, 1971

McEwen, L.M.: The effect on the isolated rabbit heart of vagal stimulation and its modification by cocaine, hexamethonium and ouabain. *J Physiol* 131: 678, 1956

McNutt, N.S., Fawcett, D.W.: The ultrastructure of the cat myocardium. *J Cell Biol* 42: 46, 1969

Masson-Pevet, M., Jongsma, H.J., Bruijne de, J.: Collagenase- and trypsin-dissociated heart cells: a comparative ultrastructural study. *J Mol Cell Cardiol* 8: 747, 1976

Mobley, B. A., Page, E.: The surface area of sheep cardiac Purkinje fibres. *J Physiol* 220: 547, 1972

Moor, H., Mühlethaler, K.: Fine structure of frozen-etched yeast cells. *J Cell Biol* 17: 609, 1963

Orci, L., Amherdt, M., Malaisse-Lagae, F., Rouiller, Ch., Reynold, A.E.: Insulin release by emiocytosis: demonstration with freeze-etching technique. *Science* 179: 82, 1973

Pollack, G.H.: Cardiac pacemaking: an obligatory role of catecholamines? A possible mechanism underlaying spontaneous pacemaking can be deduced from several recent clues. *Science* 196: 731, 1977

Reynolds, E.S.: The use of lead citrate at high pH as an electron opaque stain in electron microscopy. *J Cell Biol* 17: 208, 1963

Rhodin, J.A.G., Del Missier, P., Reid, L.C.: The structure of the specialized impulse conducting system of the steer heart. *Circulation* 24: 349, 1961

Sano, T., Yamagishi, S: Spread of excitation from the sinus node. *Circulation Res* 16: 423, 1965

Schreurs, A.W., Meijer, A.A., Bouman, L.N., Bonke, F.I.M.: Micromanipulator with an electrode driver used for microelectrode work. *Pflügers Arch* 346: 163, 1974

Smith, U., Smith, D.S., Winkler, H., Ryan, J.W.: Exocitosis in adrenal medulla demonstrated by freeze etching. *Science* 179: 79, 1973

Torii, H.: Electron microscope observations of the S.A. and A.V. nodes and the Purkinje fibres of the rabbit. *Jap Cir J* 26: 39, 1962

Tranum-Jensen, J.: The fine structure of the atrial and atrioventricular (AV) junctional specialized tissues of the rabbit heart. In: The conduction system of the heart; structure, function and clinical implications, edited by Wellens, H.J.J., Lie, K.I., Janse, M.J. Stenfert Kroese B.V. Leiden, 1976, p. 55

Trautwein, W., Uchizono, K.: Electron microscopic and electrophysiologic study of the pacemaker in the sinoatrial node of the rabbit heart. *Z Zellforsch Midrosk Anat* 61: 96, 1963

Viragh, S., Porte, A.: Le noeud de Keith et Flack et les différentes fibres auriculaires du cœur de rat. Etude au microscope optique et électronique. *CR Acad Sci* (Paris) 251: 2086, 1960

Viragh, S., Porte, A.: The fine structure of the conducting system of the monkey heart (Macaca mulatta) I. The sinoatrial node and the internodal connections. *Z Zellforsch* 145: 191, 1973

Weibele, E.R., Kistler, G.S., Walter, F.S.: Practical stereological methods for morphometric cytology. *J. Cell Biol* 30: 23, 1966

West, T.C.: Ultramicroelectrode recording from the cardiac pacemaker. *J Pharmacol Exp Ther* 115: 283, 1955

17

GENERAL COMMENTS

ANTON E. BECKER

Most investigations which correlate the structure of the human pacemaker with function fall short because of the fact that direct correlates can rarely be made. Circumstantial evidence and parallels with animal experiments are the pillars upon which most of our present day knowledge is based. Awareness of pitfalls that may accompany "facts" so obtained is essential for those working in the field. Then, however, valuable information can emerge from which the sick patient may eventually benefit.

The works presented in this chapter underline this statement and the problems encountered in correlating structure with function are exceedingly well spelled out in the contribution by Janse and co-workers (Chapter 15). It is worthwhile to pause for a while with their contribution, because it is basic to most of our knowledge of cellular electrophysiology. Most skilfully, these workers have been able to correlate cellular electrophysiology with ultrastructural morphology of the area where the micro-electrodes had been impaled. In fact their meticulous method enabled them to visualize at an ultrastructural level, the complete track of the electrode. What one of course might have predicted may still come as a shock, and this definitely applies to the colossal damage that has occurred to the cells neighbouring the track. One may only speculate to what extent this might affect our interpretations of intracellular action potential recordings and it definitely adds a new perspective to studies correlating structure and function.

A few topics have been selected for further comment, mainly because of their controversial nature.

SINUS NODE EMBRYOLOGY

At present it is still controversial whether or not the sinus node develops as a unilateral or as a bilateral structure. Patten (1956) working with chicken embryos had suggested that the sinus node developed as a paired structure, while Van Mierop and Gessner (1970) studying the mouse embryo were unable to confirm this observation. Moreover, the few workers (Robb et al., 1948; Yamauchi, 1965) which have reported on the development of the sinus node in human embryos were also unable to demonstrate a bilateral anlage. It is of interest, therefore, that the observations made by Anderson and associates (Chapter 14) in human fetuses and neonates endorse the concept that, although the sinus node can be recognized very early in development, at that stage it already is in a unilateral position. This observation, however, should not necessarily degrade a concept of bilateralness nor does it contradict the concept that the node develops from sinoatrial specialized ring tissue (Anderson et al., 1976; Wenink, 1976), since it is accepted that the greater part of these rings will disappear early in embryonic life. Arguments in favour of the "ring tissue concept" are based upon the position of the node (vide infra) which is in accordance with the anticipated "line" of incorporation of the right sinus venosus horn into the right atrium. Moreover, in the "asplenia syndrome", commonly associated with a right *and* a left superior caval vein both entering a right- and left-sided atrium, respectively, *bi*lateral sinus nodes have been described (Van Mierop and Wiglesworth, 1962; Van Mierop et al., 1964). The authors explain this observation by stating that the left sinus horn has become incorporated at a very early stage into the atrium which, according to their opinion, exhibits characteristics of a morphological right atrium. As such, the "asplenia syndrome" is considered an early developmental error which results in bilateral right-sidedness. These observations, however, may also indicate that the potential for bilateral development of the sinus node is normally present but that the development of these anlagen depends upon the development of the veno-atrial junction, rather than on unilateralness persé. It is of interest, in this respect, that in man, although the sinus node is a right-sided structure, its artery originates from either the proximal right or left coronary arteries, with only slight predominance for the right.

POSITION OF THE SINUS NODE

The position of the sinus node, laterally in the epicardial groove of the sulcus terminalis, was already pointed out by Koch in 1909. Since then the exact position of the node has become a matter of controversy, although most investigators nowadays seem to confirm Koch's original description (James, 1961; Truex et al., 1967; Lev and Bharati, 1974). Some, however, have opined a different view in describing a horse-shoe shaped sinus node (Blair and Davies, 1935), which has been portrayed with its major limb medial to the superior caval vein – right atrial junction (Hudson, 1960). The developmental and anatomical studies of Anderson and his colleagues (Chapter 14) do not endorse the latter concept, but instead support the early observations made by Koch (1909). Anderson et al. furthermore emphasize that the sinus node in the neonate and young infant is of a relatively larger size, extending more caudally towards the inferior caval vein, than in adult hearts; an observation with particular relevance for operative procedures in early infancy (Figure 1).

ARTERIAL SUPPLY TO THE SINUS NODE

Although much has been written about the arterial supply of the sinus node there still remain some matters of controversy. One of these relates to the concept proposed by James (1961) that clockwise or counter-clockwise encirclement of the right superior caval vein by the sinus node artery would influence the position of the main mass of the sinus node. These observations were not endorsed by Anderson et al. (Chapter 14), which may relate to the fact that they observed in only 4 of 8 hearts a nodal artery coursing throughout the entirety of the node. The remaining 4 specimens showed a nodal artery which upon reaching the nodal mass dissolved in several ramifications. These observations further question the significance of the concept, proposed by James (1967), that the pulsatile mechanics of the nodal artery play a role in the automaticity of pacemaker action. Knowledge of the variability of the arterial supply to the sinus node in man is of major surgical significance, since it implies that not only the region of the sulcus terminalis is a "danger area", but also the entirety of the circumference of the superior caval vein – right atrial junction.

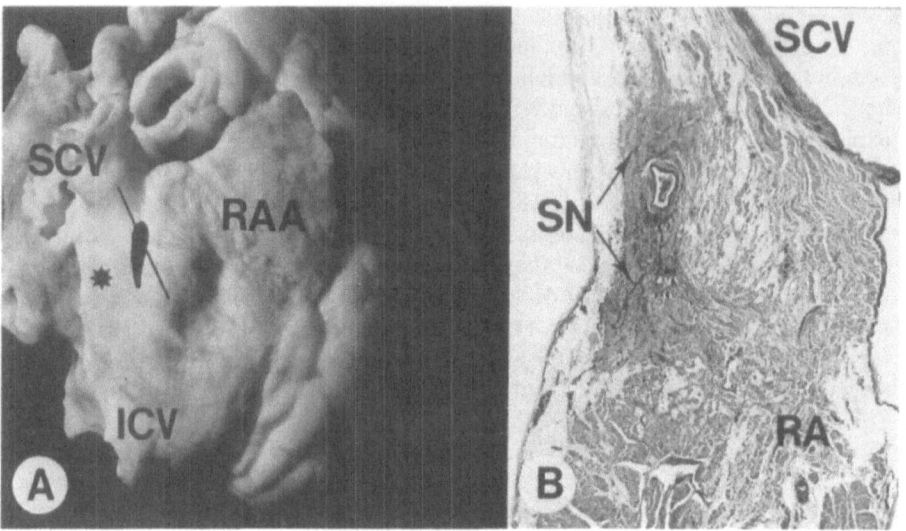

Figure 1. The human sinus node. (A) Lateral view of the right side of the heart. The lateral position of the sinus node in the sulcus terminalis has been inked (solid black). The intercaval area (asterisk) which forms the postero-lateral continuation between the superior (SCV) and inferior (ICV) caval veins is composed mainly of fibrous tissue and, therefore can play no role as a pathway for impulse propagation. The tail of the sinus node in this infant heart, comes closer to the ostium of the inferior caval vein than in the adult heart. The line drawn through the head part of the node indicates the plane of the microscopic section shown in B (and Figure 2). RAA = right atrial appendage. (B) Histological appearance of the sinus node (SN) in the sulcus terminalis covered by epicardial fat tissue and "resting" on right atrial (RA) myocardium. The sinus node artery courses through the main mass of the node. SCV = superior caval vein. Elastic tissue stain; × 7.5.

CONNECTIONS OF THE SINUS NODE

The precise way in which the cells of the sinus node make contact with surrounding cell masses is right up to this date a contentious subject. In reconstructing the node in its position in the sulcus terminalis it becomes evident that only a limited number of possibilities remain (Figure 1). For instance, the postero-lateral area between the ostia of the two caval veins, the so-called intercaval area, can play no role in propagating the sinus node impulse, since it is mainly composed of fibrous tissue. The potential sites for propagation which remain are (1) axial extensions of the head and tail parts of the node and (2) the area where the node "rests" on the crista terminalis (Figure 1). It is of interest, in this respect, that although the area of contact between nodal cells and those of the crista is large, the greater part of it is represented by contiguity between cells, rather than by actual continuity in the sense of axial cell-to-cell contacts. The latter type of contact is characterized by a "streaming" of transitional cells from the node into the crista terminalis, where the cells merge with atrial myocardium (Figure 2). These connections are of particular interest, since one may speculate whether they could serve as an anatomic pathway for re-entry phenomena within the sinus node. On the other hand, a proper understanding of the geometry of the node and its atrial connections are crucial with respect to the controversies that surround the topic of preferential internodal conduction.

Anderson and co-workers (Chapter 14) restate their opinion that histologically identifiable tracts, i.e. tracts where the cells are distinguishable from "ordinary" atrial myocardium,

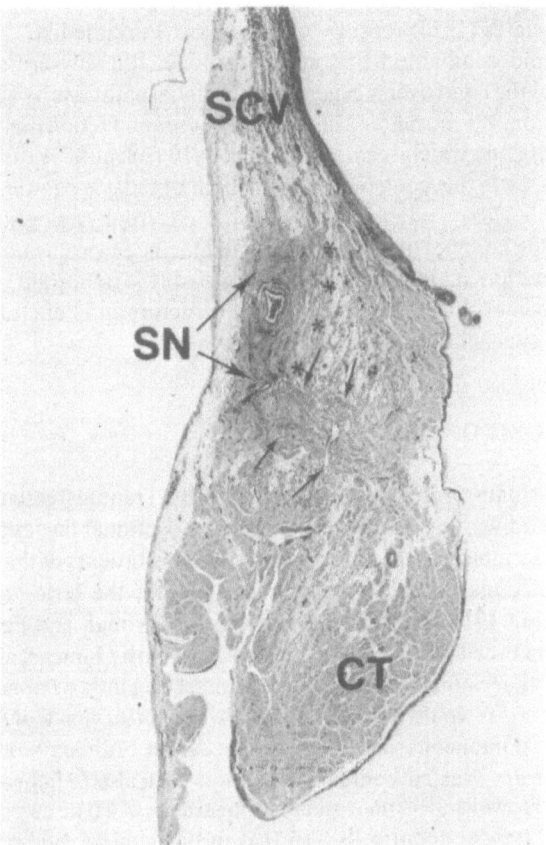

Figure 2. Histological section to show the sinus node (SN) on the epicardial aspect of the crista terminalis (CT), immediately underneath the junction between superior caval vein (SCV) and right atrium. There is a large area of contiguity between cells of the sinus node and atrial myocardial cells (asterisks). Axial cell-to-cell contact, however, is only present at the site (arrows) where transitional cells "stream" out of the node into the crista to merge with atrial myocardial cells. Elastic tissue stain; × 6.

do not connect the sinus node with the atrioventricular node. To rule out any misconception with regard to this statement, it should be re-emphasized that the authors were unable to identify histo-and cytological discrete tracts, comparable for instance to the ventricular bundle branches. This statement, however, does not interfere with a concept of electrophysiologically identifiable tracts (Spach et al., 1969; 1971). As stated previously (Becker and Anderson, 1976) the geometry of the right atrium is such that any impulse originating in the sinus node in order to reach the atrioventricular node, is bound to spread along a limited number of anatomical pathways. The way in which cell-to-cell connections between node and atrial myocardium are formed (vide supra) determines the tracts through which the sinus node impulse can be transferred to the cells in these anatomical pathways. The packing of atrial fibers in parallel bundles in these pathways, for instance in the crista terminalis, may favour rapid conduction and may thus explain the preferential routes that have been shown to exist electrophysiologically. One might then consider that the controversy is actually one of semantics. However, this seems an oversimplification, since Isa and associates (1976) recently claimed that "Purkinje-like" fibers were directly responsible for rapid conduction between both nodes, thereby criticizing a previously published review of the controversy regarding internodal pathways by Janse and Anderson (1974). In my opinion, the morphologists who study the conduction tissues of the heart and who have raised an issue which seemed buried in 1910 (Aschoff, 1910) have the responsibility also to try to settle this controversy in the light of today's knowledge of intercellular connections and in close collaboration with the electrophysiologists. The need for a re-evaluation of this complex matter is self-evident, since existence or non-existence of "specialized" tracts has major surgical implications. It is important, therefore, to state that workers which contributed to this chapter on Structure and Function of the sinus node opined that such "specialized" tracts were *non*-existent.

ULTRASTRUCTURE OF SINUS NODE

The ultrastructural data presented in this chapter by Tranum-Jensen (Chapter 13) and Masson-Pévet and co-workers (Chapter 16) are of exceptional fine quality.

First of all, the terminology used for the cellular constituents of the node is attractive, since it avoids functional implications. For this reason, the term "typical nodal cell", coined by Hayashi in 1971 and further popularized by Virágh and Porte in 1973, is preferred over the term P-cell (i.e. Pacemaker cell), suggested by James et al. (1966). Although the cell may act as the leading pacemaker cell, as most elegantly demonstrated by Masson-Pévet and co-workers, it would not necessarily always perform in that fashion. Moreover, the potential for spontaneous discharge can occur in ordinary working myocardium cells as well. The term P-cell is confusing since it is used also to indicate either Purkinje-cells or Pale cells. However, the microscopic appearance of a pale cytoplasm is considered characteristic for "typical nodal cells", so that in this context pale cells and pacemaker cells might constitute one and the same cell type. On the other hand, large "pale" cells have been described within the sinus node and these cells have been interpreted as a "special" cellular constituent, sometimes considered synonymous with Purkinje cells. Tranum-Jensen (Chapter 13) has pointed out that such cells, which he has termed "clear cells", are probably artefactual in nature, in analogy to similar cellular appearances that can occur in ischemic working myocardium. Jennings and Ganote (1974) have demonstrated that ischemia of myocardial cells may lead to excessive intracellular accumulation of water through a process of osmosis. Tranum-Jensen's hypothesis to explain the occurrence of "clear" cells within the sinus node is based on similar considerations. Rapid breakdown of glycogen storages with accumulation of metabolites, in particular lactate, could create an environment in which osmosis might change the cell into a "clear cell". This hypothesis is attractive, since similar cellular changes can be observed in other organ systems, generally referred to as "hydropic cell change". The potential reversibility of this change is a matter of dispute since the observer is not certain at which stage of cell transformation he happens to see the cell through his microscope. Basically, however, the process of "hydropic change" should be reversible in nature, although dependant upon the severity of the initial injury to the cell.

It is further pertinent to state that both light and electron microscopic studies have revealed that the sinus node has a rather homogeneous cellular composition, with prevailing nodal cells. Towards the atrial myocardium the "typical nodal cells" become replaced by a "transitional cell", which according to the ultrastructural observations regarding its cellular organelles is truly transitional between the "typical nodal cell" on the one hand and the "working atrial myocardial cell" on the other. The volume of this transitional area, however, is species dependant, being for instance broad in the rabbit heart but narrow in the sinus nodes of pigs and dogs. The transitional area in the human sinus node is narrow also, compared to the central bulk of "typical nodal cells".

One of the most fascinating aspects of the ultrastructure of "typical nodal cells", emphasized by Tranum-Jensen and Masson-Pévet et al. is the presence of caveolae, i.e. vesicular invaginations of the cell membrane. These minute structures are not specific for nodal cells but they occur in a much higher frequency in these cells than in ordinary cardiocytes. The question whether these caveolae function as endocytotic or exocytotic vesicles is a matter as yet unsettled. It is important, however, to gain a better understanding of their functional significance, in particular in view of Pollack's (1977) concept on pace-maker impulse formation. According to his views catecholamines stored within nodal cells play an important role, but in order to do so must exit from the cell and reach the outside of the cell membrane. In his concept, therefore, the caveolae function as exocytotic vesiculae. Masson-Pévet and co-workers (Chapter 16) using a freeze fracturing technique conclude that the caveolae observed are different from those described in cells with a proven neurosecretory function. They, therefore, question the exocytotic function of caveolae, but at the same time mention the work of Lorber and Bertaud (1971) who, on the other hand, considered it unlikely that these vesicles could have an endocytotic function. At the present stage the major significance of the caveolae seems to be the way they extend the total membrane surface area of the nodal cell. As such, these structures may play a crucial role in the pacemaking process, which after all seems to be a membrane bound phenomenon. It is of interest, in this respect, that Mason-Pévet et al. from their studies conclude that gap junctions or nexus between nodal cells do occur and, in fact, are more numerous than generally thought of (James, 1966; Tranum-Jensen, 1976). Again this observation made in the sinus node of the rabbit is an important contribution in an attempt to understand the basic mechanisms of impulse spread within the sinus node. Thusfar, however, none of the ultrastructural investigations have revealed anything with which spontaneous depolarization of the nodal cell can be conclusively correlated. Enhancement of our knowledge in this respect may come with the introduction of more advanced techniques that enable the study of cell membrane characteristics under experimental conditions.

SINUS NODE PATHOLOGY

It may be worthwhile to add a few lines on the pathology of the sinus node, since this also is a contentious subject. It has been shown (Lev, 1954; Davies and Pomerance, 1972) that the amount of fibrous tissue in the node increases with age. Our own studies (Becker, unpublished data) endorse this work (Figure 3). However, it is common experience that even in cases with a marked fibrosis the sinus node might have functioned normally. In a way this is not surprising since fibrosis persé would not interfere with nodal cell function nor with impulse spread, as long as the nodal cells themselves do not transfer into scleroprotein producing cells. Ultrastructural studies of nodal cells make such an event less likely, since the cells do not contain the organelles that one would consider a necessity for such a phenomenon. One may wonder, however, whether this holds true also for the transitional

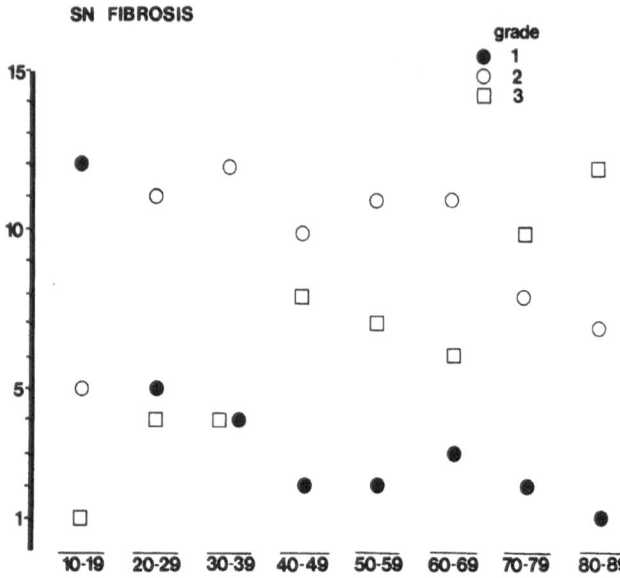

Figure 3. Graph correlating the degree of "fibrosis" within the sinus node with age. The vertical axis shows the number of cases. The horizontal axis shows the ages studied, ranging from 10 to 89 years, clustered in 8 groups each encompassing a 10 year period. In each age group 20 hearts have been studied, except for the group from 10–19 years, in which only 18 cases could be investigated. A subjective and arbitrary division has been made into 3 grades: grade 1 representing a minimal, grade 2 a moderate and grade 3 a marked fibrous component of the main nodal mass. At older age the number of cases with a marked fibrous tissue component has definitely increased over that in the younger age groups.

cells in the peripheral rim of the node. In some cases of the so-called sick sinus syndrome we have observed that the "streaming" contacts from the node with the crista terminalis were markedly fibrotic, together with parts of the "receiving" atrial myocardium; the central mass of the node being unaffected. In future studies, therefore, correlating nodal fibrosis with function one should actually specify precisely what has fibrosed since the simple qualification "fibrosis" is in itself insufficient. Another, interesting argument relative to the diseased sinus node is whether or not coronary atherosclerosis may play a role. It has been pointed out that the sinus node artery itself is only rarely involved in the atherosclerotic process (Davies and Pomerance, 1972), while other studies have denied a positive correlation between atherosclerosis of the main coronary arteries and impaired sinus node function (Engel et al., 1975).

Apart from the fact that, of course, many other conditions than ischemia alone can affect sinus node function, it also appears that the clinical parameters to establish abnormalities in sino-atrial conduction are as yet still controversial. Recently, Jordan and associates (1977) using sinoatrial conduction time as an indicator for sinus node dysfunction, conclude that coronary artery disease does play a role. From a morphologic point of view there are two considerations in this respect which should be raised and which, to my opinion, may play an important role in evaluating correlative studies on pathology and function of the sinus node. Firstly, it is a common experience for the pathologist who regularly observes post-mortem coronary angiograms to actually visualize good contrast

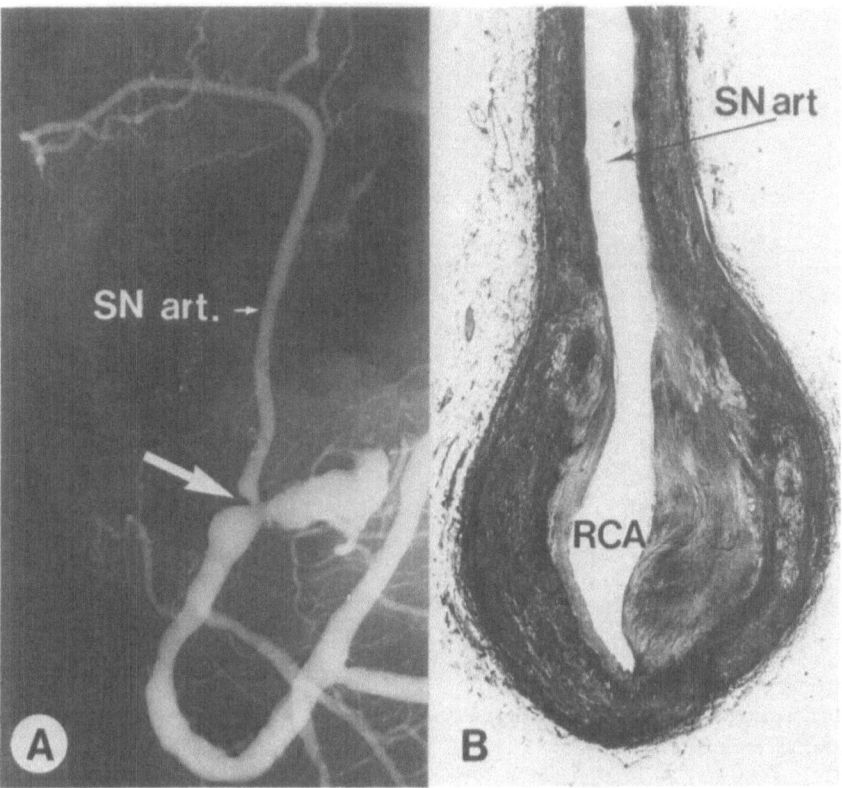

Figure 4. An example to illustrate how coronary atherosclerosis may affect the sinus node artery. (A) shows a detail of a post-mortem coronary angiogram after injection into the right coronary artery. The sinus node artery (SN-art) originates from the proximal segment of the right coronary artery. At the site of origin a severe narrowing of the lumen is present (arrow), but nevertheless a good contrast filling of the sinus node artery has been obtained. This, however, does not exclude impaired flow in vivo. Moreover, such localized stenoses can be misinterpreted on clinical angiograms, as illustrated in a histological section, (B) of this segment. The right coronary artery (RCA) shows excentric stenosis as the site where the sinus node artery originates. This type of luminal narrowing is well know to cause difficulties in angiographic recognition, since in certain views the lumen would not appear to be narrowed. Elastic tissue stain; × 14.

filling of a sinus node artery, with a non-sclerotic proximal segment of the parent coronary artery, but *with* a marked narrowing at the very origin of the sinus node artery (Figure 4). Good filling of the sinus node artery in the post-mortem angiogram does not necessarily mean that in vivo no obstruction was present. Moreover, lesions as just described may be missed on clinical angiograms or misinterpreted with respect to its significance for the sinus node artery. A second point, which is neglected, is the fact that the sinus node artery, whether it originates from the right or left coronary artery, has many anastomoses with atrial arteries from the other side, which can form significant collateral pathways for an ischemic ventricular myocardium. The possibility that such pathways may lead to a sort of "coronary steal" with ischemic effects on the pacemaker should be considered (Figure 5).

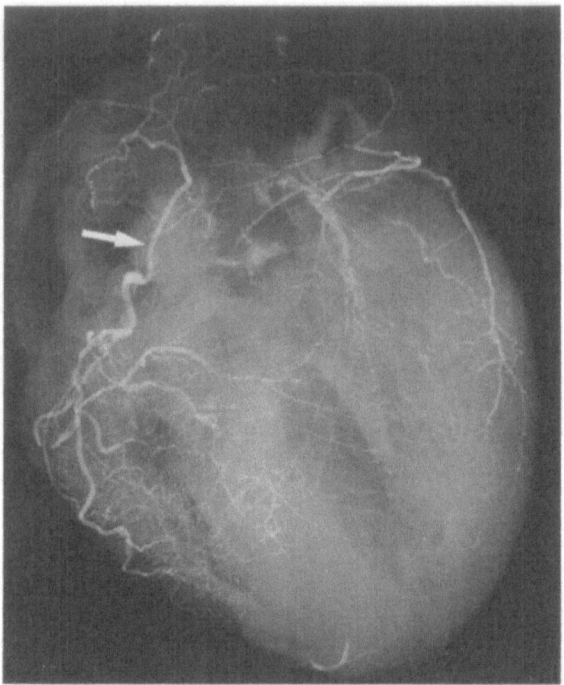

Figure 5. A post-mortem coronary angiogram, after contrast filling of the right coronary artery only, which shows an extensive collateral network through atrial arteries with participation of the sinus node artery (arrow). The collaterals "by-pass" atherosclerotic obstructions proximal in the left coronary arteries. However, the same mechanism may initiate a "coronary steal" with respect to arterial perfusion of the sinus node. These considerations are of significance in evaluating the possible role of coronary atherosclerosis for the "sick sinus node" syndrome, but as yet have not been fully investigated.

GENERAL STATEMENTS

1. The sinus node has a lateral position and in the neonate is of relatively larger size than in adults.
2. The fact that the sinus node in early human embryos can be detected as a unilateral structure does not necessarily devaluate the concept of a paired anlage.
3. The total circumference of the superior caval vein – right atrial junction should be considered a surgical "at risk" area, because of the course of the sinus node arteries.
4. The central area of "typical nodal cells" connects through a relatively narrow (in the human) zone of transitional cells to atrial myocardium; only a limited number of exits is possible.
5. "Specialized" internodal pathways, in the sense of histo- and cytologically distinct tracts connecting the sinus node with atrioventricular node, have as yet not conclusively been demonstrated.
6. Rapid internodal conduction relates to the geometry of the right atrium and the "packing" of atrial cells.

7. The sinus node has a rather homogeneous cellular composition; the central mass consists of "typical nodal cells" a term to be preferred over P-(Pacemaker) cells.
8. There is as yet no evidence that caveolae function as exocytotic organnelles; a statement not in support of a concept where catecholamines initiate spontaneous pacemaking.
9. Gap junctions or nexus are present between typical nodal cells and even in a higher number than generally thought of.
10. The role of coronary atherosclerosis as a pathogenetic factor in the so-called sick sinus node syndrome needs to be re-evaluated; localized ostial narrowing of the sinus node artery itself and the possibility of a "coronary steal" through atrial collaterals deserve consideration.
11. "Fibrosis of the sinus node" needs further specification before it can be used in arguments concerning structure and function.
12. Impalement of cells by a micro-electrode has a profound damaging effect on neighbouring cells. The significance of this needs further evaluation.

REFERENCES

Anderson, R.H., Wenink, A.C.G., Becker, A.E., Janse, M.J.: The development of the cardiac specialized tissue. In: The Conduction System of the heart. Structure, Function and Clinical Implications, edited by Wellens, H.J.J., Lie, K.I., Janse, M.J.H.E. Stenfert Kroese, B.V., Leiden, 1976, p. 1–28

Aschoff, L.: Referat über die Herzstörungen in ihren Beziehungen zu den spezifischen Muskelsystems des Herzens. *Verh Dtsch Path Ges* 14: 3, 1910

Becker, A.E., Anderson, R.H.: Morphology of the human atrioventricular junctional area. In: The Conduction System of the Heart. Structure, Function and Clinical Implications, edited by Wellens, H.J.J., Lie, K.I., Janse, M.J.H.E. Stenfert Kroese, B.V., Leiden, 1976, p. 263–266

Blair, D.M., Davies, F.: Observations on the conducting system of the heart. *J Anat* 69: 303, 1935

Davies, M.J., Pomerance, A.: Quantitative study of ageing changes in the human sinoatrial node and internodal tract. *Brit Heart J* 34: 150, 1972

Engel, T.R., Meister, S.G., Feitosa, G.S., Fischer, H.A., Frankl, W.S.: Appraisal of sinus node artery disease. *Circulation* 52: 286, 1975

Hayashi, S.: Electron microscopy of the heart conduction system of the dog. *Arch Histol Jap* 33: 67, 1971

Hudson, R.E.B.: The human pacemaker and its pathology. *Brit Heart J* 22: 153, 1960

Isa, L., Matturi, L., Rossi, L.: Contributo iso-citologico al riconoscimento delle connessioni internodali atriali. *G Ital Cardiol* 6: 1024, 1976

James, T.N.: Anatomy of the human sinus node. *Anat Rec* 141: 109, 1961

James, T.N., Sherf, L., Fine, G., Morales, A.R.: Comparative ultrastructure of the sinus node in man and dog. *Circulation* 34: 139, 1966

James, T.N.: Pulse and impulse in the sinus node. Henry Ford *Hosp Med J* 15: 275, 1967

Janse, M.J., Anderson, R.H.: Specialized internodal atrial pathways – fact or fiction? *Eur J Cardiol* 2: 117, 1974

Jennings, R.B., Ganote, C.E.: Structural changes in myocardium during acute ischemia. *Circ Res* (suppl. III), 34–35: 156, 1974

Jordan, J., Yamaguchi, J., Mandel, W.J.: Characteristics of sinoatrial conduction in patients with coronary artery disease. *Circulation* 55: 569, 1977

Koch, W.: Weitere Mitteilungen über den Sinusknoten des Herzens. *Verh Dtsch Path Ges* 13: 85, 1909

Lev, M.: Ageing changes in the human sinoatrial node. *J Gerontol* 9: 1, 1954

Lev, M., Bharati, S.: Lesions of the conduction system and their functional significance. In: Pathology Annual, edited by Sommers, S.C. Appleton-Century-Crofts, New York, 1974, p. 157–207

Lorber, V., Bertaud, W.S.: Cellular surfaces of amphibian atrial muscle. *J Cell Sci* 9: 427, 1971

Patten, B.M.: Development of the sinoventricular conduction system. *Univ Mich Med Bull* 22: 1, 1956

Pollack, G.H.: Cardiac pacemaking: an obligatory role of catecholamines? A possible mechanism underlying spontaneous pacemaking can be deduced from several recent clues. *Science* 196: 731, 1977

Robb, J.S., Kaylor, C.T., Turman, W.G.: A study of specialized heart tissue at various stages of development of the human fetal heart. *Am J Med* 5: 324, 1948

Spach, M.S., King, T.D., Barr, R.C., Boaz, D.E., Morrow, H.N., Herman-Giddens, S.: Electrical potential distribution surrounding the atria during depolarization and repolarization in the dog. *Circ Res* 24: 857, 1969

Spach, M.S., Lieberman, M., Scott, J.C., Barr, R.C., Johnson, E.A., Kootsey, J.M.: Excitation sequences of the atrial septum and AV node in isolated hearts of the dog and rabbit. *Circ Res* 29: 156, 1971

Tranum-Jensen, J.: The fine structure of the atrial and atrioventricular (AV) junctional specialized tissues of the rabbit heart. In: The Conduction System of the Heart. Structure, Function and Clinical Implications, Edited by Wellens, H.J.J., Lie, K.I., Janse, M.J.H.E. Stenfert Kroese, B.V., Leiden, 1976, p. 55–81

Truex, R.C., Smythe, M.Q., Taylor, M.J.: Reconstruction of the human sinoatrial node. *Anat Rec* 159: 371, 1967

Van Mierop, L.H.S., Wiglesworth, F.W.: Isomerism of the cardiac atria in the asplenia syndrome. *Lab Invest* 11: 1303, 1962

Van Mierop, L.H.S., Patterson, P.R., Reynolds, R.W.: Two cases of congenital asplenia with isomerism of the cardiac atria and the sinoatrial nodes. *Am J Cardiol* 13: 407, 1964

Van Mierop, L.H.S., Gessner, I.H.: The morphologic development of the sinoatrial node in the mouse. *Am J Cardiol* 25: 204, 1970

Virágh, S. Porte A.: The fine structure of the conducting system of the monkey heart (Macaca mulatta) I. The sino-atrial node and the internodal connections. *Z Zellforsch* 145: 191, 1973

Wenink, A.C.G.: Development of the human cardiac conducting system. *J Anat* 121, 617, 1976

Yamauchi, A.: Electron microscopic observations on the development of S-A and A-V nodal tissues in the human embryogenic heart. *Z Anat Entwickl Gesch* 124: 562, 1965

SECTION THREE

ELECTROPHYSIOLOGY OF THE SINUS NODE

18

A GENERAL INTRODUCTION ABOUT THE CURRENT STATUS OF THE ELECTROPHYSIOLOGY OF THE SINUS NODE

FELIX I.M. BONKE

One way to look at the sinus node – and perhaps the best – is to compare it with a black box. In this box the impulse for the heart contraction is generated and the "output" of the box is therefore the heart rate. The study of the heart rate and the influence on it of several environmental factors like changes in the ionic composition of the extra-cellular fluid and the effect of the autonomic nervous system as well as the effect of drugs, has given us an enormous amount of information.

For intact animals and for the human it is impossible to get more detailed information about the sinus node. If we disturb the function of the sinus node by premature atrial stimulation or by atrial pacing with a higher frequency than the spontaneous rate of the sinus node itself we can study the input-output relations of the black box.

Therefore, if we want to know more about the inside of this box we have to go to isolated preparations of the right atrium including the sinus node and study this area using micro-electrodes. Before discussing the electrophysiological data more in detail, it is worthwhile to realize that, 15 years before the microelectrode technique became available, Eccles and Hoff (1934) made the following prediction about the mechanism underlying the generation of the impulse in the sinus node:

"In the rhythmic mechanism there is a progressive increase in the "inner stimulus" or excitement until this reaches a threshold intensity. A beat is then set up, the excitement is abruptly depressed, and is again slowly built up to threshold at which point it sets up the next beat of the rhythmic series and so on."

This is a very original view and is proved – later on –to be very realistic.

IS ONE SINGLE CELL REPRESENTATIVE FOR THE SINUS NODE ITSELF?

The cells in the node do have contacts with low electrical resistance (nexus) as is demonstrated by several morphologists (see e.g. Tranum-Jensen, 1978; Masson-Pévet et al., 1978; Irisawa, 1978: all in this book) and there is a relatively good electrotonic interaction as demonstrated by Bonke (1973) and Seyama (1976) who found a space constant – with different methods of investigation – of 500 to 800 micron in sinus node tissue of the rabbit.

However, since the sinus node is about 2 × 5 mm (in the rabbit; there seems to be no important species difference), electrotonic interaction of all the cells in the sinus node never will be good enough to make this structure electrically homogeneous. Therefore, a group of fibers will come to a spontaneous discharge more or less simultaneously, but the fibers in the surrounding area of this group will be activated with some time delay. As a consequence, there will be a sequence of activation in the sinus node itself. The group of fibers that come to the earliest spontaneous discharge are called "the dominant or true pacemaker" and the other fibers are called "follower cells" or "latent" pacemaker fibers or "subsidiary" pacemaker fibers.

This activation pattern is studied for the rabbit sinus node in 1965 by Sano and Yamagishi and very recently by Bouman et al. (1978) and Steinbeck et al. (1978a). All these studies agree that the dominant pacemaker area is located more in the center of the sinus node, viz. about 1–2 mm apart from the crista terminalis. Normally the impulse spreads from this dominant area towards the crista terminalis and the head of the nodal structure (at the side of the vena cava superior). These studies also demonstrated that the conduction of the impulse from the dominant area directly towards the fibers in the caval area is very slow or even absent.

Thus, the sinus node is morphologically (see Tranum-Jensen, 1978, and Masson-Pévet et al., 1978) as well as electrophysiologically far from a homogeneous structure. So, one single cell of the sinus node is never representative for the sinus node as a whole. Therefore, each investigator impaling a fiber in the sinus node, has to be concerned not only about the different electrophysiological parameters of the action potential (slope of the diastolic depolarization, velocity of the depolarization phase of the action potential, total amplitude and maximal diastolic potential, duration of the action potential, etc.) but also about the relation between the cellular behaviour and the atrial activity (latency between upstroke of the action potential and the moment of activation of the crista terminalis).

WHAT IS THE EFFECT OF CHANGES IN ENVIRONMENTAL CONDITIONS ON THE FIBERS OF THE SINUS NODE?

Recently in three books the effects of several changes in ionic composition of the extra-cellular fluid and the temperature are reviewed (Brooks and Lu, 1972, West, 1972; Cranefield, 1975). I will not go into details; therefore I refer the reader to one of these books.

From the foregoing paragraph it might be obvious that it is not reasonable to use one single fiber of the sinus node as a representative example. However, in most of the studies about the effect of changes in extracellular sodium, or potassium, or calcium concentration this has been done. On the other hand, one has to realize that a continuous impalement of a single fiber is a primary condition in such a study. Therefore, the investigator has to make maximal effort to hold the microelectrode for a long period in the same fiber and change the environmental conditions in the meantime. Then this procedure will give him information about one single fiber. A series of experiments will offer him a more or less complete picture of the behavior of the several types of fibers in the sinus node under different environmental conditions. However, there is one more serious difficulty. It has been demonstrated that under several circumstances a shift of the dominant pacemaker will occur. Since the configuration of the recorded action potential not only depends on the activity of the impaled fiber itself but also on the activity of the surrounding fibers a shift of the pacemaker might influence this configuration.

Therefore, the best way to study the effect of changes in environmental conditions on the sinus node fibers is during atrial pacing (fixed pacemaker outside the sinus node) using a frequency that is only a little bit higher than the spontaneous rate of the pacemaker in the sinus node itself.

Finally, we have to realize that the interpretation of the experimental results is far from easy, since for instance several ions might influence each other. So, Isenberg (1975) demonstrated that the permeability of the membrane for potassium ions is dependent on the intracellular calcium concentration (in Purkinje fibers). From the foregoing it might be clear that electrophysiological studies about the effect of changes in environmental conditions on fibers of the sinus node are very complicated. Therefore, in my opinion a summary can be only very general and not definite.

THE EXTERNAL SODIUM CONCENTRATION

As Cranefield (1975) stated: "The effect of external sodium on the electrical activity of the sinoatrial nodal fibers is not easily summarized, in part because of the lack of systematic studies and in part because the effect is almost certainly different in true pacemaker fibers and in latent pacemaker fibers."

The amplitude of the action potential of dominant pacemaker fibers is probably very insensitive to changes in external sodium concentration; latent pacemaker fibers are more sensitive to changes in $[Na]_o$ concerning amplitude and overshoot of the action potential.

From a study of Irisawa (1972) it became clear that latent pacemaker fibers loose the ability to spontaneous discharge when $[Na]_o$ is changed from 147 mM to 102 mM. Only after a lowering of the $[Na]_o$ to 44 mM the dominant fibers will stop. Also De Mello (1961) and West (1961) demonstrated that spontaneous discharge of the sinus node will stop if the $[Na]_o$ is lowered to about 20% of normal.

THE EXTERNAL POTASSIUM CONCENTRATION

It is obvious from the literature that the fibers of the sinus node are much less sensitive to changes in the extracellular potassium concentration than myocardial fibers and Purkinje fibers. So, increased $[K]_o$ might cause inexcitability of atrial fibers, whereas the sinus nodal activity persists. Toda (1969) described that the maximal diastolic potential in nodal fibers decreased from -73 mV to -55 mV during a change of $[K]_o$ from 1.5 mM to 16.2 mM; thus about 18 mV change per tenfold change in $[K]_o$. It seems therefore, that the permeability of the membrane for potassium is relatively low in fibers of the sinus node.

The spontaneous rate of the sinus node in influenced by $[K]_o$. In almost all studies an increase in rate is found when the $[K]_o$ is increased (up to a certain level). However, "the acceleration seen as $[K]_o$ is raised, is invariably associated with a shift in the location of the pacemaker cell from one site to another" (Lu, 1970). Therefore, it seems that the fibers of the sinus node are not equally sensitive to changes in $[K]_o$; the dominant pacemaker fibers probably are less sensitive than the latent ones. Assuming that the latent pacemaker fibers depolarize more than the dominant pacemaker fibers at a certain increased $[K]_o$, the originally latent fibers might become more depolarized and therefore take over the function of pacemaker. However, another speculation might be that the dominant pacemaker fibers are depolarizing to a level where spontaneous discharge is no longer possible, whereas latent pacemaker fibers are just depolarized up till the range of membrane potential in favor of spontaneous discharge.

THE EXTERNAL CALCIUM CONCENTRATION

Generally an increase in $[Ca]_o$ increases the rate of the spontaneous discharges of the sinus node. This is true within certain limits and the interaction with the effect of $[Na]_o$ makes it very complicated. Very recently Bouman and co-workers (1978, this book) did a very careful study about the effect of $[Ca]_o$ and again I will not go into details here and refer to their paper.

THE EFFECT OF TEMPERATURE

In general an increase in temperature causes an increase in the rate of spontaneous discharges of the sinus node, whereas the node slows down if the temperature is lowered. In the isolated atrium of the rabbit the relationship between the temperature and the beat-to-beat interval is linear (at least in the range between 30°C and 40°C) and there is an interval change of about 30 msec per degree C (Bouman and Van der Westen, 1970).

The effect of temperature, however, is not the same on dominant pacemaker fibers as on latent pacemaker fibers; this causes a shift of the pacemaker site, if the temperature is lowered (see Bouman et al., 1978, this book).

THE EFFECT OF AUTONOMIC TRANSMITTERS ON THE SINUS NODE FIBERS

There are two important studies on the effect of vagal stimulation on the sinus node of the rabbit (Toda and West, 1967a, b; Bouman et al., 1968). These studies are technically very difficult since one has to make a preparation of an isolated right atrium including the sinus node and the terminal trunks of the nervus vagus. Stimulation of the vagal nerves causes a decrease of the slope of the diastolic depolarization and consequently a decrease in the rate. Furthermore, a hyperpolarization will occur in case of stronger stimulation. Also a shift of the site of the dominant pacemaker occurs. This pacemaker shift might be caused by the inequal distribution of the vagal nerve endings, but this cannot be the only reason since administration of acetylcholine to the perfusion fluid in an experiment with an isolated right atrium causes also a clear pacemaker shift.

It is assumed that acetylcholine causes in the sinus node fibers an increase of the permeability of the membrane for potassium (Harris and Hutter, 1956). The pacemaker shift, caused by ACh, might be the consequence of the removal of a difference in potassium permeability of the membrane of dominant fibers and of latent pacemaker fibers.

The effect of stimulation of the sympathetic nerves on the sinus node is an increase in the slope of the diastolic depolarization and consequently an increase of the rate (Toda, 1968; Toda and Shimamoto, 1968). It is not clear from the literature whether (nor)adrenaline has an effect on the amplitude or other parameters of the action potential. Neither is it clear whether (nor)adrenaline or stimulation of the sympathetic nerves causes a shift of the pacemaker.

THE EFFECT OF MECHANICAL STRETCH ON THE SINUS NODE

Stretch of an isolated sinus node preparation results in a more rapid rate of the pacemaker discharge and this rate declines gradually while the stretch is still maintained. The basic mechanism underlying this phenomenon is unknown. It is assumed that the membrane becomes more permeable for sodium- and calcium-ions and so depolarization will occur.

THE EFFECT OF ATRIAL PACING

If the atrial stimulation rate is only slightly above the spontaneous rate of the sinus node, the spontaneous discharge of the normal dominant pacemaker center is only slightly depressed. However, if the atrium is paced at a much higher rate than the intrinsic rate of the sinus node, a hyperpolarization of the nodal fibers occurs and after the termination of the pacing an extra long "revival" period occurs. It is postulated that high frequent atrial stimulation is liberating acetylcholine from the nerve endings and therefore causes the hyperpolarization. On the other hand, it is also possible that because of the high frequency of stimulation the active sodium pump is activated (higher intracellular sodium concentration) and thus the electrogenic action is amplified.

In conclusion, summarizing the foregoing paragraphs, it seems reasonable to suppose that the fibers, being under normal conditions the dominant pacemaker fibers of the sinus node, are different from the latent pacemaker fibers. This difference is perhaps only a qualitative one and perhaps a limited one, but still very functional.
Now we come to the question:

IS THE ACTION POTENTIAL OF THE SINUS NODE FIBERS COMPARABLE WITH THE ACTION POTENTIAL OF WORKING MYOCARDIAL FIBERS?

As stated by Cranefield (1975) one can argue about the upstroke of the dominant pacemaker that it depends on a flow of inward current through the slow channel. Therefore, the dominant pacemaker potential might be a slow response. Thus, the upstroke of the action potential is relatively insensitive to $[Na]_o$, arises in a potential range in which the "fast" channel is already inactivated, and is more or less insensitive to tetrodotoxin. On the other hand, the action potential of the sinus node fibers is very sensitive to manganese. This also is an argument in favor of the slow response character of the action potential. However, it is obvious, that not all the fibers in the sinus node are "slow response" fibers. In the latent pacemaker fibers there is a mixture of "fast channel" behavior and "slow channel" behavior. This is also shown in the experiments of Kreitner (1975 and 1978), who demonstrated that hyperpolarization of fibers in the sinus node revealed that these fibers developed TTX sensitivity and thus became fibers with a combination of "slow" response and "fast" response characteristics. This is in agreement with the results of Lipsius and Vassalle (1978).

It is therefore very attractive to assume that in the dominant pacemaker fibers there is merely a "slow" response actionpotential, whereas in the latent pacemaker fibers the actionpotential is based on a combination of a "slow" and a "fast" response.

However, if we want to know more about the ionic currents underlying the action potential of the sinus node fibers, we have to use the voltage clamp technique. The primary prerequisite for this technique is a homogeneous preparation. As we discussed already, this is not the case with the sinus node. Therefore, reliable voltage clamp of the sinus node is not possible, unless one is able to make a very small preparation of the sinus node which is still functional. It is possible to inject current via a microelectrode into one fiber of such a very small preparation and then, because of the limited number of cells, the potential decay will be only minimal. So, Noma and Irisawa (1975, 1976) were able to make a preparation of the sinus node of about 300 × 300 micron and the potential decay if current was injected in the middle of the preparation, was less than 10%. (Since the sinus node preparation is very thin the third dimension is neglected.) They demonstrated that in such a preparation, beating spontaneously, the action potentials obtained simultaneously from three different sites, were superimposable. This means that there are no signs of conduction in this very small preparation. Such a preparation is perhaps suitable for voltage clamp studies.

Noma and Irisawa (1975b) have demonstrated that in the above mentioned preparation the sinus node fibers do have a "resting" potential in the order of – 40 mV and that during the repolarization of an action potential the membrane is hyperpolarized beyond this resting value. This was already suggested by Dudel and Trautwein in 1958. As a consequence of this resting potential of – 40 mV, we might expect that the membrane of the sinus node fibers is more permeable for sodium ions than other cardiac fibers in the resting state (Trautwein and Kassebaum, 1961; Noma and Irisawa, 1975b); this is in agreement both with the fact that Mazel and Holland (1958) have shown that the intracellular sodium concentration is higher than in other cardiac fibers and with the fact that the sinus node fibers are not very much influenced by changes in the external sodium concentration (as we have discussed before). Another consequence of this "resting" potential of sinus node fibers is that these fibers will not be very sensitive to changes in the extracellular potassium concentration, as is the case.

Noma and Irisawa (1974, 1975a) have demonstrated that an electrogenic sodium pump is contributing to the membrane potential of fibers of the sinus node. If the active sodium pump is depressed by perfusion of the preparation with a potassium free solution, a depolarization occurred and upon reperfusion with a normal solution (potassium concentration 5 mM) the sodium pump is activated again causing a transient hyperpolarization. This hyperpolarization did not occur if ouabain was added to the perfusion solution. However, it is at this moment not clear whether the electrogenic sodium pump is important or not under normal conditions. From the experiments of Steinbeck et al. (1978b, this book) it turned out that the effect of ouabain on the dominant fibers of the sinus node is much less prominent than on latent pacemaker fibers. Perhaps the sodium pump is more active in the latent pacemaker fibers than the dominant ones. It is obvious that a further study is necessary about this topic.

Many studies have been done on the effect of sodium-, potassium- and calcium-ions on the configuration of the action potential, whereas the effect of several drugs is studied also. We have to realize that these studies are very difficult. Firstly, it is necessary to have a continuous impalement with a microelectrode during control (normal situation) and during the test situation (drug added, change in composition of extracellular fluid, etc.); it is far from easy to maintain a good impalement in an isolated sinus node preparation for a longer time. Secondly, such a procedure gives only information about one single cell and this is not representative for the whole sinus node (as we discussed before).

However, from all these experimental data it seems reliable to assume that the depolarization phase of the action potential is based on an inward current of sodium and calcium ions, whereas the repolarization is caused by an outward current of potassium ions. The kinetics of these currents, however, are just under investigation (see Irisawa, 1978, this book). In a recent study, Noma and Irisawa (1976) have demonstrated with voltage clamp experiments in the small sized preparation of the sinus node, that the potassium outward current is not finished after the repolarization, but is slowly decaying. This will cause in combination with the continuous "background" current (inward current of sodium and calcium ions because of the relatively high permeability of the membrane of sinus node fibers for these ions) the typical diastolic depolarization or pacemaker potential.

However, there are so many questions concerning the kinetics of the currents underlying the action potential of the sinus node fibers that – in my opinion – nothing is a proven fact at this moment about these currents. Therefore, further analysis is absolutely necessary, of which the beginning is given in section 4 of this book.

REFERENCES

1. Bonke, F.I.M.: Electrotonic spread in the sinoatrial node of the rabbit heart. *Pflügers Arch* 339: 17, 1973
2. Bonke, F.I.M.: The sinoatrial node function. In: Cardiac Pacing, edited by B. Lüderitz. Springer Verlag, Berlin, 1976, p. 5
3. Bouman, L.N., van der Westen, H.M.: Pacemaker shift in the sino-atrial node induced by a change of temperature. *Pflügers Archiv* 318: 262, 1970
4. Bouman, L.N., Gerlings, E.D., Biersteker, P.A., Bonke, F.I.M.: Pacemaker shift in the sinoatrial node during vagal stimulation. *Pflügers Archiv* 302: 255, 1968
5. Bouman, L.N., Mackaay, A.J.C., Bleeker, W.K., Becker, A.E.: Pacemaker shifts in the sinus node. Effects of vagal stimulation, temperature and reduction of extracellular calcium. This book, 1978
6. Brooks, C.Mc.C., Lu, H.H.: The sinoatrial pacemaker of the heart. Springfield, Ill., Charles C. Thomas, 1972, p. 109
7. Cranefield, P.F.: The conduction of the cardiac impulse. The slow response and cardiac arrhythmias. Mount Cosco, Futura Publishing Co., 1975
8. Dudel, J., Trautwein, W.: Der Mechanismus der automatischen rhythmischen Impulsbildung der Herzmuskelfaser. *Pflügers Arch* 267: 553, 1958
9. Eccles, J.C., Hoff, H.E.: Rhythm of heart beat: II. Disturbance of rhythm produced by late premature beats. *Proc R Soc Lond (Biol)* 115: 327, 1934
10. Harris, E.J., Hutter, O.F.: The action of acetylcholine on the movement of potassium ions in the sinus venosus of the heart. *J Physiol* 133, 588, 1956
11. Irisawa, A.: Fine fracture of the small sinoatrial node specimen used for the voltage clamp experiments. This book, 1978
12. Irisawa, H.: Electrical activity of rabbit sinoatrial node as studied by a double sucrose gap method. In: Symp. and Colloquium on the electrical field of the heart. Editor P. Rijlant, Bruxelles, Presses Académiques Européennes, 1972
13. Irisawa, H.: General comments: ionic currents underlying spontaneous rhythm of the cardiac primary pacemaker cells. This book, 1978
14. Isenberg, G.: Is potassium conductance of cardiac Purkinje fibers controlled by $(Ca^{++})_i$? *Nature* 253: 273, 1975
15. Kreitner, D.: Evidence for the existence of a rapid sodium channel in the membrane of rabbit sinoatrial cells. *J Mol Cell Cardiol* 7: 655, 1975
16. Kreitner, D.: Effects of polarization and of inhibitors of ionic conductances on the action potentials of nodal and perinodal fibers in rabbit sinoatrial node. This book, 1978
17. Lipsius, S.L., Vassalle, M.: Characterization of a two-component upstroke in the sinus node subsidiary pacemakers. This book, 1978
18. Lu, H.H.: Shifts in pacemaker dominance within the sinoatrial region of cat and rabbit hearts resulting from increase of extracellular potassium. *Circ Res* 26: 339, 1970
19. Masson-Pévet, M., Bleeker, W.K., Mackaay, A.J.C., Gros, D, Bouman, L.N.: Ultrastructural and functional aspects of the rabbit sinoatrial node. This book, 1978
20. Mazel, P., Holland W.C.: Acetylcholine and electrolyte metabolism in the various chambers of frog and turtle heart. *Circ Res* 6: 684, 1958
21. Mello de, W.C.: Some aspects of the interrelationship between ions and electrical activity in specialized tissue of the heart. In: The specialized tissue of the heart, edited by Paes de Carvalho, de Mello and Hoffman. Elsevier, New York, 1961, p. 95
22. Noma, A., Irisawa, H.: Electrogenic sodium pump in rabbit sinoatrial node cell. *Pflügers Archiv* 351: 177, 1974
23. Noma, A., Irisawa, H.: Contribution of an electrogenic sodium pump to the membrane potential in rabbit sinoatrial node cells. *Pflügers Archiv* 358: 289, 1975a
24. Noma, A., Irisawa, H.: Effects of Na^+ and K^+ on the resting membrane potential of the rabbit sinoatrial node cell. *Jap J Physiol* 25: 287, 1975b
25. Noma, A., Irisawa, H.: Membrane currents in the rabbit sinoatrial node cell as studied by the double microelectrode method. *Pflügers Archiv* 364, 45, 1976a
26. Noma, A., Irisawa, H.: A time- and voltage-dependent potassium current in the rabbit sinoatrial node cell. *Pflügers Archiv* 366, 251, 1976b
27. Sano, T., Yamagishi, S.: Spread of excitation from the sinus node. *Circ Res* 16: 423, 1965
28. Seyama, I.: Characteristics of the rectifying properties of the sinoatrial node cell of the rabbit. *J Physiol* 255: 379, 1976

29. Steinbeck, G., Allessie, M.A., Bonke, F.I.M., Lammers, W.J.E.P.: The response of the sinus node to premature stimulation of the atrium studied with microelectrodes in isolated atrial preparations of the rabbit heart. This book, 1978a
30. Steinbeck, G., Bonke, F.I.M., Allessie, M.A., Lammers, W.J.E.P.: Cardiac glycosides and pacemaker activity of the sinus node – a microelectrode study on the isolated right atrium of the rabbit. This book, 1978b
31. Toda, N.: Influence of sodium ions on the membrane potential of the sino-atrial node in response to sympathetic nerve stimulation. *J. Physiol* 196: 677, 1968
32. Toda, N.: Electrophysiological effects of potassium and calcium ions in the sino-atrial node in response to sympathetic nerve stimulation. *Pflügers Archiv* 310: 45, 1969
33. Toda, N., Shimamota, K.: The influence of sympathetic stimulation on transmembrane potentials in the S-A node *J Pharmacol Exp Ther* 159: 298, 1968
34. Toda, N., West, T.C.: Interactions of K, Na, and vagal stimulation in the S-A node of the rabbit. *Amer J Physiol* 212: 416, 1967a
35. Toda, N., West, T.C.: Interaction between Na, Ca, Mg, and vagal stimulation in the S-A node of the rabbit. *Amer J Physiol* 212: 424, 1967b
36. Tranum-Jensen, J.: The fine structure of the sinus node. This book, 1978
37. Trautwein, W., Kassebaum, D.G.: On the mechanism of spontaneous impulse generation in the pacemaker of the heart. *J Gen Physiol* 45: 317, 1961
38. West, T.C.: Effects of chronotropic influences on subthreshold oscillations in the sino-atrial node. In: The Specialized Tissue of the Heart, edited by A. Paes De Carvalho, W.C. De Mello, B.F. Hoffman, Elsevier, N.Y., 1961, p. 81
39. West, T.C.: Electrophysiology of the sinus node. In: Electrical phenomena in the heart, edited by De Mello, Academic Press, New York, 1972

19

CHARACTERIZATION OF A TWO-COMPONENT UPSTROKE IN THE SINUS NODE SUBSIDIARY PACEMAKERS*

STEPHEN L. LIPSIUS** AND MARIO VASSALLE

INTRODUCTION

There is general agreement on the fact that the upstroke of the action potential of Purkinje, atrial and ventricular muscle fibers is caused by a rapid influx of sodium through a specific fast channel (for references, see Trautwein, 1973; Cranefield, 1975; Vassalle, 1977). The depolarization induced by the fast sodium influx causes the activation of a slow inward current which is carried by calcium and/or sodium and is responsible for phase 2 of the action potential. In contrast, the excitatory currents responsible for the generation of the action potential of different sinus node cells have not been fully characterized. While the slow inward current is generally acknowledged to play a role in the shaping of the sinus node action potential configuration, the initial phase of the action potential has been attributed to sodium influx by some (Noma and Irisawa, 1974) and to the opening of a slow calcium channel by others (Brooks and Lu, 1972). It is possible that some of these discrepancies stem from the fact that the sinus node is not an homogeneous structure as it includes dominant pacemakers, subsidiary pacemakers and transitional cells. Therefore, the ionic events responsible for the activation of a sinus node cell may be different depending on the type of cell studied. In the present experiments, action potentials were recorded from subsidiary pacemakers in the guinea pig sinus node. These action potentials are characterized by the presence of a fast and a slow component in the upstroke. To gain information on the ionic species responsible for the fast and slow component of the action potential upstroke, the ionic environment was suitably changed. Also substances known to affect the currents carried by certain channels were employed. Finally, the voltage and time dependence of the components were studied by inducing extrabeats at various times during diastole.

A preliminary report has been published in abstract form (Lipsius and Vassalle, 1976).

METHODS

Male albino guinea pigs weighing 600–1000 g were sacrificed by cervical dislocation. The heart was quickly excised and placed in oxygenated Tyrode solution. The atria were separated from the ventricles and the right atrium from the left. The sinus node area was exposed by cutting away the floor of the right atrium and the wall of the superior vena cava. The sinus node was recognized by its cupped shape and whitish color. Once separated from

* This work was supported by N.I.H. Heart and Lung Institute grant no. HL17451.

** During this investigation Dr. S.L. Lipsius was an N.I.H. Postdoctoral Research Fellow supported by a National Research Service Award grant no. HL05037.

the surrounding red atrial tissue, the sinus was transferred to a tissue bath. The oxygenated (98% O_2 and 2% CO_2) Tyrode solution had the following composition (mM): NaCl 136; KCl 2.7 NaHCO$_3$ 11.9; NaH$_2$PO$_4$ 0.45; MgCl$_2$ 0.5; CaCl 2.7; glucose 5.5. Calcium and sodium concentrations were varied in different experiments.

The Tyrode solution warmed to the 35°C by flowing in tubing immersed in a large bath in which water was circulated by means of a constant temperature pump (Haake, model FS). The sinus node was held on the floor of the tissue bath by four electrode pins inserted at the periphery of the tissue. Electrical stimuli were delivered to the tissue through the pins (which were isolated except for the tips) by means of a stimulator (Grass, Model S4A) via a stimulus isolation unit (Grass, model SIU-4678). The characteristics of the stimuli were: frequency 10–15% above the spontaneous rate, voltage 20% above threshold and duration 2 msec.

Membrane potentials were recorded with microelectrodes filled with 3M KCl. The tip of one microelectrode was immersed in the perfusing solution and the other was inserted intracellularly. The potentials were displayed on a dual beam oscilloscope (Tektronix, model 565) and photographed with a camera (Nihon Kohden, model PC-2A). In a number of experiments, the maximal rate of rise of the upstroke was measured by electronic differentiation (Tektronix 3A-8).

Acetylcholine chloride (Sigma Chemical Co.) was infused in a concentration of 2.7×10^{-5} M. The amplitude of the action potential was measured from its peak to the maximum diastolic potential (E_{max}). The upstroke was measured from the take-off potential to its most positive point.

Statistical analysis of the data included the t-test for paired data and the standard error of the mean (S.E.).

RESULTS

DIFFERENT TYPES OF ACTION POTENTIALS IN THE SINUS NODE

Electrophysiologically, the pacemaker cells are distinguished into dominant and subsidiary (Figure 1). The dominant pacemakers are recognized by a pronounced diastolic depolarization, a smooth transition between diastolic depolarization and the upstroke,

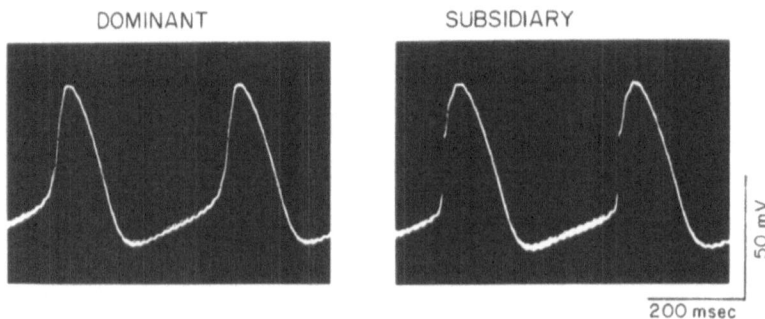

Figure 1. Action potential configuration from a dominant pacemaker cell (left panel) and a subsidiary pacemaker cell (right panel) from the same sinus node preparation.

a small maximal rate of rise and a small amplitude of the action potential. The subsidiary pacemakers, instead, show an abrupt transition between diastolic depolarization and a relatively rapid depolarization (see Brooks and Lu, 1972). However, this initial depolarization (fast component) is responsible only for the initial part of the upstroke and is followed by a slower depolarization phase (Figure 1). Sometimes the fast component continues directly into the slow component; in other instances, the fast component begins to repolarize and only then the slow component begins. In either case, the slow component is viewed as a part of the upstroke as it carries the depolarization toward more positive values. In other instances, the action potentials show characteristics which are intermediate between those of the sinus pacemaker cells and those of the atrial cells and are presumably recorded from transitional cells. These action potentials are characterized by a fast and large upstroke (as the atrial cells) and by a diastolic depolarization (as the pacemaker cells).

The results obtained in subsidiary pacemakers showing an action potential with a two component upstroke are reported below.

SOME CHARACTERISTICS OF THE TWO COMPONENT ACTION POTENTIAS

Some of the characteristics of the two component action potentias are shown in Table 1. The values were obtained from 21 impalements in 12 sinus nodes. As shown in the table, the total amplitude of the action potential averaged 74.0 ± 1.5. The fast component (measured

Table 1. Characteristics of two component action potentials.

Total ampl.	F.C.	S.C.	V_{max}	E_{max}	Take-off potential	Rate (beats/min)
72.7	41.3	15.7	31.6			175
70.2	36.3	19.4				196
65.3	29.3	21.9	25.2			190
73.8	37.5	21.8		−62.3	−48.3	198
75.2	61.8	10.1				220
64.2	34.5	15.8	38.5	−51.3	−38.7	182
77.6	50.9	15.8	30.5	−55.5	−43.7	181
81.3	52.7	18.2				220
65.3	43.7	14.5		−57.3	−48.5	225
69.7	54.5	12.1				227
65.4	35.2	19.4				221
69.1	37.5	17.0	22.9			230
73.4	25.5	31.5	30.1	−53.4	−36.4	210
81.4	59.4	8.5				202
80.2	35.8	29.1				130
78.8	24.2	38.8		−64.2	−48.5	198
64.8	27.9	27.3				204
84.2	47.3	20.6	33.7			127
75.2	31.5	27.3	20.4			152
80.0	60.6	12.1	54.5	−69.1	−57.0	190
86.7	55.8	20.0		−69.3	−55.8	166

Mean value S.E.						
74.02 ± 1.5	42.06 ± 2.6	19.9 ± 1.6	31.9 ± 3.4	-60.3 ± 2.5	-47.1 ± 2.6	191 ± 6.4

Total ampl. = total amplitude of the action potential in mV. F.C. = fast component in mV. S.C. = slow component in mV. V_{max} = maximal rate of rise in V/sec. E_{max} = maximum diastolic potential in mV. Take-off potential = potential at which the fast component began. Rate = spontaneous rate of discharge.

from the take-off potential to the abrupt termination) averaged 42.0 ± 2.6 mV (68% of the upstroke). The slow component (measured from its beginning to peak depolarization) averaged 19.9 ± 1.6 mV (32% of the upstroke). The maximal rate of rise was determined only for the fast component and it averaged 31.9 ± 3.4 V/sec. The values were obtained at an average spontaneous rate of 191 ± 6.4 beats/min.

EFFECT OF LOW CALCIUM

To explore the role of calcium influx on the two components of the upstroke, external calcium concentration was decreased to one tenth of its normal value (Figure 2).

The first panel was recorded in 2.7 mM Ca^{++} Tyrode. The two components in the upstroke are fairly pronounced, the slow components occupying about one third of the total upstroke. As seen more clearly in higher speed records, the end of the fast component was followed by a brief repolarization and then by the onset of the slow component. When $[Ca]_o$ was decreased to 0.27 mM (second panel), several changes became apparent. The slow component began after a more pronounced repolarization and increased more slowly to a smaller peak. The action potential duration increased and this (in spite of the shortening of the diastolic period) led to a small decrease in rate. In most experiments, the fast component too decreased, but it was little affected at this experiment. This figure was selected for it clearly shows that the decrease in slow component was not due to a smaller depolarization by the fast component.

In 7 experiments (9 trials), lowering $[Ca]_o$ induced the following changes. The action potential amplitude decreased from 76.9 ± 2.5 to 66.6 ± 2.4 mV (-13.4%, P < 0.001); the fast component from 43.5 ± 6.4 to 36.2 ± 6.6 mV (-16.8%, P < 0.02); the slow component from 22.6 ± 3.7 to 20.6 ± 4.5 mV (-8.9%). The time between the beginning and the peak of the slow component (time to peak) increased from 24.3 ± 2.9 to 37.7 ± 4.2 msec ($+55.1\%$, P < 0.001). The rate of discharge increased slightly from 172.4 ± 8 to 181.1 ± 11.1 beats/min, ($+5\%$, P > 0.1).

The changes induced by low calcium were reversible and the values obtained during recovery in Tyrode solution were similar to the control value. Thus in 4 experiments, during recovery the amplitude was 77.5 ± 2 mV, the fast component 43.6 ± 8.5 mV, the slow component 22.1 ± 6.6 mV, the time to peak 24.8 ± 6.0 msec and the rate of discharge 165.8 ± 15.6 beats/min.

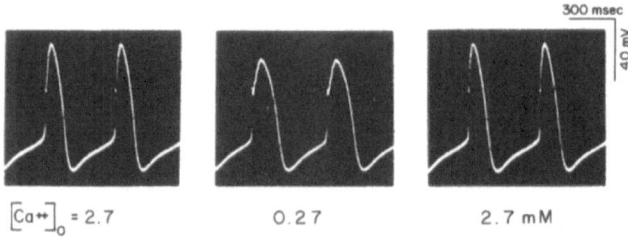

$[Ca^{++}]_o = 2.7$ 0.27   2.7 mM

Figure 2. Effect of low calcium on the action potential configuration. The first panel was recorded in 2.7 mM Ca Tyrode (control), the second in 0.27 mM Ca Tyrode (test) and the third again in 2.7 mM Ca Tyrode (recovery). All recordings are from the same cell.

The results can be explained if it is assumed that lowering $[Ca]_o$ results in 3 effects: a shift in the voltage dependence of the Na channel in a hyperpolarizing direction, a decrease in the slow inward calcium current and a decrease in potassium conductance.

THE EFFECT OF HIGH CALCIUM

High calcium should cause effects opposite to those of low calcium. In the experiment illustrated in Figure 3, the first panel was recorded in Tyrode and the second in a high calcium (8.1 mM) Tyrode. Several changes are apparent. The fast component became larger (from 31.5 to 40.0 mV) and the maximal rate of rise increased considerably (+275%); the slow component decreased in amplitude (from 21.2 to 14.5 mV) as the fast component reached more positive values. The time to peak was obviously decreased (from 38.5 to 23 msec). The action potential became shorter in high Ca. Similar results were obtained in two more experiments.

The findings can be accounted for by assuming a shift in the voltage dependence of the sodium channel in a depolarizing direction, an increase in the slow inward calcium current and an increase in g_K. These effects are opposite to those induced by low $[Ca]_o$.

EFFECT OF ACETYLCHOLINE ON THE TWO COMPONENTS

Acetylcholine causes hyperpolarization in the sinus node cells (Hutter and Trautwein, 1956) and has recently been shown to decrease the slow inward current in the atria (Ikemoto and Goto, 1975; Giles and Tsien, 1975; Ten Eick et al., 1976). Because of these two actions, acetylcholine may affect the two components in opposite directions. It could increase the fast component by increasing the take-off potential and decrease a slow component due to the opening of a slow channel. In Figure 4, the first two action potentials are control recordings and show a two component upstroke. At the arrow, acetylcholine $(2.7 \times 10^{-5}$ M) was perfused. As a consequence, there was a slowing down of the rate which allowed the diastolic depolarization to reach a more positive potential. Because of this lower take-off potential, the fast component was somewhat smaller and the slow component began at a slightly more negative potential (third action potential). Before the fourth

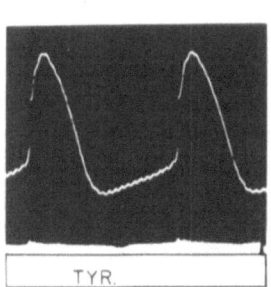
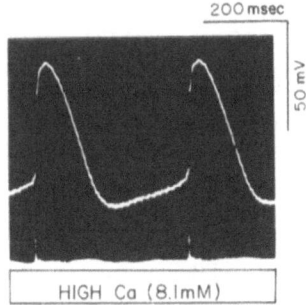

Figure 3. Effect of high calcium on the action potential configuration. The first panel was recorded in 2.7 mM Ca Tyrode and the second in 8.1 mM Ca Tyrode from the same cell.

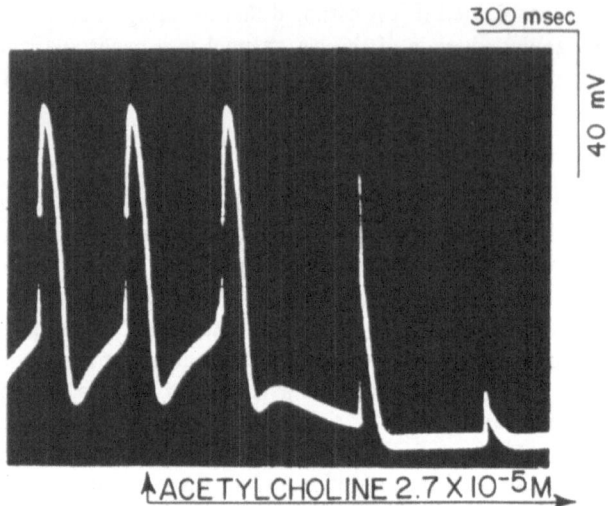

Figure 4. Effect of acetylcholine on the fast and slow component of the action potential. Acetylcholine perfusion was started at the upward arrow. Peak of the last action potential is only visible as a dot.

action potential, the acetylcholine-induced hyperpolarization was quite marked and this led to a rather pronounced increase in the fast component. The slow component did not appear at all in the upstroke and was manifest only as a phase 2 which began at more negative values and continued in the final repolarization. Following this fourth action potential, the propagated excitation clearly failed to depolarize the cell to the threshold.

In 10 experiments (11 trials), acetylcholine increased the take-off potential by 17.5 $\pm$ 1.7% (P < 0.001) and the fast component from a control value of 49.6 $\pm$ 6.0 mV to 78.4 $\pm$ 5.7 mV(+58%, P < 0.001). In 3 trials, the maximum rate of rise increased from a control value of 31.8 $\pm$ 11.8 V/sec to 79.5 $\pm$ 19.6 V/sec in the presence of acetylcholine (+150%, P < 0.05). In 4 additional experiments, the effect of acetylcholine was tested in the presence of low (0.27 mM) calcium. Acetylcholine increased the take-off potential by 13.6 $\pm$ 4.2% (P < 0.05) and the fast component from 51.9 $\pm$ 6.2 to 84.8 $\pm$ 6.0 mV (+63.4%, P < 0.05).

THE EFFECT OF NOREPINEPHRINE

In contrast to acetylcholine, norepinephrine has been shown to increase the slow inward calcium current in several tissues (see Trautwein, 1973). However, because it increases diastolic depolarization, norepinphrine decreases the take-off potential. On this basis, the slow component should be enhanced while the fast component should not increase. The results obtained in one experiment are shown in Figure 5. The first panel was recorded in low (0.27 mM) calcium Tyrode and represented the control. The slow component in this solution was 4.2 mV and the fast component 59.4 mV. On exposure to norepinephrine, the slow component increased markedly (13.2 mV, +216.7%), the action potential became larger (from 64.8 mV to 75.2 mV) and shorter (from 142.4 msec to 124.2 msec), and diastolic depolarization steeper. The reversibility of norepinephrine effects is shown by the third panel. The fourth panel was recorded in normal Tyrode and shows action potentials

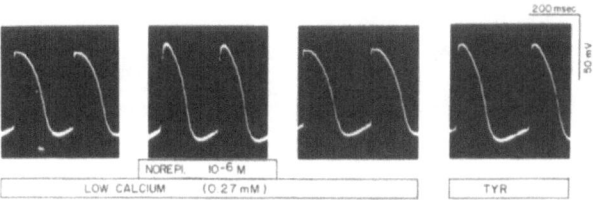

Figure 5. Effect of norepinephrine on a subsidiary pacemaker exposed to low calcium. The norepinephrine was administered during the second panel recording. The last panel was recorded in Tyrode solution.

similar (amplitude 73.9 mV, fast component 55.8 mV, slow component 10.9 mV) to those recorded in low calcium + norepinephrine. In other words, norepinephrine almost completely counteracted the effect by a tenfold decrease in $[Ca]_o$ on the action potential configuration.

In 3 tests, under the influence of norepinephrine (10^{-6} M), the action potential amplitude increased from 70.7 ± 6.2 mV to 78.6 ± 2.6 mV ($+11.1\%$); the fast component changed little (from 60.0 ± 3.0 mV to 58.8 ± 2.3 mV); and the slow component increased markedly from 5.8 ± 3.3 mv to 13.3 ± 1.4 mV ($+129.3\%$). The rate of discharge at the same time increased from 221.5 ± 16.4 to 268.5 ± 17.0 beats/min ($+21.2\%$). During recovery from norepinephrine exposure, the amplitude was 73.5 ± 4.1 mV, the fast component 57.9 ± 3.2 mV, the slow component 7.8 ± 2.2 mV and the rate 236.0 ± 16.6 beats/min.

DEPENDENCE OF THE FAST AND SLOW COMPONENTS ON THE TAKE-OFF POTENTIAL AND DURATION OF PREVIOUS DIASTOLE

The results reported above suggest that the fast component depends on sodium influx (see ACh effects) and the slow component depends on calcium influx (see calcium and norepinephrine effects). If this is so, these components should also be sensitive to other influences which affect the fast and slow channels in other tissues. For this reason, electrical stimulation was applied at various times during diastole. Earlier stimuli should enhance the fast component (because of the higher take-off potential) but not the slow component (because of the longer repriming time of the slow current). The results of this procedure are shown in Figure 6. The action potentials are shown at the top of the figure. A plot of the amplitude of the two components as a function of the take-off potential and of time is shown at the bottom of the figure. In the panels, the last action potential was induced by an electrical stimulus while the other action potentials are spontaneous. As shown by the pictures and as quantitated in the graph, there was a direct relationship between the take-off potential and the magnitude of the fast component. Thus, the fast component had its maximal amplitude when the extra action potential was elicited at E_{max}: the amplitude was then more than twice that recorded during the upstroke of the spontaneous action potential. In contrast, the amplitude of the slow component (measured in absolute value) increased as a function of the preceding interval. In the first extra beat, the slow component was smaller than the fast but in the last extrabeat it was larger than the fast component. In fact, the slow component of the last extrabeat was larger than that of the spontaneous action potentials. Furthermore, as the stimulus was applied later during diastole, the slow component reached its peak sooner. Similar results were obtained in 5 experiments.

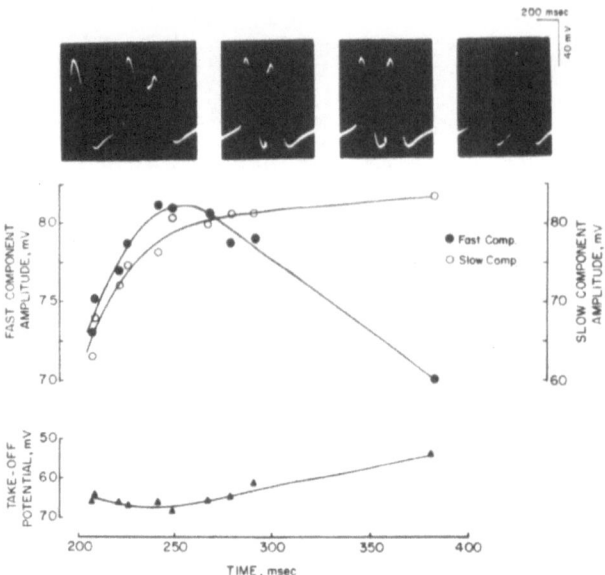

Figure 6. Effect of premature stimulation on action potential configuration. The panels show the electrical recording. In the graph, the abscissa shows the time at which the extrastimuli were delivered. The upper left ordinate is the scale for the amplitude of the fast component and the lower left ordinate is the scale for the take-off potential for the fast component. The right ordinate is the scale for the slow component.

Note: total amplitude is used as scaling for the ordinate; this means that the absolute difference between the maximum diastolic potential (E_{max}) and the maximal level reached by the fast component or the slow component.

It must be pointed out that the absolute amplitude of the fast component did not always decrease with the lower take-off potential. This might have been due to the fact that at early intervals the reactivation of the sodium system was not complete.

EFFECT OF FAST DRIVE

That there is a time-dependent lag in the reactivation of the sodium system is also suggested by the results with repetitive stimulation. As shown in Figure 7, a fast drive affects both the fast and slow components. The take-off potential of the first two driven action potentials is more negative and, as expected, the fast component is larger than for the spontaneous action potential. However, beginning with the third driven action potential, the take-off potential is constant and yet the fast component decreased gradually over several beats to reach a constant value. Because of the decrease of the fast component, the slow component began at more negative potentials and became relatively larger, although its peak reached less positive values. By the end of the drive, the peak of both the fast and the slow component had decreased with respect to control level. Although the amplitude of the action potential had declined substantially by the end of the drive, the magnitude of both the fast and slow components were still larger than control. The decrease of the total amplitude of the action potential resulted from the more negative take-

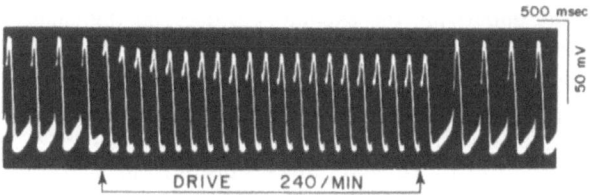

Figure 7. Effect of overdrive on action potential component. The drive was carried out during the period indicated by the arrows.

off potential. When the drive was terminated, the amplitude of the action potential recovered with the first spontaneous beat. It is of interest, however, that the fast component recovered its original value over several beats.

A five second period of fast drive at 4–5 impulses/sec was carried out in five experiments (7 trials). The control (spontaneous) action potentials were compared with the last driven beat. Drive caused a fall in total amplitude of the action potential from 81.7 ± 2.9 mV to 75.8 ± 2.8·mV (-7.3%, $P < 0.001$). The average fast component was not changed (57.9 ± 4.7 versus 57.8 ± 3.3 mV $P < 0.98$) as in some experiments actually it declined. The slow component (measured from its take-off to peak) increased from 16.2 ± 1.7 mV to 21.1 ± 2.3 mV ($+30\%$, $P < 0.2$) as the take-off for this slow component became less positive (from 66.7 ± 3.2 mV to 55.0 ± 2.5 mV, -17.5%, $P < 0.001$).

It is of interest that in an additional experiment the preparation was driven twice at a slower rate (3 and 3.5 impulses/sec): the usual effects were present with the exception that the fast component increased markedly so that the take-off potential for the slow component was far less negative and the amplitude of the slow component decreased.

Fast drive (4–5 impulses/sec) was also carried out in low (0.27 mM) calcium (3 trials). The total amplitude decreased from 76.3 ± 9.3 mV to 72.5 ± 8.5 mV; the fast component increased from 67.0 ± 5.3 mV to 72.5 ± 8.5 mV and the slow component increased from 5.6 ± 0.24 mV to 6.6 ± 1.3 mV. The amplitude of plateau (difference between the plateau peak and E_{max} decreased from 63.6 ± 7.4 mV to 55.8 ± 8.0 mV and the take-off potential for the slow component decreased from 58.4 ± 7.3 to 50.0 ± 6.8 mV.

DISCUSSION

The results of the present experiments show that: 1) subsidiary pacemakers in the sinus node have a two component upstroke; 2) the upstroke is initiated by a fast component and is completed by a slow component; 3) the fast component occupies about two thirds of the upstroke and the slow component one third; 4) the maximal rate of rise of the fast component is about 30 V/sec; 5) with a tenfold decrease in $[Ca]_o$, the fast component decreased and the slow component increased more slowly to a smaller peak; 6) with a threefold increase in $[Ca]_o$, the fast component increased and the slow component reached its maximal value sooner; 7) acetylcholine increased the take-off potential and therefore the fast component, while decreasing the slow component; 8) norepinephrine restored the slow component in low calcium Tyrode; 9) electrical stimulation early in diastole enhanced the fast but not the slow component; 10) with repeated activity, the amplitude of the action potential became smaller as both components decreased gradually to a new value.

The ionic events underlying the excitatory process in the sinus node cells are still incompletely understood. In dominant pacemaker cells, excitation is brought about only by an inward slow current (Paes de Carvalho et al., 1969; Lenfant et al., 1971; Brooks and Lu 1972; Kohlhardt et al., 1976). This slow inward current is carried by Na^+ (Noma and Irisawa 1974) and/or Ca^{++} (Brooks and Lu 1972; Noma and Irisawa 1976; Kohlhardt et al., 1976). However, the results of Noma and Irisawa (1974) showed that the maximum rate of rise of the upstroke is sensitive to the take-off potential, to temperature and to $[Na]_o$, as it is found in other cardiac tissues exhibiting a fast channel. If this introduces some uncertainties as to the characteristics of the channel responsible for excitation in dominant pacemakers, the present results show that conclusions drawn for the dominant pacemakers cannot be extrapolated to subsidiary pacemakers in the sinus node. Thus, a fast channel may be absent in dominant pacemakers but is present in subsidiary pacemaker cells. While it is clear that the maximal rate of depolarization in sinus node subsidiary pacemakers is only one twentieth of that in Purkinje fibers, it is also clear that the channel responsible for the fast component in the subsidiary pacemakers shows many of the characteristics found for that channel in other tissues of the heart. Thus, the fast component increases markedly with a more negative take-off potential, whether obtained through stimulation early in diastole or through the hyperpolarizing action of acetylcholine. After an action potential, the fast component recovers much sooner than the slow component. Also, the fast component is abolished by tetrodotoxin (TTX) and by depolarization with high $[K]_o$ (Lipsius and Vassalle, 1978). Furthermore in the presence of TTX, neither a higher take-off potential nor acetylcholine make the fast component reappear (Lipsius and Vassalle, 1978). All these findings show that the subsidiary pacemakers not only have a fast channel but that the ion carrying the current through that channel is Na^+. It is true that the magnitude of the fast component decreased in low $[Ca]_o$ and increased in high $[Ca]_o$. However, it is possible that this is an indirect effect of calcium: changes in $[Ca]_o$ shift along the voltage axis the relationship between maximum rate of rise and the membrane potential (Noma and Irisawa, 1976). In turn, a larger or smaller fast component should affect the magnitude of the subsequent slow component and the time needed to reach its peak. This indirect effect must contribute to the observed changes.

The slow component, instead, seems to be related to calcium. Thus, the slow component is made slower and smaller by lowering $[Ca]_o$, is not increased by stimulation early in diastole, is increased by stimulation late in diastole, is abolished by acetylcholine and enhanced by norepinephrine. All these findings point to an influx of calcium through a slow channel as the carrier responsible for the slow component. Thus, in different cardiac tissues, the slow inward current: becomes smaller when $[Ca]_o$ is decreased (Beeler and Reuter, 1970; Mascher and Peper, 1969; New and Trautwein, 1972), does not become larger at more negative take-off potentials (New and Trautwein, 1972), has a relatively long repriming time (Gettes and Reuter, 1974), is at least partially blocked by acetylcholine (Prokopczuk et al., 1973; Ikemoto and Goto, 1975, Giles and Tsien, 1975; Ten Eich et al., 1976) and is augmented by norepinephrine (Reuter, 1965; Vassort et al., 1969).

In discussing the importance of calcium for the slow component, two facts should be kept in mind: the first is that the slow channel has been shown to admit both Na^+ and Ca^{++} (Rougier et al., 1969) and the second is that there is an antagonism between sodium and calcium (Lüttgau and Niedergerke, 1958). Because of these interrelationships, it is not surprising that a decrease in either $[Na]_o$ or $[Ca]_o$ results in a diminution of the action potential amplitude which is less than expected (Noma and Irisawa, 1974; Noma and Irisawa, 1976).

The present experiments show another phenomenon, namely the fact that while the fast component recovers sooner than the slow component (Figure 6), repetitive stimulation reduces both the fast and the slow component (Figure 7). It seems as if the lag in the recovery of the fast component becomes cumulative with successive action potentials at fast rate.

Some of the characteristics of the sinus node action potentials seem of importance for the function of this structure. The dominant pacemakers seem to have only a slow component. Subsidiary pacemakers are activated by the process of conduction and therefore at a higher take-off potential. This results in an initial fast component of the upstroke. In turn, the fast component should accelerate conduction as the action potential moves toward the periphery of the sinus node.

Part of the characteristics of the subsidiary pacemakers is only functional. Thus, the fast component is increased by a higher take-off potential (Figure 6 and 7). The magnitude of the fast component will be thus determined by several variables such as an increase in rate of discharge or the slope of diastolic depolarization. For example, a flattening of diastolic depolarization will increase conduction velocity. The fast component will be decreased by a lower take-off potential. In fact, it may disappear altogether if the rate of discharge of the dominant pacemaker decreases so much that the diastolic depolarization of the subsidiary pacemaker slowly attains the threshold. A pacemaker shift within the sinus node must involve a change of this type. Such a transition from a subsidiary to a dominant pacemaker is readily brought about by TTX and K-induced depolarization, as mentioned above.

Part of the differences, however, is not functional. A dominant pacemaker may not develop a fast channel even if hyperpolarized by acetylcholine (Paes de Carvalho et al., 1969), exactly as it happens with the administration of acetylcholine to a subsidiary pacemaker pretreated with TTX or exposed to high K (Lipsius and Vassalle, 1978). It would seem then that while the subsidiary pacemakers can easily become dominant, the usually dominant pacemaker cells of the sinus node are unlikely to become subsidiary.

REFERENCES

1. Beeler, G. W. Jr., Reuter, H.: Membrane calcium current in ventricular myocardial fibres. *J Physiol* (*London*) 207: 191, 1970.
2. Brooks, C. McC., Lu, H. H.: The Sinoatrial Pacemaker of the Heart. Charles C. Thomas, Springfield, Illinois, 1972
3. Cranefield, P. F.: The Conduction of the Cardiac Impulse. Futura Publishing, New York, 1975
4. Gettes, L. S., Reuter, H.: Slow recovery from inactivation of inward currents in mammalian myocardial fibres. *J Physiol* (*London*) 240: 703, 1974
5. Giles, W., Tsien, R. W.: Effects of acetylcholine on membrane currents in frog atrial muscle. *J Physiol* (*London*) 246: 64P, 1975
6. Hutter, O. F., Trautwein, W.: Vagal and sympathetic effects on the pacemaker fibres in the sinus venosus of the heart. *J Gen Physiol* 39: 715, 1956
7. Ikemoto, Y., Goto, M.: Nature of the negative inotropic effect of acetylcholine on the myocardium. An elucidation on the bullfrog atrium. *Proc Japan Acad* 51: 501, 1975
8. Kohlhardt, M., Bauer, B., Krause, H., Fleckenstein, A.: Differentiation of the transmembrane Na and Ca channels in mammalian cardiac fibres by the use of specific inhibitors. *Pflügers Archiv* 335: 309, 1972
9. Lenfant, J., Mironneau, J., Aka, J. K.: Analyse des propriétés de la membrane myocardique sino-auriculaire; genèse de l'activité spontanée. *CR Acad Sc Paris* 273: 1729, Série D, 1971

10. Lipsius, S. L., Vassalle, M.: Effects of ionic changes and glycosides on sinus node action potentials. *Federation Proc* 35: 319, 1976
11. Lipsius, S. L., Vassalle, M.: Dual excitatory channels in the sinus node. *J Mol Cell Cardiol* 10: in press, 1978.
12. Lüttgau, H. C., Niedergerke, R.: The antagonism between Ca and Na ions on the frog's heart. *J Physiol* 143: 486, 1958
13. Mascher, D., Peper, K.: Two components of inward current in myocardial muscle fibers. *Pflügers Archiv* 307: 190, 1969
14. New, W., Trautwein, W.: The ionic nature of slow inward current and its relation to contraction. *Pflügers Archiv* 334: 24, 1972
15. Noma, A., Irisawa, H.: The effect of sodium ion on the initial phase of the sinoatrial pacemaker action potentials in rabbits. *Japan J Physiol* 24: 617, 1974
16. Noma, A., Irisawa, H.: Effects of calcium ion on the rising phase of the action potential in rabbit sinoatrial node cells. *Japan J Physiol* 26: 93, 1976
17. Paes de Carvalho, A., Hoffman, B. F., De Paula Carvalho, M.: Two components of the cardiac action potential. I. Voltage-time course and the effect of acetylcholine on atrial and nodal cells of the rabbit heart. *J Gen Physiol* 54: 607, 1969
18. Prokopczuk, A., Lewartowski, B., Czarnecka, M.: On the cellular mechanism of the inotropic action of acetylcholine on isolated rabbit and dog atria. *Pflügers Archiv* 339: 305, 1973
19. Reuter, H.: Über die wirkung von Adrenalin auf den cellulären Ca-Umsatz des Meerschweinchenvorhofs. *Naunyn-Schmiedebergs Archiv Pharmakol* 251: 401, 1965
20. Rougier, O., Vassort, G., Garnier, D., Gargouïl, Y.-M., Coraboeuf, E.: Existence and role of a slow inward current during the frog atrial action potential. *Pflügers Archiv* 308: 91, 1969
21. Ten Eick, R., Nawrath, H., McDonald, T. F., Trautwein W.: On the mechanism of the negative inotropic effect of acetylcholine *Pflügers Arch* 361: 207, 1976
22. Trautwein, W.: Membrane currents in cardiac muscle fibers. *Physiol Rev* 53: 793, 1973
23. Vassalle, M.: Generation and conduction of impulses in the heart under physiological and pathological conditions. *Pharmac Ther B* 3: 1, 1977
24. Vassort, G., Rougier, O., Garnier, D., Sauviat, M. P., Coraboeuf, E., Gargouïl, Y.-M.: Effects of adrenaline on membrane inward currents during the cardiac action potential. *Pflügers Archiv* 309: 70, 1969

20

PACEMAKER SHIFTS IN THE SINUS NODE: EFFECTS OF VAGAL STIMULATION, TEMPERATURE AND REDUCTION OF EXTRACELLULAR CALCIUM

L.N. BOUMAN, A.J.C. MACKAAY, W.K. BLEEKER, AND A.E. BECKER

INTRODUCTION

Shortly after the description of the sinus node by Keith and Flack in 1907, it became clear that only a small part of it generated the actual impulse. Lewis et al. (1910) first combined electrophysiological and histological methods. They determined the exact point of primary negativity in the dog heart using small surface electrodes connected to a strong galvanometer, whereafter the sinus node was demonstrated histologically. According to Lewis et al. the earliest negativity was found in the mass (head) of the node. Subsequent workers confirmed these findings (Sulze, 1913; Eyster and Meek, 1914). Although these investigators were able to locate the area of impulse formation, the exact site of pacemaker initiation could not be determined, due to limitations of the methods employed. In those days, in order to register surface negativity a relatively large group of cells showing simultaneous rapid depolarization was needed. At present it is accepted that the site of the dominating pacemaker does not fulfil these criteria. The assumption that a "presinus" existed between the superior caval vein and the sinus node (Rylant, 1930) discharging at an earlier time interval than the node itself can now be related to the same technical limitations. Further studies regarding the exact position of the pacemaker site had to wait till the activation pattern could be studied at cellular level. Recent investigations have shown that only a small part of the sinus node, containing a few thousand cells, gives origin to the cardiac impulse (West, 1955; Trautwein and Uchizono, 1963; Sano and Yamagishi, 1965; Masson-Pévet et al., chapter 16, page 195). The major part of the node seems to act as conductor like ordinary working myocardium.

It is of interest, particularly in view of the aforementioned technical limitations, that early workers already suggested that the site of origin of the impulse within the node is not fixed, but that shifts can occur either "spontaneously" or induced by one or other intervention. Sulze (1913), recording the earliest electrical activity by means of small soaked cotton threads noted that the primary negativity was localized at different places in different preparations. Meek and Eyster (1914), however, were the first who demonstrated a reversible shift of the pacemaker in one and the same node, by simultaneous measurements of the electrical activity from several sites. During weak faradic stimulation of the vagal nerves the site of primary negativity shifted to the caudal portion of the node. When vagal stimulation was ended the site of primary negativity returned to its original position. Lewis et al. (1914) came to the same conclusion by calculating conducting times. However, with the limitations of their technique it seems likely that they mainly observed changes of the activation pattern of the sinus node caused by a shift of a pacemaker. Again, West (1955) was the first to demonstrate the occurrence of a pacemaker shift at cellular level by applying acetylcholine. Subsequent workers induced pacemaker shifts by vagal stimulation (Bouman et al., 1968), sympathetic stimulation (Toda and Shimamoto, 1968) and an increase of the extracellular potassium concentration (Lu, 1970). However, the direction and magnitude of the shifts were not directly mapped.

The present investigation deals with the effects of temperature changes and alterations in the extracellular calcium concentrations on the pacemaker site. Moreover, mapping experiments have been performed, enabling us to visualize the shift of the pacemaker site, to estimate its magnitude and to correlate these data with those subsequently obtained from morphological reconstructions of the same specimen.

METHODS

GENERAL EQUIPMENT

The experiments were performed on the sinus node of adult rabbits. Under Ether or Hypnorm[R] anesthesia the hearts were excised and the sinus node – together with the intercaval region and the roof of the right atrial appendage – was isolated. The preparation was kept in a solution, the basic composition of which was derived from McEwen (1956). The preparation was fixed on wax or silicon rubber in a continuously perfused tissue bath, exposing the endocardial surface tissue.

By means of an unipolar lead an electrogram was recorded from the crista terminalis, for two reasons. Firstly it delivered via an interval counter a continuous cardiotachogram, secondly it served as reference timing when a conduction map of the sinus node was made (see further).

The electrical activity of single fibers in the sinus node was recorded in the usual way, by means of KCl/K-citrate filled microelectrodes one positioned inside the cell, the other outside in its vicinity. The exploring microelectrode was mounted on a motor driven micromanipulator on a mechanical stage, the lateral movements of which were read with vernier scales accurate to 0.01 mm (Schreurs et al., 1974). After suitable amplification the microelectrode signal was displayed on an oscilloscope and together with the amplified electrogram stored on magnetic tape for off-line analysis.

The mapping of the excitation of the sinus node and the surrounding tissue consisted of determination of the arrival time of the excitation wave at a great number of impaled cells, a small distance apart. As arrival time we chose the moment of maximal rate of rise of the recorded action potentials related to the fast deflection of the atrium electrogram. During the experiment this arrival time was estimated by means of a digital counter in order to find the site of the earliest discharge. This area was mapped with impalements at a distance of 0.1–0.2 mm. After the experiment, arrival times were calculated from the stored signals by computer analysis. The arrival times were expressed in multiples of 5 msec.

Details of the methods used have been presented previously (Bouman et al., 1968).

SPECIAL CONDITIONS

a. Vagal stimulation

In this case the preparations were made according to Opitz and Weiss (1958). In order to keep the vagal nerves intact, it was inevitable to remove much less of the adhering mediastinal tissue than otherwise. The nerves were stimulated via bipolar platinum electrodes that were kept in the perfusion fluid except during the period of stimulation. As stimuli we used rectangular pulses of 5 msec duration, frequency 10–25 Hz and intensity varying between 0.5 and 5 V.

b. Temperature change

As the electrical activity of different nodal fibers shows many differences, we always took special care that the recording microelectrode remained inside the fiber during the intervention of which we wanted to study the effect. In case of temperature change therefore a perfusion device was developed with which it was possible to switch to a new and stable temperature of the fluid inside the tissue bath within 2 minutes. Nevertheless the new temperature was maintained during at least 5 minutes to avoid the effects of temperature gradients within the tissue. The temperature of the fluid was measured by means of a thermistor in a bridge circuit of which the voltage output was digitized and read in values up to 0.1 degree centigrade. During the changes of temperature the pH of the fluid remained constant at 7.35.

c. Change of the external calcium concentration

In these experiments the perfusion fluid contained only 1.1 mmol/l $CaCl_2$ instead of the normal amount of 2.2 mmol/l. Through a mixing chamber in connection with the tissue bath the concentration of calciumchloride of the perfusion fluid could be raised rapidly up to 6.6 mmol/l. Ca^{++} concentration was measured by means of a calcium sensitive electrode (Orion 93–20).

MORPHOLOGICAL STUDIES

After completion of the electrophysiological experiments the same preparations were used for a correlative morphological investigation. The specimen were marked with small dots of alcian blue which could be used as reference points. Fixation in formalin was carried out with the specimen still attached to its silicon rubber support. After embedment in paraffin the specimen were serially sectioned at 7 micron thickness. Every tenth section was studied after being stained with an elastic tissue stain counterstained with van Gieson's stain (Lawson, 1936). A reconstruction was then made enabling us to correlate the histological findings with the excitation map obtained during the electrophysiological experiments.

RESULTS

1. NORMAL EXCITATION AND ITS STRUCTURAL BASIS

The sinus node of the rabbit consists of pale staining nodal cells (N-cells) which abut on ordinary atrial myocardium. The fibers of the N-cell group can be divided into a central compact zone, which in its periphery shows a transition into an arrangement of cells parallel to the crista terminalis. The cells themselves do not change their cytological characteristics, as judged by the light microscope. This region is contiguous with slender fibers that stream into the crista terminalis. The compact center has a roughly ellipsoid body with a maximal width of about 2 mm and a tapering end ("tail") which is a little less compact in structure.

Figure 1 shows the correlation between the activation map and the histological reconstruction of the sinus node in the same specimen. It demonstrates that the impulse starts inside the body of the compact region ("head"). The exact site of impulse formation depends on the criterium used to delineate the earliest discharging group of cells. In the

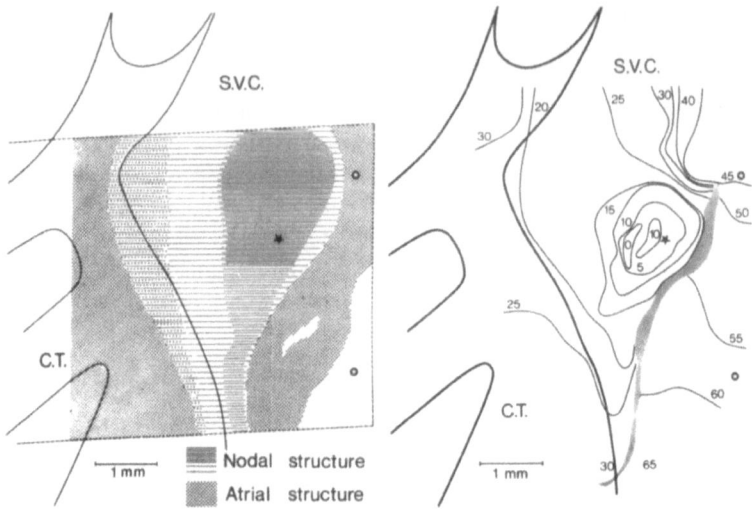

Figure 1. (*Left*) Histological reconstruction of the extension of the SA node in a rabbit heart. The core formed by a compact network of N-cells is surrounded by bundles also consisting of nodal cells. This N-cell group is surrounded by atrial cells. The lateral portion of the node partially overlies the working myocardium of the crista terminalis (C.T.). (*Right*) Excitation map of the same preparation. The impulse started low in the head of the compact centre of the node; conduction is fast in an oblique cranial direction via the area of N-cell bundles.

map, the fiber that led using the moment of V_{max} as criterium got the index 0 msec (Sano and Yamagishi, 1965). The black star in the figure marks the site where the fibers had the steepest diastolic depolarization (Paes de Carvalho et al., 1959) at the end of the diastole. From the compact body the excitation travels with rapidly increasing speed obliquely upwards to the cranial part of the crista terminalis. In other directions, conduction is slower and even can be blocked (shaded area of the excitation map in Figure 1).

2. EFFECTS OF VAGAL STIMULATION

The effects of vagal stimulation on the SA node have already been described extensively (Bouman, 1965; Bouman et al., 1968). They can be summarized as follows:
- decrease of diastolic depolarization rate
- hyperpolarization
  The maximal diastolic potential increased with more than 25 mV during strong vagal stimulation (with a high stimulating frequency). This effect was most pronounced in the normally dominant pacemaker fibers; during prolonged stimulation the hyperpolarization declined.
- desynchronization
  The amplitude of consecutive action potentials sometimes differed considerably. Small humps of a few millivolts were seen on the base line in addition to action potentials with an amplitude that was even larger than during normal action.
- sino-atrial block
  Occasionally an action potential was not accompanied by an activation of the atrium.
- shift of the site of pacemaking

Already from the recordings with a single microelectrode inside a leading pacemaker cell it can be observed that during vagal stimulation the smooth transition between diastolic depolarization and the action potential disappeared while the latency between the action potential and the atrial electrogram was shortened. Although this is suggestive for a shift of the pacemaker the proof could only be given by impalements with two micro-electrodes simultaneously. The results of such an experiment are shown in Figure 2. The intracellular recordings of the electrical activity of two fibers about 5 mm apart inside the SA node are reproduced, together with the atrial electrogram. Vagal stimulation started in panel B and was gradually increased in strength from 2 to 5 V (bottom trace). Prior to the stimulation the action potential of the fiber that gave the upper recording preceded both the action potential in the lower recording and the atrial electrogram. This sequence of excitation was maintained during weak vagal stimulation. When the strength of the stimulation was increased above 3 V (panel F) the order of excitation reversed; at that moment the beat-to-beat interval had increased with about 25%. This reversed pattern of excitation did not change anymore when the strength of stimulation was increased up to 5 V while every increase of the stimulus intensity still was followed by a corresponding increase of beat-to-beat interval. When the strength of stimulation was

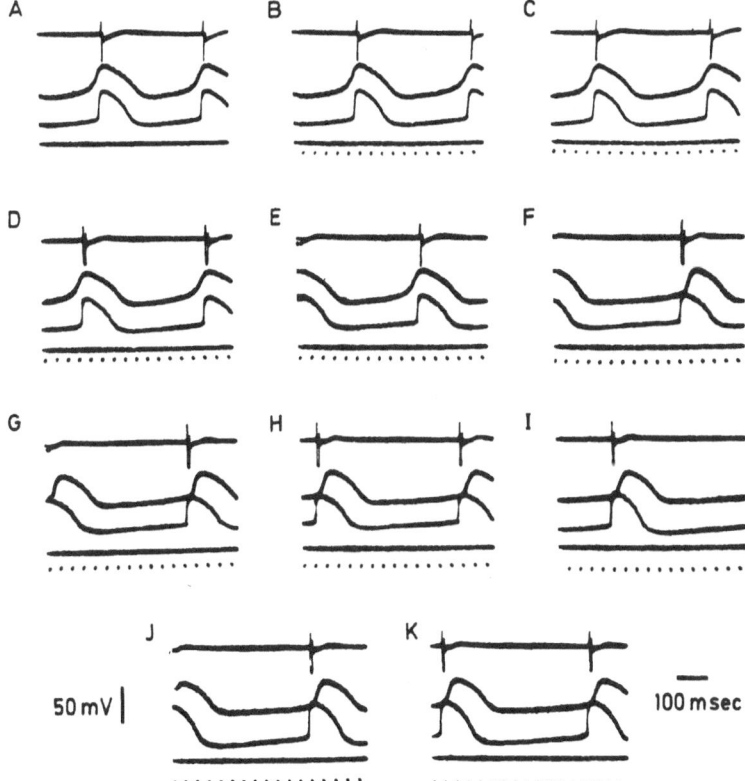

Figure 2. The effect of vagal stimulation on the activation pattern of the SA node. Upper trace: surface electrogram of right atrium; second and third trace: two different fibers in the SA node; fourth trace: intensity of vagal stimulation. (From: Bouman et al., 1968, with permission).

reduced again, the original order of excitation was restored while the beat-to-beat interval was still prolonged with about 40%.
– It was impossible to map the excitation of the SA node during the short time that the
  vagal nerves could be stimulated under those experimental conditions. We could
  neither determine the direction of the pacemaker shift, nor did we ever succeed in
  recording the transformation of a latent pacemaker fiber into a leading fiber during vagal
  stimulation.

3. DECREASE OF TEMPERATURE

The effects of a decrease of temperature can be summarized as follows. When the temperature is lowered in steps from 38°C down to 30°C the following changes can be observed
(Figure 3)
– decrease of diastolic depolarization rate
  When the prepotential is expressed as a function of the tissue bath temperature, it
  can be stated in general that the diastolic depolarization is most inhibited in fibers that
  are normally the leading fibers.
– decrease of the rapid rate of rise of the action potential
– increase of the duration of the action potential
– shift of the site of pacemaking
  Also in case of lowering of the temperature the recordings made a single microelectrode
  from a leading pacemaker cell are already suggestive for a pacemaker shift. As can be
  observed from Figure 3, the action potential of the impaled fiber preceded the atrial
  electrogram at 38°C. This order of excitation was reversed at 35°C, the atrial complex
  now being ahead of the fast depolarization phase of the action potential. When the temperature was lowered further the latency between the action potential and the atrial electrogram increased, suggesting a progressive shift of the pacemaker away from the
  recording microelectrode, but slower conduction could not be excluded. The shift was
  demonstrated directly by mapping of the excitation of the SA node at four different
  temperatures in the same preparation (see Figure 4). When temperature is lowered the
  site of earliest discharge shifted downwards to the tail of the SA node. At a temperature

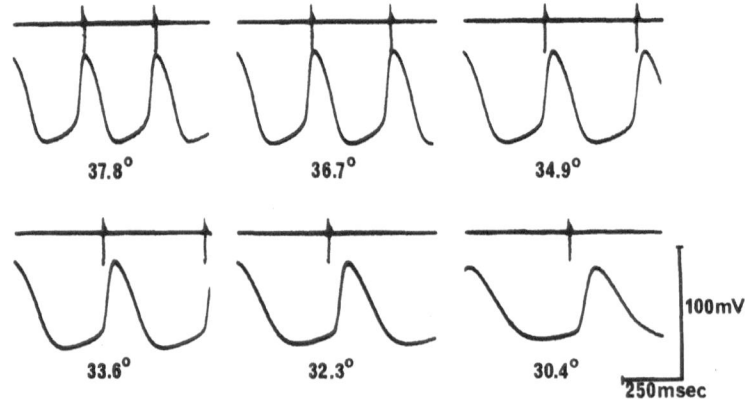

Figure 3. The effect of a stepwise lowering of the temperature on a fiber in the head of the SA node.

Temperature dependent intranodal pacemaker shift

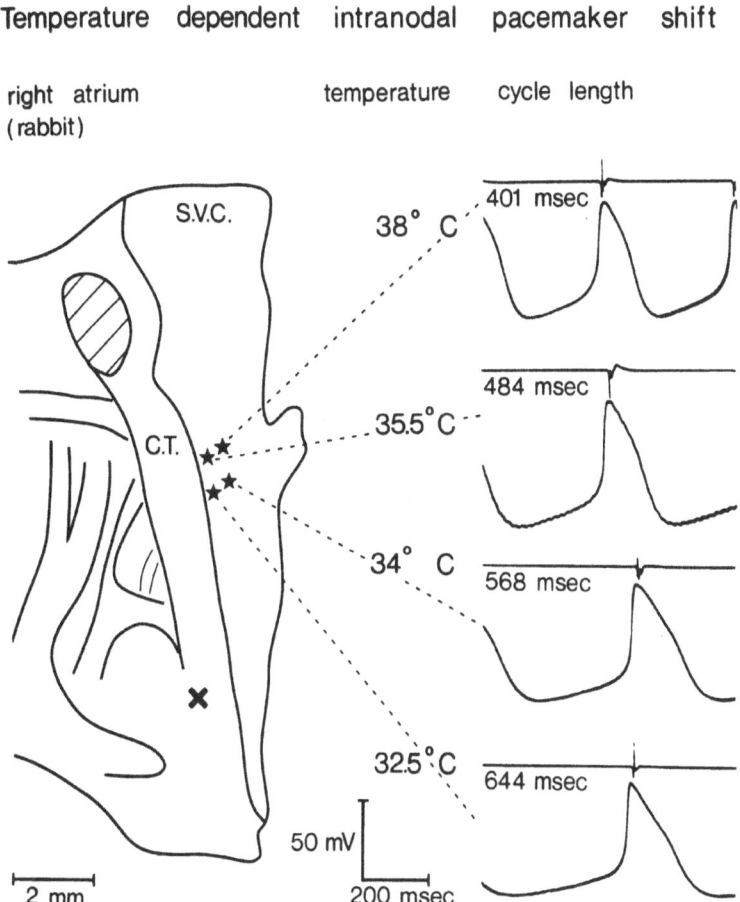

right atrium
(rabbit)

temperature   cycle length

Figure 4. Shift of the pacemaker during lowering of the temperature. At the temperatures indicated, maps were made. The black stars mark the sites of earliest discharge; on the right side the action potentials recorded at these sites. The electrogram was taken at the site indicated with a cross (X) SVC = superior vena cava; CT = crista terminalis.

of 32.5°C it was located about 1.5 mm lower than at normal temperature and more in the vicinity of the crista terminalis. Furthermore it was proven that the shift took place indeed gradually; every step of lowering of temperature was followed by another shift of the pacemaker.

4. CHANGE OF THE EXTERNAL CALCIUM CONCENTRATION

Calcium acts as a positive chronotropic agent (Seifen et al., 1964). As will be described in the next paragraph, however, this holds true only at normal temperature. At a temperature of 30°C it can induce a decrease of heart rate. When at a normal temperature (38°C) the calcium concentration of the fluid inside the tissue bath was increased from 2.2 mmol/l up to 6.6 mmol/l the following effects were observed
– shortening of the beat-to-beat interval

– increase of the rate of diastolic depolarization
– decrease of the maximal diastolic potential
– increase of the duration of the action potential
In the recordings from the leading pacemaker fibers neither the shape of the action potential nor the latency between the moment of $\dot{V}_{max}$ of the action potential and the atrial electrogram suggested a change in the pattern of excitation of the SA node.

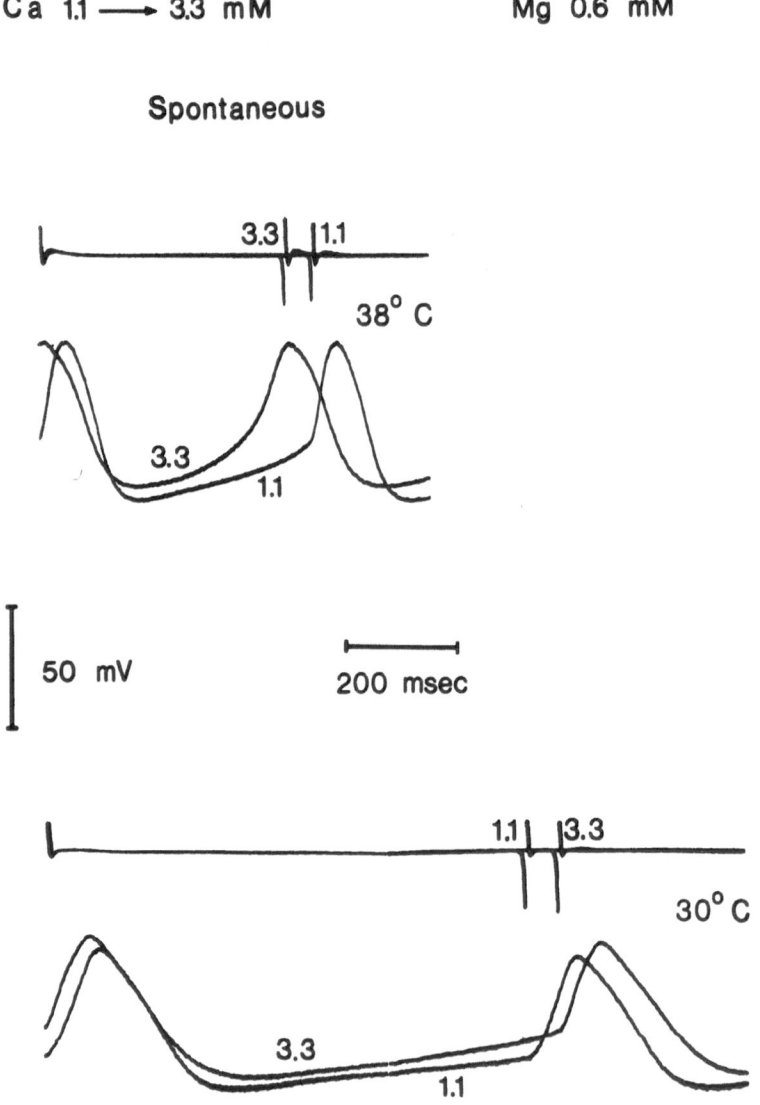

Ca 1.1 ⟶ 3.3 mM   **Mg 0.6 mM**

Spontaneous

Figure 5. The effect of a reduction of the extracellular calcium concentration from 3.3 to 1.1 mmol/l on a fiber in the head of the SA node. Upper part: at normal temperature; Lower part: at 30°C.

But when the calcium concentration was reduced to below the normal concentration, down to 1.1 mmol/l (see upper panel of figure 5), the normally leading fibers lost their pacemaking function and were discharged after the atrial reference. The abrupt transition that appeared between the diastolic and systolic depolarization phase gave another argument to assume that a shift of the pacemaker had occurred. This could be affirmed in an elaborate experiment that is summarized in Figure 6. First the leading group of fibers at the normal calcium concentration (2.2 mmol/1) was localized by extensive mapping. The fiber marked A belonged to this group; its discharge preceded the atrial time reference 28 msec. During continuous impalement the calcium concentration was decreased to 1.1 mmol/1; now the rapid discharge of this fiber came 23 msec after the atrial electrogram. At the lowered calcium concentration a new map of the excitation of the node was made. The fiber at site B was found to belong to the group of fibers leading at this calcium concentration. Its rapid discharge preceded the atrial complex 35 msec, but after increasing the calcium concentration back to 2.2 mmol/1 it lost its pacemaking function, the rapid discharge took place 21 msec after the atrial electrogram.

A very interesting phenomenon was observed in a third fiber, of which the recording is marked B', localized midway between the sites A and B. At the normal calcium concentration this fiber was discharged only shortly (7 msec) before the crista terminalis. When the calcium concentration inside the tissue bath was falling, the function of pacemaking was temporarily taken over by the group of fibers to which it belonged, the fiber now discharged 32 msec before the atrial time reference. Yet when the final calcium concentration of 1.1 mmol/1 was established, the fiber had regained its normal role in the excitation pattern, the latency was returned to only 7 msec. From this observation it can be made up that during the fall of the external calcium concentration the shift of the pacemaker took place gradually from A via B' to B.

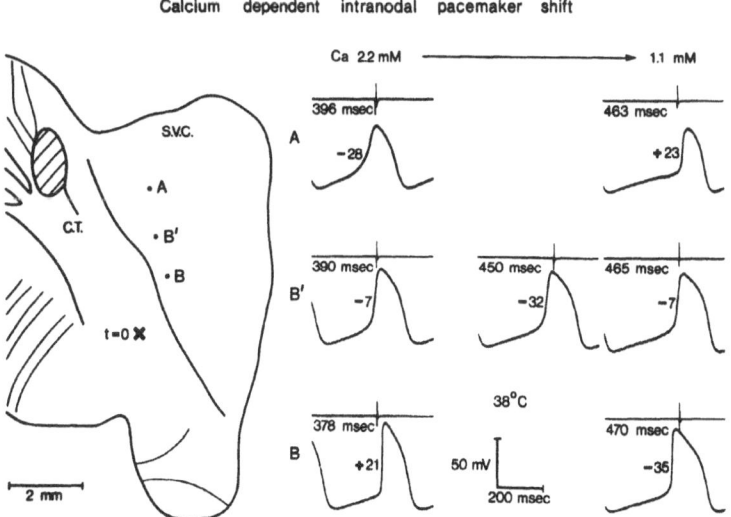

Figure 6. Calcium induced pacemaker shift. For explanation see text. SVC = superior vena cava; CT = crista terminalis; The electrogram was taken at the site indicated with a cross (X) and was used as time reference.

5. TEMPERATURE AND CALCIUM

The chronotropic action of calcium on the mammalian heart is still a matter of controversy. Seifen et al. (1964) described a positive chronotropic response of the rabbit heart on calcium excess, whereas Toda (1969) did not observe any chronotropic effect and Lenfant (1972) even found a slight decrease of heart rate in the same preparation. Close examination of the methods used by these authors revealed a possible side-effect of the temperature at which the experiments had been performed. The positive chronotropic response was obtained at normal temperature while the contradicting experiments were carried out at a temperature of 30°C.

To elucidate the possible interference of a low temperature with the chronotropic action of calcium the changes of the calcium concentration were carried out at 38°C as well as 30°C (Figure 5). As can be seen from the electrogram (upper trace) at 30°C the chronotropic action of calcium is reversed. Instead of cardiac acceleration, as shown in the upper panel (beat-to-beat interval from 470 to 425 msec), we observed a deceleration when the calcium concentration was raised; the interval increased from 840 to 900 msec.

Another peculiar thing appears from comparison of the latencies between the action potential and the atrial electrogram. All recordings of Figure 5 are from the same fiber. It was a leading fiber at a calcium concentration of 3.3 mmol/l at 38°C; the moment of $\dot{V}_{max}$ preceded the electrogram 24 msec. When the calcium concentration was reduced to 1.1 mmol/l the fiber lost its leading role, it was discharged 25 msec after the atrial time reference. So this fiber can be compared with fiber A of Figure 6. However, at low temperature (lower panel) the increase of the calcium concentration to 3.3 mmol/l is not followed by a shift back to this normally leading group, it remained discharged after the atrial reference. Furthermore it can be observed that the accelerating effect on diastolic depolarization is strongly diminished. Probably the "B-fibers" are the leading group at 30°C and calcium concentration 1.1 mmol/l as well as 3.3 mmol/l, but we did not check it by mapping yet.

In Figure 6 it can be seen that the "B-fibres" behave different from the "A-fibers" if the calcium concentration is increased: the diastolic depolarization rate is depressed while the action potential shortens in the "B-fibers", whereas in the "A-fibers" the opposite occurs. Putting those things together we conclude that at low temperature the positive chronotropic effect of calcium excess is abolished or even reversed; this is a direct consequence of the shift of the pacemaker, due to the lowering of the temperature, to fibers that have a different responsiveness to calcium.

DISCUSSION

To the well-known influences that can cause an intranodal pacemaker shift, like stimulation of the vagal nerves or accelerant nerves, the application of acetylcholine or epinephrine, and an increase of the external potassium concentration we can now add a lowering of the temperature and a reduction of the extracellular calcium concentration. We have documented that in our preparations, which were beating regularly, under normal conditions the site of the pacemaker was in the head of the compact network. The group of leading fibers is small, only a few thousands cells. Furthermore it could be shown that when the temperature is lowered there occurs a progressive shift of the pacemaker downwards into the tail of the mass of nodal cells. Histologically the tail has an architecture that is a little less compact than the head of the mass of nodal cells. Results for comparison on ultrastructural level are not available yet.

A more or less identical gradual shift in caudal direction could be observed when the external calcium concentration was reduced from 2.2 mmol/l to 1.1 mmol/l. In literature it is stated that the shift of the pacemaker observed during application of catecholamines or acetylcholine and increase of the extracellular potassium concentration, is directed to the tail also (see for review Brooks and Lu, 1972).

Generally it is believed that shifts like those described here are the consequence of differences in sensitivity to the shift inducing agents among the pacemaker fibers in different parts of the node; furthermore in case of nerve stimulation an uneven distribution of nerve endings may also play a role (Brooks and Lu, 1972). Our results, however, point to another direction which we will call the "two fibers model". Especially in case of the reduction of the extracellular calcium concentration we see that the function of pacemaking is taken over by fibers that functionally differ from the originally leading pacemaker fibers. In these fibers which we will call "tail fibers" and which are marked B in Figure 6, an increase of the calcium concentration causes a decrease of the rate of diastolic depolarization while in the original pacemaker the rate is increased. The fact that a B' fiber was found morphologically and functionally midway between A and B is reason enough to stress that the "two fibers model" is an extremely simplified representation which points to the fact that the fibers of the SA node form a functionally inhomogeneous group, the A (head) and B (tail) cell types being only the two extremes.

The effects of calcium excess on the "head fibers", namely the decrease of maximal diastolic potential and the increase of rate of diastolic depolarization, support the hypothesis that in these pacemaker fibers there is a substantial influx of Ca^{++} ions during diastole (Lu and Brooks, 1969; Kohlhardt et al., 1976; Pollack, 1977). This influx is very sensitive to changes in temperature.

The response of the "tail fibers" to an increase of the calcium concentration is so completely different, viz. a slight decrease of the rate of diastolic depolarization, that we have to assume that an influx of calcium ions plays only a minor role. Which ionic fluxes are involved in the diastolic depolarization phase in those cells is an object for mere guess. Although mapping during vagal stimulation was not possible, there is some evidence in literature that in this case also fibers in the tail take over the pacemaker function. (Meek and Eyster, 1914; Goldberg, 1975). The most simple explanation is that acetylcholine inhibits the influx of calcium ions; the observed effects are in agreement with this assumption. However, it is generally believed that the retardation of the pacemaker under the influence of acetylcholine is due to an increased potassium permeability of the membrane. This theory goes back to 1908 when Howell and Duke showed that the heart releases more potassium during vagal stimulation. It was proven directly by Harris and Hutter (1956). The finding that the potassium permeability is increased does not rule out the possibility that acetylcholine, in addition, inhibits a calcium influx. With respect to the slow channel current in the atrium the inhibiting effect of acetylcholine was already suggested in 1973 by Prokopczuk et al. and reported in frog atrium by Giles and Noble (1976). So we feel justified to suppose that the pacemaker shift during vagal stimulation is caused by the inhibition of a calcium influx which is of significant importance for the process of diastolic depolarization in normally leading pacemaker fibers.

ACKNOWLEDGEMENT

We wish to thank Mr. H. van der Westen for performing some of the temperature experiments and Miss C.E. Besselsen and Mr. M.J. Klaver for technical assistance.

REFERENCES

Bleeker, W.K., Mackaay, A.J.C., Masson-Pévet, M., Bouman, L.N.: Functional and morphological organization of the rabbit sinoatrial node. Submitted for publication. 1978

Bouman, L.N.: De werking van de nervus vagus op de prikkelvorming in de sino-auriculaire knoop. Thesis 1965

Bouman, L.N., Gerlings, E.D., Biersteker, P.A., Bonke, F.I.M.: Pacemaker shift in the sino-atrial node during vagal stimulation. *Pflügers Arch* 302: 255, 1968

Brooks, C.Mc.C., Lu, H.-H.: The sinoatrial pacemaker of the heart. Springfield, Ill., 1972

Eyster, J.A.E., Meek, W.J.: The point of primary negativity in the mammalian heart and the spread of negativity to other regions. *Heart* 5: 119, 1914

Giles, W., Noble, S.J.: Changes in membrane currents in bullfrog atrium produced by acetylcholine. *J Physiol* 261: 103, 1976

Goldberg, J.M.: Intra-SA-nodal pacemaker shifts induced by autonomic nerve stimulation in the dog. *Am J Physiol* 229: 1116, 1975

Harris, E.J., Hutter, O.F.: The action of acetylcholine on the movement of potassium ions in the sinus venosus of the heart. *J Physiol* 133: 588, 1956

Howell, W.H., Duke, W.W.: The effect of vagus inhibition on the output of potassium from the heart. *Am J Physiol* 21: 51, 1908

Keith, A., Flack, M.: The form and nature of the muscular connections between the primary division of the vertebrate heart. *J Anat and Physiol* 41: 172, 1907

Kohlhardt, M., Figulla, H.-R., Tripathi, O.: The slow membrane channel as the predominant mediator of the excitation process of the sinoatrial pacemaker cell. *Basic Res Cardiol* 71: 17, 1976

Lawson, W.H.: Elastic tissue staining; modification of Weigert-Sheridan method. *J Tech Meth* 16: 42, 1936

Lenfant, J.: Analyse des propriétés de la membrane myocardique sino-auriculaire: genèse de l'activité spontanée. Thesis, Poitiers 1972.

Lewis, Th., Oppenheimer, B.S., Oppenheimer, A.: The site of origin of the mammalian heart beat; the pacemaker in the dog. *Heart* 2: 147, 1910

Lewis, Th., Meakins, J., White, P.D.: The excitatory process in the dog's heart. *Philos Trans R Soc* 205: 375, 1914

Lu, H.-H., Brooks, C.Mc.C.: Role of calcium in cardiac pacemaker cell action. *Bull NY Acad Med* 45: 100, 1969

Lu, H.-H.: Shifts in pacemaker dominance within the sinoatrial region of cat and rabbit hearts resulting from increase of extracellular potassium. *Circ Res* 26: 339, 1970

Mc Ewen, L.M.: The effect on the isolated rabbit heart of vagal stimulation and its modification by cocaine, hexamethonium and ouabain. *J Physiol* 131: 678, 1956

Meek, W.J., Eyster, J.A.E.: The effect of vagal stimulation and of cooling on the location of the pacemaker within the sino-auricular node. *Am J Physiol* 34: 368, 1914

Opitz, H., Weiss, E.: Quantitative Untersuchungen an der inotropen Vaguswirkung auf den isolierten Kaninchen-Vorhof. *Pflügers Arch* 267: 600, 1958

Paes de Carvalho, A., de Mello, W.C., Hoffman, B.F.: Electrophysiological evidence for specialized fiber types in rabbit atrium. *Am J Physiol* 196: 483, 1959

Pollack, G.H.: Cardiac pacemaking: an obligatory role of catecholamines? A possible mechanism underlaying spontaneous pacemaking can be deduced from several recent clues. *Science* 196: 731, 1977

Prokopczuk, A., Lewartowski, B., Czarnecka, M.: On the cellular mechanism of the inotropic action of acetylcholine on isolated rabbit and dog atria. *Pflügers Arch* 339: 305, 1973

Rylant, P.: Ablation et greffe intracardiaque du noeud de Keith-Flack (sinus) chez le chien. *Arch Int Physiol Biochim* 26: 113, 1926

Sano, T., Yamagishi, S.: Spread of excitation from the sinus node. *Circ Res* 16: 423, 1965

Schreurs, A.W., Meyer, A.A., Bouman, L.N., Bonke, F.I.M.: Micromanipulator with an electrode driver used for microelectrode work. *Pflügers Arch* 346: 163, 1974

Seifen, E., Schaer, H., Marshall, J.M.: Effect of calcium on the membrane potentials of single pacemaker fibers in isolated rabbit atria. *Nature* 202: 1223, 1964

Sulze, W.: Ein Beitrag zur Kenntnis des Erregungsablaufs im Säugetierherzen. *Zeitsch f Biol* 60: 495, 1913

Toda, N., Shimamoto, K.: The influence of sympathetic stimulation on transmembrane potentials in the S-A node. *J Pharmac Exp Ther* 159: 298, 1968

Toda, N.: Electrophysiological effects of potassium and calcium ions in the sino-atrial node in response to sympathetic nerve stimulation. *Pflügers Arch* 310: 45, 1969

Trautwein, W., Uchizono, K.: Electronmicroscopic and electrophysiologic study of the pacemaker in the sinoatrial node of the rabbit heart. *Zeitsch f Zell* 61: 96, 1963

West, T.C.: Ultramicroelectrode recording from the cardiac pacemaker. *J Pharmac Exp Ther* 115: 283, 1955

21

CARDIAC GLYCOSIDES AND PACEMAKER ACTIVITY OF THE SINUS NODE – A MICROELECTRODE STUDY ON THE ISOLATED RIGHT ATRIUM OF THE RABBIT*

GERHARD STEINBECK, FELIX I.M. BONKE, MAURITS A. ALLESSIE, AND WIM J.E.P. LAMMERS

INTRODUCTION

During the last few years, the electrophysiological effects of cardiac glycosides on the specialized ventricular conducting system have been analyzed in detail by several investigators (Rosen et al., 1973a, b; Ferrier et al., 1973; Davis, 1973). From these studies it turned out that digitalis promotes a type of automaticity in Purkinje fibers distinctly different from normal pacemaker activity. In this way, Ferrier and co-workers reported in 1973 that toxic levels of cardiac glycosides induce oscillations in diastolic membrane potential of Purkinje fibers, which, if they reached threshold, induced single extrasystoles or sustained tachycardia. In contrast to normal pacemaker activity, this digitalis-produced form of automaticity is coupled to preceding closely spaced activations or oscillations. Voltage clamp studies by Lederer and Tsien (1975, 1977) suggest that the current underlying these transient depolarizations differs from normal pacemaker current.

A similar effect of digitalis was shown for the atrium of the dog by Hashimoto and Moe (1973).

On the contrary, much less is known about the electrophysiologic effects of digitalis on the sinus node. In a study on cholinergic responses in the sinus node as influenced by ouabain, Toda and West (1966) mentioned that ouabain 1×10^{-6} g/ml ($\simeq 1.5 \times 10^{-6}$ M) caused tachycardia and irregularities, a decrease of both maximal diastolic potential and action potential amplitude, and development of sinusoidal diastolic depolarization with frequent occurrence of subthreshold oscillations. Other studies are mostly concerned with the chronotropic effects of cardiac glycosides. Slowing of sinus rate is a common feature of digitalis action in patients with congestive heart failure. This does not reflect a primary therapeutic action of the drug, but occurs secondary to the improvement of the circulation (Moe and Farah, 1975). Cardiac slowing in animals has been attributed to an indirect vagomimetic (Heymans et al., 1932; Krueger and Unna, 1942; Gaffney et al., 1958; Chai et al., 1967) and antiadrenergic (Mendez et al., 1961; Nadeau and James, 1963) effect of the drug. After eliminating the effect of autonomic nerves, Ten Eick and Hoffman (1969) were unable to produce any direct negative chronotropic action of the drug on the mammalian sinus node in non-toxic concentrations. The same authors reported that prolonged exposure of ouabain 0.2–0.4 μg/ml ($\simeq 5 \times 10^{-7}$ M) in the isolated right atrium of the rabbit caused a slight increase of sinus rate. Further evidence for a positive chronotropic effect has come from in vivo or in vitro experiments on dogs, which were selectively injected with high doses of digitalis into the sinus node artery (James and Nadeau, 1963; Hashimoto and Kubota, 1974; Geer et al., 1977). Apart from some early observations made by Toda and West in 1966, and numerous studies to

* Supported by a grant of the "Deutsche Forschungsgemeinschaft" (Ste 257/1 and Ste 257/2) to G. Steinbeck.

evaluate the chronotropic effects of digitalis, no detailed electrophysiologic study is available. Because of this lack of knowledge we decided to investigate the direct electro-physiological effects of digitalis on the isolated sinus node preparation of the rabbit.

RESULTS AND DISCUSSION

The preparation and the perfusion fluid were the same as described in foregoing studies as is the case for other methodological details. See Steinbeck et al., 1978 (this book).

ATRIAL RATE AND RHYTHM

In all experiments in principle the following sequence of changes in atrial rhythm occurred. First of all, the beat to beat interval becomes shorter, meaning that the spontaneous rate of the discharges of the sinus node is increased. Thereafter, a period of irregularity in rhythm occurred, but during this period the rate increased further. This ends up with a period of regular fast rhythm. Then marked irregularity appeared in which often a number of short intervals is followed by a couple of very long intervals. If drug exposure is continued further, complete atrial arrest is occurring. In Figure 1 the effect of ouabain (1×10^{-6} M) on the isolated rabbit atrium is depicted. In this figure the four different phases, as mentioned above, are obviously present.

Figure 2 shows four examples of a recording of a surface electrogram from crista terminalis during exposure to ouabain (1×10^{-6} M) in another experiment than that of Figure 1.

The left upper panel depicts a constant rhythm with a cycle length of 410 msec during control. After 30 min drug exposure 1×10^{-6} M, a rhythm is present alternating in cycle length and configuration of the complex (left lower panel). After 40 min ouabain, a constant rapid rhythm is recorded (right upper panel). Finally, after 50 min ouabain, severe irregularity with marked changes in beat-to-beat intervals is observed.

Changes in rate and rhythm were observed in 30 preparations under the influence of ouabain 1×10^{-6} M. While there was variation from preparation to preparation with respect to basic interval, time until the drug became effective, duration of phases during which the characteristic changes were observed, we saw in each experiment the changes in atrial rate and rhythm as illustrated in Figures 1 and 2. In preliminary experiments in which lower concentrations of ouabain were applied ($5-8 \times 10^{-7}$ M), either no changes or qualitatively similar, quantitatively smaller effects were observed.

Atropine (1 mg/l) or propranolol (2 mg/l) or both, did not abolish the digitalis-induced changes of atrial rate and rhythm. It is concluded therefrom that ouabain (1×10^{-6} M) has a strong, direct positive chronotropic effect on the isolated sinus node preparation of the rabbit.

In a minority of six experiments, a slight prolongation of atrial cycles by 20–40 msec preceded the shortening of intervals as shown in Figure 1. In two experiments, in which this was studied more in detail, this biphasic effect on cycle length was observed both during administration and after withdrawal of the drug (during wash-out: prolongation of atrial interval followed by a slight decrease of cycle). Furthermore, this biphasic response persisted in these two experiments during a second digitalis exposure in the presence of atropine (1 mg/l) and propranolol (2 mg/l). Thus, ouabain (1×10^{-6} M) in

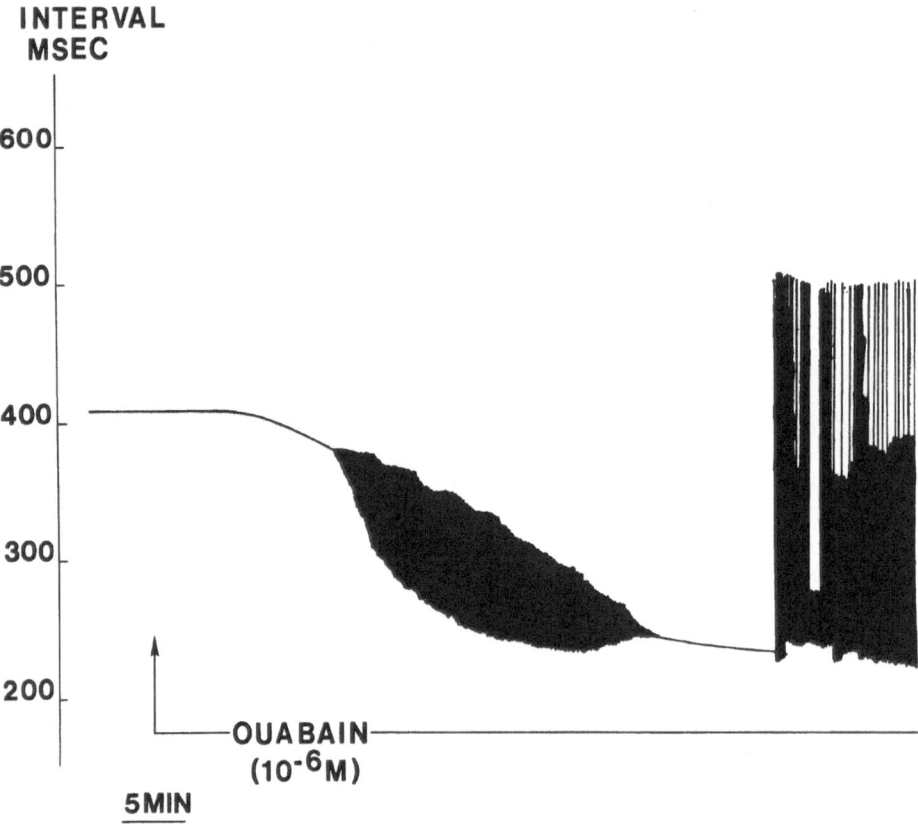

Figure 1. Effect of ouabain 1×10^{-6} M on spontaneous sinus rate in the isolated right atrium of the rabbit. For continuous on-line measurement of atrial cycles, the unipolar surface electrogram was fed into a time interval counter and following digital-analog conversion, the cycles were written on a pen recorder. Y-axis: interval between two consecutive atrial beats in msec; X-axis: time of ouabain exposure 1×10^{-6} M in min. The arrow indicates the moment the superfusion with drug-containing fluid was started. For further explanation, see text.

a minority of our experiments had a biphasic effect on atrial cycle length (slight prolongation of cycle followed by marked shortening of cycle). Biphasic effects of digitalis have also been described on Na-K-sensitive ATPase activity (Repke, 1961), on the action potential duration and membrane resistance of Purkinje fibers by Dudel and Trautwein (1958), on total steadystate current-voltage relations and reversal potential in Purkinje fibers for a K specific current (i_{K_2}, Cohen et al., 1976), and on electrical coupling between cells of ventricular muscle by Weingart (1977).

PACEMAKER LOCATION

In order to get an impression *where* the digitalis-induced rapid rhythm is originating from, the sinus node area was separated from crista terminalis by cuts parallel and close to crista terminalis: the right atrium immediately ceased to beat, the sinus node continuing with its rate of discharge as prior to the cutting procedure. Therefrom, it is concluded

EFFECT OF OUABAIN ON RHYTHM

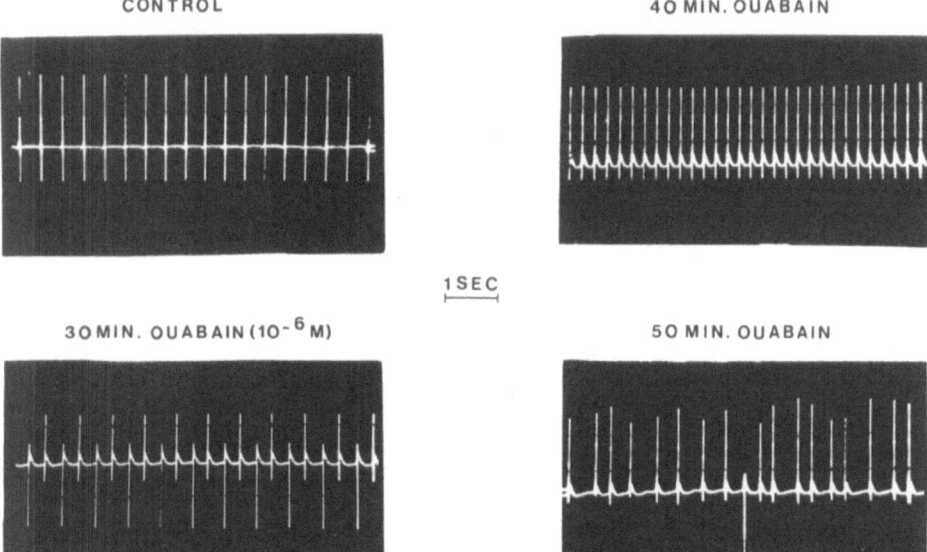

Figure 2. Representative recordings of unipolar surface electrograms of crista terminalis in the spontaneously beating right atrium during control (left upper panel) and after 30 min (left lower panel), 40 min (right upper panel), and 50 min exposure to ouabain (1 × 10⁻⁶ M) (right lower panel). For description see text.

that the rapid rhythm and the severe irregularities of rhythm were originating from the sinus node area. Therefore, we had to study this area in more detail and we had to use the microelectrode technique. However, it is very difficult to maintain a microelectrode in a cell of the sinus node when the preparation contracts vigorously because of the effect of digitalis on contractility.

In Figure 3, the results of an impalement in the area of the dominant pacemaker is given. The cycle length is 372 msec (upper panel) and the intracellular recording shows prominent diastolic depolarization with a smooth transition to the upstroke of the action potential. This upstroke precedes the atrial activity by 22 msec.

Following the administration of ouabain it was not possible to keep the microelectrode into the fiber. However, reimpalement at the same place after 41 min exposure to ouabain (6 × 10⁻⁷ M) demonstrated that the cycle length had decreased to 255 msec (phase of a constant rapid rhythm) and that the surface electrogram preceeds the activation of the fiber (lower panel of Figure 3). Besides, the shape of the atrial electrogram has changed. Since the recordings are not from the same cell it is not possible to draw firm conclusions. It is, however, obvious that under influence of ouabain the pacemaker no longer is located in this area.

An obvious question follows: *where* is the pacemaker shifting to? In an attempt to answer this question, the spread of activation was mapped during control and digitalis. For mapping we chose the period of constant rapid rhythm, as the spread of activation during this time can be assumed to be more or less constant.

CONTROL

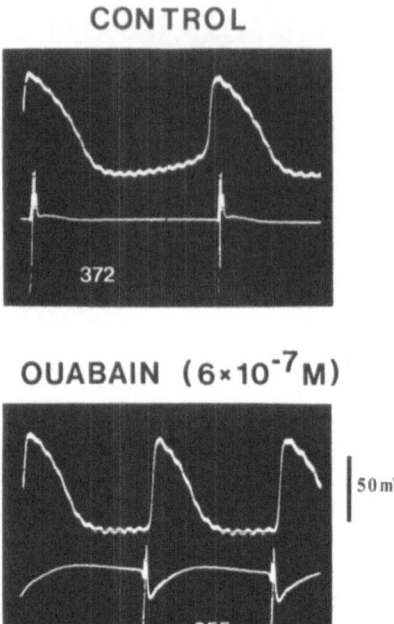

OUABAIN $(6 \times 10^{-7} M)$

Figure 3. Intracellular recording from dominant pacemaker area of the sinus node together with surface electrogram of crista terminalis during control (upper panel) and after 41 min exposure of ouabain (6 × 10^{-7} M) (lower panel); the lower panel shows a reimpalement of the same place from which the upper tracing was recorded. The interval is given in msec in between the atrial complexes.

Figure 4 shows one representative experiment. In the left hand sketch, the spread of activation is consecutively mapped during control with one micro-electrode (a detailed description of the method is also given in this book, see Steinbeck et al., 1978). An electrode brush for simultaneous recording of ten surface electrograms (1 mm interelectrode distance) is placed on crista terminalis. In this experiment, 20 msec after the discharge of the most dominant pacemaker fibers, the impulse has reached crista terminalis. Following ouabain administration, a rapid rhythm occurred with a more or less constant cycle length of 200–230 msec for a period of 10 min, during which the simultaneously recorded tenfold electrogram on crista terminalis showed a fairly constant activation pattern. The microelectrode could rapidly be impaled at 29 places in the sinus node during this period. As can be seen from the right hand sketch, earliest spontaneous discharge is observed in the sinoatrial border area at the cranial site of crista terminalis.

In eight experiments in which the spread of activation was mapped during control and digitalis, results were consistent with the one shown in detail, demonstrating a pacemaker shift towards the sinoatrial border. The exact place of the new pacemaker in vertical direction, that is either the cranial, middle, or caudal site of crista terminalis, differed from one preparation to another. In addition, in some experiments it appeared from the tenfold surface electrogram as if at least two new pacemaker centers had arisen along the sinoatrial border.

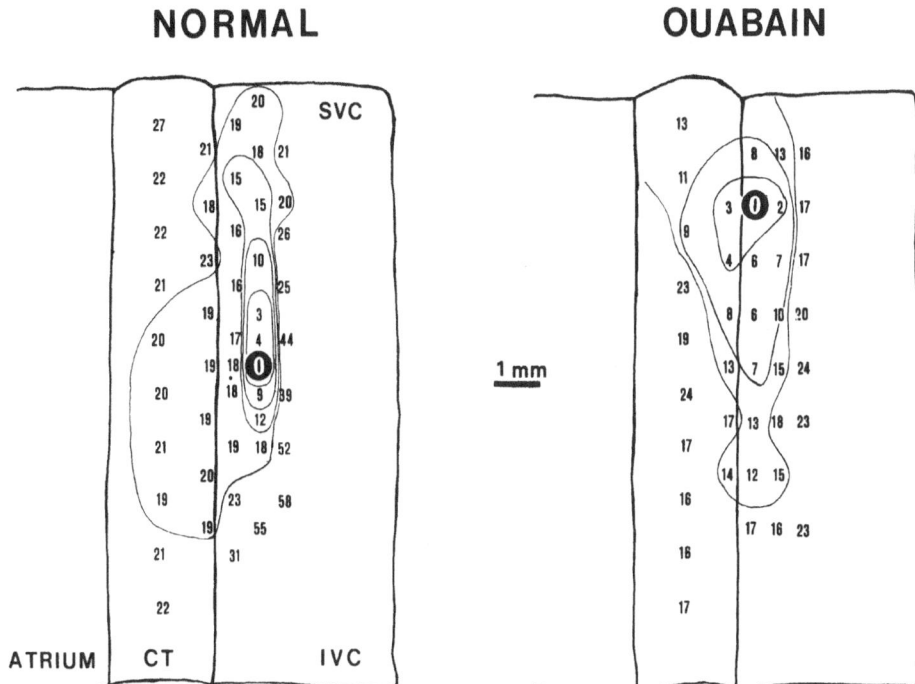

Figure 4. Map of the spread of activation in the sinus node and the crista terminalis under normal conditions (left) and during exposure to ouabain (1×10^{-6} M) (right). SVC = superior vena cava; IVC = inferior vena cava; CT = crista terminalis. The map during ouabain was made within about 10 min and the procedure was started after an ouabain administration for 60 min.

During control, the cycle length was 370 msec and constant. A total of 37 places was consecutively explored with the microelectrode. The earliest discharge of a fiber in the sinus node in relation to a reference point on crista terminalis is taken as zero. For the purpose of reference a brush of ten surface electrodes – with an interelectrode distance of 1 mm – is placed on the crista terminalis. The moment of activation of the impaled fibers is related to the "zero-moment" (earliest discharge). These activation times are indicated in the diagram. Isochronic lines were constructed 5 msec, 10 msec, 15 msec, and 20 msec after point 0. This offers a good indication for the spread of the impulse from the dominant pacemaker through the sinus node towards the crista terminalis. After 60 min exposure to ouabain a ten minute period of rapid rhythm occurred in which the beat-to-beat interval was almost constant (200–230 msec). We were able to impale at 29 sites in the sinus node and constructed a map of the spread of activation in the same way as under normal conditions. In the right hand diagram this map is given and the lines are isochronic lines for 5 msec, 10 msec, and 15 msec, respectively. It is obvious that the dominant pacemaker (indicated with "0") is shifted towards the sinoatrial border.

DIASTOLIC DEPOLARIZATION

The next question is: are any reasons apparent from the intracellular recordings *why* the dominant pacemaker site is shifting towards the sinoatrial border?

In panel A of Figure 5 an intracellular recording from an area close to the pacemaker is shown together with a surface electrogram of crista terminalis. In B, a fiber is recorded during ouabain exposure, 0.5 mm closer to crista terminalis than in A. Whereas this area

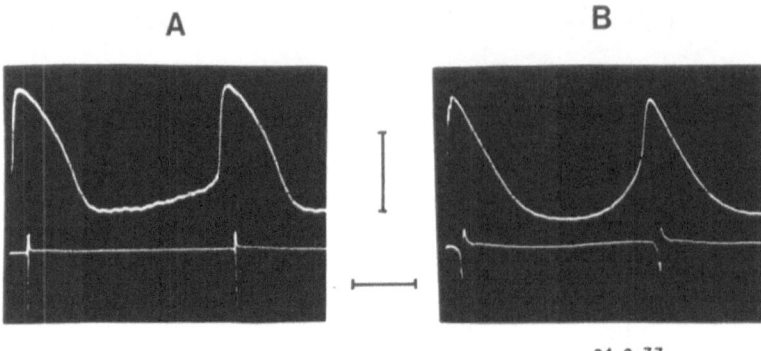

24-2-77

Figure 5. Panel A. Nearly dominant pacemaker fiber (upper trace) together with unipolar surface electrogram of crista terminalis (lower trace) during control.

Panel B. Transmembrane potential of a fiber of the sinus node located 0.5 mm closer to crista terminalis than the one recorded from in A, together with surface electrogram during digitalis exposure (ouabain 1 × 10^{-6} M for 30 min).

Ouabain produced a decrease in spontaneous atrial cycle length. Under normal conditions the fiber in B would be expected to show less diastolic depolarization than the one in A; however, diastolic depolarization is more pronounced under influence of ouabain. Note that the latency between fiber activation and activation of crista terminalis is longer in B, although this place is closer to crista terminalis than the one recorded in A. Vertical bar: 50 mV; horizontal bar: 100 msec.

would normally be expected to show less diastolic depolarization than the one recorded in A, diastolic depolarization is in fact more pronounced.

Following ouabain intoxication in another experiment, reimpalements at the same site were performed during wash-out (Figure 6). The upper panel shows a fiber at the sino-atrial border after ouabain exposure (1 × 10^{-6} M) for 60 min, together with a surface electrogram of crista terminalis. Atrial rate, action potential amplitude, and latencies between fiber and atrial activation are changing from beat to beat, indicating a continuous pacemaker shift. The same site was reimpaled following 30 min wash-out of the drug. Diastolic depolarization is still pronounced, but there is a sharp transition between phase 4 and 0. Action potential amplitude has increased (middle panel). After 60 min wash-out (lower panel), a typical latent pacemaker fiber is recorded at the same site: slow diastolic depolarization, sharp transition to a rapid upstroke, high action potential amplitude, short latency between fiber activation and activation of crista terminalis.

Figure 7 depicts the results of another experiment in which we were able to keep the microelectrode in the same fiber (0.5 mm away from crista terminalis) for 50 min of ouabain exposure (8 × 10^{-7} M).

In this fiber ouabain caused a decrease of the maximal diastolic membrane potential and an obvious increase in diastolic depolarization. Since the amount of diastolic de-polarization is strongly dependent of the distance of the fiber to the dominant pacemaker fibers, we also studied the behavior of the fiber under the situation that the preparation is electrically driven via a stimulating electrode on the crista terminalis. It is clear from Figure 7 that also in a driven situation the fiber exhibited more pronounced diastolic de-polarization after exposure to ouabain.

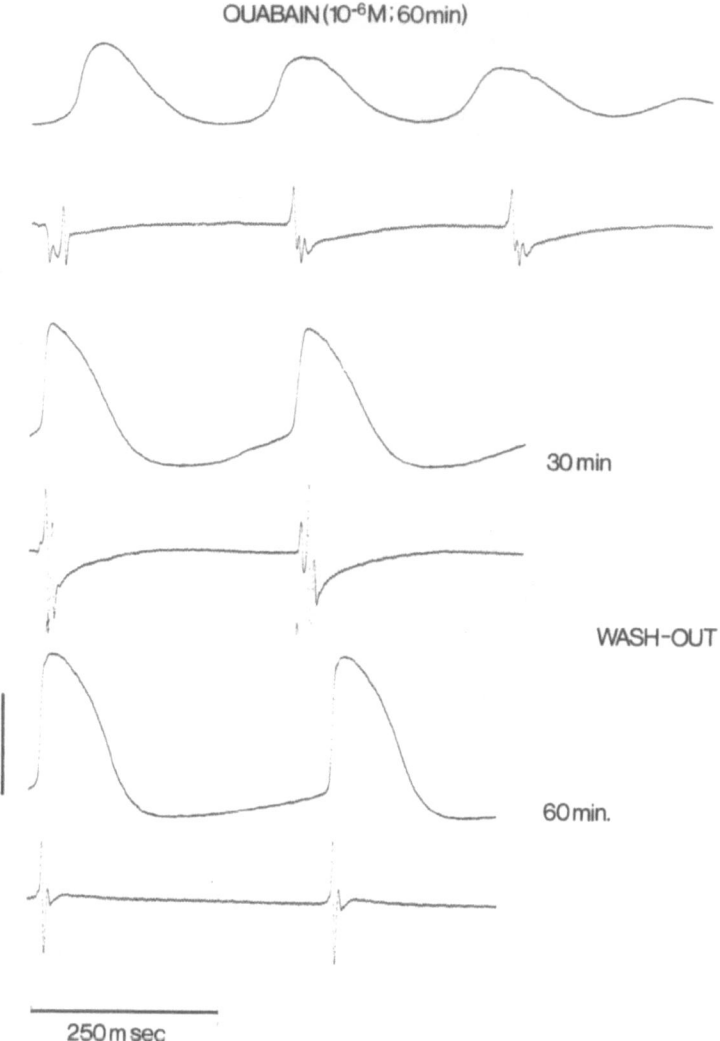

OUABAIN (10⁻⁶M ; 60min)

30 min

WASH-OUT

60 min.

250 m sec

Figure 6. In the upper panel an intracellular recording from a fiber of the sinus node, located about 0.5 mm away from the crista terminalis, is given together with a surface electrogram of the crista terminalis (lower trace) after ouabain exposure for 60 min. In the middle and lower panel recordings from the same site are given (microelectrode is reimpaled) after a wash-out period of 30 min and 60 min, respectively. The vertical bar indicates 50 mV. For further description see text.

In conclusion, Figures 5–7 demonstrate that fibers along the sinoatrial border develop pronounced diastolic depolarization whereas dominant pacemaker fibers do not (see Figure 3). As a consequence, a competition might occur between the original dominant pacemaker and groups of fibers in the border of the sinus node with this pronounced diastolic depolarization. Perhaps, this can be the reason for the arrhythmias that occur in the beginning of the ouabain exposure (Figure 1 and left lower panel of Figure 2).

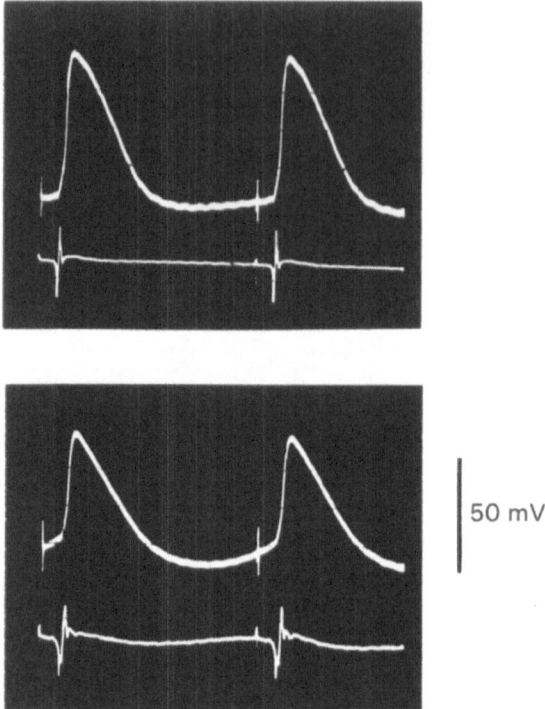

50 mV

Figure 7. Intracellular recording of sinoatrial border fiber 0.5 mm away from crista terminalis (upper trace) together with surface electrogram of crista terminalis (lower trace) during control (upper panel) and 50 min exposure of ouabain (8×10^{-7} M) (lower panel). In both instances, the preparation was electrically driven at an interval of 300 msec. The intracellular recordings are obtained from the same cell during a continuous registration. For further description see text. Vertical bar: 50 mV.

One might assume that – following the concept of "triggered activity"(Wit and Crane-field, 1976; see also Cranefield in this book) – the nomotopic sinus impulse from the dominant pacemaker center in the middle of the sinus node will trigger the appearance of an ectopic discharge of the fibers in the sinoatrial border. This could explain the alternating rhythm. With further exposure of the drug, the ectopic rhythm becomes sustained and overrides the original pacemaker, thereby producing the constant rapid rhythm (see Figure 1 and right upper panel of Figure 2).

In order to evaluate the possible role of the atrium for the production of the pacemaker shift towards the sinoatrial border, one sinus node preparation was exposed two times to the same digitalis concentration. After wash-out following the first exposure, the sinus node area was artificially separated from the atrium. Nevertheless, the rate of the rapid rhythm during the second drug exposure was fairly identical to that observed before, arguing against the assumption that the atrium by way of electrotonic effects influences the ectopic rhythm substantially.

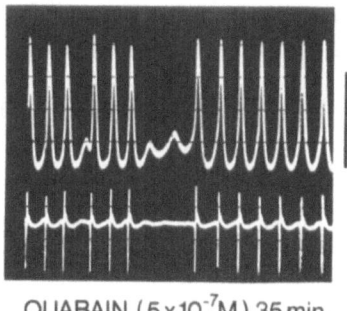

OUABAIN (5 x 10⁻⁷M) 35 min.

Figure 8. Intracellular recording of a sinoatrial border fiber (upper trace) and a surface electrogram of crista terminalis (lower trace) during a second digitalis exposure to this preparation for 35 min (ouabain concentration 5×10^{-7} M). Vertical bar: 50 mV. As time reference can be used the fact that after the sixth beat, an atrial pause appeared lasting 1100 msec. For further description see text.

SEVERE IRREGULARITY OF RHYTHM

Following prolonged exposure of toxic ouabain concentrations, severe irregularity of atrial rhythm usually occurred (see Figure 1 and right lower panel of Figure 2) with eventual occurrence of complete atrial arrest. Beat-to-beat differences amounted up to far more than 100 msec; pauses were observed with atrial intervals of approximately double or triple "basic" cycle length. The underlying electrophysiologic events could hardly be identified.

Figure 8 depicts one example. The intracellular recording is taken from a fiber of the sinoatrial border. The lower trace is a surface atrial electrogram. In the fourth beat shown, diastolic depolarization does not reach threshold, the fiber tends to repolarize until a sudden onset of activation occurs: that is, another pacemaker has taken over for this beat.

A few beats later, an atrial pause occurred lasting 1100 msec. The intracellular recording shows two subthreshold oscillations during this period. One may speculate whether this represents a failure of diastolic depolarization to reach threshold, this fiber then standing for the whole pacemaker area.

On the other hand, the oscillations might be due to the electrotonic influence exerted by a wave front coming from the non-recorded actual pacemaker, which is approaching but not capturing the impaled fiber. Thus, the intracellular recording is compatible with subthreshold oscillations as well as with a sinoatrial exit block. Both possibilities are likely to occur with continuous depolarization of the fibers caused by digitalis. To differentiate between a failure of impulse formation and intranodal impulse conduction, multiple simultaneous intracellular recordings of the pacemaker area would be necessary. In conclusion, we have shown that toxic digitalis concentrations cause an increase in rate in the isolated right atrium of the rabbit, paralleled by a pacemaker shift towards the sinoatrial border. This rapid rhythm is of focal origin, as far as one can tell from microelectrode recordings.

The explanation for the increase of rate and occurrence of a pacemaker shift lies in the fact that latent pacemaker fibers along the sinoatrial border develop strong diastolic depolarization, whereas dominant pacemaker fibers do so less or not at all. A plausible explanation for this apparent difference in sensitivity to ouabain cannot be given at present.

So-called "paroxysmal atrial tachycardia with block" has been described as a common manifestation of digitalis intoxication in man (Lown et al., 1960). The criteria given for this rhythm disorder – as far as the atrium is concerned – are quite compatible with our findings in this in vitro study. Thus, our description of the arrhythmogenic digitalis effects on the isolated rabbit right atrium, if they represent the experimental counterpart of this clinically well-known rhythm disturbance, might contribute to the understanding of this arrhythmia in man.

REFERENCES

1. Chai, C.Y., Wang, H.H., Hoffman, B.F., Wang, S.C.: Mechanisms of bradycardia induced by digitalis substances. *Am J Physiol* 212: 26, 1967
2. Cohen, I., Daut, J., Noble, D.: An analysis of the actions of low concentrations of ouabain on membrane currents in Purkinje fibers. *J Physiol (London)* 260: 75, 1976
3. Davis, L.D.: Effect of changes in cycle length on diastolic depolarization produced by ouabain in canine Purkinje fibers. *Circ Res* 32: 206, 1973
4. Dudel, J., Trautwein, W.: Elektrophysiologische Messungen zur Strophanthinwirkung am Herzmuskel. *Naunyn-Schmiedeberg's Arch Exp Pathol Pharmacol* 232: 393, 1958
5. Ferrier, G.R., Saunders, J.H., Mendez, C.: A cellular mechanism for the generation of ventricular arrhythmias by acetylstrophanthidin. *Circ Res* 32: 600, 1973
6. Gaffney, T.E., Kahn, J.B., Van Maanen, E.F., Acheson, G.H.: A mechanism of the vagal effect of cardiac glycosides. *J Pharmacol Exp Ther* 122: 423, 1958
7. Geer, M.R., Wagner, G.S., Waxman, M., Wallace, A.G.: Chronotropic effect of acetylstrophanthidin infusion into the canine sinus nodal artery. *Am J Cardiol* 39: 684, 1977
8. Hashimoto, K., Kubota, K.: Positive chronotropic effect of ouabain in the excised and blood-perfused canine SA node preparation of the dog. *Naunyn-Schmiedeberg's Arch Pharmacol* 281: 357, 1974
9. Hashimoto, K., Moe, G.K.: Transient depolarizations induced by acetylstrophanthidin in specialized tissue of dog atrium and ventricle. *Circ Res* 32: 618, 1973
10. Heymans, C., Bouckaert, J.J., Regniers, P.: Sur le mécanisme réflexe de la bradycardie provoquée par les digitaliques. *Arch Intern Pharmacodyn* 44: 31, 1932
11. James, T.N., Nadeau, R.A.: The chronotropic effect of digitalis studied by direct perfusion of the sinus node. *J Pharmacol Exp Ther* 139: 42, 1963
12. Krueger, E., Unna, K.: Comparative studies on the toxic effects of digitoxin and ouabain in cats. *J Pharmacol Exp Ther* 76: 282, 1942
13. Lederer, W.J., Tsien, R.W.: Transient inward current underlying strophanthidin's enhancement of pacemaker activity in Purkinje fibers. *J Physiol (London)* 249: 40, 1975
14. Lederer, W.J., Tsien, R.W.: Transient inward current underlying arrhythmogenic effects of cardiotonic steroids in Purkinje fibers. *J Physiol (London)* 263: 73, 1976
15. Lown, B., Wyatt, N.F., Levine, H.D.: Paroxysmal atrial tachycardia with block. *Circulation* 21: 129, 1960
16. Mendez, C., Aceves, J., Mendez, R.: Inhibition of adrenergic cardiac acceleration by cardiac glycosides. *J Pharmacol Exp Ther* 131: 191, 1961
17. Moe, G.K., Farah, A.E.: Digitalis and allied cardiac glycosides. In: The pharmacological basis of therapeutics, edited by Goodman, L.S., Gilman, A. Macmillan Publishing Co., Inc., New York (5th edition), 1975, p. 660
18. Nadeau, R.A., James, T.N.: Antagonistic effects on the sinus node of acetylstrophanthidin and adrenergic stimulation. *Circ Res* 13: 388, 1963
19. Repke, K.: Metabolism of cardiac glycosides. In: Proceedings of the First International Pharmacological Meeting, Stockholm, Pergamon Press, New York, 1961, vol. 3, p. 47
20. Rosen, M.R., Gelband, H., Hoffman, B.F.: Correlation between effects of ouabain on the canine electrocardiogram and transmembrane potentials of isolated Purkinje fibers. *Circulation* 47: 65, 1973
21. Rosen, M.R., Gelband, H., Merker, C.: Mechanisms of digitalis toxicity: effects of ouabain on phase 4 of canine Purkinje fiber transmembrane potentials. *Circulation* 47: 681, 1973
22. Steinbeck, G., Allessie, M.A., Bonke, F.I.M., Lammers, W.J.E.P.: The response of the sinus node to premature stimulation of the atrium studied with microelectrodes in isolated atrial preparations of the rabbit heart. This book, 1978

23. Ten Eick, R.E., Hoffman, B.F.: Chronotropic effect of cardiac glycosides in cats, dogs, and rabbits. *Circ Res* 25: 365, 1969
24. Toda, N., West, T.C.: The influence of ouabain on cholinergic responses in the sinoatrial node. *J Pharmacol Exp Ther* 153: 104, 1966
25. Weingart, R.: The actions of ouabain on intercellular coupling and conduction velocity in mammalian ventricular muscle. *J Physiol (London)* 264: 341, 1977
26. Wit, A.L., Cranefield, P.F.: Triggered activity in cardiac muscle fibers of the simian mitral valve. *Circ Res* 38: 85, 1976

22

EFFECTS OF POLARIZATION AND OF INHIBITORS OF IONIC CONDUCTANCES ON THE ACTION POTENTIALS OF NODAL AND PERINODAL FIBERS IN RABBIT SINOATRIAL NODE*

DANIELLE KREITNER

INTRODUCTION

Pacemaker action potentials of the mammalian sinoatrial node are well-known to have a low diastolic potential, a low rate of rise unaffected by tetrodotoxin (TTX) and to be rapidly suppressed by manganese ions (Yamagishi and Sano, 1966; Lenfant et al., 1968). These characteristics suggest a spontaneous activity resulting from the operation of the slow inward system and may be considered to be due either to the lack of fast sodium channel or to the low value of the presystolic potential which inactivates the fast sodium carrying system. The latter interpretation is plausible since in the nodal cells the value of the take-off potential is around -35 mV. According to the results obtained by Weidmann in 1955 on Purkinje fibers, the rapid sodium system is completely inactivated when the membrane potential is held at potentials lower than around -45 mV.

In order to solve this problem we have increased the membrane potential 1) with carbamylcholine (CCh), a substance known to hyperpolarize the membrane by increasing its potassium conductance (Burgen and Terroux, 1953) and 2) by using a local electrical polarization. We have thus determined whether or not the ascending phase of the sinoatrial potential becomes TTX-sensitive under these conditions. In a second part of this paper, we have studied the effects of electrical hyperpolarizations on the latent pacemaker cells.

MATERIAL AND METHODS

Young rabbits weighing between 1 and 1.5 Kg were used for this study. They were killed by a blow on the neck and the beating heart was quickly removed from the thorax. The right atrium was excised, opened according to the technique described by Paes de Carvalho et al. (1959) and immersed in an experimental chamber of 2 ml capacity. The perfusion solution was saturated with a gas mixture of 95% O_2 et 5% CO_2 and flowed continuously at a constant rate of 5 ml/min. The solution had the following composition in mM: NaCl: 130, KCl: 5.6, $CaCl_2$: 2.16, $MgCl_2$: 0.24, NaH_2PO_4: 0.6, $NaHCO_3$: 16.6, glucose: 11.1. The pH was 7.35. The temperature was kept constant at $37° \pm 0.5°C$. The preparation was mounted in the experimental chamber with two plastic ridges on which the preparation was pinned with small stainless steel needles, endocardial side uppermost. The atrial myocardium was dissected to a large extent to avoid excessive movements of the preparation.

In order to apply polarization to the nodal cells, a relatively large suction electrode

* This work was supported in part by a contract DGRST.

was built up according to the method described by Bonke (1973). As indication of a good contact between the electrode and the tissue, there should be at the end of each experiment a small hillock at the place of suction. Nevertheless, it may be assumed that the greatest part of the current flowed from the electrode to the bath through intercellular clefts and, thus, only a small amount of the injected current would cross the cell membranes. In order to control the amount of current, which indeed passed through the cell membrane, the microelectrode, after an impalement in a nodal fiber, was withdrawn until just outside the membrane. A polarizing pulse with the same amplitude was given and the potential change recorded. The difference between the potential changes measured with the microelectrode inside and outside the cell, was considered to give an indication of the amount of the extracellular shunt.

The pulses were delivered by a stimulator via a 1 MΩ resistor to obtain a constant polarizing current and 10 KΩ resistor for measuring current. The intensity of the polarizing current ranged between 3.10^{-6} and 8.10^{-5} A. The bathing solution was grounded in order to minimize the stimulus artefact on the recording system.

Conventional glass microelectrodes of about 40 MΩ were used in this study. The first derivative of the action potentials was obtained by a differentiator circuit with a time constant of 1.3 msec. A surface electrogram of the atrial appendage was simultaneously recorded as time reference by means of two Ag-AgCl wires coated with Teflon except at the tip.

RESULTS

A. NODAL RESPONSE TO CARBAMYLCHOLINE-INDUCED HYPERPOLARIZATIONS

It was first verified that the administration of TTX had no effect on the shape and only a negligible effect on the rhythm of the pacemaker action potentials (Figure 1).

Administration of CCh (Figure 2A) resulted in a decrease in the slope of the slow diastolic depolarization after 2 or 3 min causing a fall in the frequency, a reduction of the action potential duration and a change in its shape which becomes more triangular. Depending on the preparation, the value of maximum diastolic polarization increased by 2 to 8 mV while the take-off potential increased from -33 ± 3.9 mV to -40 ± 3.4 mV (n =

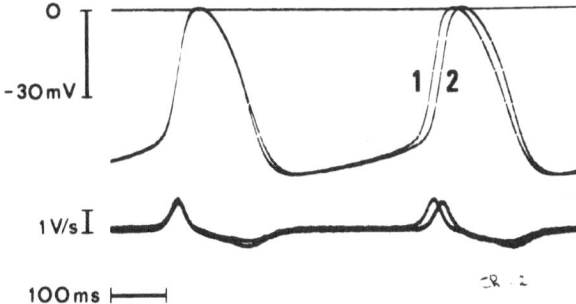

Figure 1. Lack of effect of TTX (2.10^{-6} g/ml) on the pacemaker action potential (upper trace) and its rate of rise (first derivative, lower trace). 1: control, 2: under TTX. (Kreitner (1975), reproduced by permission of J. Mol. Cell. Cardiol.).

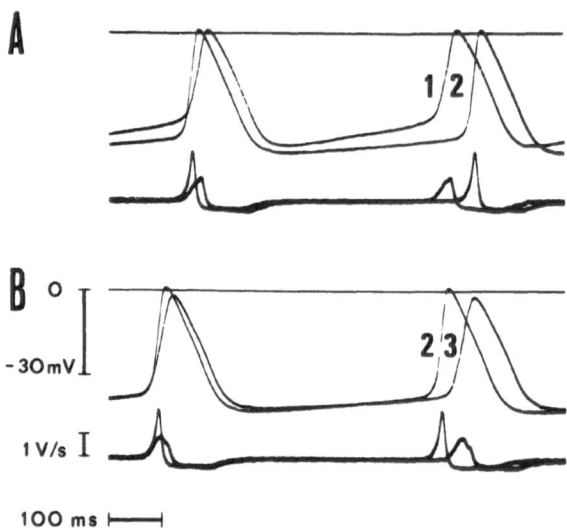

Figure 2. A) Effect of CCh (1.10⁻⁸ M) on the shape and the rhythm of the pacemaker action potentials. 1: control, 2: under CCh.

B) Effect of TTX (2.10⁻⁸ g/ml) during hyperpolarization produced by the previous administration of CCh. The increase in rate of rise of the ascending phase produced by CCh is entirely suppressed by TTX. 2: under CCh, before TTX, 3: under CCh + TTX. Upper trace = action potential; lower trace = first derivative of action potential. (Kreitner (1975), reproduced by permission of J. Mol. Cell. Cardiol.).

12. Mean and S.D.) and the rate of rise of the action potential increased by 0.95 ± 0.45 V/s ($n = 12$), the control value being 1 ± 0.14 V/s ($n = 12$).

As soon as the CCh-induced hyperpolarization was established, the addition of TTX produced in 1 to 2 min a marked reduction of the rate of rise of the ascending phase, which decreased by 0.95 ± 0.97 V/s, accompanied by a reduction of the action potential amplitude. The hyperpolarization produced by CCh remained unchanged under TTX. The slowing down of the spontaneous frequency of the preparation was more pronounced after administration of TTX, but this effect was only due to the further development of the action of CCh.

Table 1 summarizes the results obtained. It can be seen that (a) a fiber which still has, after CCh, a low take-off potential (-32 mV, preparation no. 8) remains TTX-insensitive; (b) a fiber which has, before CCh, a high take-off potential (-39, -40 mV, preparation no. 5) is normally somewhat sensitive to TTX, since its rate of rise is higher under control conditions than after TTX + CCh; (c) all the fibers that reach under CCh a take-off potential of -37 mV or more become TTX sensitive. From these observations it may be estimated that in nodal cells the sodium conductance becomes fully inactivated at a potential of about -35 to -37 mV (Kreitner, 1975), that is a somewhat lower value than in Purkinje fibers, i.e. approximately -45 mV (Weidmann (1955)).

B. NODAL RESPONSE TO ELECTRICALLY-INDUCED HYPERPOLARIZATIONS

The hyperpolarizing currents produced an increase in the amplitude of the action potentials and an increase in the rate of rise of their ascending phase. In the experiment shown in Figure 3A, the take-off potential passed from -42.5 to -45 mV while dV/dt max

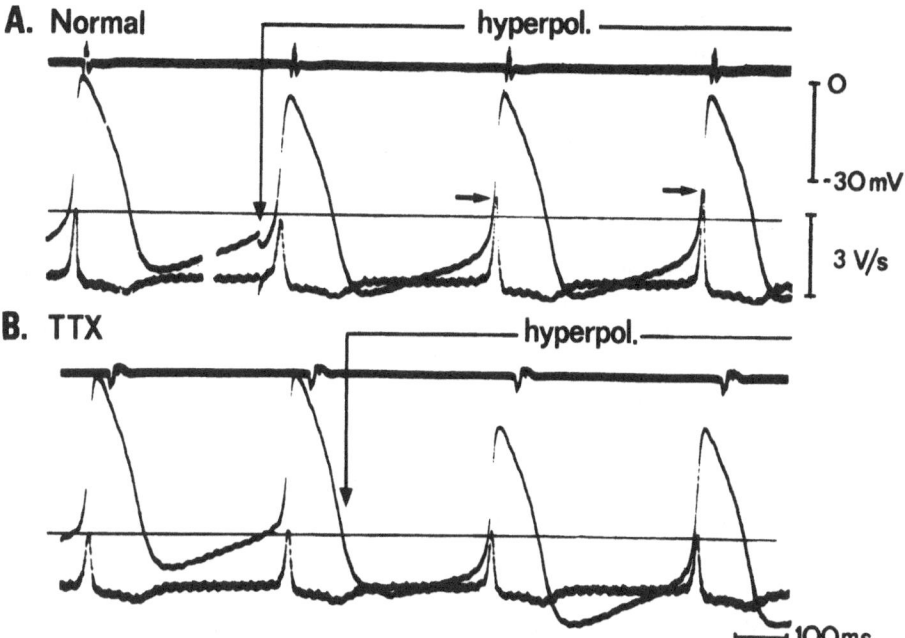

Figure 3. A) Effect of a hyperpolarizing pulse of 4.5 mV on the action potential and the first derivative of a true pacemaker cell. Hyperpolarization induces an increase in dV/dt max (horizontal arrows) in respect of the normal value (fine horizontal line).

B) After addition of TTX (6.10^{-5} g/ml) a hyperpolarizing pulse of 7 mV has no effect on dV/dt max (same impalement). Upper trace: atrial surface electrogram; middle trace: action potential; lower trace: first derivative of action potential. (Kreitner (1977), reproduced by permission of *CR Acad Sci*).

Table 1.

Preparations	Presystolic membrane potential (in mV)		Rate of rise of the ascending phase of the pacemaker action potential (in V/s)		
	Control	After action of CCh	Control	After action of CCh	After action of TTX during CCh hyperpolarization
No. 1	33	41	1.2	2.3	1.2
No. 2	29.5	37.5	1.05	1.15	–
No. 3	36	42	0.85	2.5	1.25
No. 4	35	38	0.85	1.25	–
(3 trials)	35	39	0.9	1.90	1.0
	35	40	0.95	1.35	–
No. 5	39	42	1.1	1.4	0.9
(2 trials)	40	43	1.2	2.1	1.05
No. 6	33	37	1.1	1.4	1.2
No. 7	36	44	1.2	1.7	1.2
No. 8	29	32	1.1	1.15	1.15
No. 9	33.5	37	1.0	2.0	1.0

varied from 2.6 to 3.4 V/s. On an average, over 7 trials, the former value increased by 5 ± 2.65 mV and the latter by 1 ± 0.69 V/s (mean and S.D.) (Kreitner, 1977). In some cases the latency between the time of dV/dt max and the surface electrogram was shortened as a consequence of a pacemaker shift (Bouman et al., 1968).

Under normal conditions, the administration of TTX, at concentrations ranging from 1.10^{-5} to 1.10^{-4} g/ml, produced no effect on the true pacemaker action potentials or a small decrease in dV/dt max. Figure 3B shows that a hyperpolarizing current which, before TTX, produced an increase of both dV/dt max and action potential amplitude, no longer produced these effects after administration of TTX in a concentration of 5.10^{-5} g/ml. The hyperpolarization of the membrane was not modified by TTX. On an average, over 5 trials, the decrease in dV/dt max of the hyperpolarized action potentials was 1 ± 0.94 V/s.

The results obtained in the true pacemaker cells may be summarized as follows:

a) the true pacemaker cells are normally insensitive to TTX when their take-off potential is lower than or equal to around -37 mV. They become somewhat sensitive to this substance (Figure 1B) when their take-off potential is more negative than -37 mV.

b) their sensitivity to TTX increases markedly during hyperpolarizing pulses which bring the take-off potential to around -45 mV to -50 mV.

c) even large hyperpolarizations (8 to 10 mV) do not cause a very rapid rate of rise in true pacemaker cells. Similar hyperpolarizations cause much more rapid upstrokes in most perinodal cells and in cells in the caval region, because the normal presystolic potential is higher in these cells, than in the cells in the center of the node.

C. PERINODAL RESPONSE TO ELECTRICALLY-INDUCED HYPERPOLARIZATIONS

When hyperpolarizing pulses were applied to the latent pacemaker cells close to the pacing area, the upstroke of the action potentials often exhibited a rapid TTX-sensitive first component. This rapid component increased with the hyperpolarizing current until the action potentials of the latent pacemaker cells resembled very closely the action potentials from the right superior vena cava cells (Ito et al., 1967). This can clearly be seen in Figure 4. Figure 5 shows the aspect of an action potential of a fiber of the right superior vena cava area.

It can be noticed that latent pacemaker action potentials with an upstroke exhibiting two components were often recorded spontaneously very close to the true pacemaker area.

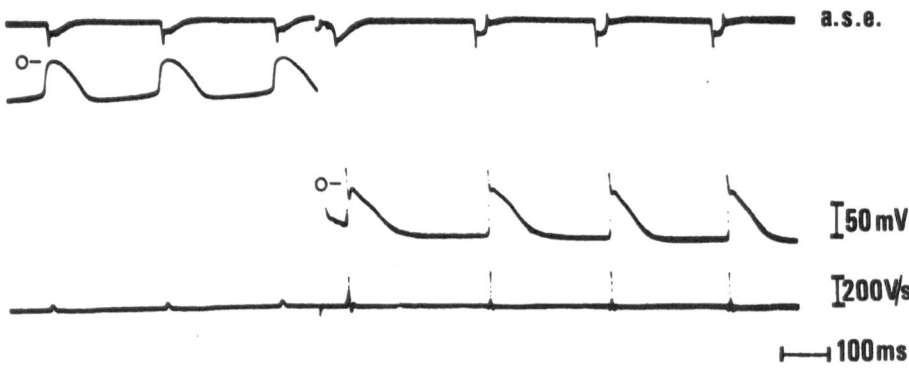

Figure 4. Effect of a hyperpolarizing pulse of 15 mV on a latent pacemaker cell. Upper trace: atrial surface electrogram; middle trace: action potential; lower trace: first derivative of the action potential.

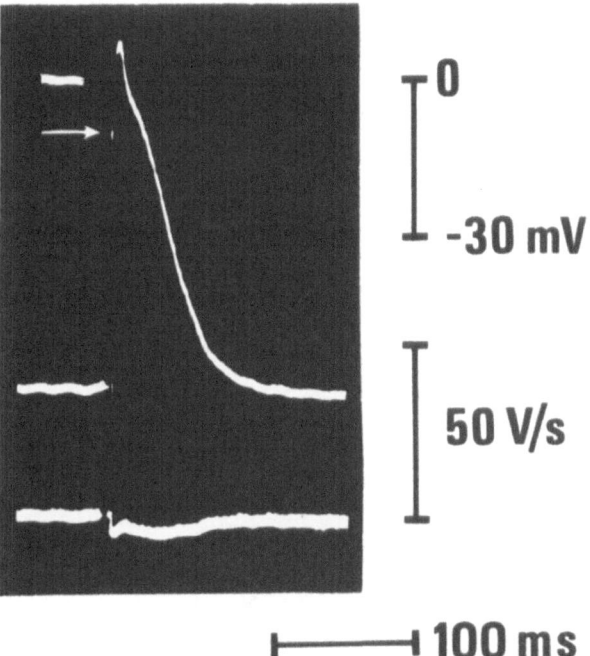

Figure 5. Aspect of an action potential of a fiber of the right superior vena cava area. Upper trace: action potential; lower trace: first derivative; arrow indicates dV/dt max.

This observation is in agreement with the one of Lipsius and Vassalle (1976) concerning subsidiary pacemaker potentials in the sinus node.

In Figure 6, dV/dt max of 4 cells from the caval area has been plotted as a function of the presystolic membrane potential during hyperpolarizing and depolarizing pulses. The normal resting potential is around − 75 mV. The curve has been drawn as best fit. Dots in the rectangle are reproduced in Figure 7. In this latter graph the dots from Figure 6 have been repeated, whereas the open circles give the values of latent pacemaker cells during hyperpolarizing and depolarizing pulses. The normal presystolic potential is around − 50 to − 60 mV. It can be seen that the voltage dependency of latent pacemaker cells exhibits about the same slope or even steeper than the cells in the caval area. This comparison has to be considered as qualitative measurements in absence of more reliable quantitative measurements.

To precise the nature of these two components, we have used inhibitors of ionic conductances. Figure 8 shows a sinocaval action potential exhibiting spontaneously two components on its upstroke. Administration of TTX, at a concentration of 2.10^{-5} g/ml, suppressed the initial rapid component while manganese ions at a concentration of 5 mM progressively depressed the slow component. These observations are in good agreement with those of Lipsius and Vassalle (1976) and allow to conclude that the upstroke of latent pacemaker action potentials results from the activation of both the rapid and the slow inward systems as in ordinary cardiac cells.

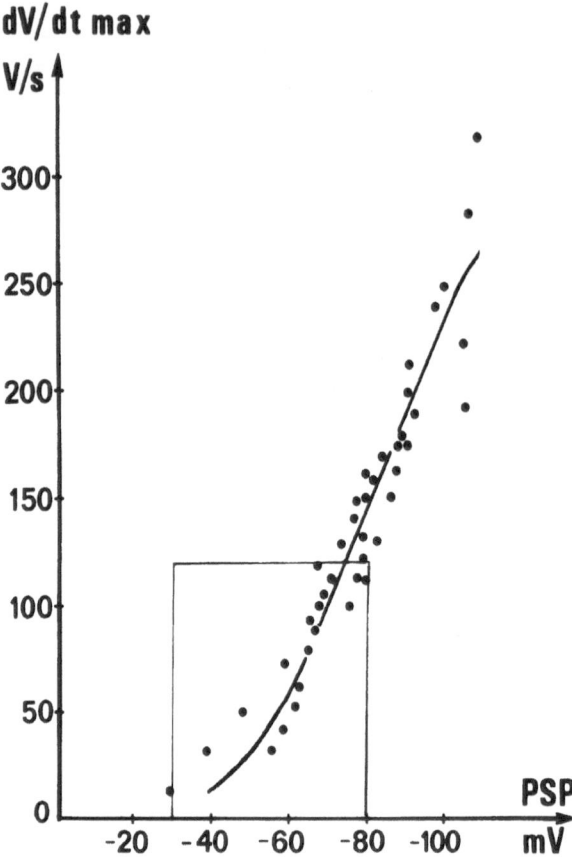

Figure 6. Upstroke velocities of 4 fibers of the caval area are plotted as a function of the presystolic potential (PSP) during hyperpolarizing and deplorizing pulses. Dots in the rectangle are reproduced in Figure 7.

DISCUSSION AND CONCLUSIONS

The increase in take-off potential obtained in our experiments on the true pacemaker cells was rather weak. The methods used do not allow to hyperpolarize the fibers more than to a presystolic potential of around − 50 mV. Because of the sigmoïd shape of the relationship between rate of rise and diastolic potential (or presystotic potential) (Weidmann, 1955), such an increased should induce a rate of rise of no more than a few volts per second. This is in agreement with our observations. The weak electrical polarization obtained may be explained principally by the structural characteristics of the nodal tissue, namely, the smallness of the cells and their complex geometrical connections, the rather small intercelular junctional areas, the low degree of electrotonic spread, and the low diastolic potential. (Sano and Yamagishi, 1965; Brooks and Lu, 1972; Bonke, 1973).

Several reports (see for instance, Kao, 1966) have stated the absolute specificity of TTX for the rapid sodium channel, although Hogan and Albuquerque (1971) have shown that TTX at low concentrations also affects the resting sodium conductance induced by batrachotoxin. Therefore, any TTX-induced slowing down in the rate of rise of an action

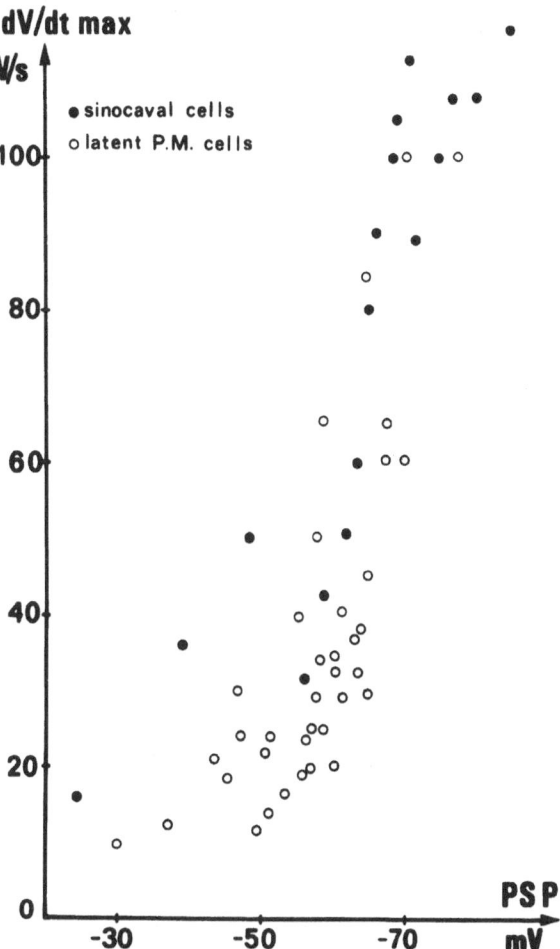

Figure 7. Maximal upstroke velocities of cells in the caval area [(solid circles, same points as in Figure 6 (rectangle)] and of latent pacemaker cells (open circles), are plotted as a function of the presystolic potential during hyperpolarizing and depolarizing pulses.

potential may be taken as evidence for the intervention of such a channel. The present work shows that the ascending phase of the true pacemaker cell action potential, which is barely sensitive or insensitive to TTX under normal conditions, becomes reliably sensitive to this substance after hyperpolarization.

The present results allow to conclude that the membrane of the true pacemaker cells possesses a rapid sodium channel normally inactivated as a consequence of the low value of the presystolic potential of this tissue.

Hyperpolarization of latent pacemaker cells induces the development of a rapid TTX-sensitive initial component of the action potential upstroke and makes them resemble cells of the right superior vena cava area.

These results suggest that the latent pacemaker cells may be regular cells from the caval area, normally depolarized, probably as a consequence of the vicinity of the true pacemaker cells.

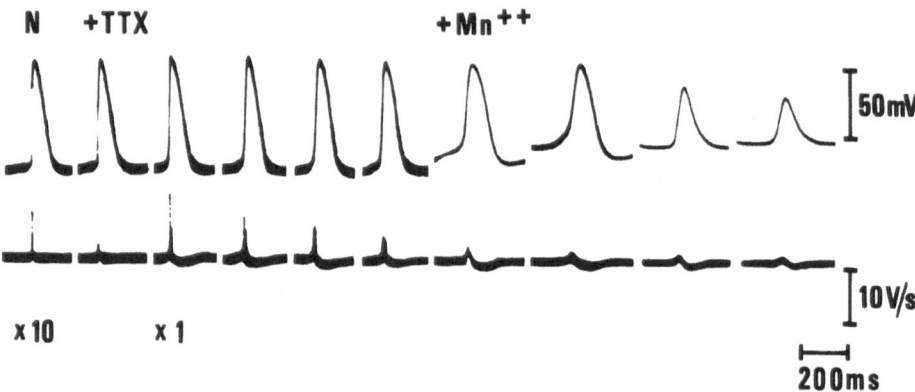

Figure 8. Effect of TTX (2.10^{-6} g/ml) and of Cl_2Mn (5mM) on the action potential of a perinodal cell. Explanations in text. Upper trace: actions potential; lower trace: first derivative, the gain of the amplifier has been increased tenfold during the action of TTX as indicated.

ACKNOWLEDGEMENTS

My thanks are due to Professor E. Coraboeuf for his constant interest and helpful suggestions. I wish to acknowledge Doctor F.I.M. Bonke for fruitful discussions and criticisms.

REFERENCES

1. Bonke, F.I.M.: Passive electrical properties of atrial fibers in the rabbit heart. *Pflügers Arch* 339: 1, 1973
2. Bonke, F.I.M.: Electrotonic spread in the sinoatrial node of the rabbit heart. *Pflügers Arch* 339: 17, 1973
3. Bouman, L.N., Gerlings, E., Biersteker, P.A., Bonke, F.I.M.: Pacemaker shift in the sinoatrial node during vagal stimulation. *Pflügers Arch* 302: 255, 1968
4. Brooks, C., Lu, H.: The sinoatrial pacemaker of the heart. Sringfield, Ill., Ch. Thomas edn., 1972
5. Burgen, A., Terroux, K.: On the negative inotropic effect in the cat's auricle. *J Physiol (London)* 120: 449, 1953
6. Hogan, P., Albuquerque, E.: The pharmacology of batrachotoxin. Effects on the heart Purkinje fibers. *J Pharmac Exp Ther* 176: 529, 1971
7. Ito, M., Arita, M., Saeki, K., Tanoué, M., Fukushima, I., Yanaga, T., Mashiba, H.: Functional properties of sinocaval conduction. *Jpn. J Physiol* 17: 174, 1967
8. Kao, C.: Tetrodotoxin, saxitoxin and their significance in the study of excitation phenomena. *Pharmacol Rev* 18: 997, 1966
9. Kreitner, D.: Evidence for the existence of a rapid sodium channel in the membrane of rabbit sinoatrial cells. *J. Mol. Cell. Cardiol.* 7: 655, 1975
10. Kreitner, D.: Effets des courants hyperpolarisants sur les potentiels d'action des cellules sinoatriales nodales et périnodales du cœur de lapin. *CR Acad Sci* 285: 1319, 1977
11. Lenfant, J., Mironneau, J., Gargouil, Y., Galand, G.: Analyse de l'activité électrique spontanée du centre de l'automatisme cardiaque de lapin par les inhibiteurs de perméabilités membranaires. *CR Acad Sci* 266: 901, 1968
12. Lipsius, S., Vassalle, M.: Effects of ionic changes and glucosides on sinus node action potentials. *Fed Proc* 35: 319, 1976
13. Paes de Carvalho, A., de Mello, W., Hoffman, B.F.: Electrophysiological evidence for specialized fibers types in rabbit atrium. *Am J Physiol 196*: 483, 1959
14. Sano, T., Yamaghishi, S.: Spread of excitation from the sinus node. *Circ Res* 16: 423, 1965
15. Weidmann, S.: The effect of cardiac membrane potential on the rapid availability of the sodium carrying system. *J Physiol (London)* 127: 213, 1955
16. Yamagishi, S., Sano, T.: Effect of tetrodotoxin on the pacemaker action potential of the sinus node. *Proc Jap Acad* 42: 1194, 1966

23

THE ACCELERATORY ACTION OF THE VAGUS ON THE SINUS NODE*

MARIO VASSALLE

INTRODUCTION

Anyone who has ever stimulated the vagus in the neck must have observed that the cessation of the stimulation is followed by a transient acceleration of the sinus node rate above the pre-stimulation control value. This sinus acceleration which follows vagal stimulation has been called "postvagal tachycardia" (Copen et al., 1968). The mechanism of the postvagal tachycardia has been studied in our laboratory in recent years. The results have appeared in several publications (Copen et al., 1968; Vassalle et al., 1970; Holder et al., 1971) one of which is in abstract form (Loeb and Vassalle, 1976). It is the purpose of the present paper to give an account of the results obtained in our laboratory on the mechanism of postvagal tachycardia. The interested reader will find a more extensive discussion of the pertinent literature in the publications cited above.

METHODS

The details of the methods employed are reported in the papers quoted above. In general outline, mongrel dogs were preanesthetized with morphine sulfate and were anesthetized with alpha-chloralose. The aortic blood pressure was recorded as well as one lead of the ECG. The animals were ventilated through a tracheal cannula. The chest was opened. A bipolar silver electrode was sewn on the epicardial surface of the right atrial appendage to record an electrogram as well as to trigger a cardiotachometer. Another electrode was sewn on the epicardial surface of the ventricles to drive these chambers. The tracings were displayed on an eight-channel switched beam oscilloscope and recorded on photographic paper.

The vagi were isolated in the neck and one or both were cut. The peripheral end was stimulated usually with stimuli of the following characteristics: 20/sec; 1–5 msec and 7–18 volts. The duration of the stimulation was 30–60 sec. The rate increment after vagal stimulation (postvagal tachycardia) was measured on the atrial electrogram trace over the 10 beat period when the increment was greatest. When the sympathetic nerves were stimulated similar parameters were used.

In most cases, the procedures were repeated several times and the results averaged. The t-test was used for comparison of the data and differences were considered statistically significant when the P value was less than 0.05. The postvagal tachycardia is usually expressed in beats/min above the control rate prior to vagal stimulation.

* The work presented in the paper was supported by grants from the N.I.H., National Heart and Lung Institute and from the American and the New York Heart Association.

RESULTS

POSTVAGAL TACHYCARDIA (PVT)

The acceleration of the sinus node after the cessation of vagal stimulation is illustrated in Figure 1. The first trace (SR) is a tachometer trace of the sinus rate; RA is an atriogram; BP is a record of aortic blood pressure and the horizontal line beneath is the zero reference line; L_2 is lead II of the electrocardiogram. The calibration for the tachometer trace (0–150 beats/min) and for the blood pressure (0–100 mmHg) are shown to the left of the respective traces.

Vagal stimulation was started at the first arrow and it caused cardiac arrest and a marked fall in blood pressure. An idioventricular escape beat is identified by a negative QRS complex. The break in the trace indicates the omission of part of the recording during the one minute vagal stimulation. At the beginning of the second section, after the last 3 idioventricular beats, the vagal stimulation was discontinued at the arrow. Within a few beats, the sinus rate increased above the control value of 96 beats/min by 39 beats/min and this acceleration was accompanied by an increase in blood pressure. When the blood pressure increased to its peak, the sinus rate transiently slowed down. However, once the pressure increase began to subside, the sinus rate increased once more to 139 beats/min. The return to control value is shown by the third section of Figure 1.

In 10 dogs, the sinus rate prior to vagal stimulation was 80.7 ± 6.1 and increased after vagal stimulation to 108.4 ± 83 beats/min (+27.7 ± 3.8 beats/min, +34%). The peak value was attained within the first 30 sec after the end of vagal stimulation of subsided in 30–60 min (Copen et al., 1968). In this series of animals, postvagal tachycardia was induced with the stimulation of the right vagus. However, it can be shown that postvagal tachycardias of comparable magnitude can be obtained with the stimulation of either vagus (Loeb and Vassalle, 1976).

THE ROLE OF REFLEX FACTORS IN POSTVAGAL TACHYCARDIA

During vagal stimulation the blood pressure falls and this must elicit a reflex that enhances sympathetic discharge and decreases the vagal discharge. The role of these reflex factors was evaluated by preventing the fall in blood pressure during vagal stimulation. This was

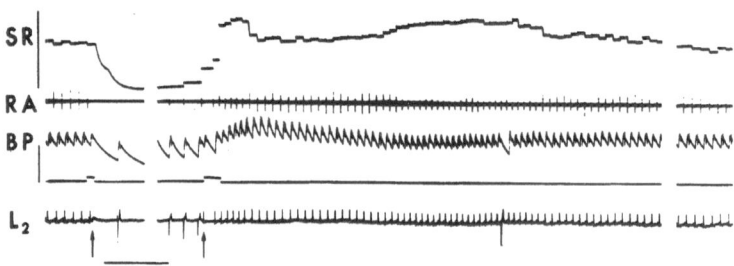

Figure 1. Acceleration of the sinus rate after vagal stimulation. The horizontal bar on the bottom is a time calibration (5 sec). The peripheral end of the right vagus was stimulated for one minute. The left vagus was intact. (From Copen et al., 1968, reproduced by permission)

done by driving the ventricles either during vagal stimulation (Copen et al., 1968) or prior, during and after vagal stimulation (Vasalle et al., 1970). The results obtained with the latter procedure are shown in Figure 2. The explanation of the lettering is the same as for Figure 1. In the upper part of the figure, vagal stimulation was carried out during the period indicated by the arrows. During the vagal stimulation there was a profound fall in blood pressure and, after the end of vagal stimulation a postvagal tachycardia of 97 beats/min. In the lower part of the figure, vagal stimulation was repeated during continuous ventricular drive. It is apparent that the vagal stimulation resulted in the complete suppression of vagal activity as shown by the tachometer trace (the small spikes on the atriogram are artifacts due to the ventricular drive). The blood pressure during vagal stimulation was maintained as the ventricles were activated by the electrical drive. The cessation of vagal stimulation was followed by a postvagal tachycardia of 89 beats/min.

In the series of Copen et al. (1968), postvagal tachycardia averaged 27.7 ± 3.8 beats/min in the absence and 28.2 ± 3.4 beats/min in the presence of ventricular drive (10 dogs). In the series of Vassalle et al. (1970), the postvagal tachycardia averaged 67 ± 13.5 beats/min in the absence and 64 ± 15.9 beats/min in the presence of ventricular drive (5 dogs).

That discharge withdrawal of the contralateral vagus played little role in postvagal

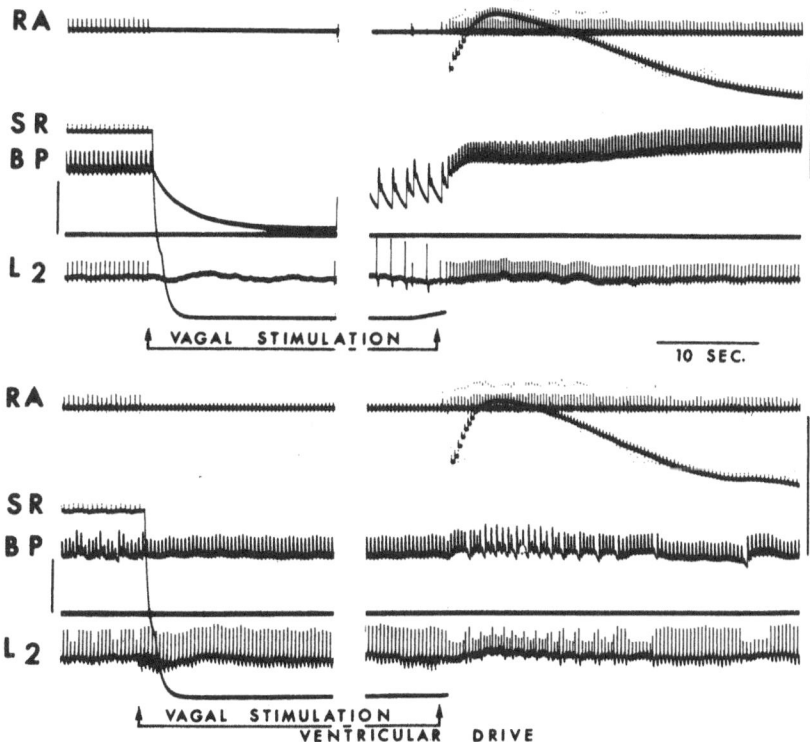

Figure 2. Postvagal tachycardia in the absence (top panel) and in the presence of ventricular drive (bottom panel). Explanation of the lettering is the same as that for Figure 1. Blood pressure calibration (0–100 mmHg) and tachometer calibration (100–200 beats/min) are the vertical bars at the left and the right of the tracings, respectively. Both vagi were cut. The connections of the right stellate ganglion had been cut except for the cardiac nerves. Duration of the vagal stimulation 1 min. (From Vassalle et al., 1970, reproduced by permission).

tachycardia was demonstrated by the fact that the tachycardia remained unchanged after the section of both vagi (Copen et al., 1968).

In another series of experiments (Vassalle et al., 1970), the role of reflex factors in postvagal tachycardia was tested by carrying out vagal stimulation before and after cardiac denervation. The denervation consisted of bilateral vagatomy and of the bilateral excision of the stellate ganglia and of the first five thoracic ganglia. In 6 experiments, postvagal tachycardia was 38 ± 5.9 before and 38 ± 7.4 beats/min after denervation. In contrast, intravenous administration of nitroglycerine provoked a reflex tachycardia of 85 ± 15.1 before and an increase of 3 ± 2.6 beats/min after denervation.

The experiments illustrated in this section show that reflex sympathetic activation or reflex vagal withdrawal are not important in the production of postvagal tachycardia.

ROLE OF CATECHOLAMINES IN POSTVAGAL TACHYCARDIA

If the withdrawal of vagal inhibition is not responsible for PVT, the mechanism of this tachycardia must involve the release of an excitatory substance. If this excitatory substance is a catecholamine, depletion of catecholamine stores by reserpine should abolish PVT. As shown in Figure 3 (upper panel), stimulation of the vagus in a reserpinized dog was

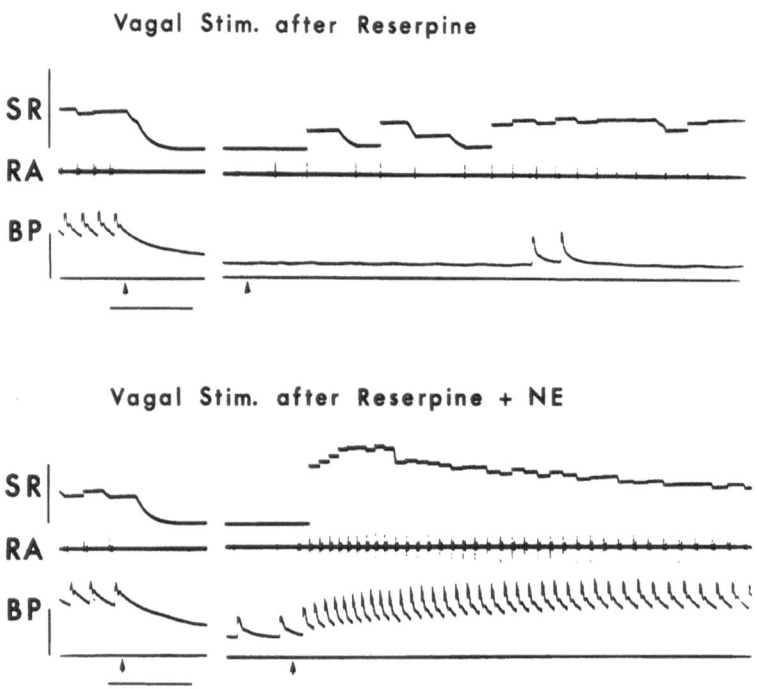

Figure 3. Effects of vagal stimulation after reserpine administration (upper panel) and replenishment with norepinephrine (lower panel). Explanation of the lettering as for Figure 1. The ECG trace has been omitted. The beginning and the end of 1 min vagal stimulation are marked by arrowheads. The vertical bars at the left of the tracing are the calibration for the tachometer trace (0–100 beats/min) and that for the blood pressure (0–100 mmHg). Horizontal bar indicates 5 sec. Right vagal stimulation. Reserpine had been given intramuscularly in a dose of 0.2 mg/kg each day for the 3 days preceding the experiment. Before the recording of the lower panel, norepinephrine (2 mg in 100 ml saline) was infused slowly intravenously. (From Copen et al., 1968; reproduced by permission).

followed by a pronounced bradycardia, not tachycardia. If the bradycardia is due only to depletion of catecholamines (and not to some other action of reserpine), administration of norepinephrine in these reserpinized dogs might restore the postvagal tachycardia. This is shown in Figure 3 lower panel (which was recorded from the same reserpinized dog): the cessation of the vagal stimulation at the second arrow was followed by a tachycardia of 49 beats/min.

In six animals treated with reserpine, vagal stimulation was followed by bradycardia in five and by a small (25 beats/min) tachycardia in one. In five of these dogs, norepinephrine was administered and postvagal tachycardia was present in each of them (Copen et al., 1968).

If, instead of depletion, norepinephrine or dopamine were applied locally on the sinus node, the duration of PVT was markedly prolonged (Loeb and Vassalle, 1976). Furthermore, block of neuronal and extra-neuronal uptake of catecholamines by desipramine and phenoxybenzamine also markedly potentiated PVT (Loeb and Vassalle, 1976). Finally, administration of propranolol, a beta blocker, reduces PVT by 66.4% (Loeb and Vassalle, 1976).

THE ROLE OF SYMPATHETIC FIBERS RUNNING IN THE VAGUS IN POSTVAGAL TACHYCARDIA

There is little question that sympathetic fibers cross over to the vagus in the neck and innervate the heart (Jung et al., 1934). Therefore, postvagal tachycardia could result from the stimulation of sympathetic fibers in the vagus rather than from that of vagal fibers. A series of experiments were done to clarify this point.

In one approach, the vagus was excited reflexly (Figure 4, upper panel, Copen et al., 1968). A balloon was placed in the carotid at the level of the carotid sinus and, at the first mark, it was rapidly inflated. The ventricles were driven at the same time in an effort to maintain the blood pressure. It is apparent that during the balloon inflation the sinus node slowed down (from 108 to 50 beats/min). After the balloon was rapidly deflated and the drive terminated, the sinus rate progressively increased to reach a value of 162 beats/min (+ 54 beats/min). Similar large increases were obtained in two more experiments.

The fall in pressure during the reflex activation was presumably due to a sympathetic withdrawal. However, once the balloon was deflated, the still lower blood pressure might have been responsible for initiating the tachycardia. To test this point, both vagi were cut. Bilateral vagotomy should abolish a tachycardia due to a reflex vagal excitation but not a tachycardia due to a reflex sympathetic discharge secondary to low blood pressure. As shown in the lower panel (taken from the same animal as in the upper panel), after bilateral vagotomy, inflation of the balloon at the mark caused a fall in sinus rate (177 to 150 beats/min) and a fall in blood pressure. When the balloon was deflated at the second mark, the sinus rate returned to a steady rate of 168 beats/min but there was no tachycardia. That the lack of tachycardia was not due to the higher control rate was shown by stimulating the vagus directly: the stimulation was followed by a tachycardia of 36 beats/min.

In another series of experiments (Holder et al., 1970), the vagus and sympathetic trunks were separated in the neck near the nodose and superior cervical ganglia. On stimulation, the vagal trunk caused bradycardia and the sympathetic caused pupillary dilatation, exophthalmos and tachycardia. Once thus identified, the trunks were cut and the peripheral end stimulated. In 17 dogs, stimulation of the vagus led to a tachycardia of 34.1 $\pm$ 5.4 beats/min and that of the sympathetic trunk to a tachycardia of 30.4 $\pm$ 3.8. It is of interest that when both trunks were stimulated together, during the stimulation there was

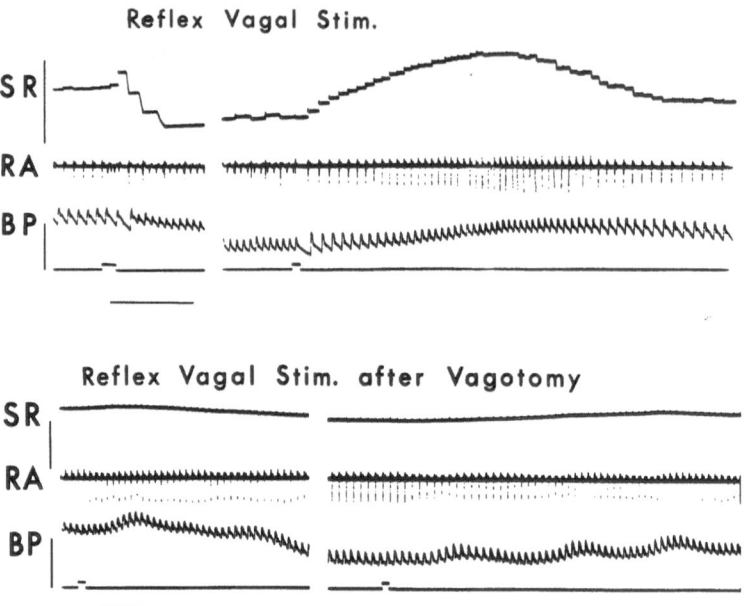

Figure 4. Changes in sinus rate during and after reflex vagal stimulation with the vagi intact (upper panel) and after bilateral vagotomy (lower panel). The first and second marks on the zero reference line indicate the inflation and deflation of the balloon in the carotid sinus. Calibration is the same as for Figure 3. The ECG trace has been omitted. The reflex stimulation was accomplished by introducing a balloon catheter into the right common artery. The balloon was placed at the level of the carotid sinus and distended with air for 30 sec. (From Copen et al., 1968, reproduced by permission).

bradycardia and after the stimulation there was a tachycardia of 38.9 ± 5.4 beats/min. The lack of summation was possibly due to the fact that acetylcholine released by the vagus interfered with norepinephrine or with the release of norepinephrine. This was tested in 3 dogs by stimulating first the vagus and then the sympathetic: the tachycardia was 65% larger than with the simultaneous stimulation of the two trunks. These experiments show that: 1) there are sympathetic fibers in the vagal trunk which accelerate the sinus node. However, the experiments also demonstrate that: 2) postvagal tachycardia persists after the separation of the sympathetic trunk; and 3) the stimulation of sympathetic fibers *during* vagal stimulation does not contribute importantly to postvagal tachycardia. In the cat the vagus and the sympathetic trunks are naturally separated: stimulation of the vagus was followed by a tachycardia of 32 ± 15.6 and that of the sympathetic trunk caused a tachycardia of 17.8 ± 7.3 beats/min. Thus, in the cat too a postvagal tachycardia can be obtained with the stimulation of the vagal trunk alone.

SELECTIVE SUPPRESSION OF POSTVAGAL AND SYMPATHETIC TACHYCARDIAS

The results obtained with the stimulation of the separated vagal and sympathetic trunks in the neck are open to the objection that possibly there were some sympathetic fibers in the separated vagal trunk. In view of this possibility, a number of different types of experiments were carried out to selectively suppress the postvagal or the sympathetic tachycardia.

In one approach (Holder et al., 1970), in five dogs, stimulation of the vagal trunk caused a PVT of 41 ± 11 and that of the separated sympathetic trunk an acceleration of 31 ± 9.7 beats/min. Bretylium, a substance which blocks the release of norepinephrine from sympathetic endings (Boura and Green, 1959), only slightly decreased PVT (33 ± 12.1 beats/min) but abolished the sympathetic tachycardia (1 ± 1.4 beats/min). When tetraethylammonium (TEA) was applied *locally* on the sinus node area (and therefore blocked only the vagal synapses), PVT was abolished (− 7 ± 3.3 beats/min). In another series of experiments, the order of administration of the drugs was reversed. As illustrated in Figure 5, locally applied TEA abolished PVT but not the sympathetic tachycardia. Subsequent administration of bretylium eliminated the sympathetic tachycardia. In 4 animals TEA abolished PVT (40 ± 12 to − 5 ± 4.4 beats/min) but did not affect the sympathetic tachycardia (29 ± 4.1 to 31 ± 4.9 beats/min). Subsequent administration of bretylium abolished the sympathetic tachycardia (2 ± 0.8 beats/min).

That bretylium did not abolish the postvagal tachycardia but abolished reflex tachycardia induced by intravenous injection of nitroglycerine was also shown by the experiments of Vassalle et al. (1970).

THE LOCATION OF THE CATECHOLAMINE STORES

The experiments with reserpine suggest that catecholamines are needed for PVT but do not clarify the point whether acetylcholine (ACh) liberates catecholamines by acting on sympathetic nerves or instead on some other structure such as chromaffin cells. Relatively small doses of reserpine markedly deplete the sympathetic neural stores but have a small

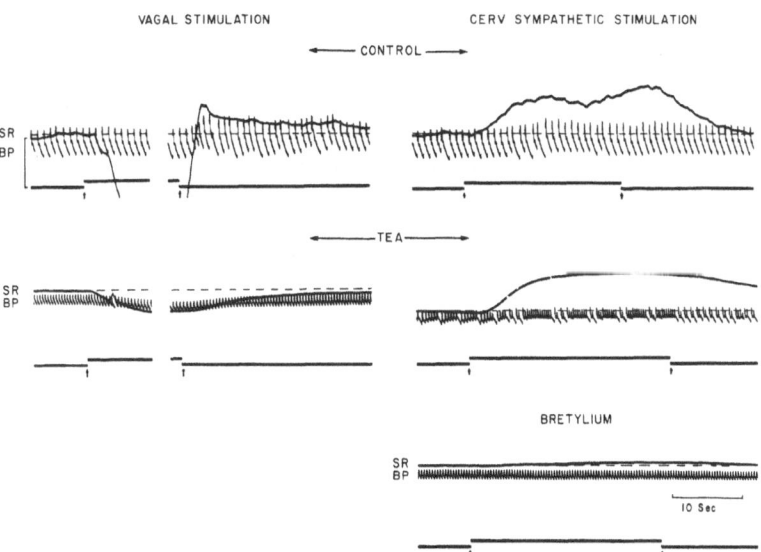

Figure 5. Changes in sinus tachycardias on stimulation of the separated vagal and sympathetic trunks before (top panels) and after TEA (middle panels) and after bretylium (bottom panel). The explanation of the lettering is as for Figure 1. Blood pressure calibration (0–100 mmHg) is the vertical line at the left of the top panels. The ventricles were driven during vagal stimulation. The ECG trace has been omitted.(From Holder et al., 1971, reproduced by permission).

effect on the adrenal medulla (Carlsson et al., 1957; Lee, 1967). Therefore in a series of experiments (Vassalle et al., 1970), a partial reserpinization was carried out by administering smaller doses of reserpine. In one of these animals, the cessation of vagal stimulation was characterized by sinus arrest. In seven other dogs, PVT averaged 24.6 beats/min. In these same dogs, stimulation of the right stellate ganglion caused an increase in rate of only 4.98 ± 4.4 beats/min. For comparison, the stimulation of the right stellate ganglion in 8 dogs was 87.6 ± 7.1 beats/min.

In another series of experiments (Vassalle et al., 1970) acetylcholine was applied locally on the sinus node area. This procedure was suggested by the finding that repeated injection ACh depletes the adrenal medulla (Butterworth and Mann, 1957). Vagal stimulation was followed by a PVT and stellate stimulation elicited a marked tachycardia. After repeated applications of ACh, the PVT was abolished but the sympathetic tachycardia was unaffected. In 6 dogs, after ACh treatment PVT decreased from 44 to 7 beats/min whereas the sympathetic tachycardia was unaltered (88 before and 94 beats/min after ACh treatment). This action of ACh was fully reversible.

In a different approach (Holder et al., 1971), the sympathetic nerves were destroyed by administration of 6-hydroxydopamine (Tranzer and Thoenen, 1967; Tranzer and Thoenen, 1968) which affects much less the chromaffin tissue of the adrenal medulla and does not affect the vagal fibers at all. As shown in Figure 6 (upper panel) recorded from a dog treated with 6-hydroxydopamine, the stimulation of the vagus caused a tachycardia of 37 beats/min while cervical sympathetic stimulation was without effect. In the lower panel, the same dog was given atropine to prevent the fall in blood pressure and the PVT was even greater (53 beats/min). The stimulation of the right stellate ganglion was without effect. Similar results were obtained in 5 cats.

The experiments with 6-hydroxydopamine show that PVT is still present when the sympathetic nerves are chemically destroyed, but do not indicate whether PVT is related to catecholamine release from extra-neuronal stores. This was tested by administering phenoxybenzamine after chemical destruction of sympathetic nerves (Loeb and Vassalle, unpublished experiments). Phenoxybenzamine is a blocker of both neuronal and extra-neuronal uptake (Iversen 1973). It was found that after 6-hydroxydopamine, PVT (but not sympathetic tachycardia) persisted, as expected. When phenoxybenzamine was administered, PVT increased.

DISCUSSION

The series of experiments reported suggests the conclusion that a sinus tachycardia: 1) follows the termination of vagal stimulation; 2) is not due to a reflex action; 3) requires the availability of catecholamines stores; 4) does not result from the stimulation of sympathetic fibers in the vagal trunk; 5) persists after the inactivation or destruction of sympathetic nerves; 6) is due to the release of ACh which in turn liberates catecholamines from extraneuronal stores.

The usual concept of neural control of the sinus node is that the vagus inhibits and the sympathetic nerves accelerate the spontaneous discharge. The experiments reported show that the vagus has excitatory as well as inhibitory actions on the sinus node. It is known that when the vagus is reflexly excited, there is a reflex withdrawal of the sympathetic discharge (Bronk et al., 1934). Therefore, the prompt restoration of the sinus node rhythm cannot be brought about by an increased sympathetic discharge. Yet, in view of

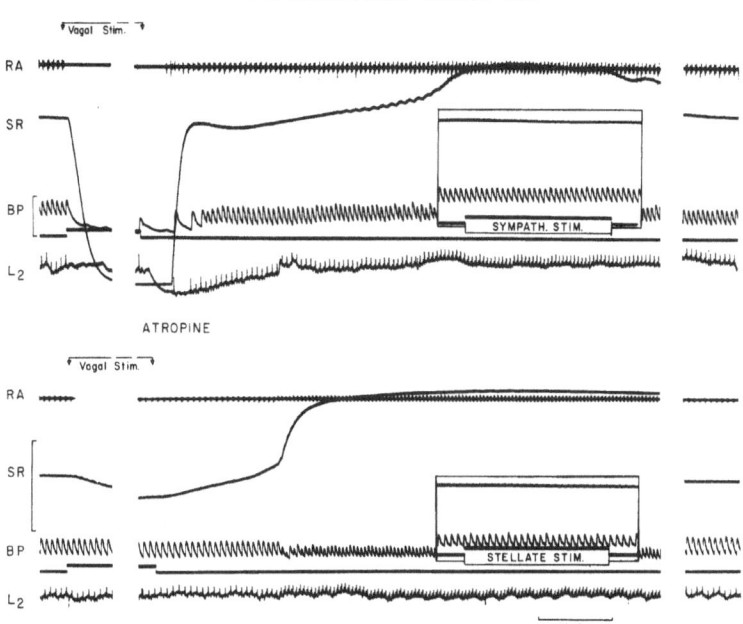

Figure 6. Effect of vagal and sympathetic stimulation in a 6-hydroxydopamine-treated dog. Explanation of the lettering is as for Figure 1. Vagal stimulation is indicated by the upper shift of the zero referenc line. In the top panel, the inset shows the lack of effect of cervical sympathetic stimulations and, in the bottom panel, the inset shows the lack of effect of stellate ganglion stimulation. The lower panel was recorded after the administration of atropine to prevent the fall in blood pressure during vagal stimulation. The vertical bar in the top panel, is the calibration for blood pressure (0–100 mmHg) and that in the bottom panel is the calibration for the tachometer trace (50–100 beats/min). (From Holder et al., 1970, reproduced by permission).

the consequences of even a short cessation of the circulation on central nervous system, it is of paramount importance that the sinus node discharge is restored quickly. In fact, not only a prompt return to control values but a temporary acceleration of the sinus node rate above control values would hasten the return of the circulation to its normal state and help to pay more quickly any oxygen debt incurred during the standstill. Thus, post-vagal tachycardia would subserve an important physiological function.

In the laboratory approach, however, the electrical stimulation of the vagus must result in an increase (not a decrease) of the reflex sympathetic discharge and also in the reflex withdrawal of the contralateral vagus. These two actions must occur, but the results show that they have a very little role in postvagal tachycardia. Thus postvagal tachycardia was unaltered when the stimulus (low blood pressure) for reflex actions was eliminated by ventricular driving (Figure 2). The unimportance of vagal withdrawal was shown by the fact that PVT was unaltered after the section of the contralateral vagus. Nor was PVT changed by cardiac denervation which practically abolished a nitroglycerin-induced reflex tachycardia of 85 beats/min.

These results point to a direct effect of the electrical stimulation of the vagus in the neck. Whatever the fibers excited by the stimulation of the vagus in the neck, the availability of catecholamines is necessary for the production of PVT. This is shown by the following findings: 1) PVT is abolished in reserpinized animals (Figure 3); 2) is restored by administration of norepinephrine in the reserpinized dogs; 3) is enhanced by local application of norepinephrine and dopamine in the sinus node area; and 4) is markedly reduced by propranolol.

These findings establish that stimulation of the vagus in the neck results in a PVT through a release of catecholamines. The following findings establish that PVT is not due to the catecholamines released by sympathetic fibers running in the vagal trunk. Thus: 1) a PVT is elicited by the reflex stimulation of the vagus (when sympathetic discharge should be reflexly *decreased*) (Figure 4); 2) PVT elicited by reflex vagal stimulation is abolished by bilateral vagotomy (Figure 4) and; 3) selective stimulation of vagal fibers in the neck (separated vagal and sympathetic trunks) elicited PVT.

That PVT occurring with the stimulation of the separated vagal trunk was not due to the stimulation of sympathetic fibers present in the separated vagus is shown by: 1) the abolition of the sympathetic tachycardia but not of PVT by bretylium and; 2) the abolition of PVT but not of the sympathetic tachycardia with TEA applied locally on the sinus node.

The possibility that ACh released by vagal fibers acted on sympathetic fibers to release catehcolamines is ruled out by the following findings: 1) the abolition of sympathetic tachycardia but not of PVT with "partial" reserpinization; 2) the abolition of PVT but not of sympathetic tachycardia with repeated application of ACh on the sinus node; 3) the abolition of the sympathetic tachycardia but not of PVT after chemical sympathectomy; 4) the enhancement of PVT after block of catecholamine reuptake with phenoxybenzamine in chemically sympathectomized dogs while sympathetic stimulation remained ineffectual.

Thus, in conclusion, PVT appears to be due to the following mechanisms. Activation of some vagal fibers leads to liberation of acetylcholine and acetylcholine in turn liberates catecholamines from extraneuronal stores. This happens during vagal stimulation. As the stimulation is terminated, acetylcholine concentration decreases more rapidly than that of the liberated norepinephrine and a transient tachycardia follows.

Where the extraneuronal catecholamine stores under vagal control are located was not determined by the experiment reported. One possibility is that the catecholamines are located in chromaffin cells. Many of the findings are compatible with such a possibility. Thus, these cells in the adrenal medulla are depleted by acetylcholine (Butterworth, 1957) and less than the sympathetic nerves by reserpine (Carlsson et al., 1957; Lee, 1967), are blocked by TEA, are little affected by bretylium (Boura and Green, 1959) and by 6-hydroxydopamine (Tranzer and Thoenen, 1967). These cells have been shown in the sinus node area (Trinci, 1907) and chromaffin cells have been described which receive a cholinergic innervation (Jacobowitz, 1967). However, too little is known at the present time about extraneuronal stores of catecholamines in the sinus node area to come to any firm conclusion.

REFERENCES

1. Boura, A.L.A., Green, A.F.: The actions of bretylium: adrenergic neurone blocking and other effects. *Brit J Pharmacol* 14: 536, 1959
2. Bronk, D.W., Ferguson, L.K., Solandt, D.Y.: Inhibition of cardiac accelerator impulses by the carotid sinus. *Proc Soc Exptl Biol Med* 31: 579, 1934
3. Butterworth, K.R., Mann, M.: The release of adrenaline and noradrenaline from the adrenal gland of the cat by acetylcholine. *Brit J Pharmacol* 12: 422, 1957
4. Carlsson, A., Rosengren, E., Bertler, Å., Nilsson, J.: Effect of reserpine on the metabolism of cate-

cholamines. In: Psychotropic Drugs, edited by S. Garattini and V. Ghetti. Amsterdam: Elsevier, 1957, p. 363

5. Copen, D.L., Cirillo, D.P., Vassalle, M.: Tachycardia following vagal stimulation. *Amer J Physiol* 215: 696, 1968

6. Holder, M.S., Anolik, M.A., Vassalle, M.: Positive chronotropic effect of vagus on sinus node. *Arch Sci Biol* 55:103, 1971

7. Irvesen, L.: Catecholamine uptake processes. *Brit Med Bull* 29: 130, 1973

8. Jacobowitz, D.: Histochemical studies of the relationship of chromaffin cells and adrenergic nerve fibers to the cardiac ganglia of several species. *J Pharmacol Exptl Therap* 158: 227, 1967

9. Jung, L., Tagand, R., Pierre, M.: Sur le trajet des éléments cardio-accélérateurs contenus dans le cordon vagosympathique du chien. *Compt Rend Soc Biol* 117: 441, 1934

10. Lee, F.L.: The relation between norepinephrine content and response to sympathetic nerve stimulation of various organs of cats pretreated with reserpine. *J Pharmacol Exptl Therap* 156: 137, 1967

11. Loeb, J.M., Vassalle, M.: The positive chronotropic action of the vagus nerve on the heart. *Fed Proc* 35: 446, 1976

12. Tranzer, J.P., Thoenen, H.: Ultramorphologische Veränderungen der Sympathischen Nervendigungen der Katze nach Vorbehandlung mit 5- und 6-Hydroxydopamin. *Naunyn-Schmiedeberg's Archiv Pharmakol exp Pathol* 257: 343, 1967

13. Tranzer, J.P., Thoenen, H.: An electron microscopic study of selective, acute degeneration of sympathetic nerve terminals after administration of 6-hydroxy-dopamin. *Experientia* 24: 155, 1968

14. Trinci, G.: Cellule cromaffini e "mastzellen" nella regione cardiaca dei mammiferi. *Mem Reale Accad Sci Ist Bologna* 4: 191, 1907

15. Vassalle, M., Mandel, W.J., Holder, M.S.: Catecholamine stores under vagal control. *Amer J Physiol* 218: 115, 1970

24

GENERAL CONCLUSIONS

W. TRAUTWEIN

In this and the previous sections the sinus node was roughly described as a cluster of cells with the special property to depolarize spontaneously in diastole, eventually to the threshold of the next action potential. The cells in the cluster are electrically coupled. Not much has been said about the passive electrical properties of the cells and of the electrical coupling. The length constant seems to be less than 1 mm. The coupling enforces a certain synchrony in the activity of the cells. In microelectrode studies, therefore, one has to keep in mind that an electrode in one cell "sees" events occurring up to one mm away. Yet it is known that the cells in the sinus node do not have all the same ability to "spontaneously" depolarize after an action potential. There is a center normally in the head of the sinus node, the pacemaker, and there are other areas in the sinus node which show diastolic depolarization at a lesser rate and which are excited by propagation. Under certain conditions the pacemaker can shift from one area to another, as shown-in this section-by mapping the spread of excitation. With the exception of the paper on post vagal tachycardia (Vassalle) this section dealt with related problems. The experiments attempted:

1. to determine the configuration of the action potential of different areas of the sinus node and
2. to study effects on the action potentials, of changes in the ionic environment, of drugs like acetylcholine, epinephrine or TTX.
3. to clarify the mechanism of the shift of the pacemaker by combined measurement of the cellular potential and of the pattern of excitation in the sinus node.

It was intended by these experimental conditions to gain some indirect information on the ionic mechanism underlying the pacemaker- and action-potentials of the sinus node.

Pacemaker potentials had been recorded extracellularly by Bozler (1943) before the microelectrode was introduced. He also found the pacemaker potential to be flatter some mm away from the earliest point of excitation. Many more details and quantitative data have been added by intracellular recordings of the pacemaker potential of the Purkinje fiber (Weidmann, 1951) and by Hutter and Trautwein (1956) in their studies on the frog sinus venosus. Both latency measurements and mapping experiments together with intracellular recordings have confirmed that the dominant pacemaker potential is characterized by the steepest diastolic depolarization recorded in the sinus node, further by a less negative maximum diastolic potential and a smooth sigmoid upstroke with a very low rate of rise. In contrast the subsidiary or latent pacemaker cells have a more negative diastolic membrane potential, less steep diastolic depolarization, and an upstroke which displays an initial rapid phase followed by a distinctly slower phase to the plateau level (Lipsius and Vassalle). The two components in the upstroke of the action potential are also seen in the rabbit sinus node (Kreitner). In rabbit these cell types could be roughly located in the compact center (head) of the sinus node where the steepest diastolic depolarization was recorded and in the tail of the node where, under normal conditions, the subsidiary pacemaker cells were observed. By mapping out the spread of excitation and correlating the activation pattern with the histological reconstruction of the sinus node it could be shown that the pacemaker is indeed located in the compact center of the sinus (Bouman et al.; Steinbeck et al.).

In an attempt to get some indirect evidence on the ionic mechanism underlying the pacemaker potential and the action potential, a relatively clear picture emerged from the studies of the upstroke. The slow upstroke of the dominant or true pacemaker action potential is insensitive to TTX but easily depressed by Mn ions, suggesting that the "slow inward" current is involved and that either there is no fast inward channel in these cells, or the fast channel is inactivated due to the low diastolic membrane potential. Hyperpolarization by carbamylcholine or by current flow increases the rate of rise of the true pacemaker action potentials. Under this condition the upstroke becomes sensitive to TTX, however, less than in latent pacemaker cells. Thus, it appears that the cells of the dominant pacemaker do have a fast sodium system, which is normally inactivated. In the latent pacemaker cells both the rapid and the slow inward current are activated during the upstroke. This was shown by the different dependence of the fast and slow component of the upstroke on the take-off level and the repriming time after preceding activation (Lipsius and Vassalle): The fast component was larger in amplitude on early stimulation (at the more negative diastolic potential) than later in diastole, whereas the slow component was larger later in diastole, presumably due to the long repriming time of the slow inward system. In line with the observation on the fast and slow channel of the action potential in subsidiary pacemaker cells are the effects of ACh and norepinephrine. According to Lipsius and Vassalle acetylcholine increases both amplitude and rate of the fast component by shifting the take-off level in a negative direction (cf. Trautwein and Dudel, 1958b). The slow component is said to be inhibited (see Figure 4 in Lipsius and Vassalle). Norepinephrine has opposite effects. The shift of the pacemaker within the sinus node which occurs during the application of ACh (as shown by Bouman et al. in mapping experiments) could result from a block of the slow inward current in the dominant pacemaker fibers, in which case previously latent pacemaker fibers operating preferably with the fast inward current would become the actual pacemaker.

The explanation of the effects of variations of the extracellular calcium concentration on the two components of the upstroke are complicated by the many effects Ca-ions exert on the excitable membrane. Changes in the extracellular calcium concentration do affect the fast component of the upstroke by shifting the steady state inactivation along the voltage axis in negative (lowering of the extracellular Ca concentration) or positive (elevation of the extracellular Ca concentration) direction. The slow component of the upstroke rises faster or slower to a more or less positive peak when $[Ca]_o$ is elevated or reduced, respectively. This differential effect of the extracellular Ca-concentration on the fast and slow component suggests that there are indeed two inward channels which pass preferentially Na (fast channel) and Ca ions (slow channel). Against the latter conclusion is the observation by Noma and Irisawa that in the sinus node of the rabbit the charge through the slow channel is mainly carried by Na-ions (voltage clamp experiments). Perhaps the finding of species differences can settle this discrepancy in the future.

In respect to the ionic movements during diastole different properties of dominant and latent pacemaker cells have been postulated by Bouman et al. in an attempt to explain the effect of elevation of the extracellular Ca-concentration on the rate of the sinus node activity and the shift of the pacemaker which occurs when $[Ca]_o$ is lowered. The stepwise shift of the pacemaker from the head downwards to the tail on stepwise lowering the extra-cellular Ca-concentration was explained by a larger (depolarizing) resting Ca influx in the dominant pacemaker cells in the head than in the latent pacemaker cells in the tail of the sinus node. This interesting but still speculative explanation implies that the mechanism for the low diastolic membrane potential in dominant as compared to latent pacemaker fibers is due to larger Ca-permeability and thus a larger Ca influx in the former cells. Dudel and Trautwein (1958) have assumed that a (depolarizing) background current together with a (repolarizing) potassium current decaying during diastole produces the pacemaker potential. The depolarizing current was supposed to be larger in true than in latent pacemaker cells since it was known that in true pacemaker cells the maximum diastolic membrane potential is less negative than in latent pacemaker cells (Hutter and Trautwein, 1956). Bouman et al. tentatively concluded that Ca influx plays the role of a depolarizing current in diastole and that this influx is blocked by acetylcholine, thereby leading to a shift of the pacemaker. Different sensitivity of the dominant and latent pace-maker fibers towards Ouabain was described by Steinbeck et al. This drug increases the diastolic depolarization of the latent fibers to such an extent that they overrule the pace-maker. The resulting shift has been shown in mapping experiments.

Summarizing the general conclusions so far, I would like to say that in the sinus node action potentials can be recorded which differ in their function and configuration. Dominant pacemaker cells occur in the head of the sinus node. They display a slow up-stroke due to the activation of the slow inward system (but with inactivated fast Na chan-nels). Latent pacemaker cells in the tail have upstrokes consisting of a fast and a slow component. Many observations suggest that the ionic movements during diastole are different in dominant pacemaker cells than in subsidiary pacemaker cells. In the former a larger Ca influx was postulated which keeps the diastolic potential at a low negative level. The different properties of these cells can explain to some extent the shifts of the pacemaker under various influences which has been shown to occur in mapping experi-ments.

Without voltage clamp experiments on the sinus node (see the next section) conclusions on the ionic movements, underlying the pacemaker- and action-potentials of the sinus node, can only be drawn on the basis of the large bulk of information obtained in recent years in voltage clamp experiments on Purkinje fibers and working myocardium. In these structures spontaneous activity of the type which occurs in the sinus node has been described under abnormal conditions and explained on the basis of the voltage- and time-dependence of the ionic currents involved (c.f. Noble, 1975). A very close model of the ionic events leading to the pacemaker in the sinus node might be the experiment shown in Figure 1 where a small trabeculum of a cat's heart was depolarized by constant current until low voltage oscillations appeared. The preparation was mounted in an apparatus which allowed to clamp the membrane voltage and to measure the resulting membrane current. When the clamp was made effective early in diastole the membrane current was either outward and falling (clamp positive to the maximum diastolic potential, E_{max}) or inward and rising (at E_{max} and -75 mV) or falling around -100 mV. The component of the net current which changes with time is a potassium current (c.f. McDonald and Trautwein, 1978) which has been activated during the preceeding action potential. If the potential is changed later in diastole the current pattern changes, indicating the activation of the slow inward current. Here, spontaneity is brough about by a depolarizing background current (supplied from an external source), a decay of a repolarizing outward potassium current, and later in diastole the activation of a depolarizing slow inward

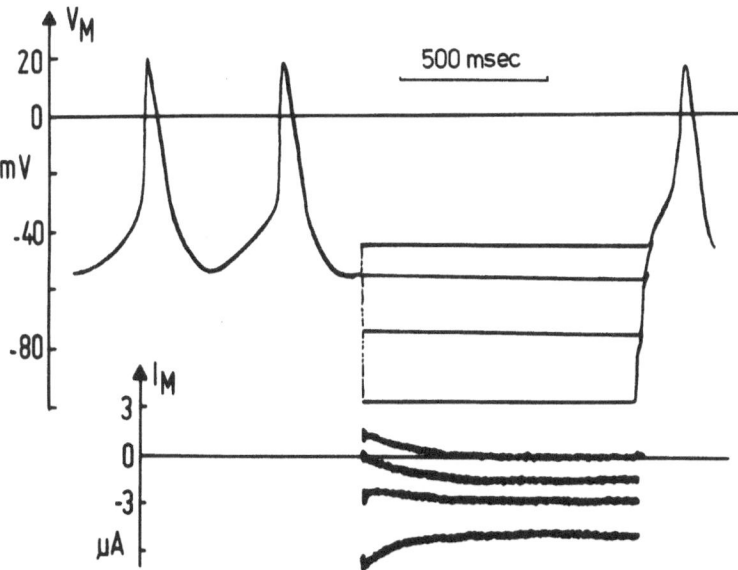

Figure 1. Trabeculum of cats ventricular myocardium has been made "spontaneously" beating by passing a small depolarizing constant current through the preparation. In order to analyse the current which produces the slow diastolic depolarizations the membrane potential was clamped four times early in diastole and the resulting membrane was recorded. Membrane potential and current responses are superimposed. Hybrid sucrose gap technique.

current. In the next section results obtained in experiments of this type carried out in the sinus node will be discussed.

The paper by Vassalle dealt with a problem which is difficult to tie in a general picture of this section. He showed that vagal stimulation produces slowing of the heart rate (inhibition) which after cessation of stimulation is followed by tachycardia. He could exclude reflex factors being responsible for the tachycardia and suggested that the excitatory substance is a catecholamine (on reserpinized dogs' postvagal bradycardia rather than tachycardia occurs; propranolol reduces the postvagal tachycardia). Somewhat unexpected is the finding that the postvagal tachycardia is not mediated via sympathetic fibers in the vagal trunc, nor seem catecholamines to be released from sympathetic nerve endings (the postvagal tachycardia is not abolished after pharmacological destruction of the sympathetic nerves). It seems likely that the ACh induced release of catecholamines occurs from extraneural stores like chromaffine cells. Such cells have been shown to occur in the sinus node and were reported to receive a cholinergic innervation. This seems to me a new and interesting explanation of postvagal tachycardia which might play a role under physiological conditions.

ACh is often been used in the experiments presented in this section and it has been said that the mode of action of this drug is both to increase the potassium permeability and to inhibit the slow inward current. I would like to add some material related to these effects of ACh. The increase in the potassium permeability has been shown in both flux experiments (Harris and Hutter, 1956, frog's sinus venosus and auricle, and Nawrath, 1977, the rat atrium) and in electrophysiological experiments in the dog atrium. One of these latter results is shown in Figure 2. Two microelectrodes for measuring the membrane potentials and for intracellular application of current square pulses remained stable

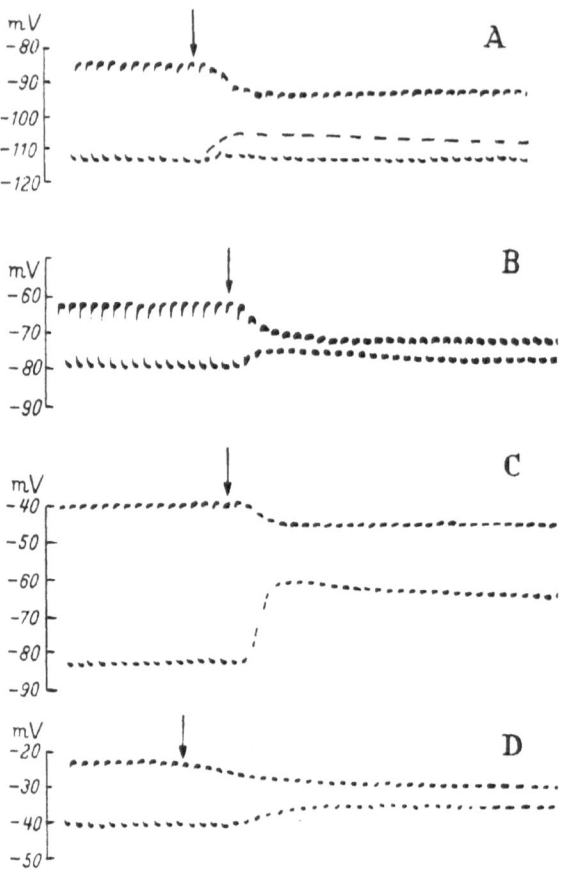

Figure 2. Experiment on a dog atrial trabeculum to show the reversal potential of the ACh effect. From A to D: Electrotonic potentials (duration 100 msec, interval 100 msec) hyperpolarized the membrane to a level 20 to 40 mV more negative than the resting potential. Potassium concentrations: A) 2.7 mM. B 11.8 mM; C 21.5 mM; D 54 mM. ACh, applied at the arrows reduced the amplitude of the electronic potential and produced hyperpolarization at the level of the resting potential in contrast to depolarization at the level of the artificially increased membrane potential. The reversal potential of the ACh effect in between the two potential levels is the less negative the higher the potassium concentration in the Tyrode's solution. The dashed line in A shows the estimated course of the potential which had to be expected when the resting potential would have been increased in a larger area of the preparation (see Trautwein and Dudel, 1958a).

(With permission of Pflügers Archiv and Springer Verlag.)

Figure 4. Effect of ACh (5×10^{-6} M) on the membrane current of a guinea pig atrial fibre. Depolarizing clamp steps lasting 800 msec were applied from a holding potential of -50 mV to the potentials indicated on each panel. Currents obtained 2 min after the introduction of ACh are identified by the dashed top trace on each panel; the center traces are the control currents. The ACh current record is offset with regard to the control record; 0 current positions are indicated on the side of the upper left panel (control solid line; ACh, dashed line). ACh increased the steady state outward current with little effect on delayed rectification, and depressed the slow inward current at each potential (from Ten Eick et al., 1976).

(With permission of Pflügers Archiv and Springer Verlag.)

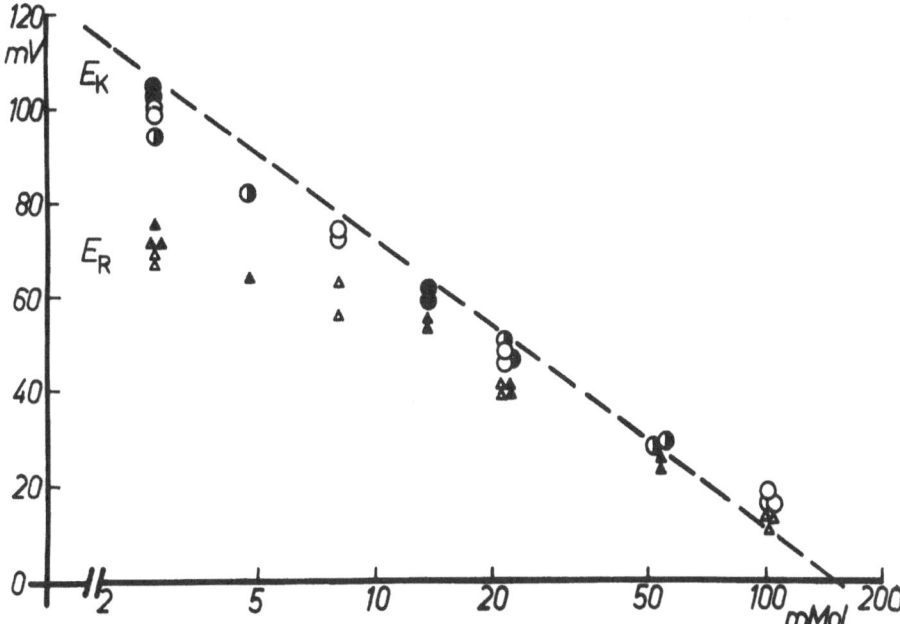

Figure 3. Dependence of the resting potential E_R ($\triangle$) and the equilibrium potentials for the ACh effect (o, ordinate) on the extracellular potassium concentration (abscissa). The dashed line indicates the potassium potential E_R according to the Nernst equation. The different symbols mark different experiments (from Trautwein and Dudel, 1958a).

(With permission of Pflügers Archiv. and Springer Verlag.)

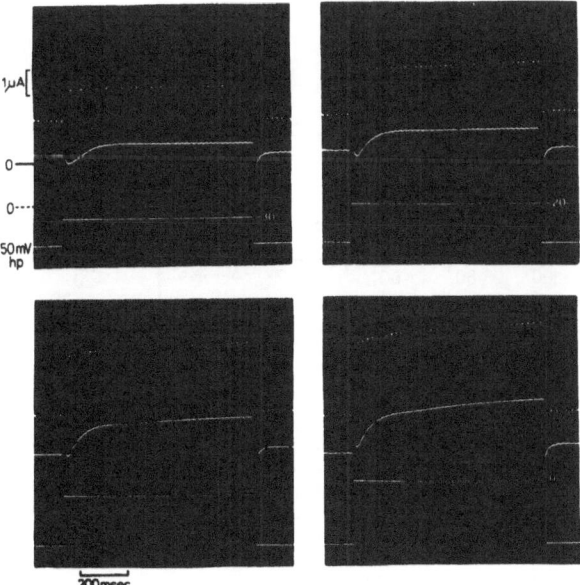

in adjacent cells of a trabeculum from a dog's atrium during four changes of the potassium concentration in the Tyrode's solution. During incubation in each of these solutions electrotonic potentials produced periodically hyperpolarization. ACh applied at the arrows reduced the amplitude of the electrotonic potential, i.e., increased the membrane conductance. The resting potential which was the less negative the higher the extra-cellular potassium concentration became more negative. In between the two potential levels is the reversal potential at which ACh produces no change in membrane potential. The reversal potential is the less negative the larger the extracellular potassium concentration. A plot of the reversal potentials vs. the logarithm of the extracellular potassium concentration indicates that the reversal potential is related to $[K]_o$ in a manner expected for a potassium electrode. The dotted line in Figure 3 has a slope of 61 mV/decade. This result suggests that ACh increases the potassium conductance in this structure, thereby producing hyperpolarization and shortening of the action potential. A close relation between the shortening of the action potential and the square of the electrotonic potential has indeed been shown (Trautwein and Dudel, 1958b).

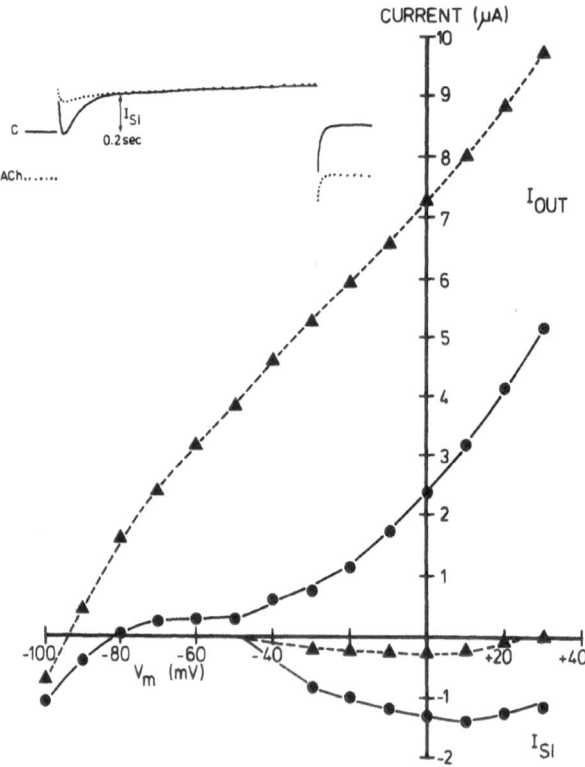

Figure 5. Voltage relations of the outward and slow inward current measured in an experiment like that shown in Figure 4. Symbols connected by dashed curved are currents recorded in presence of ACh (5 × 10⁻⁸ M). Note the suppression of the slow inward current and the large increase of the outward current in presence of ACh. The outward current was measured 800 msec after the onset of the clamp with respect to 0 current. The slow inward current of the control run was measured as difference between the peak inward directed current and the current 200 msec after the start of the pulse (see inset which shows super-imposed control (C) and ACh currents from the −10 mV step in Figure 4. (For details see Eick, et al., 1976). (With permission of Pflügers Archiv and Springer Verlag.)

Recently another interesting effect of ACh has been reported by Ikemoto and Goto (1975), Ten Eick et al. (1976), Giles and Noble (1976). Figure 4 shows the membrane currents recorded from an atrial preparation of the guinea pig in response to voltage clamp steps (bottom trace in each panel) of increasing amplitude. The control currents (middle traces) display at the beginning of the clamp step the slow inward current and later outward current. The currents recorded during administration of ACh (dashed traces) show suppression of the slow inward current and a marked increase in the outward current without a detectable change of its time course. The complete result of this experiment is shown in Figure 5. ACh increases the steady state outward current (the current amplitude at the end of the clamp pulse) and suppresses the slow inward current in the voltage range studied. The results shown in Figures 4 and 5 were obtained with a relatively high concentration of ACh (5×10^{-6} M) which reduced the amplitude of contraction to 10% of that of the control. Using lower concentrations which in a given atrial preparation reduced the force of contraction to 60–70% only, we found the slow inward current not detectably reduced whereas the outward current was increased. Thus, in atrial preparations of guinea pig the effect of ACh to increase the potassium conductance seems to be more sensitive than the inhibition of the slow inward channel. Wether this result would also be obtained in voltage clamp experiments on the mammalian sinus node remains to be seen. In frog's atrium Giles and Noble (1976) found inhibition of the slow inward current with smaller doses than required to increase the potassium conductance and this might be true for the frog sinus venosus too. It is quite possible that considerable species differences exist in regard to the ACh sensitivity of the two mechanisms.

Recently cyclic GMP has been discussed as the intracellular mediator of the cholinergic innervation. In this respect Nawrath (1977) has obtained results which suggest that the depressing effect of ACh on the slow inward current might be mediated by c GMP in contrast to the effect on the potassium permeability which seems unrelated to c GMP. He found in electrically driven rat atria that 8-bromo-cyclic GMP reduced the force and shortened the action potential (see Figure 6). Under the same experimental conditions c GMP reduced the uptake of tracer Ca but did not change the ^{42}K efflux as did ACh.

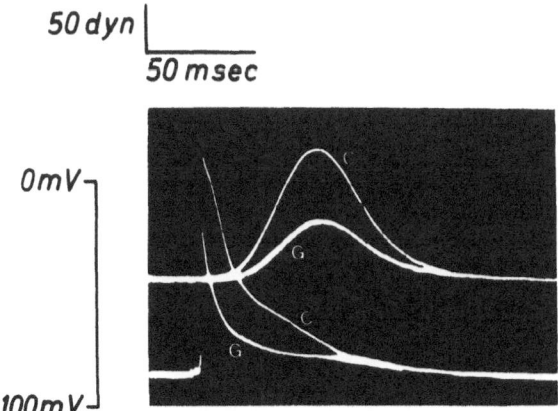

Figure 6. Effects of 10^{-4} M 8-bromo-cyclic GMP on isometric force (middle traces) and transmembrane action potential (other traces) in a rat left auricle after 60 min. C, control; G, 8-Bromo-cyclic GMP.

REFERENCES

Bozler, E.: The initiation of impulses in cardiac muscle. *Amer J Physiol* 138: 273, 1943

Dudel, J., Trautwein, W.: Der Mechanismus der automatischen rhythmischen Impulsbildung der Herz-muskelfaser. *Pflügers Arch* 267: 553, 1958

Giles, W., Noble, S.J.: Changes in membrane currents in Bullfrog atrium produced by acetylcholine. *J Physiol* 261: 103, 1976

Hutter, O.F., Trautwein, W.: Vagal and sympathetic effects on the pacemaker fibres in the sinus venosus of the heart. *J gen Physiol* 39: 715, 1956

Ikemoto, Y., Goto, M.: Nature of the negative inotropic effect of acetylcholine on the myocardium. An elucidation on the bullfrog atrium. *Proc Japan Acad* 51: 501, 1975

McDonald, T.F., Trautwein, W.: The potassium current underlying delayed rectification in cat ventricular muscle. *J. Physiol* 274: 217, 1978

Nawrath H.: Does cyclic GMP mediate the negative inotropic effect of acetylcholine in the heart. *Nature* 267: 72, 1977

Noble, D.: The initiation of the heart beat. Oxford University Press, 1975

Ten Eick, R.E., Nawrath, H., McDonald, T.F., Trautwein, W.: On the Mechanism of the Negative Inotropic Effect of Acetylcholine. *Pflügers Arch* 361: 207, 1976

Trautwein, W., Dudel, J.: Zum Mechanismus der Membranwirkung des Acetylcholin an der Herzmuskelfaser. *Pflügers Arch* 266: 324, 1958a

Trautwein, W., Dudel, J.: Hemmende und "erregende" Wirkungen des Acethylcholin am Warmblüter-herzen. Zur Frage der spontanen Erregungsbildung. *Pflügers Arch* 266: 653, 1958b

Weidmann S.: Effect of current flow on the membrane potential of cardiac muscle. *J Physiol* 115: 227, 1951

SECTION FOUR

ON THE MECHANISM OF PACEMAKING
IN THE SINUS NODE

25

IONIC CURRENTS IN RABBIT SINOATRIAL NODE CELLS

AKINORI NOMA, KAORU YANAGIHARA, AND HIROSHI IRISAWA

The voltage clamp method is the most straight forward one to examine ionic currents underlying the membrane potential changes in many excitable tissues. This method was applied to cardiac cells initially by Deck, Kern, and Trautwein (1964), and information on the ionic mechanism of the cardiac action potential was obtained by many investigators (for review, Trautwein, 1973). The cardiac rhythmic activity was also analyzed by the voltage clamp method using the Purkinje fibers (Noble and Tsien, 1968, 1969a and b). However, it was indicated that there are considerable differences in the electrical behavior between the Purkinje fiber and the cells of the sinoatrial node (S-A node) (Brooks and Lu, 1972). The maximum rate of rise of the action potential is the S-A nodal cell is significantly lower than the Purkinje fiber and the pacemaker potential is lower in the S-A nodal cell. Therefore, several attempts have been made to clamp the membrane potential of the primary pacemaker: the frog sinus venosus (Brown, Giles, and Noble, 1976) and the rabbit S-A node (Irisawa, 1972; Seyama, 1976; Noma and Irisawa, 1976a and b).

After applying three different methods: double sucrose gap, single sucrose gap, and the two-microelectrode voltage clamp method, we came to the conclusion that the two-microelectrode method applied to a small specimen is most useful for the mammalian S-A node. In this paper we will try to present a brief summary and a further mathematical analysis of the results obtained in the voltage clamp experiments by the two-microelectrode method.

SMALL S-A NODE SPECIMEN

The rabbit S-A node was cut into small pieces, approximately 0.3 × 0.3 × 0.2 mm. After the dissection the preparation did not show spontaneous activity. Some of the specimen resumed spontaneous activity within 30 min after dissection. After recovery, slow diastolic depolarization, overshoot and maximum rate of rise of the action potential were almost similar to those obtained in an undissected specimen. This small active specimen was favorable for the voltage clamp experiment because of the following four observations: 1) The spontaneous action potential, recorded simultaneously from three different points within the small specimen, coincided well. This fact suggests that virtually no conduction of excitation occurs within this specimen (Noma and Irisawa, 1976a). 2) When the electrical current was applied intracellularly through one microelectrode and electrotonic potentials were recorded with two other microelectrodes, the two electrotonic potentials coincided well. 3) The spatial homogeneity of the potential within the specimen was further tested during the voltage clamp experiments. The membrane potential outside the feedback control differed only a few millivolts from the command potential. 4) The apparent input impedance was greatly increased to 1.4–3.3 MΩ when the size of the specimen was reduced. The membrane time constant was about 12.0 msec (6 experiments) in these small Specimen.

LOW RESTING MEMBRANE POTENTIAL

The steady state current voltage curve crosses the voltage axis at -35 mV to -40 mV in the rabbit S-A node (Noma, 1976). This value is in good agreement with the membrane potential observed in temporarily quiescent S-A node specimen under various experimental conditions (Noma and Irisawa, 1975). On the other hand, the equilibrium potential for K was -100 mV at 2.7 mM $[K]_o$ when it was indirectly measured by the reversal potential of the outward current tail (Noma and Irisawa, 1976b). These facts indicate a considerable amount of leakage current at the resting potential level as has been suggested by Dudel and Trautwein (1958) and by Trautwein and Kassebaum (1961). Supporting this concept is the fact that the resting potential was reduced only by 5 to 10 mV by increasing $[K]_o$ from 2.7 to 25 mM. This insensitivity of the cell membrane to $[K]_o$ is also present in embryonic heart cells showing spontaneous activity (DeHaan and Gotlieb, 1968; Sperelakis, 1972).

INWARD CURRENTS

It is well known that the maximum rate of rise of the S-A node action potential is approximately 5 V/sec and is blocked by Mn and D 600, but insensitive to TTX (for review, see Brooks and Lu, 1972). These facts strongly suggested that the slow inward current system contributes to the S-A node action potential. A slow inward current was indeed recorded in the voltage clamp experiment in the S-A node. Figure 1A gives the voltage clamp record, where the holding potential was -40 mV and the membrane was clamped at 0 mV during 0.1 sec. When the membrane potential was clamped at -40 mV immediately after an action potential, an outward current tail was recorded, which decayed within 3 sec and was followed by a steady inward-going current. The depolarizing pulse was applied at this phase, and the membrane potential (upper trace) and the current (lower trace) were shown at the high time resolution in Figure 1B. The slow inward current on depolarization slowly inactivated; the net inward current continued for about 30 msec. A slowly increasing outward current during depolarization and an outward current tail on repolarization were observed.

When the membrane potential was held negative to -40 mV, a fast inward current was recorded prior to the slow inward current in several successful experiments. The fast inward current was suppressed by 10^{-7} g/ml TTX and was insensitive to 5×10^{-7} g/ml D 600, a methoxyderivative of verapamil (Figure 2). On the other hand, the slow inward current was suppressed by D 600, but was insensitive to TTX (Figure 2). The fast inward current was fully inactivated when the holding potential was less than -40 mV, while the slow inward current was fully inactivated with the holding potential positive to -20 mV. In most of our preparations the transition from phase 4 (diastolic depolarization) to phase 0 (upstroke of the action potential) takes place at about -35 mV. Therefore, most of the fast inward current may be inactivated during the later part of the slow diastolic depolarization. Therefore, the slow inward current may play a major role in the spontaneous action potential in the S-A node cell. The fast inward current is present as a latent

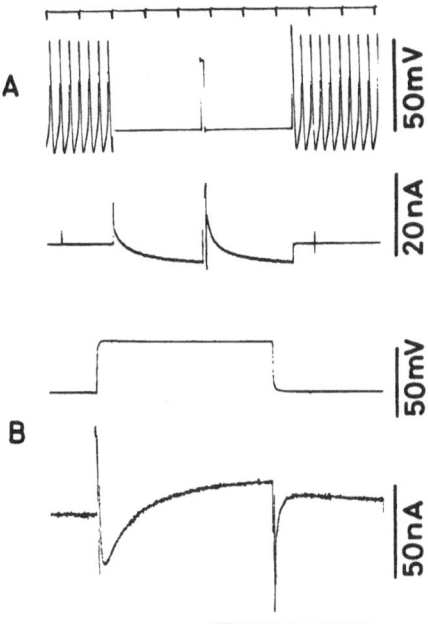

Figure 1. Voltage clamp record in cells of the SA node.

A) top tracing is the marking of 1 sec. Middle tracing is the potential record. Holding potential was −40 mV. Lower tracing is the current record. The small notch at the beginning of the voltage pulse is due to the inertial movement of the recording pen.

B) High speed tracings of the potential (upper curve) and the current (lower curve) of the same voltage clamp as in A. The clamp pulse was 0 mV. Bar indicates 0.1 sec.

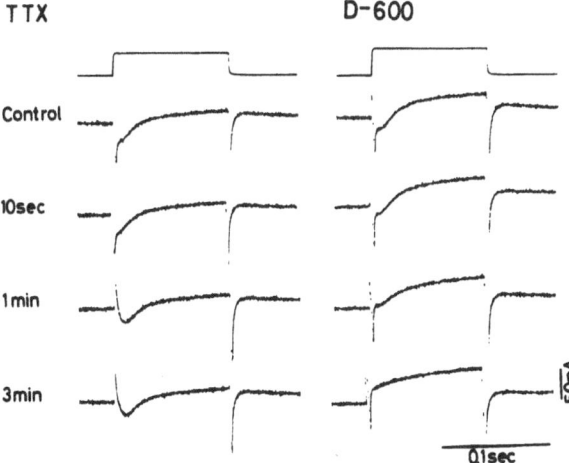

Figure 2. Effects of TTX and D 600 on the fast and slow inward currents of cells of the SA node. Top tracings are the voltage record, holding potential was −40 mV and the clamp was to −10 mV. Lower four tracings are the current record before, and 10 sec, 1 min and 3 min after the application of 1×10^{-7} g/ml TTX (left column) and of 5×10^{-7} g/ml D 600 (right column).

current system in the S-A node cell. These findings are in good agreement with the fact that the action potential is not affected by TTX under normal conditions (Yamagishi and Sano, 1966), but becomes sensitive during hyperpolarization under the effect of carbomyl-choline (Kreitner, 1975).

The pharmacological characteristics of the slow inward current in the S-A node cell are in accord with those of the slow inward current in other cardiac cells, which is carried by Ca, or by both Ca and Na (for review see Trautwein, 1973; Reuter, 1973). In the S-A node the slow inward current may mainly be carried by Na, since the net inward current is abolished on Na removal. However, the contribution of other cations on the slow inward current of the rabbit S-A node cell was suggested by the following observations: 1) the magnitude of the slow inward current in 30% $[Na]_o$ was about 32% of control in normal Tyrode solution. This value is larger than the theoretical value of 18% (at $-$ 10 mV with E_{Na} = 40 mV) (Noma, et al., 1977). 2) The intersection of the slow inward current with the voltage axis was shifted only by about 20 mV in negative direction when $[Na]_o$ was decreased to 30%. 3) The overshoot potential of the S-A node action potential was increased by 12 mV for a ten-fold increase in $[Ca]_o$ in the range of 0.1 to 5.0 mM (Noma and Irisawa, 1976c). 4) Recently, it was found that action potentials were generated by Ba in a Na-free solution.

These findings suggest that the slow inward current system of the S-A node cell is not very selective, since several ions, like Na, Ca and Ba can pass through the slow inward current system. A slow inward current carried by both Na and Ca has been demonstrated in the frog atrium (Rougier et al., 1969; Tarr, 1971), in the Purkinje fiber (Vitek and Trautwein, 1973) and in the mammalian ventricle (Ochi, 1970; Mascher and Peper, 1969; Reuter and Scholz, 1977).

OUTWARD CURRENT TAIL

Figures 1 and 2 show the activation of the outward current during depolarization and a slowly decaying outward current tail on repolarization to the holding potential of -40 mV. The outward current tail decreased exponentially after a relatively short depolarizing pulse of 0.1 to 0.5 sec, indicating that a single current system is responsible for this current tail (Noma and Irisawa, 1976b). The reversal potential of the outward current tail in the S-A node cell was recorded from specimen bathed in various $[K]_o$. The data was fitted by a straight line with a slope of -58 to -60 mV for a ten fold increase in $[K]_o$, indicating that the outward current tail is carried highly selectively by K ions.

In describing the kinetics of the K outward current tail, the Hodgkin-Huxley equations were used, and the rectifying properties were related to the voltage dependency of $\bar{g}$ in the same manner as has been done for the K currents in the Purkinje fiber (McAllister et al., 1975). Since the outward current tail is mainly responsible for the slow diastolic depolarization, the tail current is defined as pacemaker current (I_p) and its kinetic variable as p. The following equations were used:

$$I_p = \bar{g}_p \cdot p \cdot (E - E_k) \tag{1}$$

$$dp/dt = \alpha_p \cdot (1 - p) - \beta_p \cdot p \tag{2}$$

$$p_\infty = \alpha_p/(\alpha_p + \beta_p) \tag{3}$$

$$\tau_p^{-1} = \alpha_p + \beta_p \tag{4}$$

Figure 3 gives the time- and voltage-dependent kinetics of I_p. Based on these experimental data, the rate constant α_p and β_p were determined as follows:

$$\alpha_p = 5.6 \times 10^{-3} \exp(E/11.78) \tag{5}$$

$$\beta_p = 2.55 \times 10^{-4} (40 + E)/(\exp[(40 + E)/13.3] - 1) \tag{6}$$

The curve given in Figure 3A is the reconstructed curve showing the relationship between p_∞ and the membrane potential. The U-shaped curve given in Figure 3B is the computed relation between the τ_p^{-1} and the membrane potential, while the negative slope curve is β_p and the positive slope curve is α_p.

The K outward current system of cells of the S-A node showed the inward-going rectification as the K current systems in the Purkinje fibers (McAllister et al., 1975) and in calf ventricular fibers (McGuigan, 1974). When $\bar{g}_p$ was calculated using equation 1 by the magnitude of the tail current, the E_K, and the decrease of the kinetic variable p, the relationship between $\bar{g}_p$ and the membrane potential showed an inward-going rectification (Noma and Irisawa, 1976b). By fitting the experimental data (closed circles in Figure 4A) $\bar{g}_p$ was expressed as a function of the membrane potential. In this calculation it was

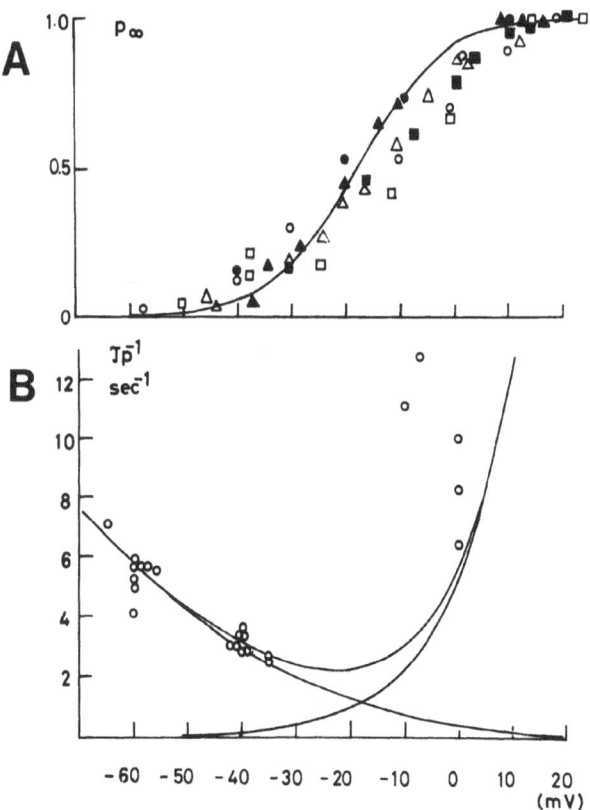

Figure 3. Time- and voltage-dependent kinetics of I_p. Upper graph: voltage dependence of fractional activation (p_∞) in the steady state measured by the magnitude of the outward current tail with a holding potential of −50 to −60 mV. Different symbols indicate different experiment. Lower graph: voltage dependence of τ_p^{-1}. See text for further explanation.

assumed with hyperpolarization $\bar{g}_p$ would approach some limited value and that with depolarization $\bar{g}_p$ would decrease to a minimum value. The relationship between $\bar{g}_p$ and the membrane potential was given as,

$$\bar{g}_p = A/(1 + \exp[(51 + E)/11.61]) \qquad (7)$$

where A is a constant, depending on the size of the specimen, and the curve in Figure 4A was drawn assuming that the A is equal to unity. The computed curve is closely in accordance with the experimental data. Figure 4B shows the fully activated current volt-age relation calculated from equations 1 and 7 with p = 1. It is clear that the I_p system shows an inward-going rectification.

RECONSTRUCTION OF THE OUTWARD CURRENT TAIL

Using the above equations, outward current tails were reconstructed on clamping back to $-20, -31, -42, -55, -68, -78$, and -90 mV, after 2 sec depolarization to 0 mV. The value of I_p was 0.922 when the membrane potential was clamped at 0 mV as long as 2 sec (A was assumed as 1.762×10^{-5} mho). A series of outward current tails, as shown in Figure 5B, was obtained in this way. In Figure 5A the experimental data, obtained under similar experimental conditions as the simulation program except for the duration of the repolarization, which was only 0.5 sec, is given. The calculated current pattern is quite similar to the experimental data.

RECONSTRUCTION OF THE PACEMAKER POTENTIAL

We have the following concept of the ionic mechanism of the pacemaker potential. The outward current is activated during the preceding action potential and decays slowly on repolarization. The slow decay of the outward current associated with the relatively large inward-going background current may be the major cause of the slow diastolic depolar-ization. This was strongly suggested in one of the experiments of foregoing report (Noma and Irisawa, 1976b), where the clamp circuit was switched off at various times during the

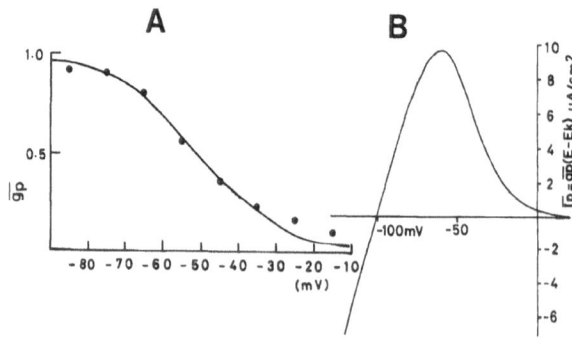

Figure 4. A) Relationship between $\bar{g}_p$ and the membrane potential.
  B) Relationship between $\bar{I}_p$ and the membrane potential. See text for further description.

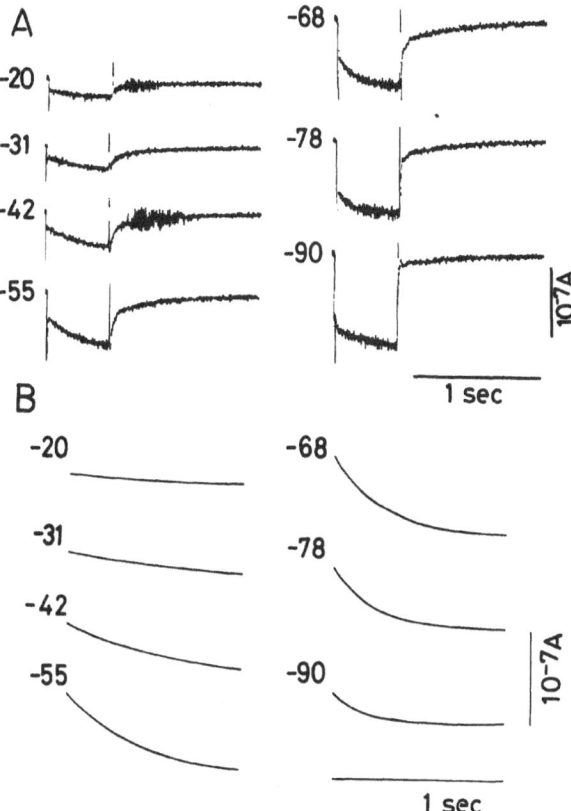

Figure 5. A) Outward current tails recorded in a specimen bathed in the normal Tyrode solution (redrawn from Noma and Irisawa, 1976b).

B) computed outward current tails on repolarization from 0 mV to membrane potentials shown at the left hand of each trace.

outward current tail, and the following membrane potential change was recorded. In this experiment the membrane was clamped at − 10 mV for 0.5 sec and thereafter clamped back to the holding potential of −40 mV. When the clamp circuit was turned off after the disappearance of the outward current tail (2.4 sec after the end of the test pulse) a spontaneous action potential was generated after a quiescent period of about 0.5 sec. Switching off the clamp circuit during the outward current tail, resulted in a hyperpolarization of the membrane followed by a slow diastolic depolarization, which magnitude increased in accordance with the increase in the outward current tail (Figure 12 in Noma and Irisawa, 1976b).

This membrane potential change was reconstructed using kinetics of the I_p. Since kinetics of the other current components are still not available, a "background current" was assumed, which may be carried by Na (Trautwein and Kassebaum, 1961; Noma and Irisawa, 1975) and Cl (Seyama, 1976). In this calculation, the value of the conductance for the total background current (I_{bg}) was determined from the resting potential of − 40 mV, at which $I_p + I_{bg} = 0$. The following equations were used for calculation in addition to the equations 1–7.

$$-C \cdot dV/dT = I_i \tag{8}$$

$$I_i = I_p + I_{bg} \tag{9}$$

$$I_{bg} = g_{bg} \cdot (E - E_{rest}) \tag{10}$$

Figure 6A shows the computed membrane potential change and Figure 6B the decay of p after switching off the clamp circuit. The value of p was 0.611 at the end of the clamp pulse, which was 0.5 sec in duration and to − 10 mV. When the clamp circuit was switched off, the membrane is hyperpolarized by I_p and the outward-going I_{bg}. The I_{bg} is then gradually reduced as the membrane potential approached the resting potential, and after crossing the resting potential level, the I_{bg} is in an inward-going direction. However, I_p will increase rapidly due to the inward-going rectification at about −30 mV, resulting in an obvious hyperpolarization of the membrane. At about −70 mV, the values of I_p and I_{bg} approximated each other closely and the maximum diastolic potential will then be reached.

Thereafter, I_p will gradually deactivate (a′, b′, and c′ in Figure 6B) and inward-going I_{bg} will become predominant, depolarizing the membrane toward the resting potential.

It is clear in Figure 6 that this system never discharges spontaneously. On the other hand, S-A node cells discharge spontaneously under the condition where almost no outward current tail remains as in Figure 12 in Noma and Irisawa's paper (1976b). The dotted line in Figure 6d shows a calculated action potential. However, in order to clarify the role of the slow inward current system, completing the later phase of the pacemaker potential, determination of the kinetics of the slow inward current system is awaited.

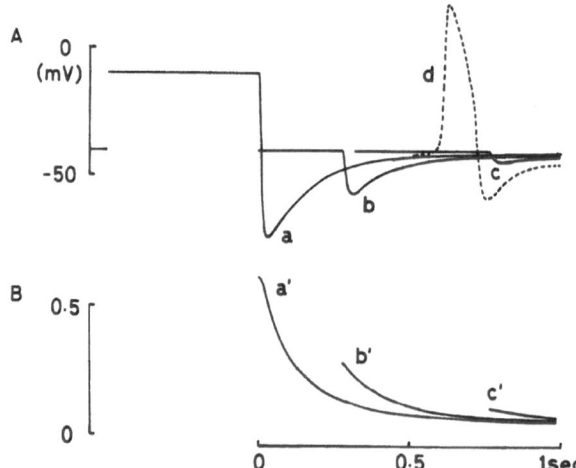

Figure 6. Computed membrane potential changes (A) after the clamp was switched off: (A) immediately at the end of the clamp pulse, (B) 280 msec, (C) 780 msec after the end of the clamp pulse, respectively. Corresponding changes in the kinetic variable p are shown in B (a′, b′, and c′). Dotted line in A-d indicates the action potential which was reconstructed with the preliminary kinetics of the membrane currents in the S-A node cell.

ACKNOWLEDGEMENT

This work was supported by grants from the Ministry of Education, Science and Culture of Japan, Japan Heart Foundation and the Mitsubishi Science Foundation.

REFERENCES

1. Brooks, C.McC., Lu, H.H.: The sinoatrial pacemaker of the heart. Springfield, Ill., Charles C. Thomas, 1972
2. Brown, H.F., Giles, W., Noble, S.J.: Voltage clamp of frog sinus venosus. *J Physiol (London) (abstract)* 258: 78, 1976
3. Deck, K.A., Kern, R., Trautwein, W.: Voltage clamp technique in mammalian cardiac fibres. *Pflügers Archiv* 280: 50, 1964
4. DeHaan, R.L., Gottlieb, S.H.: The electrical activity of embryonic chick heart cells isolated in tissue culture singly or interconnected cell shiets. *J gen Physiol* 52: 643, 1968
5. Dudel, J., Trautwein, W.: Der Mechanismus der automatischen rhythmischen Impulsbildung der Herz-muskelfaser. *Pflügers Archiv* 267: 553, 1958
6. Irisawa, H.: Electrical activity of rabbit sino-atrial node as studied by a double sucrose gap method. In Symposium and colloquium on the electrical field of the heart. P. Rijlant (ed.), Bruxelles, Presses Acade-miques Europeenes, 1972
7. Kreitner, D.: Evidence for the existence of a rapid sodium channel in the membrane of rabbit sinoatrial cells. *J Mol and Cell Cardiology* 7: 655, 1975
8. Mascher, D., Peper, K.: Two components of inward current in myocardial muscle fibers. *Pflügers Archiv* 307: 190, 1969
9. McAllister, R.E., Noble, D., Tsien, R.W.: Reconstruction of the electrical activity of cardiac Purkinje fibres. *J Physiol* 251: 1, 1975
10. McGuigan, J.A.S.: Some limitations of the double sucrose gap, and its use in a study of the slow outward current in mammalian ventricular muscle. *J Physiol* 240: 775, 1974
11. Noble, D., Tsien, R.W.: The kinetics and rectifier properties of the slow potassium current in cardiac Purkinje fibres. *J Physiol* 195: 185, 1968
12. Noble, D., Tsien, R.W.: Outward membrane currents activated in the plateau range of potentials in car-diac Purkinje fibres. *J Physiol* 200: 205, 1969a
13. Noble, D., Tsien, R.W.: Reconstruction of the repolarization process in cardiac Purkinje fibres based on voltage clamp measurements of membrane current. *J Physiol* 200: 233, 1969b
14. Noma, A.: Mechanisms underlying cessation of rabbit sinoatrial node pacemaker activity in high potas-sium solutions. *Jap J Physiol* 26: 619, 1976
15. Noma, A., Irisawa, H.: Effects of Na$^+$ and K$^+$ on the resting membrane potential of the rabbit sinoatrial node cell. *Jap J Physiol* 25: 287, 1975
16. Noma, A., Irisawa, H.: Membrane currents in the rabbit sinoatrial node cell as studied by the double microelectrode method. *Pflügers Archiv* 364: 45, 1976a
17. Noma, A., Irisawa, H.: A time- and voltage-dependent potassium current in the rabbit sinoatrial node cell. *Pflügers Archiv* 366: 251, 1976b
18. Noma, A., Irisawa, H.: Effects of calcium ion on the rising phase of the rabbit sinoatrial node cells. *Jap J Physiol* 26: 93, 1976c
19. Noma, A., Yanagihara, K., Irisawa, H.: Inward current of the rabbit sinoatrial node cell. *Pflügers Archiv* 372: 43, 1977
20. Ochi, R.: The slow inward current and the action of manganese ions in guinea-pig's myocardium. *Pflügers Archiv* 316: 81, 1970
21. Reuter, H.: Divalent cations as charge carriers in excitable membranes. *Prog Biophys mol Biol* 26: 1–43, 1973
22. Reuter, H., Scholz, H.: A study of the ion selectivity and the kinetic properties of the calcium dependent slow inward current in mammalian cardiac muscle. *J Physiol* 264: 17, 1977
23. Rougier, O., Vassort, G., Garnier, D., Gargouil, Z.M., Coraboeuf, E.: Existence and role of a slow in-ward current during the frog atrial action potential. *Pflügers Archiv* 308: 91, 1969
24. Seyama, I.: Characteristics of the rectifying properties of the sino-atrial node cell of the rabbit. *J Physiol* 255: 379, 1976
25. Sperelakis, N.: Electrical properties of embryonic heart cells. In: Electrical Phenomena in the Heart, edited by W.C. De Mello. Academic Press New York, p. 1–61, 1972

26. Tarr. M.: Two inward currents in frog atrial muscle. *J Gen Physiol* 58: 55, 1971
27. Trautwein, W.: Membrane currents in cardiac muscle fibers. *Physiol Rev* 53: 793, 1973
28. Trautwein, W., Kassebaum, D.G.: On the mechanism of spontaneous impulse generation in the pace-maker of the heart. *J Gen Physiol* 45: 317, 1961
29. Vitek, M., Trautwein, W.: Slow inward current and action potential in cardiac Purkinje fibres. *Pflügers Archiv* 323: 204, 1971
30. Yamagishi, S., Sano, T.: Effect of tetrodotoxine on the pacemaker action potential of the sinus node. *Proc Japan Acad* 42: 1194, 1966

26

FINE STRUCTURE OF THE SMALL SINOATRIAL NODE SPECIMEN USED FOR THE VOLTAGE CLAMP EXPERIMENT

AYA IRISAWA

Recently, much histological work concerning the sino-atrial (S-A) node of various animals has been published (Hayashi, 1962; Torii, 1962; Trautwein and Uchizono, 1963; Kawamura and Hayashi, 1966; James et al., 1966; Viragh and Porte, 1969; Kawamura, 1974; Irisawa, 1976; Tranum-Jensen, 1976; Masson-Pévet et al., 1978; Tranum-Jensen, 1978). Almost all observations of these authors agree with respect to the following points: 1) The myocardial cells in the S-A nodal region were classified in three types: the nodal cell, the intermediate type of cell and the atrial type of cell. 2) Fundamental structures within the three types of cells, such as myofibrils, mitochondria, sarcoplasmic reticulum and cell junctional organization, differ only quantitatively. 3) The location and arrangement of those structures in the cell differ from one type to the other.

In the present study the interest was focused especially on the connection between the cells, since some authors were not sure about the existence of nexus connections between nodal cells (Trautwein and Uchizone, 1963; James et al., 1966) although the electrophysiological data suggested that low resistance pathways between the nodal cells as well as the intermediate cells are present (Bonke, 1973; Seyama, 1976). Furthermore, it appeared to be necessary to have more precise criteria of both the nodal and the intermediate type of cell, especially in relation with the configuration of the preparation that was used for voltage clamp experiments by Irisawa and Noma and co-workers.

METHOD

After the rabbit was killed by a blow in the neck, the right atrium was isolated. Several thin strands – less than 1 mm in width – of the sinus node were made by dissecting the preparation perpendicularly to the crista terminalis (Figure 1). After dissecting almost all the remaining muscular parts of the crista terminalis, a strand of 0.3–0.5 mm in length was chosen for a physiological experiment. For histological examination a strand adjacent to this latter was taken.

The small specimen were fixed by 4% glutaraldehyde in 0.1 M cacodylate buffer (pH 7.4) and post fixed by 1% OsO_4 solution in s-collidin buffer (pH 7.35). Blocks were stained with 1% $KMnO_4$-aceton solution at the end of dehydration in graded aceton series. Specimen were embedded in Epon-812 mixture. Less than 1 μM thick sections, stained with with toluidine blue alkaline solution, were used for light microscopic examination. Ultrathin sections were stained with uranyl acetate and lead, examined by the electron-microscope, Hitachi HS 7 and JEM 100-S.

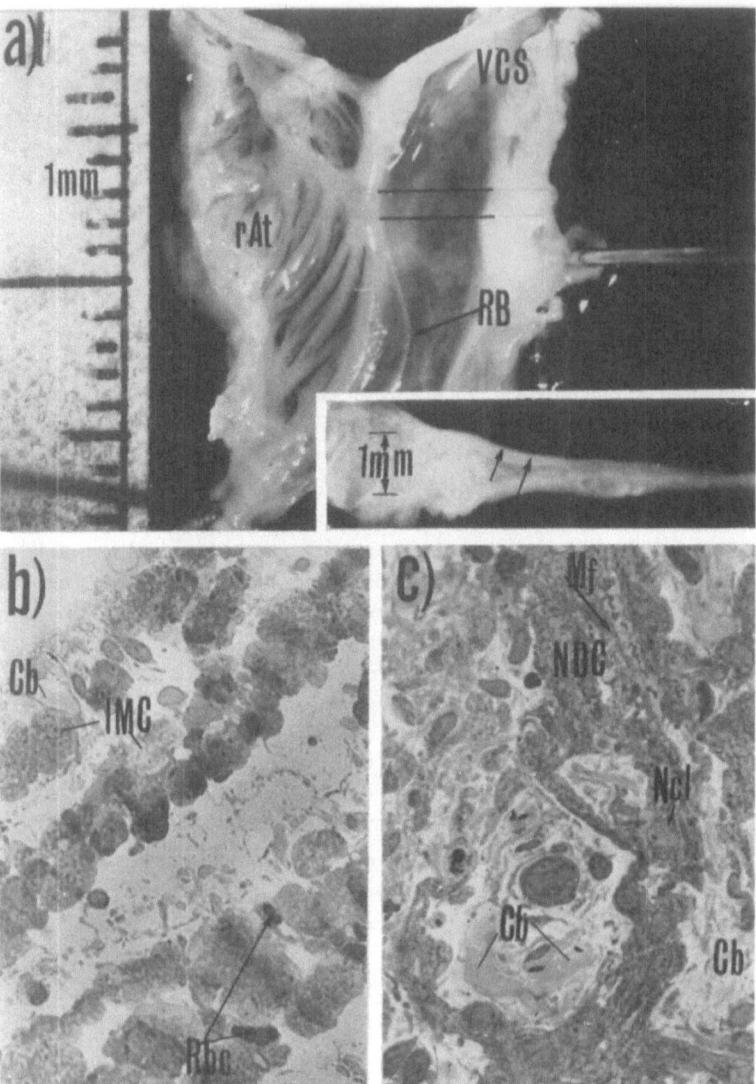

Figure 1. a: Photograph of a right atrium preparation. Specimen cut perpendicular to the crista terminalis is shown by the two parallel lines. Inset shows one of such pieces of S-A node. Present histological examination was made between the two arrows. Figures 1b and c show examples of light microscopic view of the intermediate type and the nodal type, respectively. (×1000).

Abbreviation in Figures

Bm	basement membrane	Nex	nexus
Cb	collagen bundle	NDC	nodal cell
Cf	collagen fibril	Ncl	nucleus
Ds	desmosome	Sc	subsarcolemmal cisterna
Ecs	extracellular space		(peripheral coupling)
Gly	glycogen granules	Pv	pinocytotic vesicles
Gv	Golgi vesicles	Rbc	red blood cell
IMC	intermediate cell	rsr	rough surface sarcoplasmic reticulum
Mf	myofibrils	tfc	thin filaments
Mt	mitochondria	VCS	Vena cava superior
Nb	nerve bundle	VCI	Vena cava inferior

RESULTS AND DISCUSSIONS

Serial sections have been made through the specimen. Samples for electron microscopy were taken non-selectively during advancement of the sectioning.

LIGHT MICROSCOPIC VIEW

Several thin muscle strands separated by broad connective tissue spaces, containing vascular- and nervous-elements, were observed. Some clusters of these muscle cells were located very close to the endocardium, but the majority of them was not, in this level of the section (Figure 1b). This might be the reason why the microelectrode can easily penetrate at some sites but not in others during the electrophysiological experiments. Some cells appeared clearer than others, because of the paucity of cellular elements.

Towards the atrial septum, the diameter of the strand becomes thinner and its collagenous space surrounding bilaterally the clusters of cells becomes wider. At this level of section, a part of the cell cluster forms a network and looses the parallel orientation. Sectioning further in the same direction, another type of cell begins to appear among these cell clusters. These cells have a small number of mitochondria, a round nucleus and a few irregularly oriented myofibrils. As the sectioning is advancing further, the network of this type of cells becomes denser (Figure 1c). The specialized contact organization, such as intercalated discs, is not found (James et al., 1966).

It is difficult to define the cell boundary between adjacent cells under the light microscope, because the gap between two facing membranes is often very narrow, less than 200 Å, and because of the polyhedral orientation. These two types of cells correspond to the "intermediate" and "nodal" type of previous authors.

ELECTRONMICROSCOPICAL VIEW

The typical nodal cells are characterized by their small irregular shape with the polyhedral mutual contacts, a few single myofibrils with a few myofilaments, and very short filamentous structures running at random through the myoplasm (Figures 3 and 5). A deep invagination of the sarcolemma was not found (James et al., 1966). There are no T-tubules in nodal cells. Desmosomal attachments are often found in both the nodal and the intermediate type of cells (Figures 2 and 3).

The short nexus appeared between the nodal cells in either end to end (Figure 5), or side by side (Figures 3, 4, 6) configuration. Because nexus are short and thin and relatively rare in nodal cells, they have seldom been found previously. Frequent occurrence of desmosomes and lack of nexus in nodal cell sections raised once a hypothesis that the desmosome plays a role as low resistance pathway between nodal cells (James et al., 1966). The present findings of nexus in the nodal cell, support the electrophysiological findings of Bonke (1973) and Seyama (1976), estimating the space constant of nodal cells to be about 0.5 and 0.8 mm, respectively. Recently, Tranum-Jansen (1976, 1978), Masson-Pévet (1978), Viragh and Porte (1973), Kawamura (1974) and Irisawa (1976) also reported on the existence of nexus connection between nodal cells. Sarcoplasmic reticulum in the nodal cell is not abundant and its distribution within the cell is not well organized. They do not form lace-like networks surrounding myofibrils, but there are many subsarcolemmal cisterna (Figures 3 and 4).

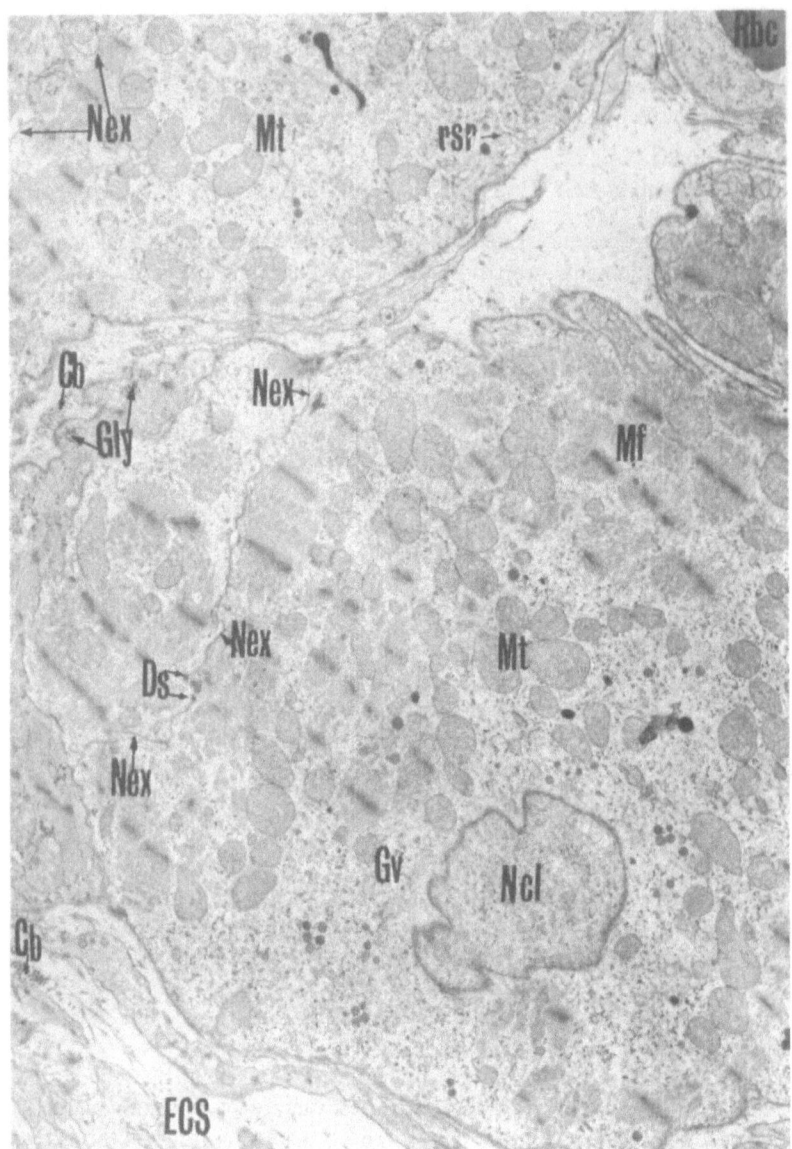

Figure 2. Electronmicrograph of an intermediate type of cell. 5 nexuses and 2 desmosomes are found along the cell boundary. Myofibrils and mitochondria are less frequent than in the working myocardium × 6600. For abbreviations see legend Figure 1.

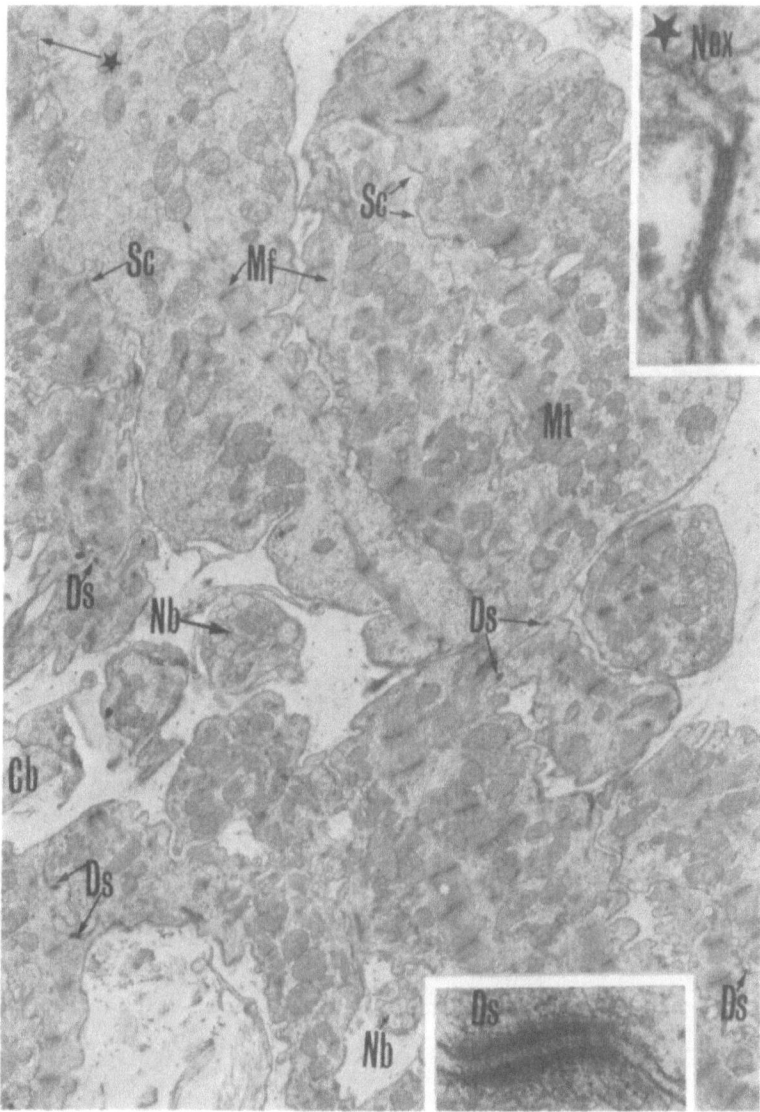

Figure 3. A part of nodal cell cluster. There are a few thin myofibrils running at random to the cell axis. The adjacent cells contact each other with small processes. × 5000.

One small nexus contact (asterisk and arrow at the upper left corner) is enlarged and shown in the inset in right upper corner, × 200,000

Higher magnification of desmosome in the inset right lower corner is also shown. x 100,000. For abbreviations see legend Figure 1.

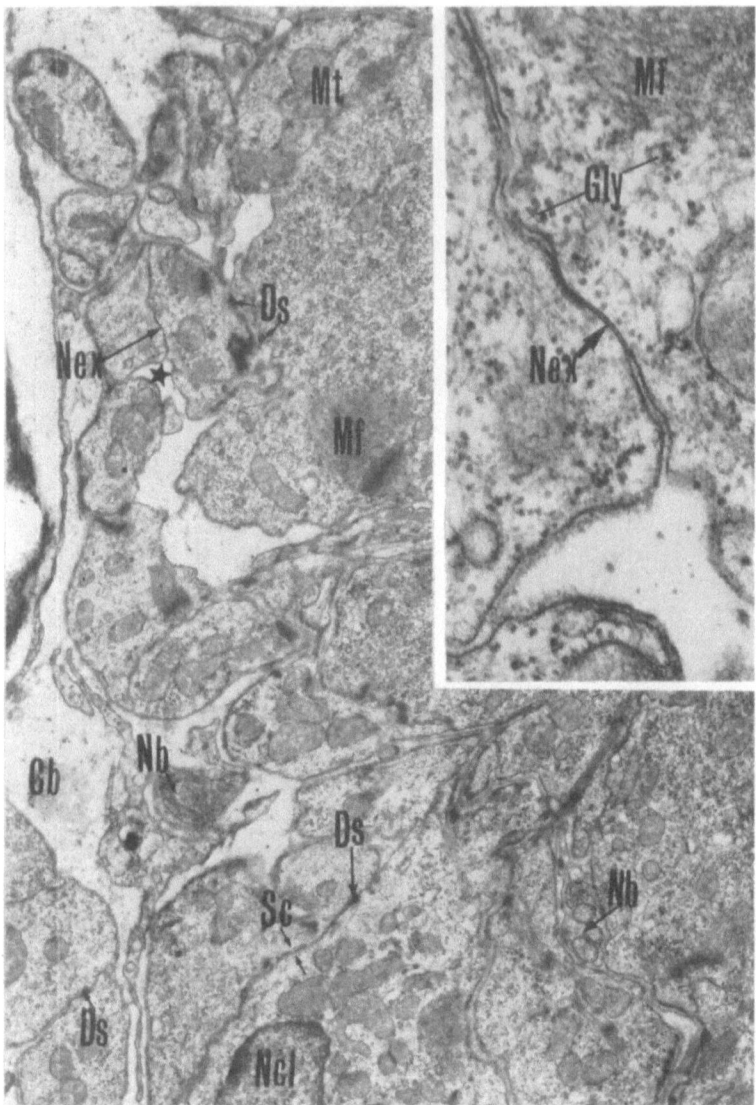

Figure 4. An oblique section of a nodal cell. A few myofibrils running at random, therefore their length and their running directions cannot be estimated. Nexus between adjacent cells is short, in case of side by side connection. (×13,000). Inset is an enlarged picture of cell junctions (×68,000). For abbreviations see legend Figure 1.

Numerous pinocytotic vesicles or surface vesicles corresponding to the vacuoles nominated by Tranum-Jensen (1976) are also found (Figures 5 and 6). Both subsarcolemmal cisterna and pinocytotic vesicles can be seen either at the free surface, covered with basement membrane, or intracellular. Electron-density of the content of the vesicles differs from that of the basement membrane itself. Whether these vesicles might be a site of Ca-exchange as has been discussed for smooth muscle (Devine et al., 1972) or might increase the membrane capacity (Tranum-Jensen, 1976) has to be studied further.

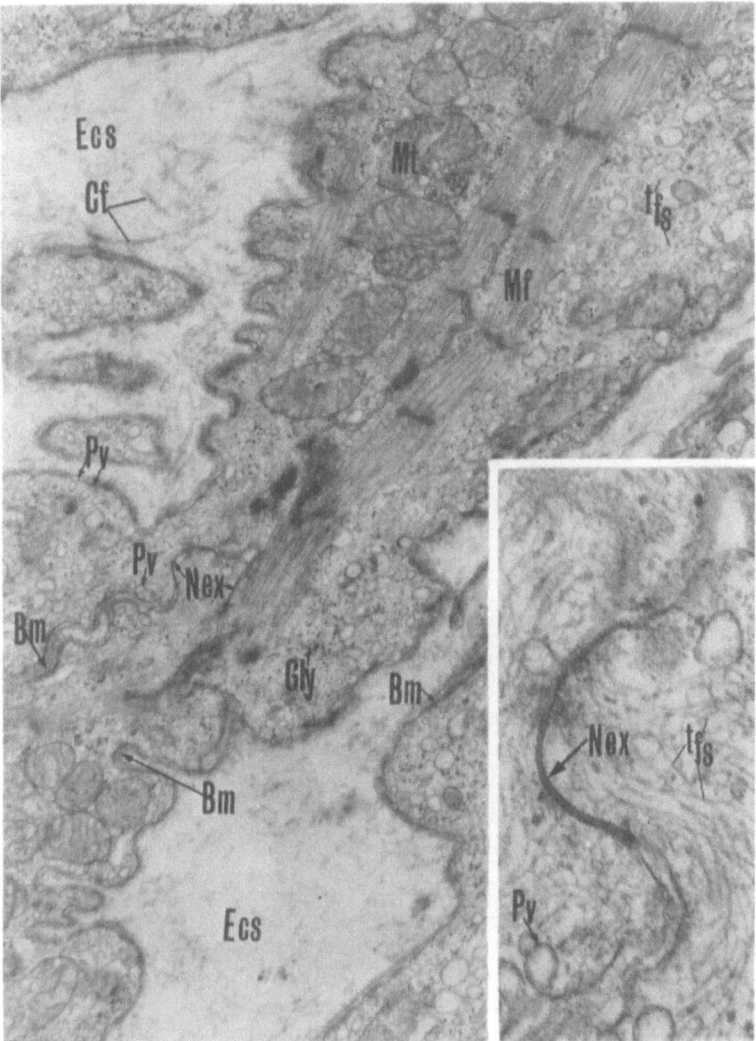

Figure 5. A longitudinal section of nodal cells. At the cell junction two nexus connections are observed (end to end). Many pinocytotic vesicles and subsarcolemmal cisterna are also seen. 24,000 (inset ×94,000). For abbreviations see legend of Figure 1.

CONCLUSION

S-A node specimen within the limited area, which have been employed in the physiological experiments, contained mainly two types of myocytes. They seem to have the same morphological features of the nodal and intermediate type of cells, respectively, as classified by others. In the present study, nexus connections between nodal cells as well as between the intermediate type of cells, were found, in nodal cells less frequent than in intermediate cells.

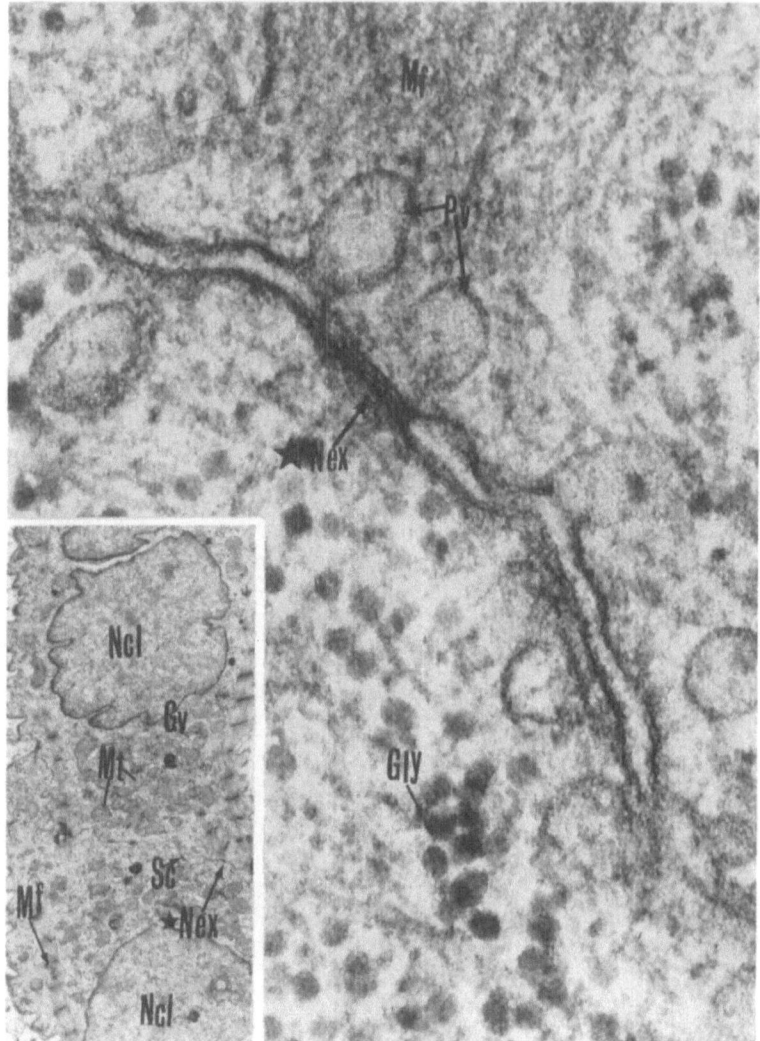

Figure 6. Very small nexus between nodal cells. Nexus occupies very small portion of the whole cross sectional area of the cell. Pinocytotic vesicles are also observed in the same cell boundary. × 250,000. The inset picture shows the two adjacent nodal cells having the nexus junction. × 5400. For abbreviations see legend of Figure 1.

ACKNOWLEDGEMENT

This study was supported by the Ministry of Education, Science and Culture of Japan, The Japan Heart Foundation and the Mitsubishi Science Foundation.

REFERENCES

Bonke, F.I.M.: Electrotonic spread in the sinoatrial node of the rabbit heart. *Pflügers Archiv* 339: 17, 1973
Devine, C.E., Somlyo, A.V., Somlyo, A.P.: Sarcoplasmic reticulum and excitation-contraction coupling in mammalian smooth muscles. *J Cell Biol* 52: 690, 1972

Irisawa, A.: The fine structure of the sinoatrial node of the rabbit heart. (abstract) In the 8th Natl. Mtg. of the Intr. Study Group for Research in Cardiac Metabolism, p 151, 1976

James, T.N., Sherf, L., Fine, G., Morles, A.R.: Comparative ultrastructure of the sinus node in Man and Dog. *Circulation* 34: 139, 1966

Hayashi, K.: An electron microscope study of the conduction system of the cow heart. *Jap Circ J* 26: 765, 1962

Kawamura, K., Hayashi, K.: Electron microscope study of the cardiac conduction system. *Jap Circ J* 30: 149, 1966

Kawamura, K.: Sino-atrial node and atrio-ventricular node. In: Conduction system (in Japanese), edited by Sano, T. Igaku Shoin Co., Tokyo, p. 22, 1974

Masson-Pévet, M., Bleeker, W.K., Mackaay, A.J.C., Gros, D., Bouman, L.N.: Ultrastructural and functional aspects of the rabbit sino-atrial node. This book, 1978

McNutt, N.S., Fawcett, W.: The ultrastructure of cat myocardium. II. Atrial muscle 42: 46, 1969

Seyama, I.: Characteristics of the rectifying properties of the sino-atrial node cell of the rabbit. *J Physiol* 255: p. 379, 1976

Torii, H.: Electron microscope observation of the S-A and A-V nodes and Purkinje fibers of the rabbit. *Jap Circ J* 26: 39, 1962

Tranum-Jensen, J.: The fine structure of the atrial and atrio-ventricular (AV) junctional specialized tissues of the rabbit heart. In: The conduction system of the heart, Structure, Function and Clinical implications, edited by Wellens, H.J.J., Lie, K.I., Janse, M.J. Stenfert Kroese, Leiden, p. 296, 1976

Tranum-Jensen, J.: Fine structure of the sinus node. This book, 1978

Trautwein, W., Uchizono, K.: Electron microscopic and electrophysiological study of the pacemaker in sino-atrial node of the rabbit heart. *Zeitsch Zellforsch* 61: 96, 1963

27

MEMBRANE CURRENTS UNDERLYING RHYTHMIC ACTIVITY IN FROG SINUS VENOSUS

HILARY BROWN, WAYNE GILES, AND SUSAN NOBLE

In the early 1950s, intracelluar microelectrode recordings demonstrated conclusively that the myogenic rhythm of the heart originates in the sinus venosus of amphibia and the sino-atrial region of mammals (Trautwein and Zink, 1952; Brady and Hecht, 1954; del Castillo and Katz, 1955; Hutter and Trautwein, 1955; West, 1955). Subsequently, a large number of microelectrode studies have described the changes in the pacemaker depolarization and the action potential which are produced by polarizing current pulses, by autonomic transmitters and by changes of ionic environment (see Brooks and Lu, 1972; West, 1972).

However, in order to make a quantitative study of the membrane currents underlying spontaneous pacemaker activity in cardiac muscle it is necessary to hold the membrane potential of sinus tissue constant at known values while simultaneously monitoring the current flow. This, the voltage clamp technique, has proved difficult to apply to natural pacemaker cells presumably because of their small size and irregular arrangement (Virágh and Porte, 1973). Thus, until 1976, only one preliminary report of voltage clamp experiments on primary pacemaker tissue had appeared (Irisawa, 1972). Recently, however, certain changes in technique have allowed rabbit sino-atrial node cells (Seyama, 1976; Noma and Irisawa, 1976a and b) and frog sinus venosus tissue (Brown et al., 1976, 1977b) to be successfully voltage clamped.

In this paper we describe the voltage clamp of the sinus venosus of the American bullfrog *R. catesbeiana* using a double sucrose gap technique. Since its success depends largely upon the nature of the sinus tissue used, it is important to describe the dissection procedure itself and the criteria applied to distinguish sinus from atrial cells.

It has long been assumed that the junction between frog sinus venosus and frog atrial cells is very distinct and lies at the boundary between trabecular and non-trabecular regions visible in isolated, opened frog sino-atrial preparations. We have found that the physiological transition is not strictly correlated with the anatomical one and that a band of trabecular cells surrounding the borders of the "anatomical" sinus and running into the atrial wall and interatrial septum exhibit all the accepted properties of primary sinus tissue. Thus application of tetrodotoxin (TTX) to the sinus venosus and atria of a frog heart, opened up and beating in a dissection dish, shows this band of tissue to be highly TTX-resistant to doses of TTX which render the atria completely quiescent. It is from this region that our preparations come.

The distal ends of such trabeculae (dimensions c̄. 150 μm × 3–4 mm) are tied with fine nylon thread and cut, after which they can be seen to beat spontaneously and at a different rate from the rest of the atrium. After a suitable "healing over" period (30–60 min) the preparations are ligatured again at their proximal ends, freed from the heart and mounted in a five-chambered, double sucrose gap perfusion bath (for details see Brown et al., 1976a). Chambers 1 and 5 of the bath are perfused with Ringer's solution in which all the sodium has been replaced by potassium. This depolarizes the membranes in these regions to approximately zero mV eliminating all electrical signals from them and at the same time giving an estimate of the resting potential of the trabeculum. Chambers 2 and 4 are perfused with isotonic sucrose solution which prevents extracellular current flow between chambers 1 and 5 and the central test chamber, chamber 3. Chamber 3 is initially perfused with normal Ringer's solution. Under these conditions the type of electrical response corresponding to the leading trace, a, shown in Figure 1A is frequently recorded across the sucrose gap. It can be seen that this preparation fulfils the first criterion required of sinus tissue, namely that of spontaneity, and that the action potential upstroke is preceded by a marked diastolic depolarization, the pacemaker depolarization. The second criterion used to distinguish primary sinus tissue in its insensitivity to tetrodotoxin (TTX) (see Yamagishi and Sano, 1966; Brooks and Lu, 1972). In Figure 1A, the following trace, b, shows the effect of perfusing the preparation with Ringer's solution to which TTX at a concentration of 2.0×10^{-6} g/ml has been added. Some hyperpolarization occurs (see Brown et al., 1977b), but apart from this the electrical activity is nearly identical to that of trace a. Thus the maximum rates of rise of the action potentials (shown by the magnitude of the vertical lines in Figure 1B) are 9.1 and 8.9 V/s, respectively.

Such behaviour indicates that the tissue in the test compartment is primary pacemaker tissue and this type of preparation has been used for voltage clamp experiments. Preparations in which the electrical activity was abolished by TTX were discarded since it was judged that in these cases only pacemaker cells of the "follower" type were present (i.e. pacemaker cells in which the chief depolarizing current is the "fast" sodium current). In the frog, trabecular preparations respond much better to the voltage clamp than do "man-

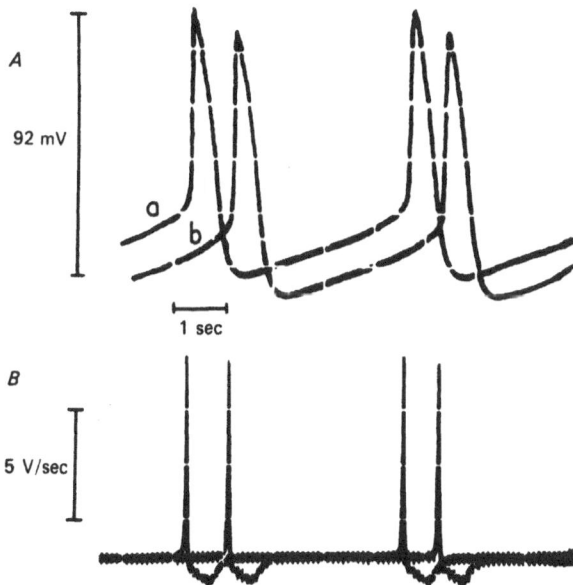

Figure 1. A) Electrical responses recorded across a sucrose gap from an isolated pacemaker preparation before (trace a) and after (trace b) application of TTX (2.0 −⁶ g/ml).

B) Maximum rate of rise (dV/dt) of the action potentials. The similarity of the voltage responses in the presence and absence of TTX indicates primary pacemaker activity.

(With permission of The Physiological Society.)

made" strips of sinus tissue dissected directly from the "anatomical" sinus (contrast mammalian tissue: Irisawa, 1972; Seyama, 1976). We have found that in trabecular preparations of frog sinus the leakage current flowing through the sucrose gaps, as estimated by attenuation of electrical signals, is much less than in "man-made" strips and it would seem that the resting space constant, λ, though not directly measurable in preparations showing spontaneous electrical activity, must approach those values measured by Bonke (1973) and Seyama (1976) in rabbit sino-atrial node (500–800 μm). Even so, it is not always possible to clamp the inward current: we obtained controlled development of inward current as a function of potential in only some preparations.

An example of a voltage clamp experiment in which the inward current of a primary pacemaker preparation was successfully controlled is shown in Figure 2. In this experiment the holding potential selected was – 70 mV (equal to the apparent maximum diastolic potential of the fibre) and upon this, rectangular depolarizations of 800 msec duration were superimposed. The maximum inward, or minimum outward current recorded in response to each depolarization was measured (see arrows on insets A and B) and plotted as a function of potential, giving the curve shown by the filled symbols. The crosses in Figure 2 show the effect on the current-voltage relationship of adding 4 mM Mn^{++} to the perfusate: the inward depolarizing current was virtually abolished by Mn^{++} ions (compare inset records A and B). This result suggests that the properties of the current channel concerned resemble those of the slow inward (Ca^{++}/Na^+ channel which has been extensively investigated in other regions of the heart: Reuter and Beeler, 1969; Rougier et al., 1969; Reuter, 1973). Coupled with the observation that repetitive activity is abolished by Mn^{++} ions in spontaneously active frog pacemaker tissue (Babskii et al., 1972), this leads to the con-

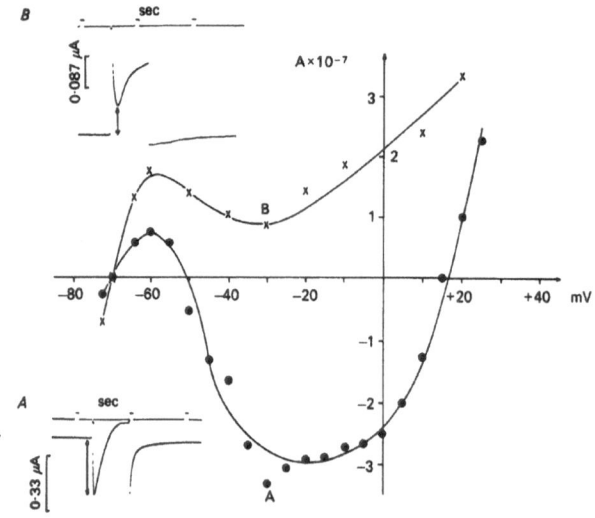

Figure 2. Current-voltage relationship of the slow inward I_{si} current in a TTX-insensitive pacemaker preparation from *Rana catesbeiana*. Filled circles ($\bullet$): current measured in TTX (2.0×10^{-6} g/ml) Ringer's solution. Crosses ($\times$): current after the addition of 4 mM Mn^{++}.

The insets show the actual voltage clamp current records from which points A and B were plotted. The arrows on these records indicate the measurement made, which in each case was at the point of peak inward, or minimal outward current.

(With permission of The Physiological Society.)

clusion that the major depolarizing current in TTX-insensitive sinus tissue is the slow inward (Ca^{++}/Na^+) current I_{s_i}.

In the experiment shown in Figure 2 it will be noticed that net inward current was not recorded until the membrane had been depolarized by about 20 mV, but this is a rather atypical finding, probably due to the presence of a fairly large leakage current. Net inward current can often be seen when the membrane is depolarized by as little as 5–10 mV from the maximum diastolic level, as illustrated in Figure 3. Here, a spontaneously active, TTX-insensitive preparation was voltage clamped to the maximum diastolic potential and small, square depolarizing clamp pulses were applied. A pulse of +4 mV (Figure 3B,a) induced some inward current (which, as the trabeculum was in TTX (2.0×10^{-6} g/ml), must have been I_{s_i}). A clamp pulse of +5 mV from the maximum diastolic potential, (Figure 3B,b),

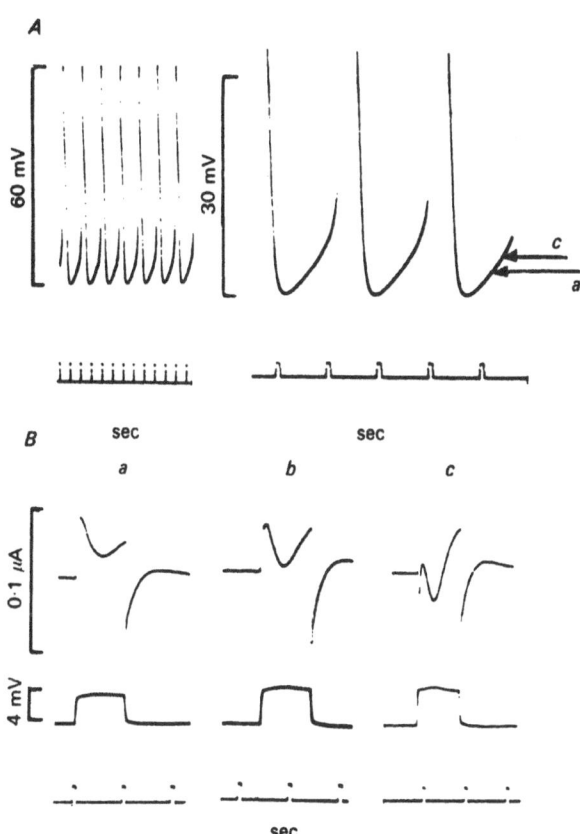

Figure 3. A) Spontaneous activity of a sinus preparation in TTX-Ringer's solution. Left: lower gain record. Right: higher gain record to show the pacemaker depolarization in more detail. Levels to which voltage clamp pulses a and c below depolarized the membrane are marked against the pacemaker potential.

B) The preparation was then clamped at the maximum diastolic potential and depolarizing voltage clamp pulses of +4, +5 and +6 mV applied (a, b and c). The corresponding current records are shown above each voltage clamp pulse and illustrate the onset of slow inward current, I_{s_i}. Although voltage control for the +5 and +6 mV is not complete, the threshold of the slow inward current is evident (see text).
(With permission of The Physiological Society.)

brought in more I_{s_i} and at $+6$ mV positive to the maximum diastolic potential, the current became net inward (Figure 3B,c).

As can be seen from the top trace in Figure 3A, the onset of I_{s_i} occurred during the latter half of the pacemaker depolarization. The importance of the activation of I_{s_i} during the pacemaker depolarization will be discussed below when a model of pacemaking is presented in connection with Figure 8.

The infrequency with which adequate control of the inward current can be achieved in voltage clamp experiments on sinus makes it difficult to investigate the important subject of the mode of action of autonomic transmitters on this tissue. This difficulty can, to some extent, be circumvented by using changes in the maximum rate of rise of the sinus action potential (dV/dt) as a monitor of the effect of such substances on I_{s_i} in TTX-resistant sinus tissue. Figure 4A shows the effect on a frog sinus preparation of carbachol 5×10^{-7} M in TTX-Ringer's solution. There was a decrease in rate of spontaneous firing and a marked reduction in the maximum dV/dt of the upstroke accompanied the reduction in action-potential height (Figure 4B). There was, however, no hyperpolarization of the maximum diastolic potential, nor did this occur until the dose of carbachol was increased to more than 1.0×10^{-6} M. Since E_K for frog sinus tissue lies probably 30 mV negative to the maximum diastolic potential, a selective increase in potassium permeability would cause appreciable hyperpolarization, so this result indicates that cholinomimetic substances can reduce I_{s_i} in frog sinus at doses too low to increase K^+ permeability substantially.

Figures 4C and D show the opposite effect on addition of adrenaline: an increase in maximum dV/dt of the upstroke is correlated with an increase in action potential height and a slight increase in firing frequency. Thus it appears that cholinomimetic substances and catecholamines respectively decrease and increase the second inward current in frog sinus tissue. This is not surprising in view of their similar effects in atrial tissue which have been clearly demonstrated under voltage clamp conditions to which atrial tissue is so much more amenable (Rougier et al., 1969; Giles and Noble, 1976). It was suggested by Paes de Carvallo (1969) that acetylcholine could reduce the inward depolarizing current in rabbit sinoatrial node, and Kohlhardt et al. (1976) have shown that isoproterenol increases the upstroke velocity and overshoot of the rabbit sinoatrial pacemaker cell.

There have been many previous indications that the kinetic and voltage-dependent characteristics of the depolarizing current channel in primary sinus muscle must be similar to that carrying the slow inward current in other cardiac tissues, although the ionic specificity of this channel may be different (see Noma and Irisawa, 1974). A more open question, however, concerns the nature and interactions of all the currents underlying the pacemaker depolarization in sinus tissue. Clearly an outward current or currents must be involved and voltage clamp analysis of sinus cells would be expected to reveal the presence of delayed rectification. Figure 5 shows how one of the outward currents can be recorded and its reversal potential determined. The voltage protocol is shown in the upper half of the figure: from a holding potential of -50 mV (10 mV positive to the maximum diastolic potential) small (20 mV) depolarizations were applied for 2 sec. These test pulses were designed (as will be explained in association with Figure 6 below) to activate only one of the outward currents. After each test pulse the membrane voltage was returned to progressively more hyperpolarized levels ranging between -50 and -85 mV. The bottom half of Figure 5 shows the current records obtained both during and following the depolarizing pulses. During the 20 mV depolarizations, a transient, rapidly-inactivated inward current (the slow inward current, I_{s_i}) is followed by the virtually exponential onset of an outward current. After the depolarising pulse, decay of outward current was recorded at -50, -55, -60, -65, -70 and, minimally, at -75 mV. At -80 mV the current

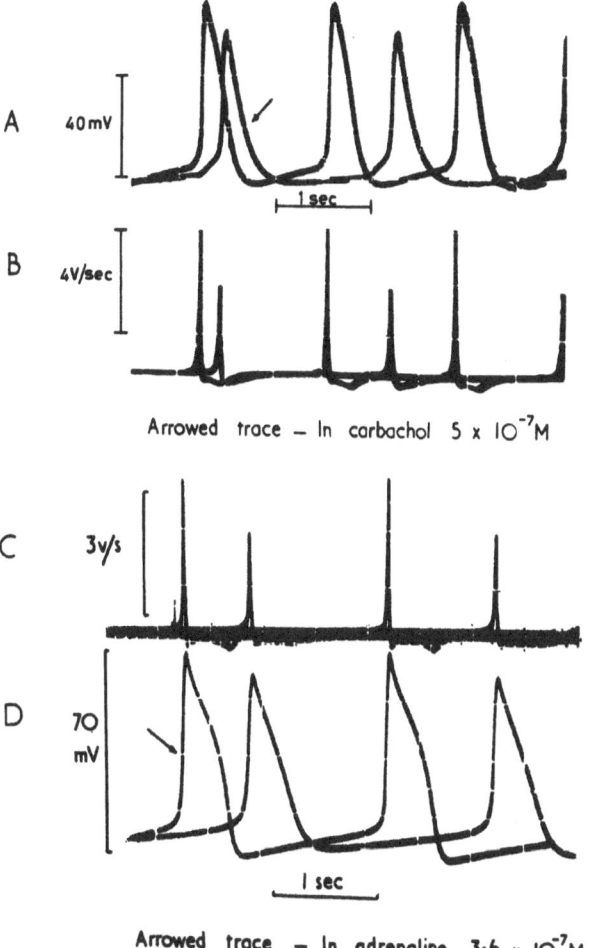

Arrowed trace — In carbachol 5 x 10^{-7}M

Arrowed trace — In adrenaline 3·6 x 10^{-7}M

Figure 4. Frog sinus; sucrose gap recordings.
A and *B*: Effects of carbachol (5 × 10^{-7} M) in TTX Ringer's solution on spontaneous electrical activity and dV/dt.
C and *D*: Effect of adrenaline (3.6 × 10^{-7} M) in TTX-Ringer's solution on dV/dt and spontaneous electrical activity.

trace is almost flat and at -85 mV the current trace has definitely changed sign and become the decay of an inward current.

Since potassium-sensitive microelectrode studies indicate a potassium equilibrium potential in frog sinus tissue of close to -88 mV (Walker and Ladle, 1973), a simple interpretation of the result shown in Figure 5 is that the decay of a virtually pure potassium current activated by the frog sinus action potential, controls the rate of development of the diastolic depolarization in the natural pacemaker region of the frog heart, as it does in the mammalian sino-atrial node (Noma and Irisawa, 1976b), and in the mammalian Purkinje fibre (Noble and Tsien, 1968).

A decay of outward current alone would not, however, produce depolarization and, as already stated, more than one current system must be involved in generating the pace-

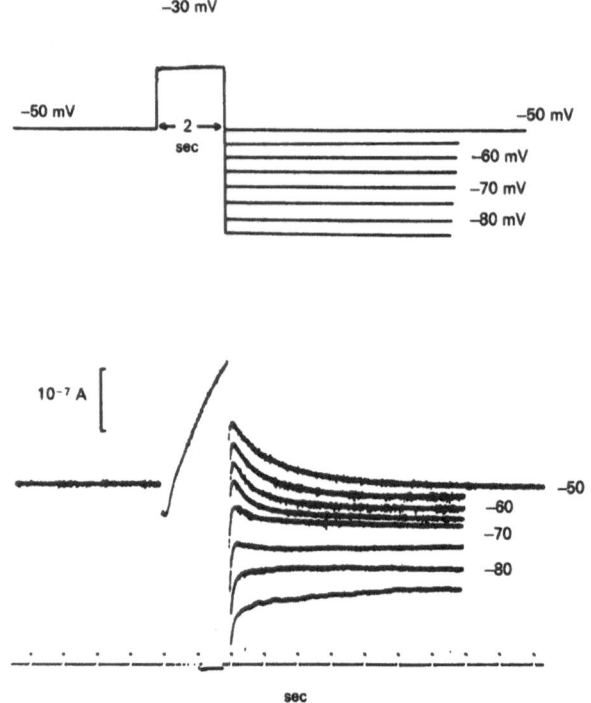

Figure 5. Voltage clamp records obtained in a TTX-insensitive pacemaker preparation. A constant, small (20 mV) depolarizing clamp pulse was first applied (from −50 mV to −30 mV) for 2.0 sec, and each depolarization was succeeded by a long (10 sec) hyperpolarizing clamp to the potential levels indicated. The corresponding currents are shown below. Note current reversal near −80 mV.

(With permission of The Physiological Society.)

maker response. Furthermore, analysis of the outward currents in frog atrium has shown that *two* components of time-dependent outward current are present in this tissue (Brown et al., 1976a, b). Are two components of outward current normally activated in frog sinus muscle?

Figure 6 shows that the answer to this question is almost certainly yes. Here the activation curves for the two components of delayed rectification, i_{slow} and i_{fast}, found to be present in frog sinus cells, are shown. The activation curves were obtained from analysis of outward current "tails" recorded in response to a range of depolarizing and hyperpolarizing voltage clamp pulses in a trabeculum having a very good survival time. Since the presence of potassium ion accumulation made the analysis rather complicated (see Noble, 1976), it is not described here in detail. A full account of the methods used together with an assessment of their reliability is published elsewhere (Brown et al., 1977).

In Figure 6A the activation curve of the current whose reversal potential measurement was illustrated in Figure 5, i_{slow}, is shown by the filled symbols. The time constant of deactivation of this current lies between 1.5 and 3.5 sec at −40 mV. By contrast, the current whose activation is represented by the crosses in Figure 6A, has a rapid deactivation time: $\tau_{i_{fast}}$ lies between 300 and 700 msec at about −40 mV. It is difficult to obtain an estimate of the reversal potential of i_{fast} since it is never activated alone. However,

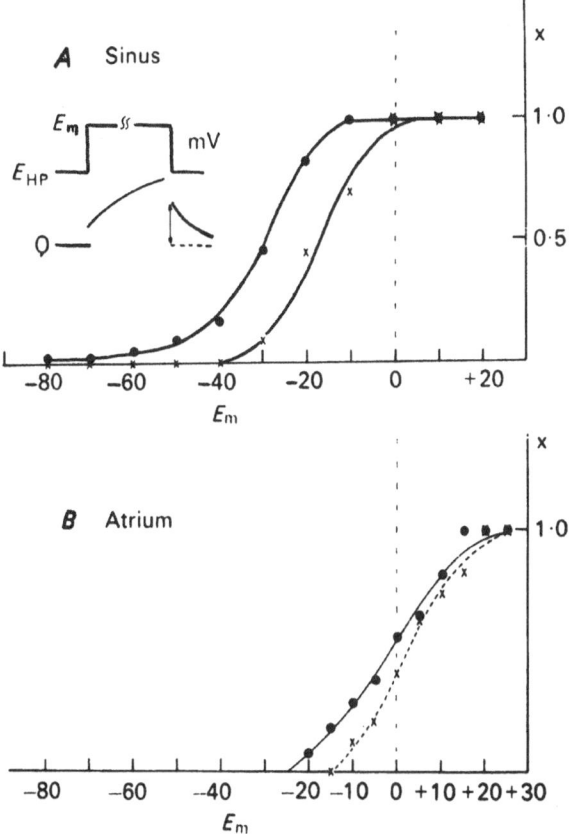

Figure 6. Activation curves for the two components of delayed rectification present in frog sinus (A) and in frog atrial wall (B) preparations. The inset in (A) shows the method used to obtain these curves which is more fully explained in the text.

A) Frog sinus. The filled circles represent the activation curve for the more slowly decaying component of delayed rectification (i_{slow}), the crosses that for the more rapidly decaying component (i_{fast}).

B) Frog atrium. Activation curves for the outward currents in atrium, filled circles: slowly decaying component ($i_{x_{slow}}$); crosses: rapidly decaying component ($i_{x_{fast}}$). From Brown, Clark and Noble, 1976b. The relatively positive activation range of these outward currents is characteristic of frog *atrial wall* (quiescent) trabeculae and contrasts sharply with the corresponding activation ranges observed in *sinus* (spontaneous) preparations.

(With permission of The Physiological Society.)

experiments in which the voltage clamp was imposed immediately following an action potential (see Brown et al., 1977b) indicate a reversal potential positive to that for i_{slow} but nevertheless fairly close to E_K.

When the activation curves for these two components of delayed rectification in sinus muscle are compared with those obtained earlier for the outward, time-dependent atrial wall currents, $i_{x_{fast}}$ and $i_{x_{slow}}$ (shown in Figure 6B), it is striking that at zero mV, whereas the atrial outward current activation curves have reached only 55% and 40% activation, both i_{slow} and i_{fast} in sinus are fully activated. Considering the small size of the sinus action potential as compared with the atrial action potential, this result is to be expected if both the i_{slow} and i_{fast} currents are as important in repolarization in sinus as $i_{x_{slow}}$ is in atrium.

In atrium the role of the more rapidly deactivating component of delayed rectification, $i_{x_{fast}}$, is obscure. It can play no part in repolarization since even following large depolarizations, none of this current appears in current "tails" following pulses of less than about 700 ms duration. It is never seen in the current record when the induced atrial pacemaker response is clamped directly (see Brown et al., 1976a). We were therefore interested to see whether the onset of the more rapidly deactivating sinus current, i_{fast}, parallels the very sigmoid onset of $i_{x_{fast}}$ in atrium.

To do this we analysed current records obtained when the voltage clamp was applied to a spontaneously active preparation at different times during the diastolic depolarization. The method is shown in Figure 7A. In Figure 7B and C are shown semi-logarithmic plots of outward currents recorded by clamping a preparation to its maximum diastolic

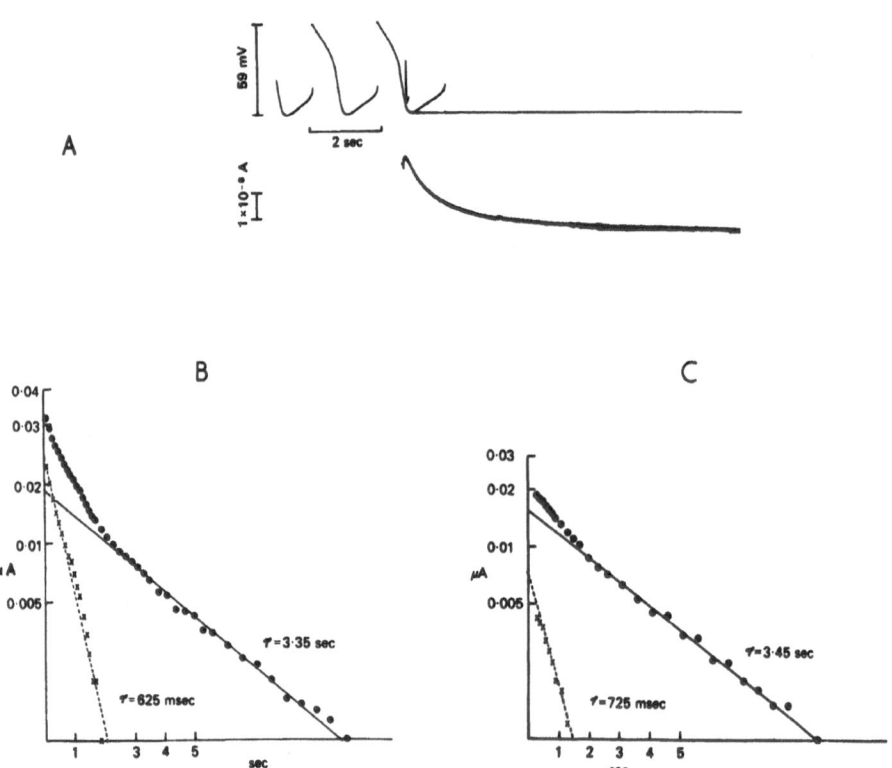

Figure 7. A) Illustration of the method used to apply the voltage clamp to a spontaneously active preparation during the diastolic depolarisation.

B) Semilogarithmic analysis of two of the outward "pacemaker" currents, obtained as shown in A. The clamp was switched on 1.0 sec (B) and 2.25 sec (C) after the upstroke of the previous action potential. Each current tail can be successfully separated into two exponentially decaying components. The time constant of decay of the more slowly deactivating component (i_{slow} – filled circles) is fairly constant (3.45 – 3.3 sec) while that of i_{fast} (crosses) is more variable (575–725 msec). The ratio of the magnitudes of i_{slow} to i_{fast} varies from 1.47 in B to 0.47 in C, suggesting that during the unclamped section of the pacemaker depolarisation they decay as separate, independent processes with the time constants shown.

(With permission of The Physiological Society.)

potential (-46 mV) at two different times after the upstroke of the previous action potential. In Figure 7B (voltage clamp switched on 1.0 sec after the action potential upstroke) the semi-logarithmic plot of the outward 'pacemaker' current has been divided into a more slowly decaying component ($\tau = 3.35$ sec) which, by subtraction, leaves a more rapidly decaying component ($\tau = 625$ msec). Clamping the preparation at other times during the pacemaker depolarization (e.g. at 2.25 sec after the previous action potential upstroke, as shown in Figure 7C) reveals in each case two exponentially decaying outward current components with similar time-constants of decay to the faster and slower components shown in Figure 7B.

Thus, it seems that both of the time-dependent outward currents, i_{fast} and i_{slow} are deactivating *throughout* the duration of the diastolic depolarization and furthermore that they are decaying in the manner expected of independent components, for the ratio of the amplitudes of i_{fast} and i_{slow} decreases the longer the pacemaker depolarization has continued before the clamp is applied. This result also indicates that the onset of the sinus i_{fast} current cannot be as sigmoid as its atrial counterpart, i_{xfast}. This has been confirmed using more conventional voltage clamp methods (Brown et al., 1977b).

Interesting as this result is in assigning a definite function to the i_{fast} sinus current, it is unlikely to make a great difference when qualitatively formulating a possible sinus pacemaker model. Since the properties of the inward and outward sinus currents are quite distinct from those of the frog atrial wall, frog and mammalian ventricle and mammalian Purkinje fibres, it may be helpful to summarize their probable rôles in the generation of the sinus pacemaker depolarization by presenting such a model.

Figure 8 shows in diagrammatic form the way in which the ionic currents change during the pacemaker potential. At the end of the action potential (point A) the net ionic current must be outward for repolarization to occur. At this time the net time-dependent and background outward (potassium) current is larger than the net inward current. How is this situation reversed so that pacemaker depolarization may begin? It seems clear that deactivation of the two time-dependent outward currents, i_{slow} and i_{fast}, unmasks the background inward current. This process is represented in Figure 8 by the locus connecting points A and B. The potential at this time is fairly constant (as the direction of change switches from hyperpolarizing to depolarizing) and the current locus between A and B therefore follows closely the current change during a voltage clamp to the maximal diastolic potential.

If the potential remained at the A–B level, the current would become strongly inward as i_{fast} and i_{slow} decay completely. Since this potential is negative to the threshold of the slow inward current, I_{si}, the inward current responsible for the early phase of depolarization must be the time-independent inward (background) current. The ionic nature of this current in sinus tissue is still unclear, although part of it is almost certainly attributable to sodium since TTX often hyperpolarizes the membrane (see Figure 1A) as does sodium removal (Trautwein and Kassebaum, 1961; Seyama, 1976). It is the presence of this background inward current that ensures that the pacemaker potential will develop spontaneously even after a prolonged voltage clamp at the level of the maximum diastolic potential (see Noma and Irisawa, 1976a, Figure 6).

As the pacemaker potential continues to slowly depolarize the cell, the net inward current remains fairly constant for a period of time (B–D in Figure 8) during which the membrane depolarizes at a nearly constant rate. This is because the depolarization itself increases the outward current driving force, so that although the time-dependent potassium *conductance* is decaying, the potassium *current* may remain constant. This is

represented in Figure 8 by the fact that the locus moves into current decay tails corresponding to voltage clamps *positive* to the maximum diastolic potential. The family of decay tails
drawn in the lower panel of Figure 8 is based on the kind of results shown in Figures 5 and 7.

When the threshold for activation of I_{s_i} is exceeded, the inward current increases and
the net ionic current becomes strongly inward in spite of the increase in outward current
produced by depolarization (locus D–E). If for any reason the inward current is insufficiently large, the increase in outward current (resulting both from the depolarization
directly and via its effect on the degree of activation of i_{fast} and i_{slow}), may prevent firing
and an oscillation may occur (D–E′) instead of an action potential. This type of behaviour
has been seen in frog sinus tissue when I_{s_i} is reduced by acetyl-choline or its cholinesterase

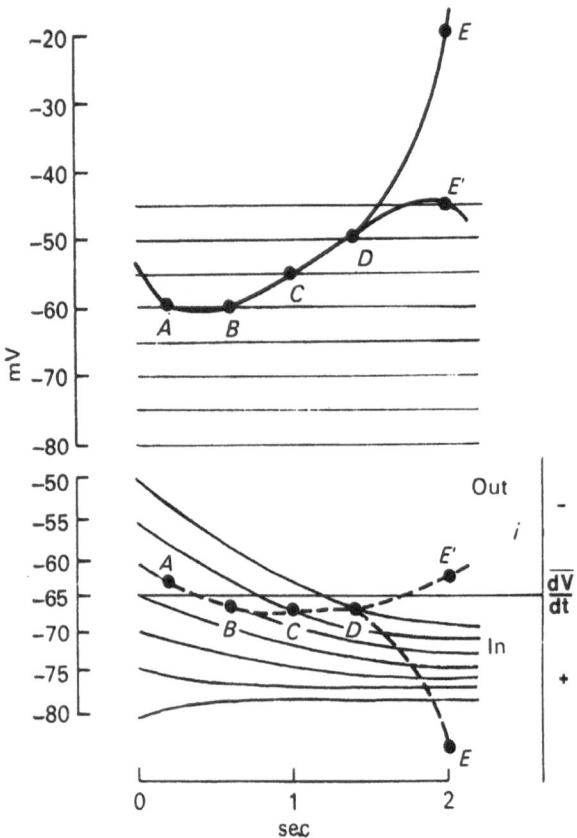

Figure 8. Diagram illustrating possible functional roles of ionic currents in the development of the sinus
pacemaker potential.

Top: pacemaker potential (points A to E) and an oscillation (A to E′).

Bottom: continuous lines represent a family of current decay curves similar to the current decay tails
shown in Figure 5. The points A to E represent the ionic current during the corresponding points on the
pacemaker potential. Points A to D occur on the corresponding voltage clamp current decay tails. Since
$I = -C_m (dV/dt)$, the ionic current points are also proportional to $-dV/dt$. Points E and E′ do not lie on any
of the decay tails since they occur outside their range of applicability. In the case of E, the activation of
the slow inward current (I_{s_i}) has occurred. In the case of E′ it is probable that by this time i_{slow} is re-
activating since its activation curve lies within the pacemaker range. See text also.

(With permission of The Physiological Society.)

insensitive derivative, carbamylcholine (Brown et al., 1977a). Subthreshold pacemaker oscillations have also been observed in the mammalian sino-atrial node when $[Na^+]_o$ is reduced to about half normal (West, 1961).

Most previous hypotheses for the initiation of the cardiac impulse within sinus tissue have been based on data obtained from the mammalian Purkinje fibre which shows pacemaker activity over a much more negative range of potentials (-90 to -60 mV) than does the sinus (-40 to -60 mV). The earlier investigations (Weidmann, 1951; Trautwein and Kassebaum, 1961; Vassalle, 1966) culminated in the quantitative analysis by Noble and Tsien (1968) of the membrane current activated in the pacemaker range of the Purkinje fibre. They were able to reconstruct the pacemaker response on the basis of the decay of an outward potassium current (i_{K_2}) superimposed on a steady-state background inward current. More recently, attempts to reconstruct the effects of raised $[Ca^{++}]_o$, which lengthens the diastolic interval, have made it likely that, in Purkinje fibre pacing, time-dependent activation of the rapid sodium inward current is also an essential feature in the 100 or 200 msec of the pacemaker depolarization which immediately precedes the rapid upstroke (McAllister et al., 1975).

In principle, therefore, the present hypothesis for the generation of the pacemaker depolarization in the Purkinje fibre is quite similar to our model for pacemaking in sinus tissue, but there are two important differences. The time-dependent inward current (the rapid sodium current) which is activated during the diastolic depolarization in the Purkinje fibre is TTX-sensitive, whereas I_{si}, of sinus tissue is not. In addition, an important characteristic of the Purkinje fibre i_{K_2} current is that it shows inward-going rectification positive to about -75 mV, including a negative slope at potentials positive to -60 mV. Although little information is yet available concerning the rectifier properties of the sinus time-dependent outward currents, their clearly observable onset at positive potentials (i.e. at $+20$ mV) makes it extremely improbable that the negative slope characteristic exists.

REFERENCES

Babskii, E.B., Berdiaev, S.J., Khorunchi, V.A.: Manganese ion action on the automaticity of frog cardiac pacemakers. *Doklad Acad Sci (U.S.S.R.)* 209; 996, 1972

Bonke, F.I.M.: Electrotonic spread in the sino-atrial node of the rabbit heart. *Pflügers Archiv ges Physiol* 339: 17, 1973

Brady, A.J., Hecht, J.: On the origin of the heartbeat. *Am J Med* 17: 110, 1954

Brooks, C.McC., Lu, H.H.: *The sinoatrial pacemaker of the heart.* Springfield, Illinois. Charles C. Thomas, 1972

Brown, H.F., Clark, A., Noble, S.J.: Identification of the pacemaker current in frog atrium. *J Physiol* 258: 521, 1976a

Brown, H.F., Clark, A., Noble, S.J.: Analysis of pacemaker and repolarisation currents in frog atrium. *J Physiol* 258: 547, 1976b

Brown, H.F., Giles, W.R., Noble, S.J.: Voltage clamp of frog sinus venosus. *J Physiol* 258: 78, 1976

Brown, H.F., Giles, W.R., Noble, S.J.: Cholinergic inhibition of frog sinus venosus. *J Physiol* 267: 38, 1977a

Brown, H.F., Giles, W.R., Noble, S.J.: Membrane currents underlying rhythmic activity in frog sinus venosus, *J Physiol* 271, pp. 783–816, 1977b

Del Castillo, J., Katz, B.: The membrane potential changes in frog's heart produced by inhibitory nerve impulses. *Nature* 175: 1035, 1955

Giles, W., Noble, S.J.: Changes in membrane currents in bullfrog atrium produced by acetylcholine. *J Physiol* 261: 141, 1976

Hutter, O.F., Trautwein, W.: Effect of vagal stimulation on the sinus venosus of the frog's heart. *Nature (Lond.)* 176: 512, 1955

Irisawa, H.: Electrical activity of rabbit sino-atrial node. In: *Symposium on the Electrical Field of the Heart,* edited by Rijlant, P. Brussels: Presses Académiques Européennes, 1972

Kohlhardt, M., Figulla, H.R., Tripathi, O.: The slow membrane channel as the predominant mediator of the excitation process of the sino-atrial pacemaker cell. *Basic Res in Cardiol* 71: 17, 1976

McAllister, R.E., Noble, D., Tsien, R.W.: Reconstruction of the electrical activity of cardiac Purkinje fibres. *J Physiol* 251: 1, 1975

Noble, D., Tsien, R.W.: The kinetic and rectifier properties of the slow potassium current in cardiac Purkinje fibres. *J Physiol* 195: 185, 1968

Noble, S.J.: Potassium accumulation and depletion in frog atrial muscle. *J Physiol* 258: 578, 1976

Noma, A., Irisawa, H.: The effect of sodium on the initial phase of the sinoatrial pacemaker action potentials in rabbits. *Japan J Physiol* 24: 617, 1974

Noma, A., Irisawa, H.: Membrane currents in rabbit sinoatrial node cells studied by the double micro-electrode method. *Pflügers Archiv ges Physiol* 364: 45, 1976a

Noma, A., Irisawa, H.: The time- and voltage-dependent potassium current in the rabbit sino-atrial node cell. *Pflüg Archiv ges Physiol* 366: 251, 1976b

Paes de Carvahlo, A.: The two components of the cardiac action potential. p. 71–80 in *Research in Physiology*, a liber memoralis in honor of C.McC. Brooks, edited by Kao, F.F. Koizumi, K., Vassalle, M. Bologna: Aulo Guggi, Publisher, 1971

Reuter, H.: Divalent cations as charge carriers in excitable membranes. *Prog Biophys* 26: 1, 1973

Reuter, H., Beeler, G.W. Jr.: Calcium current and activation of contraction in ventricular myocardial fibres. *Science (N.Y.)* 163: 399, 1969

Rougier, O., Vassort, G., Garnier, D., Gargouil, Y.M. Coraboeuf, E.: Existence and role of a slow inward current during the frog atrial action potential. *Pflügers Archiv ges Physiol* 308: 91, 1969

Seyama, I.: Characteristics of the rectifying properties of the sinoatrial node cell of the rabbit. *J Physiol* 255: 379, 1976

Trautwein, W., Kassebaum, D.G.: On the mechanism of spontaneous impulse generation in the pacemaker of the heart. *J Gen Physiol* 45: 317, 1961

Trautwein, W., Zink, K.: Über Membran- und Aktionspotentiale einzelner Myokardfasern des Kalt- und Warmblütherzens. *Pflügers Archiv ges Physiol* 256: 68, 1952

Vassalle, M.: Analysis of cardiac pacemaker potential using a "voltage clamp" technique. *Am J Physiol* 210: 1335, 1966

Viràgh S., Porte, A.: The fine structure of the conducting system of the monkey heart (Macaca mulatta). I. The sino-atrial node and the internodal connections. *A Zellforsch* 145: 191, 1973

Walker, J.L., Ladle, R.O.: Frog heart intracellular potassium activities measured with potassium micro-electrodes. *Am J Physiol* 225: 263, 1973

Weidmann, S.: Effect of current flow on the membrane potential of cardiac muscle. *J Physiol* 115: 227, 1951

West, T.C.: Ultramicroelectrode recording from the cardiac pacemaker. *J Pharmacol exp Thera* 115: 283, 1955

West, T.C.: *Electrophysiology of the sinoatrial node*, p. 191–216 In: Electrical phenomena in the Heart, de Mello, W.C., New York, Academic Press, 1972

Yamagishi, S., Sano, J.: Effect of tetrodotoxin on the pacemaker action potential of the sinus node. *Proc Japan Acad* 42: 1194, 1966

28

INVOLVEMENT OF THE CHLORIDE IONS IN THE MEMBRANE CURRENTS UNDERLYING PACEMAKING ACTIVITY IN FROG ATRIAL TRABECULAE

JACQUES LENFANT AND NOËL GOUPIL

INTRODUCTION

When chloride ions are replaced by foreign anions several striking effects are produced in the spontaneous activity of the cardiac muscle. In sheep and dog Purkinje fibers, when chloride is replaced by nitrate, the spontaneous activity initially slows down and then accelerates. By readmission of chloride solution a further increase in frequency occurs before the original rhythm is attained. With a large impermeant anion such as methylsulphate replacing chloride the reverse effects are obtained (Hutter and Noble, 1961). In the sinus node of the rabbit, the initial effect of replacing chloride by acetate is to increase the slope of the diastolic depolarization and to cause some arrhythmias. Then the diastolic depolarization slows down and there is a concomitant decrease of the frequency (DeMello, 1963). The effects of the substitution of chloride by other anions have been attributed to the sensitivity of certain phases of the cardiac action potential to changes in membrane conductance. The contribution of the chloride ions to the total membrane conductance increased with depolarization (Carmeliet, 1961). However, it has recently been reported that a part of changes in the membrane resistance of the Purkinje fiber in chloride-free media was due to a simultaneous decrease in potassium conductance (Carmeliet and Verdonock, 1977).

More detailed information concerning the role of the chloride ions in the cardiac pacemaking activity can be expected from voltage clamp studies on frog atrial trabeculae. In fact this preparation may be induced to show a repetitive activity like that of the mammalian sinus node by applying a steady depolarizing current (Brown and Noble, 1969). The ionic mechanisms involved in development of the pacemaker activity can be described as follows: the slope of the diastolic depolarization depends upon the deactivation of a slow component of the outward current, the decay of which allows a background inward current to depolarize the membrane to the firing threshold (Brown et al., 1976a). A slow time-dependent inward current is responsible for the depolarization and the plateau of the responses (Brown and Noble, 1969; Lenfant et al., 1972). The activation of the slow component of the outward current is implicated in the repolarization of the action potential (Brown et al., 1976b). The present investigation is designed to test the effects of replacing chloride by methylsulphate on the ionic mechanisms underlying the repetitive activity.

METHODS

The experiments have been carried out at about 20°C on single trabeculae which were isolated from the auricle of the frog (*Rana esculenta*). The preparation was mounted in a double sucrose gap apparatus derived from the one described by Rougier et al. (1968).

Solutions used had the following composition in mM: NaCl 110, KCl 2.5, CaCl$_2$ 1.8. The solutions were buffered to pH 7.8 with 10 mM trishydroxymethylaminomethane maleate. In chloride-poor solutions NaCl was replaced by equimolar amounts of sodium methylsulphate. This anion has been chosen because it seems to be the best substitute which does not significantly reduce the concentration of ionized calcium (Hutter and Noble, 1960; Christoffersen and Skibsted, 1975). In some conditions, tetrodotoxin (10^{-3} mM) and manganese chloride (2.5 mM) were used to inhibit the fast and the slow inward currents, respectively. In presence of manganese-chloride, potassium-chloride was also replaced by equimolar amount of potassium methylsulphate. The following nomenclature was used: V (mV) variations of the membrane potential referred to the resting potential which has been taken as zero. The positive values of V corresponded with depolarizations, the negative ones with hyperpolarizations; 1 (A) membrane current: the outward currents (efflux of cations or influx of anions) were positive, the inward currents (influx of cations or efflux of anions) were negative.

RESULTS

EFFECTS OF CHLORIDE REPLACEMENT BY METHYLSULPHATE ON THE REPETITIVE ACTIVITY

Spontaneous activity in a frog atrial trabecula can be induced by small current pulses depolarizing the membrane 30 to 50 mV positive to the resting potential (Lenfant et al., 1972). Figure 1a shows such an activity induced by a depolarizing current of 0.3 microAmpere. It is characterized by responses of small amplitude and slow rise time and by a diastolic instability of membrane potential: from the maximum value of diastolic potential reached immediately after recovery from the preceding excitatory event, the membrane is gradually

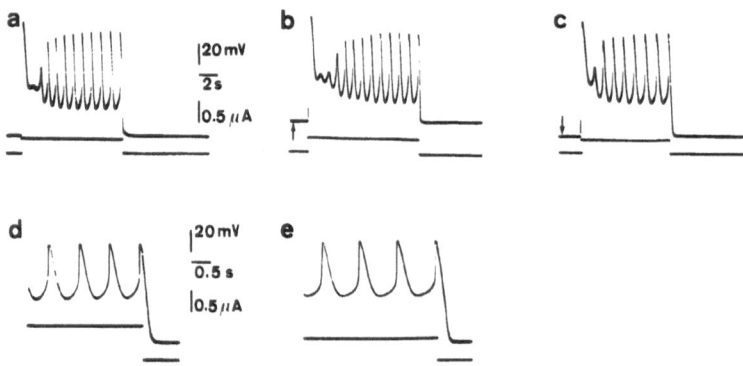

Figure 1.a: Repetitive activity induced by a depolarizing current of 0.3 microAmpere intensity in normal solution. b: Repetitive activity induced by the same depolarizing current after 3 min methylsulphate exposure. c: The same spontaneous activity after 15 min methylsulphate solution. d: Repetitive activity induced by a depolarizing current of 0.8 microAmpere intensity and recorded at higher sweep speed in chloride solution. e: Spontaneous responses induced from the same value of maximum diastolic potential after 15 min methylsulphate solution.

Note: The transient depolarization of the membrane in the non-clamped situation in panel b. For clarity this is indicated by arrows in b and c (again normalized, compare a).

depolarized during the later diastolic period. The replacement of chloride by methylsulphate depolarizes the membrane in resting conditions by about 15 mV (Figure 1b, arrow). The repetitive activity is induced by the same depolarizing current pulse after 3 min methylsulphate exposure. The maximum diastolic potential becomes more positive, the amplitude of the responses decreases, the slope of the diastolic depolarization and the rhythm increase (Figure 1b). However, the resting depolarization is not maintained and the potential returns to its original value in 13–15 min (Figure 1c, arrow). In this case the maximum diastolic potential remains more positive than in normal solution. The amplitude of the responses is decreased and the diastolic slope is reduced leading to a rhythm slower than that recorded in chloride solution (Figure 1c). By returning to chloride solution these changes are reversible after a transient hyperpolarization of the resting potential. Figure 1d illustrates the repetitive activity induced by a depolarizing current pulse of 0.8 micro-Ampere and recorded at higher sweep speed in normal solution. In presence of methylsulphate, after the transient depolarization of the resting potential, the current pulse is reduced in order to induce the repetitive activity from the same maximum diastolic potential than that in normal solution (Figure 1e). In these conditions, the amplitude of the repetitive response does not change but its duration is prolonged, the slope of the diastolic phase is reduced and the rhythm is decreased.

EFFECTS OF CHLORIDE REPLACEMENT BY METHYLSULPHATE ON THE SLOW INWARD CURRENT

Figure 2a shows the maximum intensity of the slow inward current elicited in a chloride-tetrodotoxin solution by a depolarizing pulse of $+80$ mV amplitude and of 180 msec duration. 15 min after the replacement of chloride by methylsulphate the time course of the current is not significantly changed but the intensity is slightly increased (Figure 2b). In Figure 2c the current-voltage relationship of the slow inward current is plotted in tetrodotoxin solution. In presence of methylsulphate the whole curve is shifted downwards (thus to more negative values). Figure 2d illustrates the current-voltage relationship obtained after substraction of the currents recorded in manganese-tetrodotoxin solutions, (See methods). In presence of chloride the approximate reversal potential corresponding to the apparent intersection of the current curve with the voltage axis is $+110$ mV. The replacement of chloride by methylsulphate does neither significantly affect the evolution of the current with membrane potential nor the reversal potential value.

EFFECTS OF CHLORIDE REPLACEMENT BY METHYLSULPHATE ON THE DEACTIVATION OF THE DELAYED OUTWARD CURRENTS AND ON THE STEADY-STATE BACKGROUND CURRENTS

In presence of tetrodotoxin and manganese ions a pulse of 80 mV amplitude and of 1.5 sec duration is induced from the resting potential: the preparation is then repolarized to different potential levels. Figure 3a illustrates such an experiment where a delayed outward current is activated during the pulse. When the membrane is repolarized to $+40$ mV and 20 mV the result is a decaying outward current. In case of a repolarization to the resting potential, a decaying inward current is observed. This suggests that the reversal potential is probably near $+10$ mV. 15 min after the replacement of chloride by methylsulphate the outward current, which is activated during the pulse and the tail currents occurring after repolarization, seems to be decreased (Figure 3b). In order to study this phenomenon, the

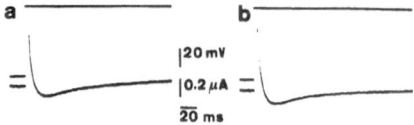

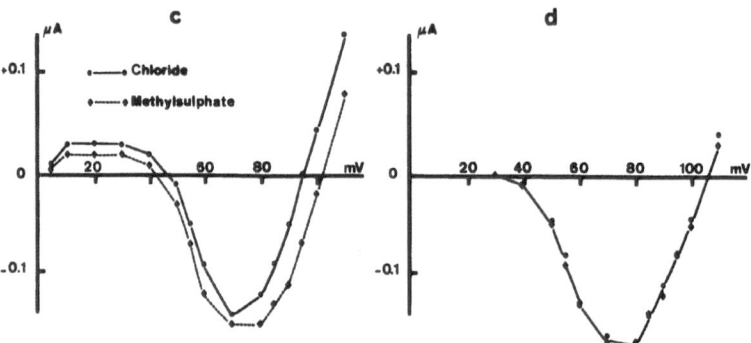

Figure 2. a: Slow inward current initiated by a +80 mV depolarizing impulse in chloride-TTX solution. b: The same record 15 min after methylsulphate-TTX exposure. c,d: Current-voltage relations for the peak slow inward current in chloride-TTX and in methylsulphate-TTX solution before (c) and after (d) subtracting the currents recorded in TTX-manganese solutions.

values of the total current before (i_o) and after (i_{ss}) the deactivation are plotted against different values of repolarization. Figure 3c shows the curves obtained in a chloride-containing solution. The arrows indicate the direction and the magnitude of the deactivation at a given potential. The curves cross each other at about + 10 mV which represents the reversal potential of the delayed system. In methylsulphate-solution the steady state current i_{ss} is decreased at any potential (Figure 3d). The values of the current i_o are slightly reduced. There is no clear change of the reversal potential.

DISCUSSION

The present experiments demonstrate that the replacement of chloride ions by methylsulphate ions induces a transient depolarization of the resting potential. Similar results have been obtained by Hodgkin and Horowicz (1959) on the skeletal fiber in sulphate solution. In the frog atrium, Ladle and Walker (1975) have shown that the chloride equilibrium potential is less negative than the resting potential and therefore the chloride ions are not passively distributed. Thus in the resting condition there exists a continuous efflux of chloride ions tending to a depolarization. In methylsulphate solution the transient depolarization of the membrane potential may be obtained by a transient increase of the efflux of chloride ions. According to Hodgkin and Horowicz (1959) water leaves the fiber in order to preserve osmotic equilibrium. The return to the original value of the resting potential involves a loss of potassium chloride and of water in amounts such that the internal potassium concentration is virtually unchanged.

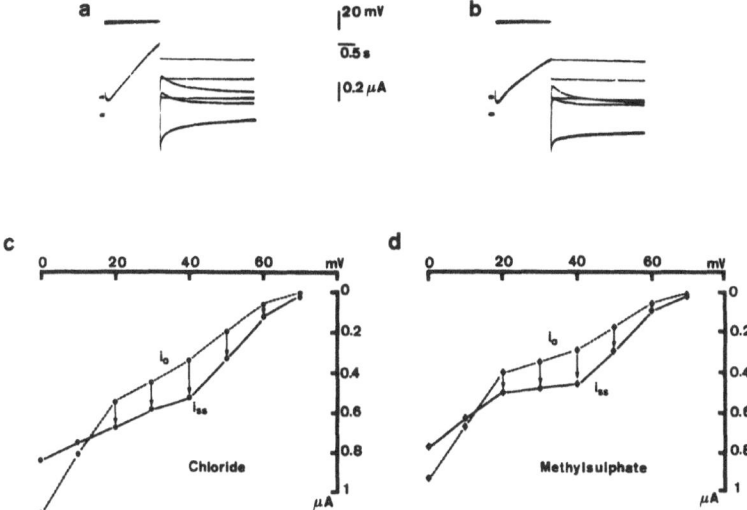

Figure 3. a,b: Outward current associated with a +80 mV depolarizing pulse starting from the resting potential and returning to different holding potentials in chloride (a) and in methylsulphate (b) solution. c,d: Current-voltage relations for the current tails illustrated in a and b. The interrupted lines represent the maximum current obtained by extrapolating the slow decline at t = 0 (i_o). The solid lines represent the steady-state current (i_{ss}). The o-point on the voltage-axis represent the resting potential.

Note: In a and b the two traces have to be separated. The upper trace gives the potential change with straight lines after the pulse indicating the clamp back to 40 mV and 20 mV above the resting potential and to the resting potential itself. The lower trace gives the corresponding current changes.

In presence of methylsulphate the repetitive activity first accelerates and then slows down. Such effects have been observed by Hutter and Noble (1961) in the Purkinje fiber and by DeMello (1963) in the sinus node of the rabbit. In the present study the reduction of the spontaneous rhythm can be explained as follows. The decay of the outward current between +30 and +50 mV, illustrated in Figure 3, might change the net ionic current from outward to inward and generates in this way the slow depolarization responsible for pacemaking (Hauswirth et al., 1972). The decrease of the deactivation observed in methylsulphate solution would have an accelerating effect since a smaller outward current will take shorter to decay and should therefore lead to a reduced interval between action potentials. However, the reduction of the steady-state current (i_{ss}) obtained with methylsulphate may lead to further decrease in the slope of the diastolic depolarization observed in Figure 1c. The initial increase of the diastolic slope and of the rhythm observed during the transient depolarization (Figure 1b) may be due to a transient increase of the steady-state inward current Ladle and Walker (1975) have calculated a chloride equilibrium potential value of about − 30 mV in the frog atrium which would correspond to the potential value of about + 50 mV in the present experiments. Because of the relatively positive values of the chloride reversal potential it is suggested that the chloride ions may play a role together with the deactivation of the delayed outward current in the potential range between + 30 and + 50 mV (i.e. between about − 10 mV and − 30 mV). The replacement of chloride ions by methylsulphate ions does not change the net current-voltage relationship for the slow inward current. This explains why the amplitude of the repetitive responses induced from the same maximum diastolic potential in chloride and in methylsulphate solution is unaffected (Figures 1d and 1e). The prolongation of the response duration observed in poor-chloride solution may be due to the decrease of the time-independent outward current, or to the decrease of the time-dependent outward current or to both. Finally, from the present investigations it appears that a time independent chloride component contributes to the evolution of the repetitive activity in depolarized frog atrium. According to the results obtained by DeMello (1963) and on the sinus node of the rabbit, it is suggested that the same ionic mechanism may be involved in the genesis of the spontaneous activity of the mammalian heart.

REFERENCES

Brown, H.F., Noble, S.J.: Membrane currents underlying delayed rectification and pace-maker activity in frog atrial muscle. *J Physiol (Lond)* 204: 717, 1969

Brown, H.F., Clark, A., Noble, S.J.: Identification of the pacemaker current in frog atrium. *J Physiol (London)* 258: 521, 1976a.

Brown, H.F., Clark, A., Noble, S.J.: Analysis of pace-maker and repolarization currents in frog atrial muscle. *J Physiol (London)* 258: 547, 1976b.

Carmeliet, E.E.: Chloride ions and the membrane potential of Purkinje fibres. *J Physiol (London)* 156: 375, 1961.

Carmeliet, E.E., Verdonck, F.: Reduction of potassium permeability by chloride substitution in cardiac cells. *J Physiol (London)* 265: 193, 1977

Christoffersen, G.R.J., Skibsted, L.H.: Calcium ion activity in physiological salt solutions: influence of anions substituted for chloride. *Comp Biochem Physiol* 52: 317, 1975

De Mello, W.C.: Role of chloride ions in cardiac action and pacemaker potentials. *Amer J Physiol* 205: 567, 1963

Hauswirth, O., Noble, D., Tsien, R.W.: Separation of the pacemaker and plateau components of delayed rectification in cardiac Purkinje fibres. *J Physiol (London)* 255: 211, 1972

Hodgkin, A.L., Horowicz, P.: The influence of potassium and chloride ions on the membrane potential of single muscle fibres. *J Physiol (London)* 148: 127, 1959

Hutter, O.F., Noble, D.: The chloride conductance of frog skeletal muscle. *J Physiol (London)* 151: 89, 1960

Hutter, O.F., Noble, D.: Anion conductance of cardiac muscle. *J Physiol (London)* 157: 335, 1961

Ladle, R.O., Walker, J.L.: Intracellular chloride activity in frog heart. *J Physiol (London)* 251: 549, 1975

Leant, J., Mironneau, J., Aka, J.K.: Activité répétitive de la fibre sino-auriculaire de grenouille: analyse des courants membranaires responsables de l'automatisme cardiaque. *J Physiol (Paris)* 64: 5, 1972

Rougier, O., Vassort, G., Stämpfli, R.: Voltage clamp experiments on frog atrial heat muscle fibres with the double sucrose gap technique. *Pflügers Archiv ges Physiol* 301: 91, 1968

29

WHICH IONS ARE IMPORTANT FOR THE MAINTENANCE OF THE RESTING MEMBRANE POTENTIAL OF THE CELLS OF THE SINOTRIAL NODE OF THE RABBIT?

ISSEI SEYAMA

INTRODUCTION

The cell of the sinoatrial (SA) node have a resting potential of -30 to -50 mV. This is a relatively low value compared to working myocardium. The response of the cells of the SA node to change in the extracellular potassium-concentration was small, viz. below 5 mM. Changes of the $[K]_o$ only have a slight effect on the membrane potential whereas an increase of $[K]_o$ from 25 to 50 mM causes a change of 21.5 mV per tenfold change in $[K]_o$ (Noma and Irisawa, 1975).

However, if the concentration of sodium ions in the extracellular fluid is diminished strongly, the cells of the SA node are hyperpolarized and more sensitive to changes in $[K]_o$ viz. the membrane potential changing 40–50 mV per tenfold change in $[K]_o$ (Irisawa et al., 1975). These observations might be explained by the fact that the membrane of the SA nodal cells is relatively well permeable for sodium ions at the resting potential. The role of anions, especially chloride ions, seems to be of only minor importance for the resting potential (de Mello, 1963). To elucidate the mechanism of the resting membrane of cells of the SA node, we studied the relative conductance ratio between potassium sodium and chloride ions.

METHODS

PREPARATIONS

Hearts were isolated from albino rabbits weighing 2–2.5 kg under pentobarbital anaesthesia (20 mg/kg). After separating the SA node from the right atrium, a strand preparation perpendicular to the crista terminalis was prepared and the epicardial side was removed with a razor blade. Furthermore, this strand preparation was ligated at two sites by a silk thread. Final dimension of the preparation was $300 \times 300\,\mu$. In most cases, these small preparations spontaneously resumed beating after immersing in normal Tyrode solution for 10–60 min and generate action potentials similar to those observed in intact SA node. This small piece of preparation has provided several useful conditions to study the electrical activity of SA nodal cells: 1) no appreciable conduction was observed within this preparation, and, therefore, the phenomenon of pacemaker shift could be avoided. 2) Since two-thirds of the SA node was also removed from the epicardial surface, diffusion delay in exchanging the composition of external solution could be minimized. 3) Due to a lack of conduction in this preparation, there is no electrical interference caused by asynchronous electrical activity of neighbouring cells. 4) The microelectrode could remain within a cell for as long as 1–2 hours, probably because there is only a minimal movement of these small preparations. The input impedance of the cell increased continuously for about 10 min after the penetration of the microelectrode, and concomitant with this increase the amplitude of the action potential enhanced gradually. These findings suggest that the sealing around the microelectrode becomes better during this interval, a fact which has been never observed in a large SA node specimen.

ELECTRICAL MEASUREMENT

Conventional microelectrodes, filled with 3 M KCl, were used. The resting potential was monitored by both an oscilloscope and a strip chart recorder. The reference electrode was clamped at ground potential by a feed-back circuit (Hagiwara et al., 1971).

SOLUTIONS

The normal Tyrode solution had the following composition: NaCl 136.8, KCl 2.7, $CaCl_2$ 1.8, $MgCl_2$ 0.5, HEPES 5.0 in mM. In preparing SCN Tyrode solution and acetate Tyrode solution, salt of normal Tyrode solution was replaced by a corresponding SCN or acetate salt. The compositions of the various Tyrode solutions are given in Table 1 and 2. pH was adjusted to 7.4. The rate of perfusion of solution was 3 ml/min and the chamber volume was 0.4 ml. Temperature was kept constant at 37°C.

RESULTS

EFFECT OF CHANGES IN $[K]_o$ ON THE RESTING MEMBRANE POTENTIAL OF CELLS OF SA NODE IN NA-FREE TYRODE SOLUTION

The small response of the resting membrane potential of quiescent SA nodal cells to changes in $[K]_o$ from 1 to 50 mM was reconfirmed in a separate experiment. The slope per tenfold change in $[K]_o$ from 10.8 to 50 mM was 12.3 mV. Because the sealing condition of the microelectrode differs from penetration to penetration, all data in one series were collected continuously from one cell in all experiments. When Na was removed from the external medium at 2.7 mM $[K]_o$ the cells hyperpolarized to various potential levels in 10 min. In the cells that were hyperpolarized by 10–15 mV, the effect of changes in $[K]_o$ was studied. In a concentration range from 1 to 10.8 mM $[K]_o$ the slope of membrane potential per tenfold change of $[K]_o$ was from 10 to 29 mV. Beyond 10.8 mM $[K]_o$ the slope per tenfold change became 44 ± 2.5 mV (5 cells, see Figure 1). Upon transfer into Na-free medium at 2.7 mM $[K]_o$, some cells showed an extensive hyperpolarization of more than 30 mV. This hyperpolarization might be explained by an increase in K-permeability because of the Na-Ca exchange mechanism (Irisawa and Noma, 1976). Therefore, data used to obtain the slope in Na-free medium did not include those from the cells having extensive hyperpolarization.

EFFECT OF CHANGES IN $[K]_o$ ON THE RESTING MEMBRANE POTENTIAL OF CELLS OF THE SA NODE IN NA-FREE MEDIUM WITH CONSTANT $[K]_o[Cl]_o$ PRODUCT

If the sodium ions are removed from the external medium, both potassium and chloride ions remain current carriers. When the external medium is then changed in such a way

Table 1. Compositions of various Na-free Tyrode solutions (in mM).

	$[K]_o \cdot [Cl]_o = 389$				$[Cl]_o = 144.2\ mM$				
$[K]_o$ in mM	2.7	10.8	25	50	1	2.7	10.8	25	50
Tris base	150.56	250.61	242.86	192.86	152.06	150.56	142.46	128.26	103.26
Tris HCl	136.90	20.65	–	–	136.90	136.90	136.90	136.90	136.90
KCl	2.7	10.8	15.57	7.79	1.0	2.7	2.7	2.7	2.7
$CaCl_2$	1.8	–	–	–	1.8	1.8	1.8	1.8	1.8
$MgCl_2$	0.5	–	–	–	0.5	0.5	0.5	0.5	0.5
K acetate	–	–	9.43	42.21	–	–	8.10	22.30	47.30
Ca acetate	–	1.8	1.8	1.8	–	–	–	–	–
Mg acetate	–	0.5	0.5	0.5	–	–	–	–	–

pH was adjusted by glacial acetic acid.

Table 2. Compositions of various $[Cl]_o$ Tyrode solution (in mM).

	Na-free $[Cl]_o = 144.2$ mM (A)	Na-free Cl-free (B)
Tris base	150.56	287.46
Tris HCl	136.90	–
KCl	2.7	–
CaCl₂	1.8	–
MgCl₂	0.5	–
K acetate	–	2.7
Ca acetate	–	1.8
Mg acetate	–	0.5

pH was adjusted by glacial acetic acid.
The mixing proportion to make an appropriate $[Cl]_o$ solution.

	(A)	(B)
100 mM-Cl	0.69 parts	0.31 parts
30 mM-Cl	0.21	0.79
10 mM-Cl	0.069	0.931
1 mM-Cl	0.007	0.993

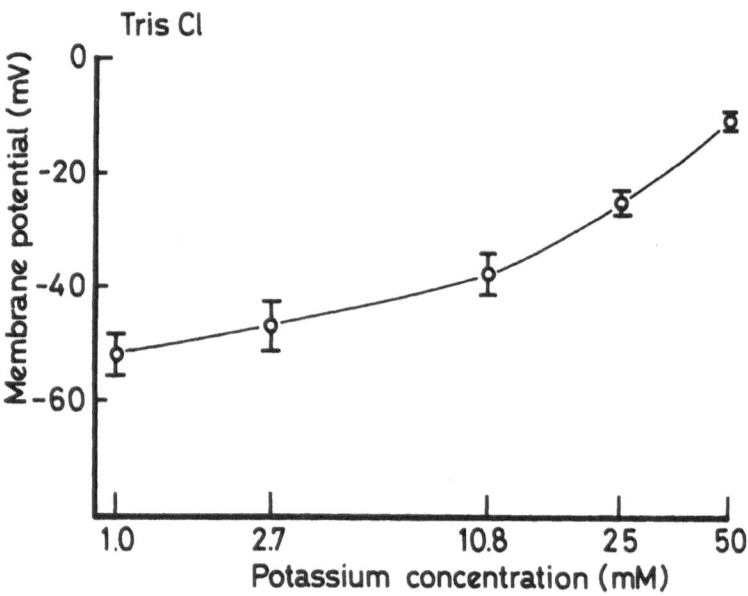

Figure 1. Relation between membrane resting potential and log $[K]_o$ in Na-free Tyrode solution. Open circles and vertical bars indicate mean of 5 cells and S.E. of mean, respectively.

that the product of $[K]_o \times [Cl]_o$ stays constant (this means that an increase of $[K]_o$ is accompanied by a decrease of $[Cl]_o$), the result will be a change of the membrane potential. If both ions are equally active or equally important for the maintenance of the membrane potential, an increase of the external potassium concentration would then cause a decrease

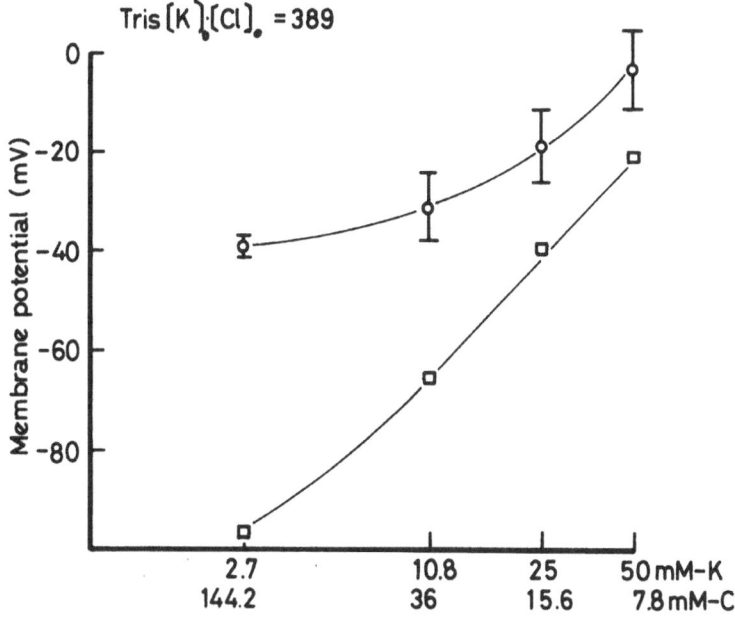

Figure 2. Relation between membrane potential and log $[K]_o$ or $-\log [Cl]_o$ in Na-free solution with $[K]_o \times [Cl]_o = 389$. Open circles and vertical bars indicate mean of 5 cells and S.E. of mean, respectively. Open squares indicate the response of a cell showing extensive hyperpolarization to changes in $[K]_o$.

of the membrane potential of 61 mV per tenfold change of $[K]_o$. Beyond 10.8 mM $[K]_o$ the slope of the change in membrane potential was estimated to be 54 ± 3.1 mV (5 cells), as shown in Figure 2. In this figure the data of a cell that hyperpolarized extensively in Na-free medium, is also shown by the open squares. Such a cell behaves almost as a perfect potassium electrode.

EFFECT OF CHANGES IN $[K]_o$ ON THE RESTING MEMBRANE POTENTIAL OF CELLS OF THE SA NODE IN SCN TYRODE

To study the relative importance of anions and especially of chloride ions for the maintenance of the membrane potential at rest, the preparation was bathed in a Tyrode without chloride ions. The latter ions were replaced by SCN ions. The membrane is much more permeable for SCN ions than for Cl-ions, viz. a factor of 2.9 as reported by Seyama (1977). After the change from normal Tyrode to SCN–Tyrode, SCN ions will enter the cells and cause a hyperpolarization. This hyperpolarization is about 30 mV and only transient. As shown in Figure 3, the membrane returned to a potential level, about 5 mV more polarized than under normal Tyrode. This difference of membrane potential might be explained by the fact that chloride ions are no longer available to contribute to the stabilization of the resting potential.

It is assumed that the SCN-ions are distributed between the intracellular compartment and the extracellular fluid according to the membrane potential. Then, in case of SCN-Tyrode, the membrane potential is mainly established by the distribution of the sodium

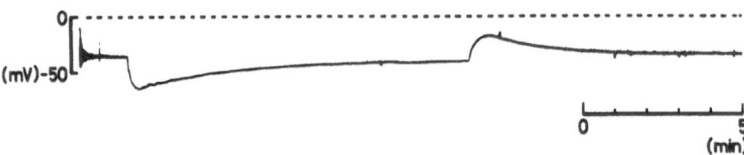

Figure 3. Change in resting membrane potential upon the substitution of Cl ions by SCN ions. The change in Tyrode took place at the beginning of the trace.

and the potassium ions. The membrane potential can be expressed under these circumstances, as

$$V = \frac{g_K \cdot E_K + g_{Na} \cdot E_{Na}}{g_K + g_{Na}}$$

where E_K and E_{Na} indicate the equilibrium potential for potassium and sodium, respectively, whereas g_K and g_{Na} indicate the conductance for these ions. According to de Mello (1961) E_K is taken as -102 mV and we assumed E_{Na} to be about $+50$ mV. The membrane potential of cells in SCN-Tyrode had a mean value of -45 mV. It can be calculated that $g_{Na} = 0.58 \, g_K$. We also studied the effect of changes in the extracellular potassium concentration in case of perfusion with SCN-Tyrode. It turned out that in the range of 10.8 mM to 50 mM $[K]_o$, the membrane potential is changed with 25 ± 1.5 mV per tenfold change in $[K]_o$ (Figure 4). This is more than in normal Tyrode (Noma and Irisawa, 1975).

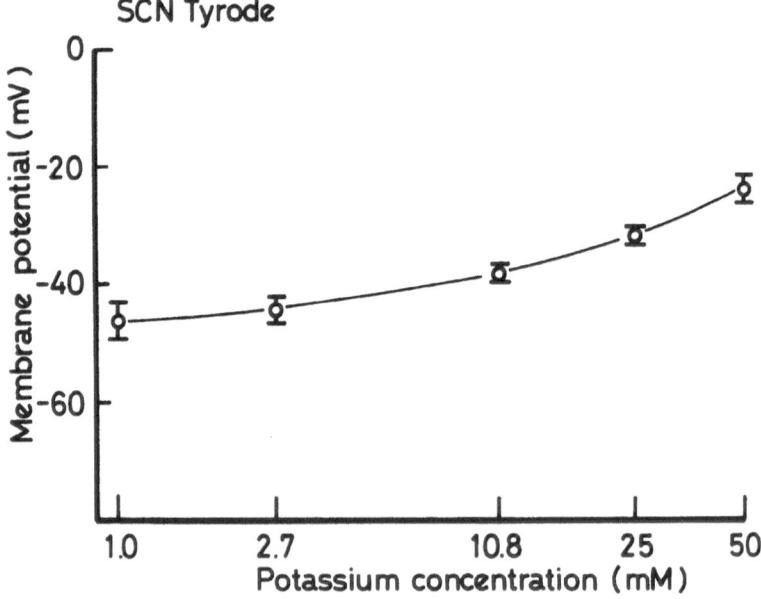

Figure 4. Relation between membrane resting potential and log $[K]_o$ in SCN Tyrode solution. Open circles and vertical bars indicate mean of 5 cells and S.E. of mean, respectively.

THE CONTRIBUTION OF CHLORIDE IONS TO THE RESTING MEMBRANE POTENTIAL

The membrane is more permeable for chloride ions than for acetate ions. Seayama (1977) demonstrated that the ratio acetate: chloride is about 0.7. If a preparation is brought from normal Tyrode to acetate Tyrode (Tyrode in which the chloride ions are substituted by acetate ions) one might expect an initial hyperpolarization because the acetate ions are diffusing into the cells. However, chloride ions will leave the cell and this might cause a depolarization. The latter is seldom observed. In Figure 5 (upper panel) an example is shown in which a quiescent preparation of the SA node developed a transient hyperpolarization followed by spontaneous activity after the change from normal Tyrode to acetate Tyrode.

After eliminating sodium ions from the external medium the substitution of chloride by acetate produced a transient depolarization. This is shown in the middle panel of Figure 5. In this case a spontaneous beating preparation became quiescent in Na-free Tyrode; the change to Na-free, acetate Tyrode caused a transient depolarization. The amount of transient depolarization is dependent on the proportion of chloride substitution and we, therefore, studied the change in membrane potential in relation to the chloride concentration (varying the amount of substitution of chloride by acetate). It turned out that the membrane potential changed -6.8 mV per tenfold change of the $[Cl]$.

We also did experiments in which the preparation was brought into Na-free Tyrode in which the potassium concentration was enhanced to 50 mM. The substitution of chloride by acetate ions did not cause a transient depolarization (in five cases) as shown in the lower panel of Figure 5, whereas in three cases a small transient hyperpolarization was found.

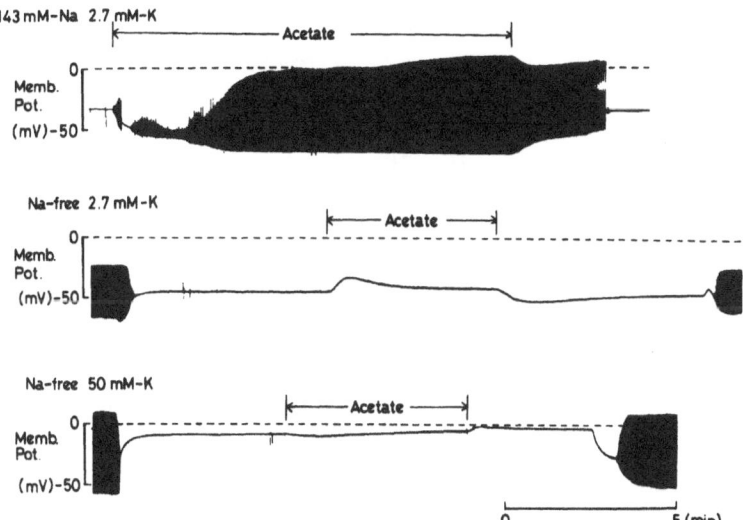

Figure 5. Change of the membrane potential caused by substitution of Cl by acetate under various conditions. Top panel shows the replacement of Cl by acetate in the presence of Na. This particular preparation, which was quiescent in normal Tyrode solution, generated spontaneous beating during the perfusion of acetate Tyrode solution.

Middle panel shows a transient depolarization caused by substitution of Cl by acetate at 2.7 mM $[K]_o$ in the absence of Na ion. Since the movement of the pen of the recorder was limited to one side, part of the action potential was not shown. Bottom panel shows a lack of transient depolarization upon substitution of Cl by acetate at 50 mM $[K]_o$ in the absence of Na.

To obtain the relative conductances of potassium and chloride, the equation, originally developed by Hodgkin and Horowicz (1959) and modified by Brown et al. (1970) for the condition of different equilibrium potentials for potassium and chloride, was used. Since in sodium-free medium, the slope of the change of the membrane potential at different $[K]_o$ (for $[K]_o$ beyond 10.8 mM) at constant $[Cl]_o$ is 44 mV per tenfold change of $[K]_o$ and the slope of the change of the membrane potential at different $[Cl]_o$ ($[Cl]_o$ between 10 and 100 mM) at constant $[K]_o$ is -6.8 mV per tenfold change of $[Cl]_o$ (see Figure 6), the following equations can be used for a small change from the equilibrium state:

$$\frac{dV}{d \log[K]_o}[Cl]_o = 61\ T_K$$

$$\frac{dV}{-d \log[Cl]_o}[K]_o = 61\ T_{Cl}$$

where T_K and T_{Cl} are the transport members for potassium and chloride ions, respectively. It can be calculated that $T_K = 0.72$ and $T_{Cl} = 0.11$; therefore $g_{Cl} = 0.15\ g_K$.

If the membrane properties and the intracellular ionic composition of cells of the SA node are not influenced by the fact that the preparation is superfused with solutions that contain various abnormal anions, the relative conductance ratio for the membrane of these nodal cells at the resting membrane potential can be expressed for Na, K, and Cl as follows:

$$g_K:g_{Na}:g_{ce} = 1:0.58:015.$$

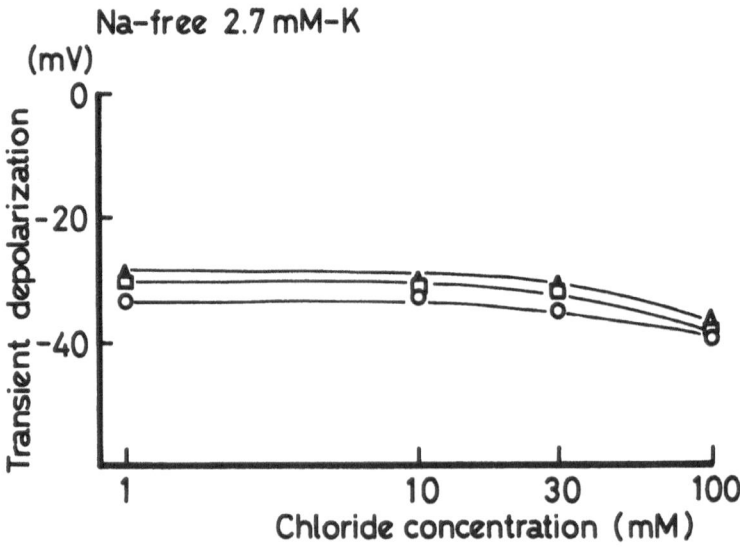

Figure 6. Relation between transient depolarization and $\log[Cl]_o$ in Na-free, 2.7 mM $[K]_o$ Tyrode of which the chloride concentration is changed by substitution of Cl by acetate. Each symbol belongs to one cell.

DISCUSSION

From the measurement of the relative conductance ratio, it can be concluded that both sodium and potassium ions are important for the membrane potential of quiescent SA nodal cells.

The earlier observation that the slope per tenfold change of $[K]_o$ in Na-free solution is much larger than in normal Tyrode solution (Irisawa et al., 1975) supports this conclusion. We have calculated that the conductance of the membrane of cells of the SA node for chloride is about 9% of the total membrane conductance at rest. Hutter and Noble (1961) suggested that Cl ions carry at most 0.3 of the total membrane current in resting membrane condition of Purkinje fibers. Carmeliet (1961) mentioned that the contribution of chloride to the resting membrane conductance might be small in Purkinje fibers. Recently, Fozzard and Lee (1976) also estimated that the ratio between chloride and potassium conductance is 0.17 in ventricular myocardium. However, in skeletal muscle, the chloride conductance forms 68% of the total membrane conductance (Hodgkin and Horowicz, 1959). Variation of $[Cl]_o$ at a wide concentration range of $[K]_o$ could produce large transient potential changes, showing that chloride ions are very important for the maintenance of the resting membrane potential in skeletal fibers. On the contrary, in the SA nodal cell, the membrane permeability to Na is high and the proportion of Cl conductance to the total membrane conductance is small. Therefore, no transient depolarization of the membrane could be observed when the SA node was transferred from a normal solution into acetate solution; only in the absence of sodium a transient change in membrane potential was observed. These observations are in agreement with the low conductance ratio between K and Cl ions. In Purkinje fibers the potassium conductance of depolarized membranes is increased and one expects therefore that the relative chloride conductance is even smaller in such circumstances. If the same is true for cells of the SA node, then the absence of transient depolarizations in case of substitution of chloride by acetate in a Tyrode that was sodium-free and contained a high potassium concentration (50 mM) (see Figure 5, lower panel) might be explained.

REFERENCES

Brown, A.M., Walker, J.L. Jr., Sutton, R.B.: Increase chloride conductance as the proximate cause of hydrogen ion concentration effects in Aplysia neurons. *J Gen Physiol* 56: 559, 1970

Carmeliet, E.: Chloride ions and the membrane potential of Purkinje fibres. *J Physiol* 156: 375, 1961

De Mello, W.C.: Some aspects of the interrelationship between ions and electrical activity in specialized tissue of the heart. In: The specialized tissues of the heart, edited by Paes de Carvalho, A., de Mello, W.C. and Hoffman, B.F. Elsevier Publishing Co., Amsterdam, p. 95, 1961

De Mello, W.C.: Role of chloride ions in cardiac action and pacemaker potentials. *Am J Physiol* 205: 567, 1963

Fozzard, H.A., Lee, C.O.: Influence of changes in external potassium and chloride ions on membrane potential and intracellular potassium ion activity in rabbit ventricular muscle. *J Physiol* 256: 663, 1976

Hagiwara, S., Toyama, K., Hayashi, H.: Mechanisms of anion and cation permeations in the resting membranes of a barnacle muscle fiber. *J Gen Physiol* 57: 408, 1971

Hodgkin, A.L., Horowicz, P.: The influence of potassium and chloride ions on the membrane potential of single muscle fibres. *J Physiol* 148: 127, 1959

Hutter, O.F., Noble, D.: Anion conductance of cardiac muscle. *J Physiol* 157: 335, 1961

Irisawa, H., Noma, A.: Contracture and hyperpolarization of the rabbit sinoatrial node cell in Na-depleted solution. *Jap J Physiol* 26: 133, 1976

Irisawa, H., Seyama, I., Noma, A.: Resting and action potentials of rabbit sinoatrial node cells. In: Developmental and physiological correlates of cardiac muscle, edited by Lieberman, M. and Sano, T. Raven Press., New York, p. 287, 1975

Seyama, I.: The effect of anions on the membrane properties of sino-atrial node cell of the rabbit. *J Physiol Soc Japan* 39: 1977

30

DOES SPONTANEOUS ACTIVITY ARISE FROM PHASE 4 DEPOLARIZATION OR FROM TRIGGERING?

PAUL F. CRANEFIELD

There are many ways in which cardiac tissue can become and remain rhythmically active; some require the presence of phase 4 depolarization and others, such as sustained circus movement of excitation, do not. In my monograph, "The Conduction of the Cardiac Impulse" (Cranefield, 1975), I used the term "sustained rhythmic activity" to embrace all of those forms of rhythmic activity without respect to their cause. There are also many ways in which one may divide examples of sustained rhythmic activity but one seems fundamental: the division into tissues that show spontaneous activity and those that do not. We have long been accustomed to identify spontaneous activity with the presence of phase 4 depolarization. The terms spontaneous activity or automatic activity should, in my opinion, be used in a purely descriptive way without reference to an actual or assumed mechanism. A heart, or a preparation containing cardiac tissue, is spontaneously active if, and only if, having for any reason become quiescent, it invariably again becomes rhythmically active *without the intervention of any outside agent* such as an applied stimulus. This agrees with a definition of "spontaneous" found in the Oxford English Dictionary: "Spontaneous. 3. Of natural processes. Occurring without apparent external cause; having a self-contained cause or origin." The Oxford English Dictionary similarly defines "automatic" as "Self-acting, having the power of motion or action within itself." It will be noted that I have emphasized the appearance of rhythmic activity in a quiescent preparation as an essential characteristic of spontaneity or automaticity. I have done that in part because there are at least two kinds of sustained rhythmic activity that are not automatic exactly because they never carry a preparation from quiescence to sustained rhythmic activity. Their "rhythmicity" must be initiated by at least one impulse that originates in a way different from the train of impulses that follow it. I refer, of course, to sustained circus movement of excitation and to triggered activity in which each action potential arises from a preceding after-potential.

Let us consider a quiescent heart, one in which the SA node is, for some reason, inactive and in which no other automatic focus is present and active. If we excite such a heart by an applied electrical stimulus we may, in principle, set up a circus movement of excitation. Certainly we know that if we drive such a heart *twice*, the first stimulus may initiate a normal activation of the heart and the second may initiate rhythmic activity sustained by circus movement around a pathway involving the AV node. That activity may persist for a long time and might even be life-saving! But note that if it stops, it will not start again so that this form of self-sustained rhythmic activity is *not spontaneous*. Let me, for the sake of argument, suggest a way in which it could be combined with an automatic mechanism, i.e. with a sort of "physiological" demand pacemaker. Let us assume that there are a few cells in the heart which maintain a high resting potential when activated regularly and rapidly but which tend to depolarize when quiescent and tend, when depolarized, to develop oscillatory activity that can reach threshold and initiate one or two action potentials which are capable of re-starting the circuit of reentrant excitation. We would now have a system in which sustained rhythmic activity is the normal state of affairs but in which that activity is sustained by circus movement. Should that circus movement stop, it would not start itself again but it could, after a pause, be started again by impulses that arose in a different way. And so the system *as a whole* would be automatic but the mechanism (and focus) of the automatic activity is different from that which gives rise to the usual rhythmic excitation of that heart. In this hypothetical heart the "normal" rhythmic activity is caused by circus movement; "automaticity" is seen only rarely, serves to "re-start" the circus movement, and arises from oscillations in membrane potential seen only if the "normal" rhythmic activity stops for a time.

The above example may seem overly artificial but it does, I hope, make it clear that automaticity and sustained rhythmic activity are not the same thing. Automaticity always leads to sustained rhythmic activity; the presence of sustained rhythmic activity does not imply the presence of automaticity.

The form of activity that I have referred to as triggered activity leads us to a rather more subtle example, one in which we find that rhythmic activity is sustained by and depends upon phase 4 depolarization, i.e. by the very property that we have for so long associated with the activity of automatic fibers of the sort seen in the SA node and in the ventricular conducting system. Triggered activity of this sort is seen in fibers in which each action potential is followed by an early after-hyperpolarization which is, in turn, followed by a delayed after-depolarization (Figure 1). If the after-depolarization reaches threshold it will give rise to another action potential. The delayed-after depolarization that follows that action potential may give rise to yet another action potential, and if this goes on and on, the fiber in which all this occurs will be a focus of sustained rhythmic activity. What is more, each action potential grows out of what appears to be (and indeed is) phase 4 depolarization. At the end of each action potential the membrane potential does not remain constant but moves away from the maximum diastolic potential towards and to the threshold potential. If we impale a fiber while it is showing this sort of rhythmic activity there will be nothing to suggest that this smooth phase 4 depolarization is really made up

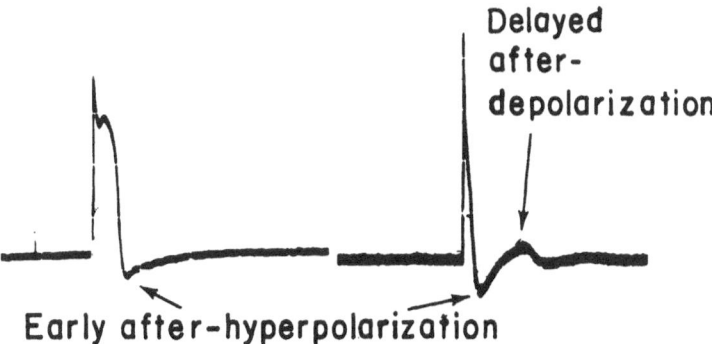

Figure 1. The first action potential is followed by an early after-hyperpolarization that carries the membrane potential negative to the level of the resting potential and then returns to that level. The second action potential is followed by an early after-hyperpolarization which is in turn followed by a delayed after-depolarization. The delayed after-depolarization carries the membrane potential positive to the level of the resting potential. (Canine Purkinje fibers exposed to Na-free, Ca-rich, TEA-containing solutions; based on Figure 1-6 of Cranefield, 1975).

of the decay of an after-hyperpolarization which leads into a delayed after-depolarization. There will, i.e., be nothing to suggest this *unless* the rhythmic activity stops. If it stops we may note an oscillatory after-potential the early part of which is hyperpolarizing and the late part of which is depolarizing with respect to the subsequent "resting" potential (Figure 2). We will also find that such a fiber, once quiescent, will remain quiescent until it is once again excited by some external stimulus (or driven at a critical rate, see Cranefield, 1977). This sort of behavior has been identified in fibers of the simian mitral valve (Wit and Cranefield, 1976) and in fibers of the canine coronary sinus (Wit and Cranefield, 1977) and in a number of other preparations (for review see Cranefield, 1977).

Preparations of this sort show sustained rhythmic activity but they are not spontaneous, i.e. they will not, if quiescent, spontaneously become rhythmically active. We must, therefore, conclude that the finding of phase 4 depolarization in a rhythmically active fiber does not show that the activity of that fiber is spontaneous or automatic. On the other hand we may ask whether there is some way in which we might "add" the property of automaticity to such a preparation, just as we added it to the preparation the activity of which was sustained by circus movement of excitation?

We might, indeed, add the same property to this system that we added to the system in which sustained rhythmic activity arose from sustained circus movement, namely the ability of a quiescent fiber to develop oscillatory changes in membrane potential, oscillations that grow in amplitude until they evoke an action potential. This kind of automaticity might be found in a fiber that is not triggerable, in which case the action potential that arises in the automatic fiber could propagate into the triggerable focus and there evoke sustained rhythmic activity. On the other hand the triggerable fiber might, after a period of quiescence, itself develop oscillatory activity and generate the action potential that is necessary to initiate a train of action potentials that arise from after-potentials, i.e., initiate triggered sustained rhythmic activity. We have, in fact, seen this sort of behavior in Purkinje fibers exposed to Na-free, Ca-rich solutions. An example is shown in Figure 3, in which it might be noticed that the oscillatory prepotentials are very small compared with the early after-hyperpolarization that follows the first and subsequent action potentials. In terms of their size and shape there is no real similarity between the oscillatory prepotentials which initiate the first action potential and the after-potentials which sustain the later rhythmic activity. Figure 4 shows the essential equivalence of an

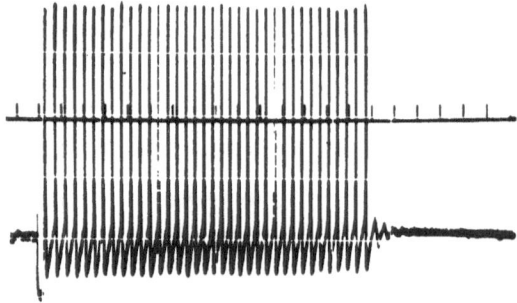

Figure 2. The termination of sustained rhythmic activity reveals that although it appears to depend on "spontaneous" phase 4 depolarization, the resting potential is markedly positive to the maximum diastolic potential and the rhythmic activity is actually sustained by after-potentials. The "phase 4 depolarization" consists of the decay of an early after-hyperpolarization and the depolarizing phase of a delayed after-depolarization. (Canine Purkinje fibers exposed to Na-free, Ca-rich, TEA-containing solution; previously unpublished).

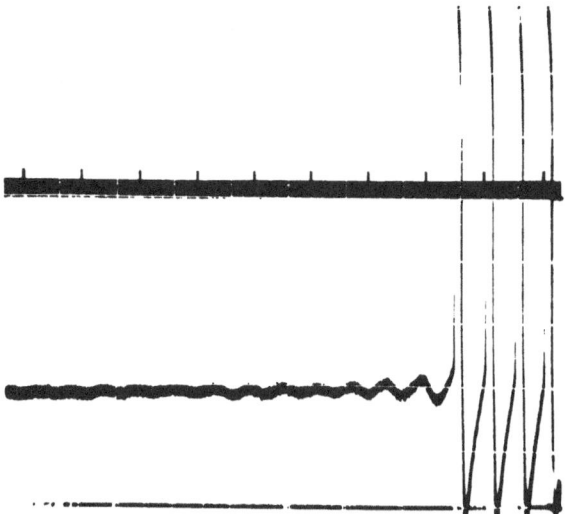

Figure 3. Initiation of sustained rhythmic activity by oscillatory changes in membrane potential. The oscillations appear to carry the fiber from quiescence to activity. After the first action potential, however, the activity is sustained by phase 4 depolarization that does not resemble the oscillatory activity that led to the first action potential. (Canine Purkinje fiber exposed to Na-free, Ca-rich, TEA-containing solutions; from Figure VI-22 of Cranefield, 1975).

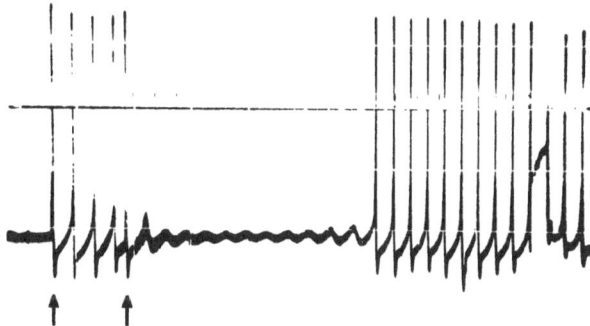

Figure 4. At the beginning of the record the fiber is quiescent. The first stimulus (first arrow) initiates an action potential that is followed by 3 non-driven action potentials. At the second arrow an applied stimulus evokes a premature action potential that is followed by quiescence. Oscillatory changes in membrane potential at first diminish and then increase in amplitude until an action potential is evoked. The action potentials that follow appear to grow out of after-potentials, having been triggered by the oscillatory change that evoked the first action potential. (Canine Purkinje fibers exposed to Na-free, Ca-rich, TEA-containing solution; from Figure VI-23, Cranefield, 1975).

applied stimulus and an oscillatory prepotential in triggering activity: each serves to evoke an initial action potential the after-potential of which in turn evokes the next action potential. (Figure 4 also shows another phenomenon sometimes seen in triggerable fibers, the cessation of activity following a premature impulse.)

There are many triggerable fibers that will remain quiescent indefinitely long, i.e. until driven; there are others that always resume activity in the manner just described. The latter fibers are automatic but their automaticity resides in their tendency to develop oscillatory prepotentials. In this connection I would call attention to Vassalle's finding (Vassalle, 1965) that Purkinje fibers which pass from quiescence to "spontaneous" activity when $[K]_o$ is reduced from 5.4 mM to 2.7 mM do so in a manner very like that just described, i.e. they develop low amplitude oscillatory prepotentials one of which evokes an action potential. The first action potential and the preceding prepotential closely resemble those seen in Figure 3.

There is another way in which activity may appear in Purkinje fibers, namely a very slow and gradual depolarization (which in no way resembles ordinary phase 4 depolarization) may bring membranes to the threshold potential. The action potential thus evoked is followed by an after-hyperpolarization the decay of which does in fact resemble ordinary phase 4 depolarization and which may lead into sustained rhythmic activity. This sort of behavior is exactly what is seen during the resumption of activity after a period of overdrive suppression (Figure 5).

Before turning to the SA node I should again make it clear that I do not claim that there is no such thing as an automatic fiber. On the contrary, I suggest that there is a class of fibers that show sustained rhythmic activity when "triggered" and I divide that class of fibers into automatic and non-automatic. Non-automatic triggerable fibers must be driven (by applied stimuli or by a propagated impulse) so that an initiating action potential can give rise to the after-hyperpolarization and after-depolarization that give rise to the next action potential. The automatic fibers drive themselves and thus trigger themselves but their automaticity resides in a property (very gradual depolarization or oscillatory prepotentials) which may be quite different from the property (development of afterpotentials) which gives rise to their subsequent sustained rhythmic activity.

There are some situations in which rhythmic activity apparently sustained by classic

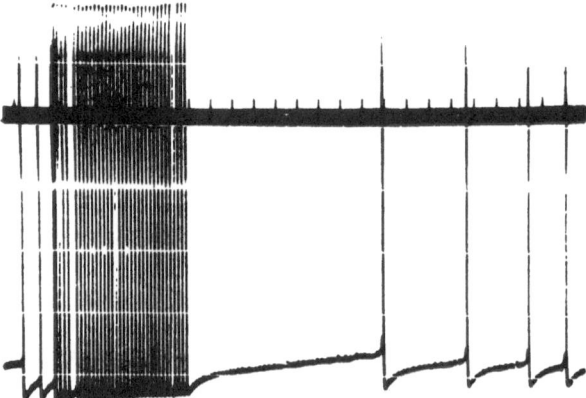

Figure 5. At the begining of the trace the fiber is quiescent. After two stimuli at a low rate the fiber was driven rapidly; the drive was then stopped. Note the long and gradual depolarization preceding the first non-driven action potential. Note that all subsequent action potentials arise from phase 4 depolarization that may be regarded as an after-potential, at least in so far as it occurs in a range of voltage almost wholly negative to the original resting potential, a range into which the membrane potential is carried by an early after-hyperpolarization that follows each action potential. (Canine Purkinje fiber exposed to normal Tyrode's solution; from Figure VI-20, Cranefield, 1975).

phase 4 depolarization is unquestionably really triggered activity sustained by after-potentials (mitral valve, coronary sinus, Purkinje fibers exposed to Na-free solutions). There are other situations in which that may be so (Purkinje fibers recovering from over-drive suppression, Purkinje fibers becoming active as $[K]_o$ is lowered). Is there any evidence to suggest that the rhythmic activity of fibers of the SA node is triggered? It is well known that "depressed" fibers of the SA node often resume normal activity after a period of subthreshold oscillatory changes in membrane potential (see West, 1961; Brooks and Lu, 1972). And, indeed, fibers of the SA node may return to activity after a period of over-drive suppression in the same way that Purkinje fibers do, i.e. via a slow and gradual depolarization that differs considerably from the ordinary phase 4 depolarization seen when such fibers demonstrate their normal "spontaneous" activity (see Brooks and Lu, 1972, Figure 52). A further suggestive finding is that of Lu, Lange and Brooks (1965), namely that when the SA node was divided into two parts the pacemakers of the "lower" node often did not become rhythmically active until they had been driven one or more times by applied stimuli. Finally, preliminary studies by Wit and myself have revealed some interesting properties of cells of the rabbit SA node exposed to 0.5 mg/l of verapamil. In such preparations the action potential is somewhat reduced in amplitude but the nodal cells remain rhythmically active and appear to be essentially normal unless they are driven at a rapid rate. After such a period of "overdrive", the rhythmic activity stops and the membrane potential shows only low-voltage oscillations. Such cells remain quiescent until they are driven whereupon, as in all the examples of triggered activity mentioned above, sustained activity, apparently caused by after-potentials, is evoked (Figure 6). The behavior of this preparation seems to be an interesting model for certain kinds of behavior of the "sick sinus", such as "tachycardia-bradycardia" behavior (Ferrer, 1974). It also supports my argument that at least some of the "spontaneous" activity of the SA node may actually be triggered.

Before concluding, we should examine in more detail the relationship between "conventional" phase 4 depolarization and the after-potentials seen in triggerable fibers. It was pointed out some 20 years ago by Dudel and Trautwein (1958) that there is a striking similarity between "conventional" phase 4 depolarization and the decay of an early after-hyperpolarization of the sort shown above in Figure 1. It may also be noted that marked early after-hyperpolarization is not characteristic of the action potentials of all fibers. It is not, e.g., a notable feature of the action potentials of the contractile cells of the atrium or ventricle (cf. Trautwein and Kassebaum, 1961); it is, however, prominent in cells that are supposedly automatic, such as those of the SA node and of the ventricular conducting system. On the other hand, it is perfectly possible for an early after-hyper-polarization to decay to the resting potential (as in the first action potential in Figure 1 above) without either evoking an action potential or being followed by and merging with a delayed after-depolarization. It is possible that an essential characteristic of triggerable fibers is that the action potentials of those fibers are followed not only by an after-hyperpolarization but also by a delayed after-depolarization (Figure 1). In such fibers the amplitude of the delayed after-depolarization increases with increasing drive rate or with premature excitation. The non-driven, triggered rhythm arises only when the delayed after-depolarization is large enough to reach threshold. It may be, therefore, that the presence of an early after-hyperpolarization is not sufficient grounds for regarding the phase 4 depolarization it causes as being identical with that seen in triggerable fibers in which the later part of the phase 4 depolarization corresponds to the beginning of a delayed after-depolarization. On the other hand, if the threshold potential is only a very

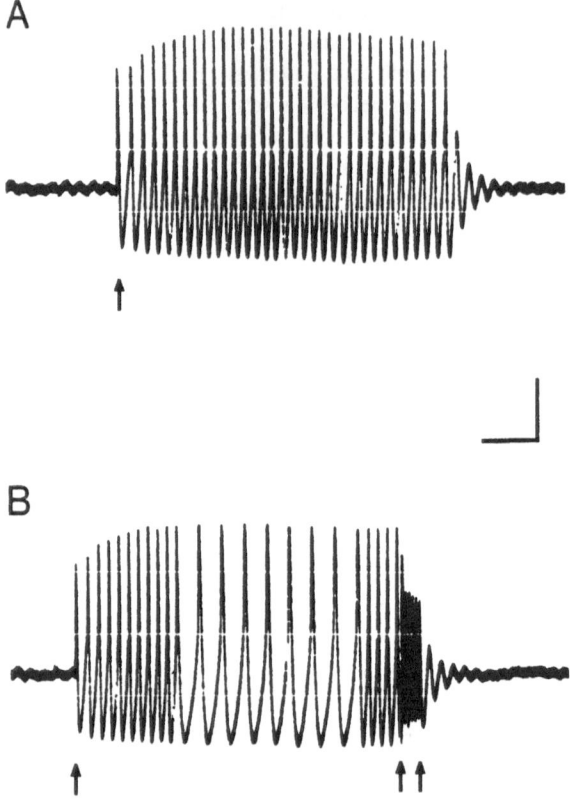

Figure 6. Activity in rabbit SA node exposed to verapamil (0.5 mg/l). In A, the rhythmic activity of the preparation had stopped following a period of overdrive and the preparation had been quiescent for a prolonged period. The first action potential (arrow) was evoked by an applied stimulus; the rest of the action potentials were non-driven. The activity stopped spontaneously, revealing an early after-hyperpolarization followed by a sub-threshold delayed after-depolarization which was, in turn, followed by damped oscillations in membrane potential. In B, the preparation became quiescent at the end of a 2 min period of stimulation at 150/min and had remained quiescent for several minutes until a single stimulus (arrow) triggered the preparation into activity that was maintained until it was again suppressed by a period of rapid overdrive (seven stimuli applied between second and third arrows). During the middle of the record the sweep speed was increased to show the shape of the action potential in more detail. The vertical calibration in A corresponds to 7.5 mV in both A and B; the horizontal calibration in A represents 5 sec both in A and at the beginning and end of B and represents 2 sec during the middle of B. (A.L. Wit and P.F. Cranefield, previously unpublished).

few mV positive to the "resting" potential, the decay of an early after-hyperpolarization, perhaps "assisted" by a minute delayed after-depolarization might in fact suffice to initiate the next action potential. In any event, whether rhythmic activity which is sustained by phase 4 depolarization does or does not require the presence of delayed after-depolarizations, it is seen only in fibers that do develop early after-hyperpolarizations, and the decay of those early after-hyperpolarizations always merges smoothly into the upstroke of the action potential of a "true pacemaker." Another way of saying this is, of course, that if an automatic fiber is quiescent, its resting potential is always substantially positive with respect to the maximum diastolic potential seen during activity. That is another way of saying that an *after-potential* plays an important role in causing rhythmic activity sustained by phase 4 depolarization. And that in turn brings me back to my original position that no such after-potential can precede the *first* action potential in such a fiber. What precedes the first action potential is a slow and gradual depolarization or an oscillatory pre-potential and it is in those phenomena that the property of automaticity resides. Thus I do not lump together (at least with any confidence) "traditional" phase 4 depolarization and triggered activity of the sort requiring delayed after-depolarizations. Or rather, I do lump them together, but only to the extent that each displays an early after-depolarization, an event that can occur only following an action potential, and to the extent that some event other than "traditional" phase 4 depolarization initiates the first in any series of action potentials.

It is not, I think, a verbal quibble to suggest, as I have done, that at least some of the fibers traditionally regarded as automatic do not derive their automaticity from their familiar phase 4 depolarization, but from some other property such as the ability to show a slow gradual depolarization or oscillatory prepotentials. On the one hand the ionic mechanisms that cause after-potentials and thus permit triggering may be quite different from those that cause oscillatory prepotentials or the very slow and gradual depolarization that leads to the first action potential. The most obvious difference is that the early after-hyperpolarization is almost certainly caused by the same increase in potassium conductance that plays a role in repolarization, an increase which is, in turn, almost certainly initiated by the action potential itself. (That is why the early after-depolarization is, in the strictest sense, an *after-potential*, i.e., a change in membrane potential that follows and is caused by the preceding action potential.) On the other hand, we often wish to use drugs to initiate a rhythm or to interrupt a tachycardia. If true automaticity derives from causes different from those which sustain rhythmic activity once it has been triggered, then we must allow for that when we search for drugs that can initiate, modify or terminate rhythmic activity.

ACKNOWLEDGEMENTS

My studies of triggered arrhythmias have been conducted in collaboration with R.S. Aronson, Andrew L. Wit, Jay R. Wiggins and David C. Gadsby, to all of whom I am deeply indebted.

The research upon which the results reported in this article are based has been supported by a grant from The National Institutes of Health (HL-14899).

REFERENCES

Brooks, C.McC., H.-H.: Lu, *The Sinoatrial Pacemaker of the Heart*. Springfield, Charles C. Thomas, 1972

Cranefield, P.F.: *The Conduction of the Cardiac Impulse. The Slow Response and Cardiac Arrhythmias*. Mount Kisco, Futura Publishing Co., 1975

Cranefield, P.F.: Action potentials, after-potentials and arrhythmias. *Circ Res* 41: 415, 1977

Dudel, J., Trautwein, W.: Der Mechanismus der automatischen rhythmischen Impulsbildung der Herzmuskelfaser. *Pflügers Arch* 267: 553, 1958

Ferrer, M.I.: *The Sick Sinus Syndrome*. Mount Kisco, Futura Publishing Co. 1974

Lu, H.-H., Lange, G., Brooks, C.McC.: Factors controlling pacemaker action in cells of the sinoatrial node. *Circ Res* 17: 460, 1965

Trautwein, W., Kassebaum, D.G.: On the mechanism of spontaneous impulse generation in the pacemaker of the heart. *J Gen Physiol* 45: 317, 1961

Vassalle, M.: Cardiac pacemaker potentials at different extra- and intracellular K concentrations. *Am J Physiol* 208: 770, 1965

West, T.C.: Effects of chronotropic influences on subthreshold oscillations in the sino-atrial node. In: *The*

Specialized Tissues of the Heart. A. Paes de Carvalho, W.C. De Mello and B.F. Hoffman (eds.). New York, Elsevier, 1961

Wit, A.L., Cranefield, P.F.: Triggered activity in cardiac muscle fibers of the simian mitral valve. *Circ Res* 38: 85, 1976

Wit, A.L., Cranefield, P.F.: Triggered and automatic activity in the canine coronary sinus. *Circ Res* 41: 435, 1977

31

ON THE POSSIBLE MECHANISM UNDERLYING SPONTANEOUS PACEMAKING

G.H. POLLACK

Notwithstanding years of study, the mechanism by which the heart beat is initiated remains uncertain; so uncertain, in fact, that Brooks and Lu (1972) in their excellent review concluded that the mechanism underlying spontaneous pacemaking in the sinus node remains a "mystery."

Actually, there appear to be two mysteries. The most obvious, perhaps, is the mechanism by which each of the many cells in the sinus node depolarizes and repolarizes spontaneously during each heartbeat. The more subtle, but equally intriguing mystery is the manner by which the independent activities of individual cells are coordinated such that the sinus node does not issue forth a barrage of independent, uncoordinated signals to the heart, but an effectively synchronous burst.

Some avenues of approach to the solution of these two mysteries have recently been offered (Pollack, 1977). Here, in a more informal way, I would like to recapitulate some of the important pieces of evidence which have led to the formulation of these hypotheses, describe the hypotheses, explore their physiological consequences, and finally touch on their possible implication *vis-à-vis* the genesis of certain cardiac arrhythmias.

CLUES

That catecholamines exert a powerful modulatory influence on pacemaking frequency has been evident for many years. In the mid-fifties, with the advent of microelectrodes, the positive chronotropic action of catecholamines was demonstrated to arise out of an enhancement of the rate of spontaneous depolarization of the pacemaker cells (Hutter and Trautwein, 1956; West et al., 1956). It now appears that this modulatory effect on the rate of spontaneous depolarization is perhaps only one aspect of a more fundamental role; catecholamines may in fact, be *required* for the generation of spontaneous depolarization.

Before considering the evidence for this, it is relevant to note that catecholamine stores in the sinus node are not restricted to sympathetic nerve terminals. In dog hearts that had been denervated both surgically and chemically (with 6-hydroxydopamine), the sinus node was found to have retained about half the epinephrine present in non-denervated controls (Spurgeon et al., 1974). The authors implicated an extraneural storage site, possibly in cells analogous to the catecholamine containing chromaffin cells of the adrenal medulla. Fluorescence histochemical studies (Miyagishima, 1975) confirm a rather widespread distribution of catecholamines in the sinus node; the distribution pattern is consistent with localization within *each* pacemaking cell. Intracellular storage would not be surprising in light of the "conspicuously numerous" subsarcolemmal vesicles found in these cells (James et al., 1966), vesicles also seen by other investigators (Ruska, 1965; Trautwein and Uchizono, 1963; Challice, 1966; Cheng, 1971; Viragh and Porte, 1973) and described by some as bearing structural similarity to those in the chromaffin cells of the adrenal medulla that store catecholamines.

That the presence of endogenous catecholamines is *required* for pacemaking has been demonstrated in a series of elegant studies by Tuganowski and colleagues. Tuganowski et al. (1973) exposed isolated rabbit sinoatrial node to reserpine, an agent which depletes catecholamine stores. Reserpine (10 μM) reduced the spontaneous rate and brought beating to a halt in 5 to 25 minutes. When catecholamines were added to the bath containing the reserpine, beating resumed within 1 to 3 minutes. In another series of experiments the node was exposed to α-methyl tyrosine (1 mM), a specific inhibitor of catecholamine synthesis. Spontaneous activity ceased in 1 to 4 hours. When catecholamines were added to this bath, beating resumed in 2 to 5 minutes. Although these results implicate a catecholamine requirement in pacemaking, the investigators considered the alternative possibility that the termination of spontaneous activity was not due to catecholamine depletion but to some indirect or nonspecific effect of these inhibitors. When the preparations were pretreated with reserpine to deplete catecholamine stores, and washed with fresh Tyrode's solution to restore beating, the time required for α-methyl tyrosine to inhibit beating was reduced 100-fold. This provided powerful evidence that these agents did indeed inhibit beating by depleting endogenous catecholamines.

More recently, the catecholamine requirement has been underscored by the observation that inhibition of adenylate cyclase, the enzyme responsible for catalyzing the formation of the "second messenger" of catecholamines, cAMP, abolished pacing. Exposure of the isolated sinus node to haloperidol or chlorpromazine was found to inhibit spontaneous activity (Tuganowski, 1977). These effects could be reversed by exposure of the preparation to dibutyryl cyclic AMP, a derivative of cAMP which can diffuse through the plasma membrane. Thus, both catecholamines and cyclic AMP, the first two elements in the beta adrenergic pathway, not only modulate spontaneous activity, but appear to be *required* in some way for pacemaking to occur.

A POSSIBLE ROLE OF ENDOGENOUS CATECHOLAMINES

Although the storage site of catecholamines appears to be located *within* the cell, the action of catecholamines on pacemaker (and other) cells is on the *outside* of the membrane (Yamasaki et al., 1974; Lefkowitz et al., 1973; Reuter, 1974). If endogenous catecholamines play an obligatory role in pacemaking, a way must be identified for the catecholamines to leave the cell. Diffusion is the simplest possibility. On the other hand, the numerous exocytotic figures seen on the membranes of these pacemaking cells (James et al., 1966) raises the intriguing possibility that the catecholamines are stored within the subsarcolemmal vesicles, and discharged from the cell into the extracellular space by exocytosis. The discharge process would then be analogous to that found in neurosecretory tissues.

Could catecholamine discharge and subsequent binding to the outside of the plasma membrane lead to spontaneous pacemaking? This appears possible. Consider first the elements involved in catecholamine discharge. There is little doubt that intracellular Ca^{++} is required, since Ca^{++} influx into the cell is a necessary condition for exocytosis in perhaps all neurosecretory systems studied so far (Douglas, 1968; Cochrane et al., 1975). Ca^{++} entry also tends to depolarize the cell. Although the complexity of the mechanism by which Ca^{++} entry mediates vesicle discharge presumably transcends mere cellular depolarization (Dean, 1975), there nevertheless appears to be a good correlation between cellular depolarization and vesicle discharge rate: In the neuromuscular junction, perhaps the best studied secretory system, the rate of discharge varies exponentially with the degree of cellular depolarization (del Castillo and Katz, 1954). Even when the presynaptic cell is fully polarized (about -90 mV), there remains some random, spontaneous discharge of vesicles, the manifestation of which is the miniature end plate potential. As an initial supposition, it seems reasonable to assume that if vesicle discharge did, indeed, occur from sinus node cells, the properties of the discharge system would be similar to those described above. Principally, this means that the rate of catecholamine discharge from the cell increases as the cell is depolarized by Ca^{++} entry.

Secondly, consider the action of the binding of catecholamines to the outside of the cell membrane. Among the most fundamental actions is the increase of calcium flux into the cell (Grossman and Furchgott, 1964; Reuter, 1965). This appears to occur through the beta-adrenergic pathway, illustrated in Figure 1. Catecholamines stimulate the production of cAMP by activation of adenylate cyclase; this causes phosphorylation of a membrane protein, which results in an increase of calcium conductance (Greengard, 1976; Wollenberger, 1975).

In view of the fact that an ultimate action of catecholamines is the promotion of Ca^{++} influx, and an action of Ca^{++} influx is the promotion of catecholamine discharge, which in turn increases the availability of catecholamines for further action on the outside of the membrane, one has at hand the elements of a positive feedback, or regenerative, system. Spontaneous depolarization and repolarization could then occur by the following scheme (Figure 2A):

(i) Vesicles begin discharging catecholamines spontaneously into the extracellular space; the discharge rate is low at first because the cell is relatively polarized (-50 to -60 mV), and intracellular Ca^{++} is relatively low.

(ii) Catecholamines discharged into the extracellular space diffuse away from the discharge site; those molecules which bind to the outside of the cell membrane activate adenylate cyclase, thereby increasing cAMP, bringing about the phosphorylation of membrane proteins, and transiently opening calcium channels; this allows Ca^{++} to enter and further depolarize the cell.

(iii) The more the cell is depolarized by Ca^{++} entry, the higher the rate of catechola-

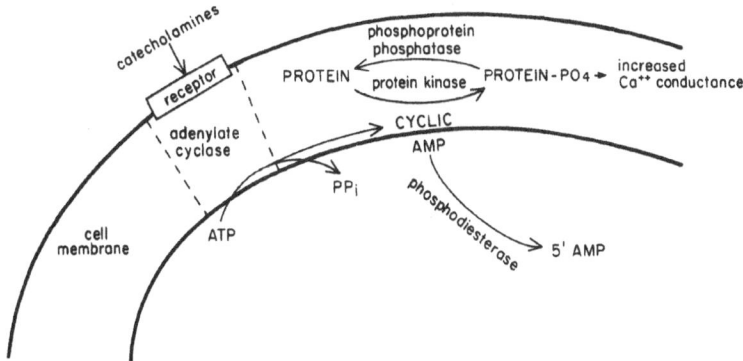

Figure 1. The mechanism by which catecholamines appear to increase calcium influx into the cell. (Modified from Greengard, 1976).

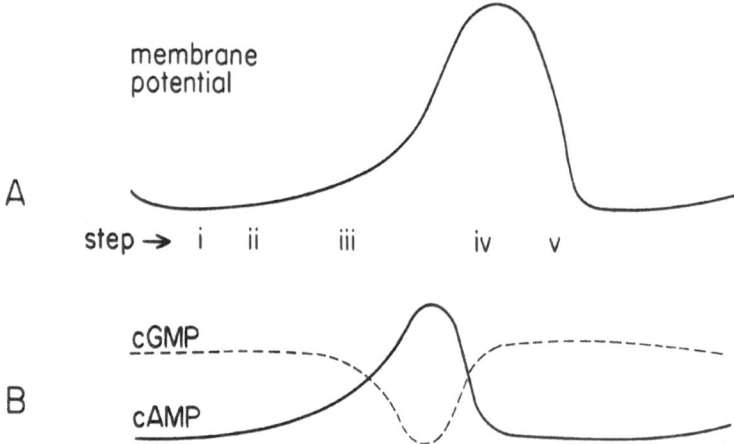

Figure 2. A) The time course of the pacemaker potential in primary pacemaking cells. The cycle is broken into five phases, during which the events described in the text may take place. *B*) The time course of the concentration of intracellular cyclic AMP expected from the proposed model. Reciprocal fluctuation of cyclic GMP may also occur as it does in another cardiac tissue.

mine discharge; this positive feedback loop results in a depolarization which has the shape of a rising exponential; ultimately all catecholamines in the releasable pool are discharged.

(iv) With no further catecholamine-mediated adenylate cyclase activity, cAMP returns to baseline levels, and there is no further opening of calcium channels; thus the cell stops depolarizing.

(v) As the cell repolarizes by Ca^{++} extrusion, the vesicles reform and are replenished with catecholamines; when replenishment is adequate, spontaneous discharge commences and the cycle begins once again.

This scheme accounts for the obligatory role of the beta adrenergic pathway in pacemaking. If catecholamines are depleted, or if adenylate cyclase activity is blocked, pacemaking stops; exogenous catecholamines can restore beating by supplementing endogenous stores. Beating can also be stopped by any agent which hyperpolarizes the cell (e.g. acetylcholine) to the point where the rate of spontaneous discharge becomes inadequate to initiate the cycle.

An important implication of the proposed scheme is that the concentration of cAMP is expected to oscillate during the pacemaking cycle, as shown in Figure 2B. During steps i and ii and most of step iii, the level of cAMP increases, since catecholamine-mediated adenylate cyclase activity increases. When further catecholamine binding ceases, cAMP production is no longer stimulated. Phosphodiesterase activity then breaks down cAMP and causes a diminution of the pool. Baseline levels of cAMP are reached during step iv, and with no further adenylate cyclase activity, cAMP remains at this level until the cycle begins again.

Although the concentrations of cyclic AMP during the cardiac cycle have not yet been measured in pacemaker tissue, they have been found to oscillate in frog ventricular tissue (Brooker, 1973; Wollenberger et al., 1973). In these studies the level of cyclic AMP increased in the early part of the cycle, returned approximately to baseline levels prior to repolarization and remained there until the beginning of the following cycle, a time course similar to the one in the proposed scheme (Figure 2B).

Maintenance of stable cycling requires that the processes mediating depolarization be prevented from occurring during the phase of repolarization; thus Ca^{++} influx must not be allowed to occur beyond step iii. While this can be achieved in the scheme through phosphodiesterase-mediated diminution of the cyclic AMP level, two additional factors may augment this mechanism and thereby enhance cycling stability.

The first is the acceleration of phosphodiesterase activity during step iii. The relatively low activity found at low Ca^{++} concentrations increases when the Ca^{++} concentration is elevated above 1 μM to a greatly enhanced activity at 10 μM (Teo and Wang, 1973). Because there is good reason (though no conclusive evidence) to believe that intracellular Ca^{++} rises to these concentrations at the peak of the cardiac cycle (Katz, 1970; Winegrad, 1971), it is possible that a greatly enhanced phosphodiesterase activity in step iii may drive cycle AMP down to baseline levels rapidly.

The second factor may involve cyclic GMP, the other important cyclic nucleotide found in the cardiac cell. In accordance with the so-called "yin-yang" hypothesis (Goldberg et al., 1973) cyclic GMP antagonizes the action of cyclic AMP. This probably occurs by dephosphorylation of proteins through activation of phosphoprotein phosphatase (Sandoval and Cuatrecasas, 1976). The intracellular concentration of cyclic GMP oscillates during the cardiac cycle of frog ventricle with a time course similar, but a direction opposite, to that of cyclic AMP (Wollenberger et al., 1973); this may occur through the conversion of one cyclic nucleotide into the other (Simon, 1976). Should cyclic GMP and cyclic AMP fluctuate reciprocally in pacemaker cells as well (Figure 2B), the effect of the cyclic GMP fluctuations would be to enhance phosphorylation at the time in the cycle that the processes mediating Ca^{++} influx required activation (steps i to iii), and to prevent phosphorylation at the time these processes required inhibition (steps iv and v). Oscillations of cyclic GMP, if they occurred, would therefore serve to increase cycling stability.

Elements of the pacemaking cycle which are least clear are those occurring in step v. Repolarization might occur by a delayed efflux of K^+ as it does in many other cells; a K^+-Ca^{++} pump would then be required to maintain steady state concentrations of these ions. A simpler possibility is that repolarization occurs as a direct consequence of Ca^{++} being pumped out of the cytosol. A Ca^{++}-dependent ATPase is known to exist in the membrane of the catecholamine vesicles of chromaffin cells (Kirschner, 1974), and an analogous one might exist in vesicles of the sinus node. If the process of exocytosis involves a continual turnover of vesicle membrane and plasma membrane (Heuser and Reese, 1973), then a Ca^{++}-dependent ATPase should also exist in the cell membrane; this could mediate Ca^{++} extrusion from the cell. This area requires further study.

PHARMACOLOGIC TESTS OF THE PROPOSED SCHEME

Figure 3 shows the elements of the proposed scheme in some detail. Listed toward the left of the figure are the various classes of agents expected to stimulate or inhibit certain of the processes along the proposed pathway. The expected effect on beating frequency of each of these is indicated at the far left. For example, phosphodiesterase inhibitors (such as caffeine or theophylline) should increase the amount of cAMP, thereby accelerating spontaneous depolarization and increasing beating frequency. Exogenous cyclic GMP, either added directly, or indirectly through administration of acetylcholine (George et al., 1973), should activate phosphoprotein phosphatase, diminishing the degree of protein phosphorylation and Ca^{++} influx, thereby diminishing spontaneous rate.

The actions of some of the agents listed in Figure 3 have been discussed above. A fuller

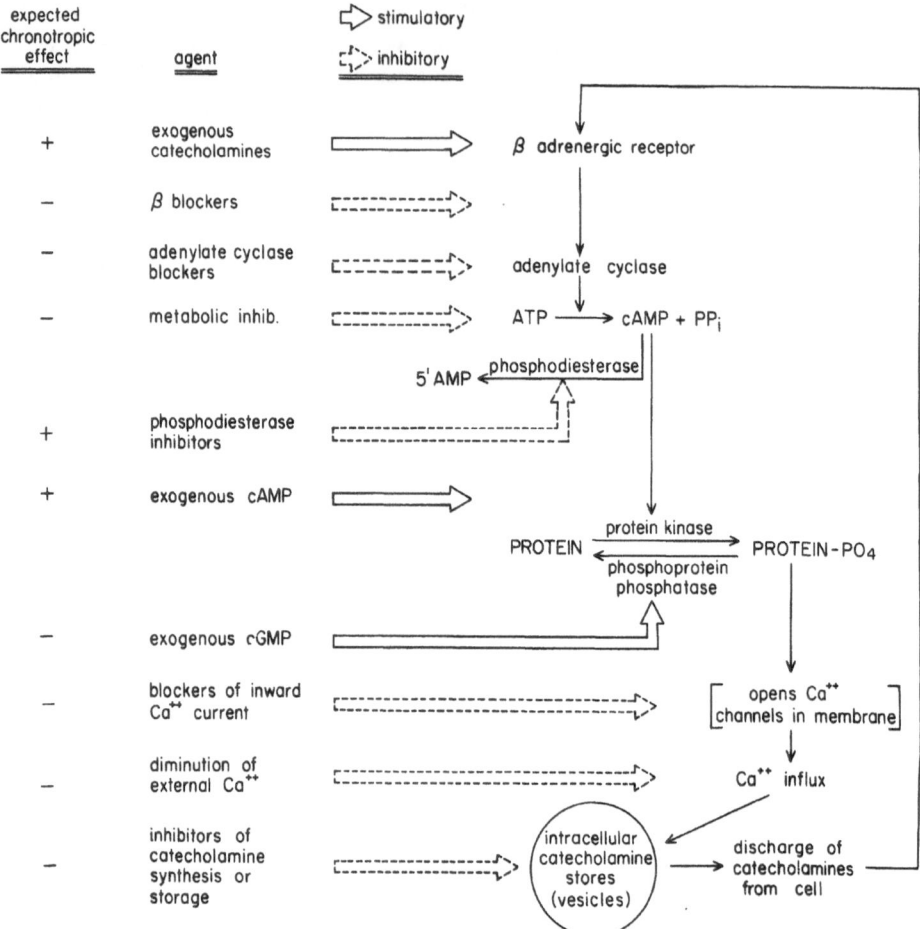

Figure 3. Details of the proposed mechanism of generation of the pacemaker potential. By inhibiting or accelerating certain processes, the agents listed at the left of the figure should give rise to increases or decreases of pacing frequency. The expected responses are confirmed experimentally, as detailed in the text and in the paper by Pollack (1977).

treatment is found in a previous paper (Pollack, 1977). In general, all agents listed in Figure 3 exert a chronotropic effect which is in the expected direction. While this by no means proves that the hypothesis is valid, it indicates that it is at least a reasonable working hypothesis.

SYNCHRONIZATION AND POPULATION DYNAMICS

The second "mystery" of cardiac pacemaking is the mechanism underlying intercellular synchronization. Many pacemaker cells comprise the sinus node. Each one begins depolarizing at a rate largely independent of the other pacemaking cells, so that there is a spectrum of initial rates of depolarization ranging from the fastest (primary) to the slower (secondary, latent, or follower) pacemaking cells (Hoffman and Cranefield, 1960). But such evidently independent cellular activity does not last throughout the pacemaking cycle; as the primary pacemaker cell undergoes full, regenerative depolarization, the secondary pacemaking cells are soon made to follow suit, so that a synchronous output emerges from the sinus node to the atrium.

How is the "turn-on" signal communicated from the primary pacemaking cell to latent pacemaking cells? One possibility is that communication is electrically mediated, i.e., by way of currents flowing between cells. In most cardiac tissues gap junctional channels interconnect contiguous cells, channels which are widely held to represent the sites of current flow between cells (Dewey and Barr, 1962; McNutt and Weinstein, 1970). Thus depolarization of one cell establishes a potential gradient between contiguous cells, thereby driving current through the gap junctional channels; this depolarizes the contiguous cells sufficiently that they reach threshold, fire, and sustain propagated activity. There is some evidence based upon voltage clamp studies (Noma and Irisawa, 1976; Brown, Giles and Noble, 1977) and upon measurements of space constant (Bonke, 1973) that sinus node cells communicate electrically; however, other considerations indicate that whatever electrical communication might exist is probably far too weak to sustain propagation through the sinus node.

One consideration is based on the very fact that during the phase of spontaneous depolarization the pacemaking cells depolarize at different rates. Long-lasting potential gradients of substantial magnitude develop between neighboring pacemaker cells during this period (Figure 4), an observation difficult to reconcile with the presumption of tight electrical coupling. Along similar lines of thought, the maximum diastolic potential in sinus node cells is lower than the resting potential in nearby atrial cells, raising once again the question of how such long-lasting gradients could be sustained if the cells were tightly coupled.

Morphologically, the cellular architecture does not lend itself well to electrical coupling. The gap junctional channels of intercellular communication are rare or absent in the sinus node (James et al., 1966; Cheng, 1971; Viragh and Porte, 1973). This does not rule out the possibility that another type of intercellular communication channel peculiar to the sinus

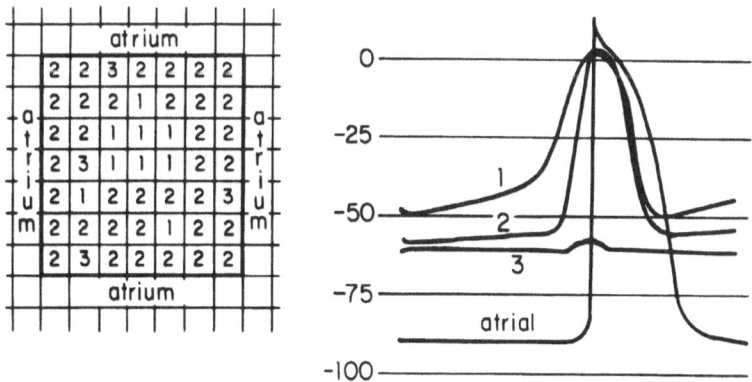

Figure 4. Left. Schematic representation of the arrangement of pacemaking cells in ths sinus node. Primary pacemaking cells (1) are located generally, but not exclusively, near the center of the sinus node. Latent or secondary pacemaking cells (2) are located closer to the periphery of the node. Some cells may show no regenerative activity (3). *Right.* Observed waveshapes of depolarization among the various types of cell.

node might one day be identified; however, its properties would have to be remarkable. The required intercellular conductance would have to be much higher than between, say, atrial cells in order that the high intercellular currents required to sustain propagation could flow. Sinus cells are remarkably insensitive to depolarizing current, some cells failing to respond to depolarizing currents raised to levels sufficient to destroy the cell (Ushiyama and Brooks, 1974).

A possibility worth considering is one in which communication occurs mechanically. For example, it has been proposed that propagation through the AV node occurs by a stretch-induced depolarization mechanism: proximal cells are excited, depolarize, contract, and thereby stretch more distally placed cells. Stretch depolarizes these latter cells, causing them to contract and stretch cells which are still more distally placed, and so on (Pollack, 1974). Could such a mechanism apply in the sinus node?

The required contractile machinery is present in sinus node cells, though the myofilament packing density is relatively lower than in "working" myocardium (James et al., 1966). Contractile activity of the sinus node has been observed and measured (Irisawa and Noma, 1976). Since the primary pacemaking cells depolarize first, presumably they also contract first. Neighboring latent pacemaker cells, as yet unactivated, should offer little resistance to stretch; if stretch could abruptly accelerate their slow spontaneous rate of depolarization, propagation could be sustained. In such a way an excitation signal from a primary pacemaking cell could propagate through the sinus node and synchronize the action of the constituent pacemaking cells.

Pacemaking cells do appear to be sensitive to stretch. For example, in mammalian sinus node stretch increases the frequency of discharge (Deck, 1964), an effect which is mediated by an increase in the rate of spontaneous depolarization. This action can be sufficiently strong to induce spontaneous depolarization in those cells within the sinus node in which activity had been absent prior to stretch (Brooks and Lu, 1972). In cells of many species throughout the animal kingdom, particularly in the more primitive phyla, the distension caused by filling of the cardiac chambers is often the physiologic "trigger" of pacing; i.e., unless sufficiently stretched some pacemakers will not pace.

Returning to the proposed mechanism of spontaneous pacemaking, we can identify a possible mechanism by which stretch might accelerate depolarization. Consider, again, the analogy to other vesicle discharge systems. At the myoneural junction, where the effect of stretch is best documented, stretch increases the presynaptic vesicle discharge rate (Hutter and Trautwein, 1956). The action is instantaneous (Ypey, 1975), and the sensitivity to stretch is exquisite: stretch of 10–15%, depending upon the frequency of stimulation, increases the probability of vesicle discharge by five to ten times (IJpeij et al., 1974).

If an analogous situation existed in pacemaking cells, the means by which stretch induces depolarization would be evident. Stretch of a latent pacemaking cell would provoke a more intense discharge of catecholamines, thereby providing the means by which its rate of depolarization could be accelerated. Through such a mechanism the action of the latent cells could by synchronized to the action of the more primary cells.

One powerful feature of such a communication mechanism is its inherent safeness. As the number of depolarized cells increases, a progressively larger fraction of the cells stretches the remaining diminishing fraction; consequently the "gain" increases progressively. Once a critical fraction of the cells is contracting, stretch of the remaining cells should be sufficiently vigorous that their full activation is inevitable. Synchronization is thereby achieved by an effectively regenerative mechanism. Yet the safeness inherent in the redundancy of multiple independent pacemaking cells is retained. If the communication occurs this way, nature will have created an elegant mechanism.

The stretch mechanism explains the paradox of independent cellular behavior during the early phase of the cycle, as well as the highly coordinated behavior later in the cycle. During the early phase, the cells are sufficiently polarized that contraction would not be expected to occur; consequently, synchronization is effectively turned off, and the cells behave independently. Later in the cycle, as cells depolarize further and the communication mechanism turns on, the independent behavior of individual cells gives way to synchronized behavior.

The mechanism also accounts for the fact that the speed of propagation through the sinus node is about two orders of magnitude lower than through cardiac tissues where intercellular propagation is electrically mediated (Sano and Yamagishi, 1965). Propagation by stretch is limited in speed by the time required to activate the myofilaments and by the maximum velocity with which the cells can contract, factors which are not relevant in electrically mediated propagation.

ARRYTHMIAS

Sinus arrhythmias, according to the proposed hypothesis, can be caused either through some action on the mechanism of spontaneous cellular depolarization, or through some action on the mechanism of intercellular synchronization. Sinus tachycardia, often the result of excessive sympathetic drive, is readily explained in terms of increased supply of catecholamines. Sinus bradycardia, usually the result of excessive vagal tone, is explained in terms of the inhibitory effect of acetylcholine, as described above.

The cyclic variation of heart rate during the respiratory cycle – an increase during inspiration and a decrease during expiration – is generally attributed to cyclic variations of vagal tone. An alternative possibility stems from the direct effect of stretch. The sinus node is probably stretched during inspiration as a result of the reduced intrathoracic pressure, and consequently should depolarize more rapidly and discharge at a relatively elevated frequency.

"Sick sinus syndrome," otherwise known as sinus block, is likely the manifestation of diminished efficacy of communication. It is a condition in which not every depolarization generated by primary pacemaking cells propagates sufficiently to reach the atrium. According to the hypothesis, the efficacy of communication depends upon the vigor of contraction, the susceptibility to stretch, and the level of catecholamines in the latent pacemaking cells. Sick sinus syndrome often occurs in the elderly, where contractile strength may be reduced, where increased connective tissue deposition is likely to limit cellular stretch, and where diminished enzymatic activity could reduce the rate of catecholamine synthesis.

The conditions leading to sinus block should be pharmacologically evocable by agents which impair contractility, inhibit catecholamine synthesis, or block catecholamine discharge. The effects of some of these agents have already been explored. Impaired communication results from the application of acetylcholine, vagal stimulation, Mn^{++}, electrical overdrive, hypothermia, propranolol and reserpine, (Brooks and Lu, 1972; Bouman et al., 1968; Sano and Yamagishi, 1965; Lu et al., 1965). Conversely synchronization is improved by stretch (Brooks and Lu, 1972), an agent which should increase both contractility and the rate of vesicle discharge.

Could stretch be a useful clinical tool to alleviate sick sinus syndrome?

REFERENCES

Bonke, F.I.M.: Electronic spread in the sinoatrial node of the rabbit heart. *Pflügers Arch* 339: 17–23, 1973

Bouman, L.N., Gerlings, E.D., Biersteker, P.A., Bonke, F.I.M.: Pacemaker shift in the sino-atrial node during vagal stimulation. *Pflügers Arch Europ J Physiol* 302: 255–267, 1968

Brooker, G.: Oscillation of cyclic adenosine monophosphate concentration during the myocardial contraction cycle. *Science* 182: 933–934, 1973

Brooks, C.M., Lu, H-H.: The Sinoatrial Pacemaker of the Heart, Thomas, Springfield, Ill., 1972

Brown, H.F., Giles, W., Noble, S.J.: Membrane currents underlying rhythmic activity in frog sinus venosus. *J Physiol (London)*, 271: 783–816, 1977

Challice, C.E.: Studies on the microstructure of the heart. I. The sinoatrial node and sino-atrial ring bundle. *J Royal Microscopical Soc* 85: 1–21, 1966

Cheng, Y-P.: The ultrastructure of the rat sino-atrial node. Anatomica Nipponica, 46: 339–358, 1971

Cochrane, D.E., Douglas, W.W., Mouri, T., Nakazato, Y.: Calcium and stimulus-secretion coupling in the adrenal medulla: Contrasting stimulating effects of the ionophores X-537A and A23187 on catecholamine output. *J Physiol* 252: 363–378, 1975

Dean, P.M.: Exocytosis modelling: An electrostatic function for calcium in stimulus-secretion coupling. *J Theor Biol* 54: 289–308, 1975

Deck, K.A.: Dehnungseffekte am spontanschlagenden, isolierten Sinusknoten. *Pflügers Arch ges Physiol* 280: 120–130, 1964

del Castillo, J., Katz, B.: Changes in end-plate activity produced by presynaptic polarization. *J Physiol (London)* 124: 586–604, 1954

Dewey, M.M., Barr, L.: Intercellular connection between smooth muscle cells: the nexus. *Science*, N.Y. 137: 670–672, 1962

Douglas, W.W.: Stimulus-secretion coupling: The concept and clues from chromaffin and other cells. *Br J Pharmac* 34: 451–474, 1968

George, W.J., Wilkerson, R.D., Kadowitz, P.J.: Influence of acetylcholine on contractile force and cyclic nucleotide levels in the isolated perfused rat heart. *J Pharmacol Exp Ther* 184: 228–235, 1973

Goldberg, N.D., Haddox, M.K., Hartle, D.K., Hadden, J.W.: *In* Proceedings of the Fifth International Congress on Pharmacology, R.A. Maxwell and G.H. Achson (eds.), Karger, Basel, 1973, p. 146

Greengard, P.: Possible role for cyclic nucleotides and phosphorylated membrane proteins in postsynaptic actions of neurotransmitters. *Nature* 260: 101–108, 1976

Grossman, A., Furchgott, R.F.: The effects of various drugs on calcium exchange in the isolated guinea-pig left auricle. *J Pharmacol Exp Ther* 145: 162–172, 1964

Heuser, J.E., Reese, T.S.: Evidence for recycling of synaptic vesicle membrane during transmitter release at the frog neuromuscular junction. *J Cell Biol* 57: 315–344, 1973

Hoffman, B.F., Cranefield, P.F.: *In* Electrophysiology of the Heart, McGraw-Hill, New York, 1960

Hutter, O.F., Trautwein, W.: Vagal and sympathetic effects on pacemaker fibers in sinus venosus of heart. *J Gen Physiol* 39: 715–733, 1956

IJpeij, D., Kerkhof, P.L.M., Bobbert, A.C.: Muscle length and neuromuscular transmission in the frog. *Pflügers Arch* 347; 309–322, 1974

Irisawa, H., Noma, A.: Contracture and hyperpolarization of the rabbit sinoatrial node cells in Na-depleted solution. *Jap J Physiol* 26: 133–144, 1976

James, T.N., Sherf, L., Fine, G., Morales, A.R.: Comparative ultrastructure of the sinus node in man and dog. *Circulation* 34: 139–163, 1966

Katz, A.M.: Contractile proteins of the heart. *Physiological Reviews* 50: 63–158, 1970

Kirshner, N.: Function and organization of chromaffin vesicle. *Life Sci* 14: 1153–1167, 1974

Lefkowitz, R.J., O'Hara, D.S., Warshaw, J.: Binding of catecholamines to receptors in cultured myocardial cells. *Nature New Biology* 244: 79–80, 1973

Lu, H-H., Lange, G., Brooks, C.M.: Factors controlling pacemaker action in cells of the sinoatrial node. *Circulation Research* 17: 460–471, 1965

Miyagishima, Y.: Studies on catecholamine (CA) of the heart – fluorescence histochemical method. *Jap Circ J* 39: 361–375, 1975

McNutt, N.S., Weinstein, R.S.: The ultrastructure of the nexus. A correlated thin-section and freeze-cleave study. *Cell Biol* 47: 666–688, 1970

Noma, A., Irisawa, H.: Membrane currents in the rabbit sinoatrial node cell as studied by the double microelectrode method. *Pflügers Arch* 364: 45–52, 1976

Pollack, G.H.: AV nodal transmission: A proposed electromechanical mechanism. *J Electrocardiology* 7: 245–258, 1974

Pollack, G.H.: Cardiac Pacemaking: An obligatory role of catecholamines? *Science* 196: 731–738, 1977

Reuter, H.: Localization of BETA adrenergic receptors, and effects of noradrenaline and cyclic neuclotides on action potentials, ionic currents and tension in mammalian cardiac muscle. *J Physiol* 242: 429–451, 1974

Reuter, H.: Uber die wirkung von adrenalin auf den cellulären Ca-umsatz des meerschweinchenvorhofs. *Naunyn-Schmeidebergs Arch Pharmakol Exp Path* vol. 251: 401–412, 1965

Ruska, H.: *In* International Symposium on Electrophysiology of the Heart, B. Taccardi and G. Marchetti (eds.), Pergamon, New York, 1965, p. 1–19

Sandoval, I.V., Cuatrecasas, P.: Opposing effects of cyclic AMP and cyclic GMP on protein phosphorylation in tubulin preparations. *Nature* 262, 1976

Sano, T., Yamagishi, S.: Spread of excitation from the sinus node. *Circ Res* 16: 423–430, 1965

Simon, M.: Conversion of guanosine 3′, 5′-monophosphate to adenosine 3′, 5′-monophosphate in frog myocardial tissue. *Biochem Biophys Res Commun* 68: 1219–1225, 1976

Spurgeon, H.A., Priola, D.V., Montoya, P., Weiss, G.K., Alter, W.A. III: Catecholamines associated with conductile and contractile myocardium of normal and denervated dog hearts. *J Pharmacol Exp Ther* 190: 466–471, 1974

Teo, T.S., Wang, J.H.: Mechanisms of activation of a cyclic adenosine 3′5′-monophosphate phosphodiesterase from bovine heart by calcium ions. Identification of the protein activator as a Ca^{2+} binding protein. *J Biol Chem* 248: 5950–5955, 1973

Trautwein, W., Uchizono, K.: Electron microscopic and electrophysiologic study of the pacemaker in the sino-atrial node of the rabbit heart. *Z Zellforsch* 61: 96–109, 1963

Tuganowski, W., Krause, M., Korczak, K.: The effect of diputyryl 3′5′-cyclic AMP on the cardiac pacemaker, arrested with reserpine and α-methyl-tyrosine. *Naunyn-Schmiedeberg's Arch Pharmacol* 280: 63–70, 1973

Tuganowski, W.: The influence of adenylate cyclase inhibitors on the spontaneous activity of the cardiac pacemaker. *Arch int Pharmacodyn* 225: 275–286, 1977

Ushiyama, J., Brooks, C.M.: Intercellular stimulation and recording from single cardiac cells in the rabbit atrium. *J Electrocardiology* 7(2): 119–126, 1974

Viragh, Sz., Porte, A.: On the impulse conducting system of the monkey heart (macaca mulatta) II. The atrio-ventricular node and bundle. *Z Zellforsch* 145: 363–388, 1973

West, T.C., Landa, J.: Transmembrane potentials and contractility in the pregnant rat uterus. *Amer J of Phys* 187: 333–337, 1956

Winegrad, S.: Studies of cardiac muscle with a high permeability to calcium produced by treatment with ethylenediaminetetraacetic acid. *J Gen Physiol* 58: 71–93, 1971

Wollenberger, A.: The role of cyclic AMP in the adrenergic control of the heart. *In* Contraction and Relaxation in the Myocardium, W.G. Nayler (Ed.). Academic Press, New York, 1975

Wollenberger, A., Babskii, G.B., Krause, E.G., Genz, S., Blohn, D., Bogdanova, E.V.: Cyclic changes in levels of cyclic AMP and cyclic CMP in frog myocardium during the cardiac cycle. *Biochem Biophys Res Commun* 55: 446–452, 1973

Yamagishi, S., Sano, T.: Effect of temperature on pacemaker activity of rabbit sinus node. *Amer J Physiol* 212: 829–834, 1967

Yamasaki, Y., Fujiwara, M. and Toda, N.: Effects of catecholamines injected into sinoatrial nodal cells on their electrical activity. *Japan J. Pharmacol* 24: 383–391, 1974

Ypey, D.L.: Feedback of isotonic muscle contraction on neuromuscular impulse transmission in the frog. *Pflügers Arch* 355: 291–306, 1975

GENERAL COMMENTS: IONIC CURRENTS UNDERLYING SPONTANEOUS RHYTHM OF THE CARDIAC PRIMARY PACEMAKER CELLS

HIROSHI IRISAWA

To understand the ionic mechanism underlying the pacemaker potential one has to know the kinetic properties of the current system and which ions are involved in these currents. This information will only become available if the voltage clamp technique is used and this was not possible in the sinus node until very recently (Irisawa, 1972; Noma and Irisawa, 1976a,b; Seyama, 1976; Brown et al., 1976). In very small isolated specimen of the area of the sinus node there is a fairly equal potential distribution within the specimen (see Figure 1); therefore electrotonic spread can be ignored. There are two other advantages of the small sized preparation: firstly, because of the removal of the connective tissue from the epicardial surface the diffusion is favored and secondly, a stable impalement with a microelectrode during a couple of hours is possible. Therefore the small preparations of the sinus node turned out to be useful for voltage clamp experiments using the double microelectrode technique.

IONIC CURRENTS IN PACEMAKER CELLS

In the Purkinje fiber several currents are involved – during the action potential – according to the kinetic properties of the ionic channels (the threshold of activation and the potential range in which the current system is activated and also the time constant of the decay of a current after activation of the current system with a voltage clamp to various levels of the membrane potential). So, McAllister, Noble and Tsien (1975) postulated that there are two transient inward currents – a fast current and a secondary slow current – and five outward currents – K_1, K_2, X_1, X_2 and a chloride current. There is also a time independent background current or leakage current. In the Purkinje fiber, the principal mechanism for the pacemaker depolarization (diastolic depolarization) is the time dependent decay of I_{K_2}, which allows – in combination with a partial activation of I_{Na} – the membrane to depolarize.

The results of the experiments with the voltage clamp method on the mammalian sinus node and sinus venosus of the frog are comparable to those on the Purkinje fiber. There are differences, but they are mainly quantitative. So, even the fast inward current, playing a major role for the maximal rate of rise of the action potential in the Purkinje fiber, was found also in sinus node cells (Noma et al., 1977) although its magnitude was very small. This is demonstrated in Figure 2. At the end of a hyperpolarizing clamp the rate of rise of the depolarization phase of the action potential is increased (trace 3 of panel A); this was not the case after the addition of 10^{-7} gr/ml TTX (trace 3 of panel B). Since the fast inward current is almost completely inactivated at -40 mV, the physiological significance of this current for the automaticity of pacemaker cells in the sinus mode may be small. However, there are also cells in the area of the sinus node which exhibit a rate of rise of the action

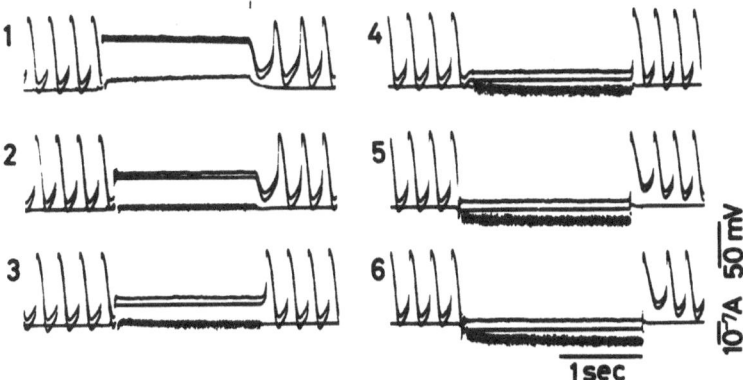

Figure 1. Evaluation of the spatial homogeneity under the voltage clamp conditions.

The top and middle traces are recordings by a microelectrode. The second electrode is not impaled perfectly and therefore the amplitude of the action potential was about 13% smaller than the one recorded by the other electrode. Besides this difference, the action potentials are superimposable and there is no sign of conduction delay between these two sites of impalement.

The third trace is the current record. The membrane potentials under clamp condition were -8, -29, -40, -56, -68 and -71 mV in the order from 1 to 6 respectively. Note that during the clamps 1 and 2 the current is outward and during clamp steps shown in 4, 5 and 6 the current is inward. During a clamp to -40 mV (see 3) no current is measured.

(From Noma, Jap. J. Physiol., 26, 619, 1976; with permission of the publisher)

potential of 10–20 V/sec. In these cells – transitional cells – the fast inward current may play a more important role than in the cells in the center of the node. Certainly, in relation to the conduction of the impulse through the sinus node area the role of the fast inward current should not be ignored.

The secondary slow inward current is very important for the rising phase of the action potential of the nodal fibers (Noma et al., 1977; Brown et al., 1978). It seems that both sodium and calcium ions are the current carriers. The activation and inactivation of the slow inward current may be governed by the gating variables of d and f respectively and they are similar to those described for the Purkinje fiber (McAllister et al., 1975) and for the ventricular myocardial fiber (Beeler and Reuter, 1977). At a membrane potential lesser than the resting potential d increases, whereas f increases at a potential higher than the resting potential. It will be essential to investigate further the kinetic properties of d and f on the nodal fibers for the reconstruction of the pacemaker action potential although such a study is difficult.

There is a time independent leakage current which is inward at membrane potentials more negative than -40 mV and outward at membrane potentials more positive than -40 mV (Noma et al., 1977). There appeared to be another inward current in sinus node fibers which is both time and voltage dependent. This current is activated in response to hyperpolarizing clamp pulses to a membrane potential of more than -50 mV and showed to have a time constant of more than 2 seconds. This "ultra slow" inward current has been first observed by Seyama (1976); this current is partly abolished after removal of chloride ions from the extracellular solution or in a sodium depleted solution (Noma et al., 1977). Therefore this current system is considered to be a mixed current and it might have some physiological significance for the slow diastolic phase if the nodal fibers become hyperpolarized beyond the level of -50 mV.

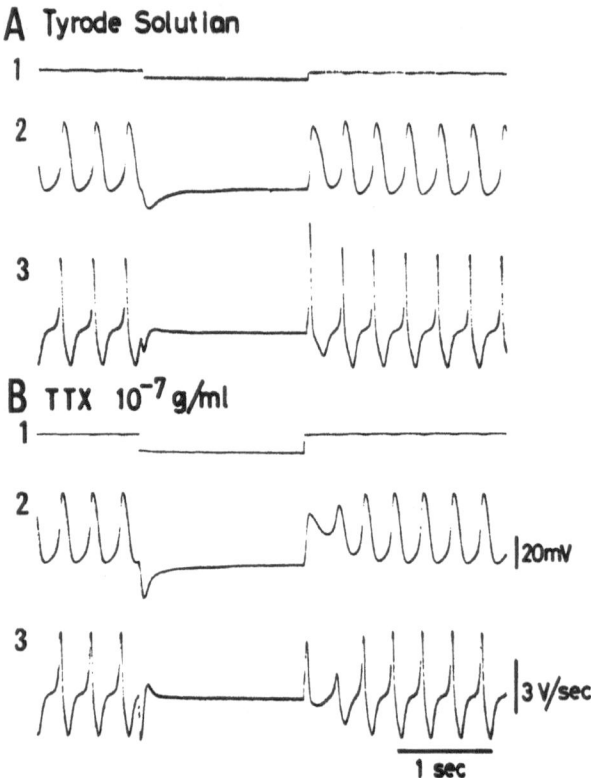

Figure 2. Effect of TTX on the action potential (2) and the maximum rate of rise (3) of the action potential, during and after current application (1). Control rate of rise was 3.8 V/sec which increased to 5.0 V/sec at the break excitation. After 10^{-7} g/ml TTX application, control rate of rise reduced a little bit (3.4 V/sec), the maximum rate of rise at the break excitation also reduced to 2 V/sec.

After depolarization an outward current is activated. The gating variable of this outward current (p) is zero at a membrane potential of about -50 mV and approaches 1 at about 0 mV in the sinus node. (In the sinus venosus of the frog these values are -40 mV and 0 mV.) The time constant of the decaying outward current is about 300 msec in the sinus node (600 msec in the sinus venosus of the frog). This decay of the outward current is mainly responsible for the hyperpolarization following the repolarization. Since there is a remarkable similarity between the I_{K_2} (Purkinje fiber) and I_p (sinus node fiber) it seems reasonable to assume that there are qualitative similarities between these tissues. However, many questions are still unsolved and the quality of the voltage clamp method in sinus node preparations has to be improved before these questions can be solved.

POSSIBLE IONIC MECHANISMS UNDERLYING THE PACEMAKER ACTIVITY OF THE SINUS NODE CELLS

The foregoing discussion indicated that the basic mechanisms underlying the spontaneous activity in cells of the sinus node might be qualitatively similar to those postulated for the Purkinje fiber. As discussed by Noma et al. (1978, this book; see their Figure 6) a pacemaker current I_p is activated after depolarization. However, this current is very small at a potential of -10 mV and – even if the gates are fully opened – this current will not be important until the membrane potential is approaching the resting potential (this will happen since during depolarization the background current is outward and favors repolarization).

At potentials more negative than -30 mV the conductance for this I_p is increasing and therefore I_p increases. Because at potentials more negative than -40 mV the background current is inward, I_p and $I_{background}$ are then working in an opposite direction. Therefore as soon as I_p and $I_{background}$ are equal, the membrane potential will be stable and this is the maximal diastolic potential.

The deactivation of I_p will cause that the membrane depolarizes towards the resting potential. At the higher membrane potentials the ultraslow inward current is also activated and will help to depolarize the membrane.

According to this explanation, the initial depolarization (upstroke of the action potential) is a prerequisite condition to cause a positive feedback oscillation.

SOME CHARACTERISTICS OF THE MEMBRANE OF NODAL CELLS

From voltage clamp studies it became clear that the current-voltage relationship in the sinus node showed a stable point at about -40 mV (see Figure 3B). This value might be called "resting potential" although there is no "rest" in spontaneously active cells. At this potential the membrane is relatively less sensitive to changes in $[K]_o$ and Seyama has demonstrated a conductance ratio for K:Na:Cl of 1:0,6:0,15 (Seyama, 1978, this book) indicating the importance of the sodium permeability to the resting membrane potential. Because of this relatively high sodium permeability, an active sodium pump is necessary to maintain the intracellular sodium concentration more or less constant. It appeared that this sodium pump can work electrogenic (Noma and Irisawa, 1974, 1975).

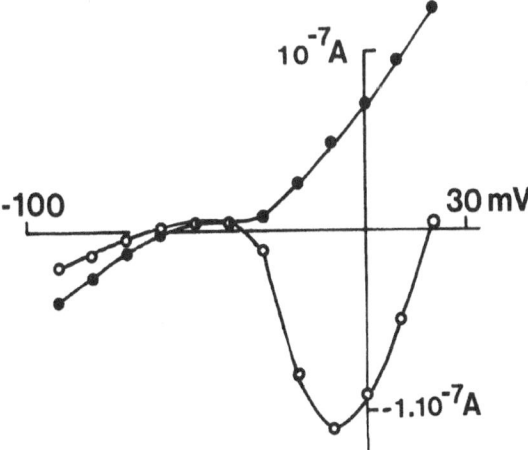

Figure 3. Current voltage relationship at 10 msec after the onset of the voltage step (open circles) and at 500 msec after the onset of the pulse (closed circles).

In pacemaker tissues this pumping mechanism is common in both vertebrates and invertebrates. Figure 4 shows several examples in which the preparation was exposed to a potassium free solution prior to a solution containing potassium ions; in all cases a hyperpolarization is effected by this change and this is probably due to the electrogenic activity of the pump that is reactivated by the return to normal K solution.

The possibility of a sodium-calcium exchange mechanism must be considered also. Such a mechanism has been observed in various cardiac tissues (Reuter, 1974; Bremner et al., 1977), but this exchange is probably more pronounced in sinus node fibers. This is shown in Figure 5. In Figure 5A spontaneous activity of the sinus node preparation stopped after change to a sodium-free perfusion solution and the membrane is depolarizing. However, if the preparation is pretreated with ouabain (high concentration, 10^{-5} M, for a short time) spontaneous activity stopped also in a sodium-free solution but now a hyperpolarization occurred. In a Na-free solution an increased mechanical tension occurred, but this contracture was enhanced strongly after pretreatment with ouabain (Figure 5B). This behavior might be explained in the following way: If the extracellular solution does not contain sodium ions, there is a gradient for sodium from inside to outside; the sodium

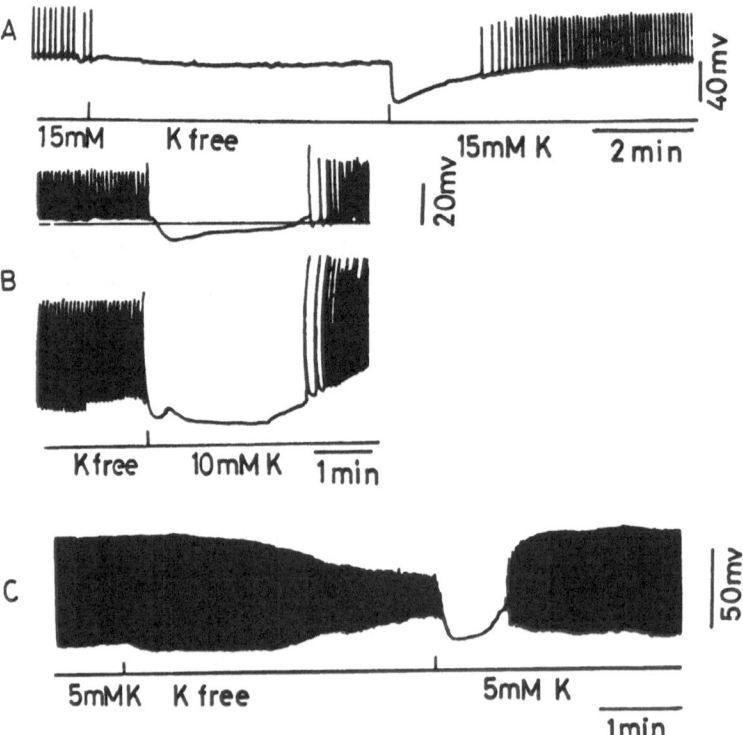

Figure 4. Three examples of experiments in which a preparation showing spontaneous activity is brought in a potassium-free solution and after some time is perfused again with a normal solution. During the perfusion with K-free solution the active Na-K pump is inactivated and after the return to the normal solution this pump starts its activity again. *A*) Mantis shrimp cardiac ganglion (Livengood and Kusano, 1973). *B*) Mussel heart (Modiolur demisur); top trace is a recording of the membrane potential and the bottom trace is a recording of the mechanical activity (Wilkens, 1972). *C*) Rabbit sinus node (Noma and Irisawa, 1975a)

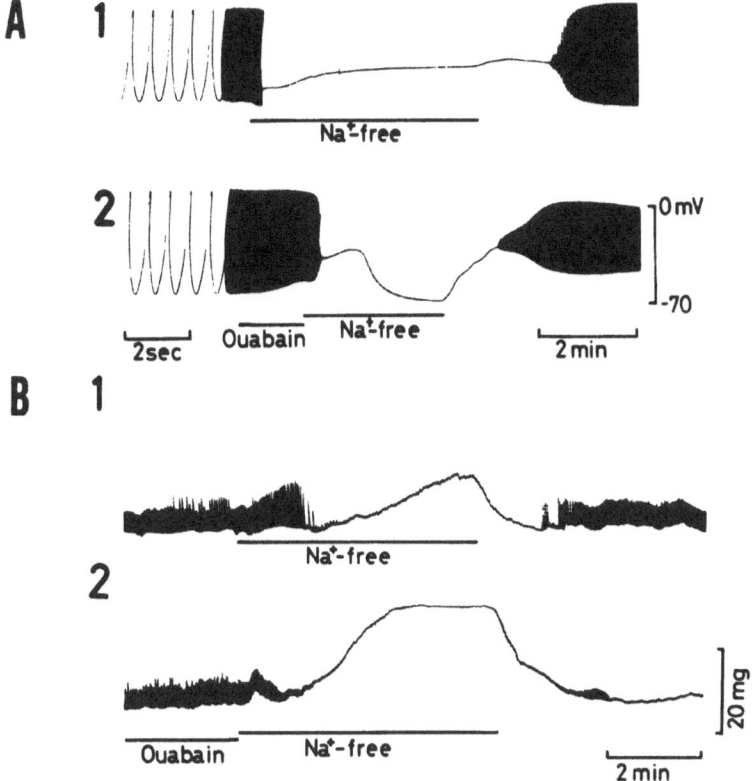

Figure 5. A) Recording of the membrane potential in a strip of the sinus node of the rabbit. In A1 the effect of a period of perfusion with sodium free solution is shown; in A2 first the preparation was perfused with a normal solution containing 10^{-5} M ouabain during a period of 1.5 min and thereafter with a Na-free solution. After this pretreatment with ouabain a marked hyperpolarization of the membrane was recorded during perfusion with a Na-free solution.

B) Recording of the mechanical activity of the same strip. Note that a contracture of the muscle occurred in Na-free solution and that contracture is intensified clearly after the pretreatment with ouabain (in this case 5×10^{-6} M).

(This figure is a combination of figures 7 and 8 of the publication of Irisawa and Noma in Jap. J. Physiol., 26, 133, 1976. With permission of the publishers.)

ions diffusing out of the cell, will be replaced by calcium ions and this exchange both will prevent the hyperpolarization and will cause an increase in the intracellular calcium concentration resulting in a contracture. After pretreatment with ouabain the intracellular sodium concentration is increased and therefore the Na-efflux in Na-free solution will be enlarged. Probably the Na-Ca exchange is not 2:1 and so the amount of calcium ions in exchange is not enough to prevent a hyperpolarization, but on the other hand more than without the pretreatment with ouabain; this will cause a stronger contracture.

Subthreshold oscillations in the membrane potential are occurring in the sinus node fibers. Because the membrane resistance is relatively high near the "resting" potential, any small change of the current will cause a sizeable fluctuation of the membrane potential.

These subthreshold oscillations were observed by West (1961), Vassalle (1965), Brooks and Lu (1972) and Noma and Irisawa (1975b) and in Figure 6 an example is given. These

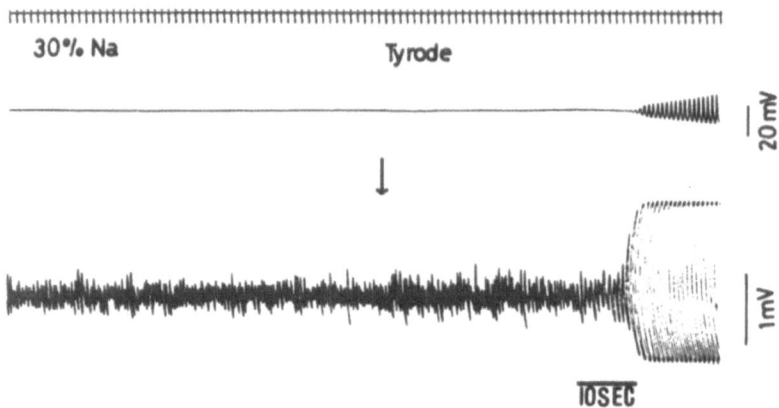

Figure 6. Miniature fluctuation of the membrane potential in a sinus node cell. Upper trace is the membrane potential recorded with normal amplification, the lower trace is an amplification of the upper trace. A continuous miniature oscillation was observed when the membrane became quiescent in 30% Na-Tyrode solution. At the arrow, Tyrode solution was perfused and the miniature oscillation gradually increased and merged to a subthreshold oscillation.

small fluctuations were always observed in the sinus node if the preparation loosed it spontaneity. They remained present under Ca-free and Na-free conditions and also after application of verapamil (or D-600) or manganese. These facts suggest that an inward current of Ca- and Na-ions is not directly responsible for these fluctuations, but it is not excluded that fluctuation of the permeability of the resting membrane for sodium and calcium is contributing.

In aggregates of cultured heart cells a similar fluctuation of the membrane potential is found (De Haan and De Felice, 1977). Since the fluctuations smoothly merged to subthreshold oscillations, they might be the basis of spontaneous activity (Cranefield, 1978, this book).

REFERENCES

Beeler, G.W., Reuter, H.: Reconstruction of the action potential of ventricular myocardial fibres. *J Physiol* 268: 177, 1977

Brown, H.F., Giles, W., Noble, S.J.: Voltage clamp of frog sinus venosus. *J Physiol* 258: 78, 1976

Brown, H.F., Giles, W., Noble, S.J.: Membrane currents underlying rhythmic activity in Frog sinus venosus. 1978 in this book

Brooks, C.McC., Lu, H.H.: The Sino Atrial Pacemaker of the Heart. Springfield, Ill. Charles C. Thomas, 1972

Bremner, F., Fry, C.H. McGuigan, J.A.S.: Action of ouabain on Nafree contraction in mammalian ventricular muscle. *J Physiol* 268: 30P, 1977

Cranefield, P.F.: Does spontaneous activity arise from phase 4 depolarization or from triggering? 1978, in this book

DeHaan, R.L., DeFelice, L.J.: Oscillatory properties and excitability of the heart cell membrane. To be published in: Periodicities in Chemistry and Biology, (edited by Eying, H. Academic Press, 1977

Irisawa, H.: Electrical activity of rabbit sino-atrial node as studied by a double sucrose gap method. In: *Proc Satel Symp of 25th Intern Congr Physiol Sci* The electrical field of the heart. Bruxelles Presses Academiques Européenes, 1972, p. 242.

Irisawa, H., Noma, A.: Contracture and hyperpolarization of the rabbit sinoatrial node cells in Na-depleted solution. *Jap J Physiol* 26: 133, 1976

Livengood, D.R., Kusano, K.: Modulation of the crustacean heart rate by an electrogenic Na-pump. Neurobiology of Invertebrates, Tihany, 1971, 213, 1973

McAllister, R.D., Noble, D., Tsien R.W.: Reconstruction of electrical activity of cardiac Purkinje fibers. *J Physiol* 251: 1, 1975

Noma, A., Irisawa, H.: Electrogenic sodium pump in rabbit sinoatrial node cell. *Pflügers Archiv* 351: 177, 1974

Noma, A., Irisawa, H.: Contribution of an electrogenic sodium pump to the membrane potential in rabbit. *Pflügers Archiv* 358: 289, 1975a

Noma, A., Irisawa, H.: Effects of Na^+ and K^+ on the resting membrane potential of the rabbit sinoatrial node cell. *Jap J Physiol* 25: 287, 1975b

Noma, A., Irisawa, H.: Membrane currents in the rabbit sinoatrial node cell as studied by the double micro-electrode method. *Pflügers Archiv* 364: 45, 1976a

Noma, A., Irisawa, H.: A time- and voltage-dependent potassium current in the rabbit sinoatrial node cell. *Pflügers Archiv* 366: 251, 1976b

Noma, A., Yanagihara, K., Irisawa, H.: Inward current of the rabbit sinoatrial node cell. *Pflügers Archiv* in press, 1977

Noma, A., Yanagihara, K., Irisawa, H.: Ionic currents in rabbit sinoatrial node cells 1978, in this book

Reuter, H.: Exchange of calcium ions in the mammalian myocardium. Mechanisms and Physiological significance. *Circ Res* 34: 599, 1974

Seyama, I.: Characteristics of the rectifying properties of the Sino-atrial node cell of the rabbit. *J Physiol (London)* 255: 379, 1976

Seyama, I.: Which ions are important for the maintenance of the resting potential of the cells of the sinoatrial node of the rabbit. 1978, in this book

Vassalle, M.: Cardiac pacemaker potentials at different extra- and intra-cellular K concentrations. *Am J Physiol* 208: 770, 1965

West, T.C.: Effects of chronotropic influences on subthreshold oscillation in the sinoatrial node. in: The Specialized Tissues of the Heart, edited by A. Paes de Carvalho, W.C. DeMello and B.F. Hoffman. New York, Elsevier, 1961, p. 81

Wilkens, L.A.: Electrophysiological studies of the heart of bivalve molluscs *Modiolus demissus*. I. ionic basis of the membrane potential. *J Exp Biol* 56: 273, 1972

SECTION FIVE
DOES THE SINUS NODE PLAY A ROLE IN REENTRANT ARRHYTHMIAS?

33

CLINICAL EVIDENCE FOR SINUS NODE REENTRY*

ANTHONY N. DAMATO

INTRODUCTION

The responses of the sinus node to premature atrial stimulation can be variable depending on several factors. Some though not all of the factors which can influence the post-extrasystolic response of the sinus node include: 1) degree of prematurity of the atrial extrasystole; 2) arrival time of the extrasystolic impulse at the sinus node region; 3) whether the extrasystolic impulse gains access into or is blocked at the sinus node; 4) the intranodal pathway(s) and speed of conduction of the extrasystolic impulse within the sinus node; 5) how the extrasystolic impulse influences normal automaticity of the sinus node; 6) the exit time of the extrasystolic impulse; 7) the relative state refractoriness between the sinus node and the atrium itself; 8) the degree of vagal tone acting on the sinus node.

Late occurring extrasystoles may fail to disturb automaticity of the sinus node. The post-extrasystolic sinus beat appears at its expected time and the sum of the intervals of the foreshortened and post-extrasystolic cycles equals two sinus cycles. This has been referred to as a "fully compensatory pause." Extrasystoles which are more premature generally result in what has been termed "less than compensatory pauses," i.e., the sum of the foreshortened and post-extrasystolic intervals equals less than two sinus cycles. Very early extrasystoles may produce two additional responses. An atrial extrasystole may have so-called entrance block into the sinus node. Sinus rhythm is undisturbed by the extrasystole and the sum of the foreshortened and post-extrasystolic intervals equals one sinus cycle length. In the second type of response to very early atrial extrasystoles, the post-extrasystolic sinus beat(s) appears earlier than expected i.e., the sum of the foreshortened and post-extrasystolic intervals is less than one sinus cycle. This latter response has been assumed to be a manifestation of reentry within or immediately around the sinus node. Sinus node reentry may present as one or more consecutive beats, as an accelerated atrial rhythm (see below) or as a tachycardic rhythm. It is the purpose of this report to review some of the indirect evidence which suggests that reentry does occur in the region of the sinus node bearing in mind that the phenomenon has not yet been unequivocally proven to exist.

METHODS

Methods used to study atrial responses subsequent to premature stimulation of the atria in both man and the intact animal heart have been previously described (Paulay et al., 1973a, b; Narula, 1974; Weisfogel et al., 1975).

* This work was supported in part by the Bureau of Medical Services, National Heart, Lung and Blood Institute, Project HL 12536-07.

DEFINITION OF TERMS

A_1 = Atrial depolarization of either a spontaneous sinus beat or a paced atrial beat

A_2 = Atrial depolarization of an induced atrial premature beat

A_3, A_4, A_5, etc = Subsequent atrial beats

A_1-A_1 = Atrial interval measured during sinus rhythm or atrial pacing

A_1-A_2 = Coupling interval measured from the last sinus or paced beat (A_1) to the atrial premature depolarization (A_2)

A_2-A_3 = Interval measured from the induced atrial premature depolarization (A_2) to the subsequent atrial beat (A_3)

A_1-A_3 = Sum of the A_1-A_2 and A_2-A_3 intervals

A_3-A_4, A_4-A_5, etc = Intervals between atrial depolarization subsequent to A_3

S = Stimulus

S_1 = Basic pacing stimulus

S_2 = Premature stimulus

RESULTS

Figure 1 illustrates the effects of premature stimulation of the low right atrium at different coupling intervals on the return sinus cycle. In panels A and B, premature stimulation of the low right atrium at A_1-A_2 intervals of 410 and 315 msec, respectively, results in delayed appearance of the post-extrasystolic sinus beat (A_3). The sinus node response is considered less than compensatory since the A_1-A_3 interval is less than two sinus cycles. At an A_1-A_2 coupling interval of 235 msec (panel C), the post-extrasystolic beat (A_3) appears earlier than expected. The A_1-A_3 interval (680 msec) is significantly less than the A_1-A_1 interval (850 msec). A_3 is considered to be a sinus node reentrant beat; the P wave morphology, high to low sequence of atrial activation and morphology of the intra-atrial electrograms are all similar to sinus beats (A_1). At times the P wave morphology of sinus node reentrant beats is slightly different from sinus P waves. This difference has been attributed to either aberrant intra-atrial conduction or a different exit site of the reentrant impulse from the sinus node. At an A_1-A_2 coupling interval of 210 msec (panel D) the atrium is refractory and sinus rhythm is undisturbed. Delivery of a stimulus at several times diastolic threshold during the refractory period fails to elicit a post stimulus response.

Figure 2 demonstrates, in the same patient, that sinus node reentry can be elicited from different sites of premature atrial stimulation. Appropriately timed stimulation of the high right atrium (panel A) or of the low right atrium (panel B) results in a sinus node reentrant beat (A_3). It is to be noted in Figure 1 and panel B of Figure 2 that even though the site of premature stimulation produces a low to high sequence of atrial activation, A_3 consistently has a high to low sequence of activation. This suggests that A_3 is not the result of local reentry at the site of premature stimulation. However, the site of premature atrial stimulation can at times very much affect the occurrence of sinus node reentry. This is illustrated in Figure 3 which is taken from an intact animal heart experiment. When the tip of the right atrial appendage was stimulated at an A_1-A_2 interval of 130 msec (panel a), activation at the region of the sinus node occurred 220 msec after the last sinus activation (A_1). Sinus node reentry did not occur. As illustrated in panel B, activation of the base of the right atrial appendage, even at a longer coupling interval (180 msec), resulted in

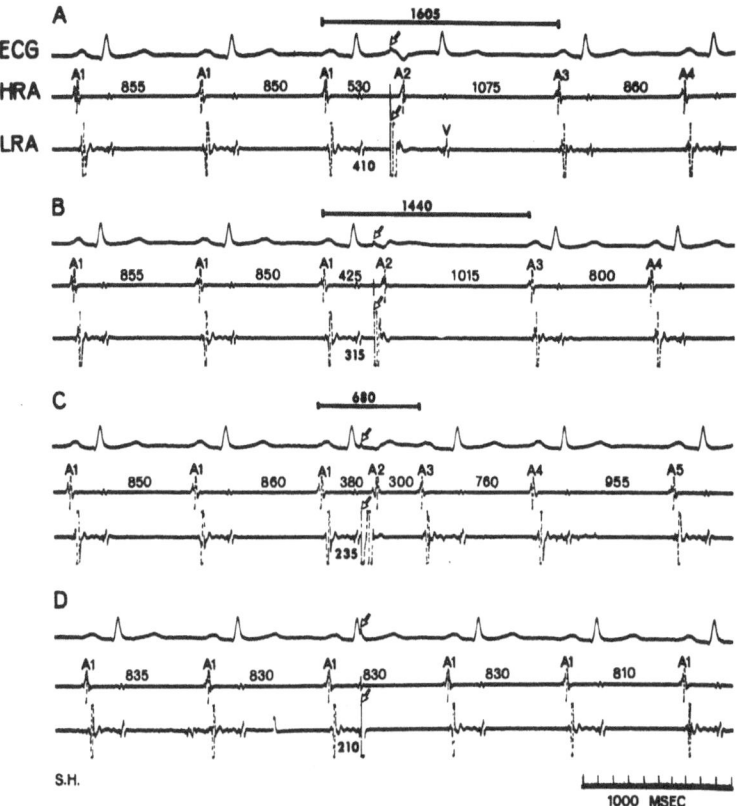

Figure 1. Effects of premature stimulation of the low right atrium on the return sinus cycle. In each panel the tracings from top to bottom are ECG lead 2, a high right atrial electrogram (HRA) and a low right atrial electrogram (LRA). A₁ represents spontaneous sinus beats. A₂ is the induced premature atrial depolarization. A₃-A₄ etc are the post-extrasystolic sinus beats. The open arrow indicates the stimulus artifact. The intra-atrial cycle lengths are indicated on the HRA tracing. The A_1A_2 coupling interval is indicated on the LRA tracing. The sum of the foreshortened and the immediate post-extrasystolic intervals (A_1-A_3) intervals are indicated above the ECG tracings. Similar abbreviations will be used for subsequent figures. Note that premature stimulation of the low right atrium produces a low to high sequence of atrial activation while all the post-extrasystolic response (A_3) produce a high to low sequence of activation similar to A_1.

earlier activation in the region of the sinus node (200 msec), following which sinus node reentry occurred (A_3). It would appear that the arrival time of the extrasystolic impulse at the region of the sinus node is an important determinant of sinus node reentry.

Figure 4 depicts sinus node reentry presenting as an accelerated atrial rhythm which is defined as an atrial rate faster than the basic sinus rhythm but less than a rate of 100 min. In this example, the cycle length of the accelerated atrial rhythm gradually increases until the cycle length of sinus rhythm is reestablished. This gradual transition to sinus rhythm is to be contrasted with the findings illustrated in Figure 5. Spontaneous termination of a sinus node reentrant tachycardia is usually followed by a sinus pause which is greater than the basic sinus cycle length.

Premature atrial stimulation is the more frequent means by which sinus node reentry can be induced. At times, sinus node reentry can be elicited by continuous atrial pacing or

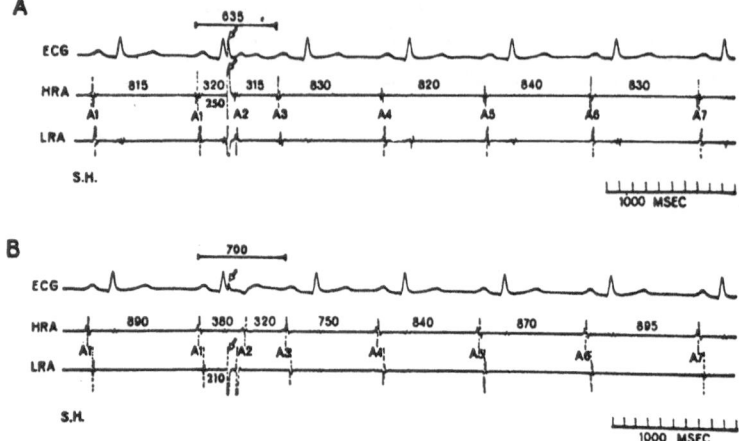

Figure 2. Same patient as Figure 1 showing sinus node reentry (A₃) occurring when appropriately timed extrasystoles are introduced into the high (panel A) and low (panel B) right atrium. In both instances A₃ has a high to low sequence of atrial activation.
(From Paulay, K.L. et al., Am. Heart J. 85:323, 1973).

ventricular pacing with 1:1 retrograde capture. Figure 6 depicts sinus node reentry occurring during continuous atrial pacing.

Another feature of sinus node reentry is illustrated in Figure 7. It is to be noted that following the initiation of a sinus node reentrant tachycardia by a single atrial extrasystole (A₂), the post-extrasystolic tachycardia is sustained despite the fact that not all of the atrial impulses propagate to the ventricular specialized conducting tissue or ventricular muscle.

In our experience, sinus node reentrant tachycardias are rarely sustained for prolonged periods of time. They generally terminate spontaneously and are easily terminated by carotid sinus pressure or other maneuvers which increase vagal tone. Figure 8 illustrates termination of a sinus node reentrant tachycardia in man by carotid sinus pressure.

The effects of vagal stimulation on experimentally induced sinus node reentry are further illustrated in Figures 9 and 10. Figure 9A shows the early appearance of A₃ from the sinus node region following premature stimulation of the coronary sinus region. In panel B, premature stimulation at the same coupling during vagal stimulation at relatively high voltage fails to elicit the sinus node reentrant beat.

The effects of graded vagal stimulation (0–10 volts) on the A₂-A₃ interval are shown in panels A–G of Figure 10. The escape time following ten basic drive beats without premature stimulation was also determined at every voltage level. At above 4 volts there was a progressive increase in the A₂-A₃ interval during graded vagal stimulation. The relationships between voltage strength, the A₂-A₃ intervals, the sum of the A₁-A₂ and A₂-A₃ intervals and the escape times are depicted in Figure 11. When the curve representing the sum of the A₁-A₂ and A₂-A₃ intervals was below the curve of the escape time the phenomenon of sinus node reentrance block for A₂ could be excluded. Thus, vagal stimulation at levels which do not affect inherent sinus node automaticity can very much influence the appearance time of a sinus node reentrant beat.

Other indirect evidence supporting the concept of sinus node reentry is derived

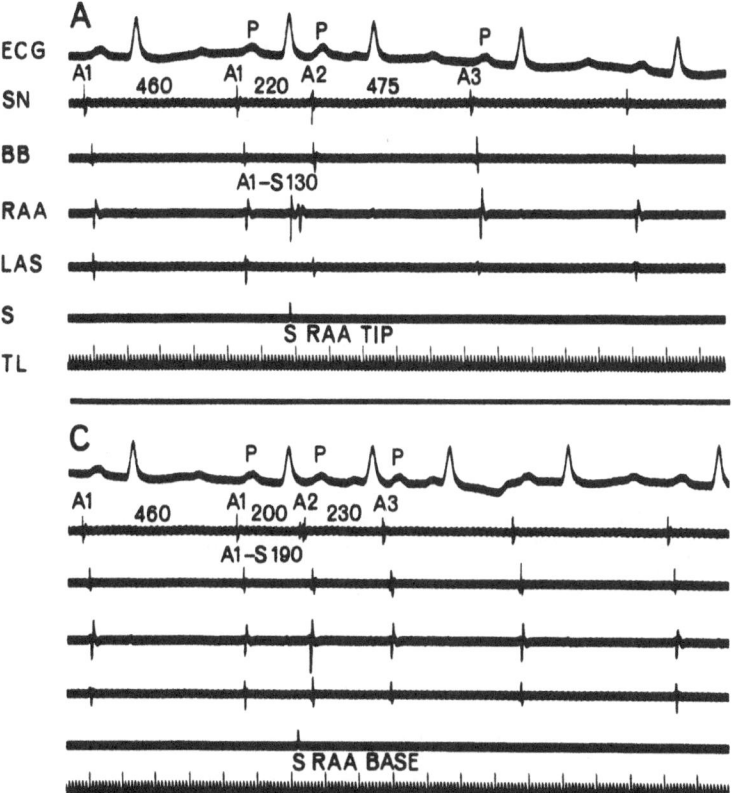

Figure 3. Intact animal heart experiment demonstrating the importance of activation time at the sinus node region. Tracings from top to bottom are ECG lead 2, electrograms recorded from regions of the sinus node (SN), Bahmann's bundle (BB), right atrial appendage (RAA) and low atrial septum (LAS). S denotes the stimulus artifact and TL are time lines at 10 and 100 msec. In panel A, the tip of the right atrial appendage was stimulated at a coupling interval of 130 msec and in panel B the base of the right atrium was stimulated at a coupling interval of 190 msec.
(From Paulay, K.L. et al., Circ. Res. 32:455, 1973).

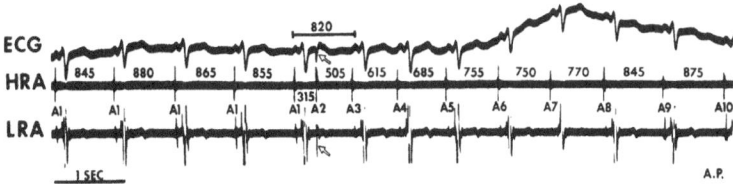

Figure 4. Stimulation of the high right atrium at a coupling interval of 315 msec results in an accelerated atrial rate which gradually returns to a spontaneous sinus rate.
(From Paulay, K.L. et al., Am. Heart J. 85:323, 1972).

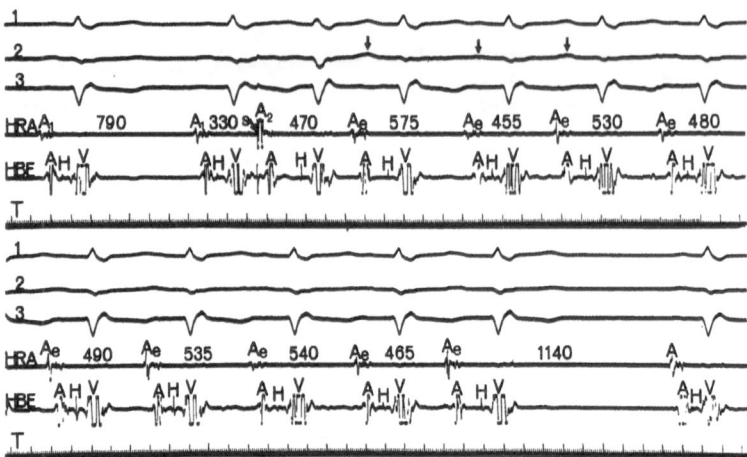

Figure 5. Spontaneous termination of sinus node reentrant tachycardia. Tracings from top to bottom are ECG leads 1, 2 and 3, a high right atrial electrogram (HRA), a His bundle recording (HBE) and time lines at 10 and 100 msec. A sinus cycle length was 790 msec. A sinus node reentrant tachycardia is initiated by a premature atrial depolarization (A₂) introduced 330 msec after a series of sinus beats (A₁). Following spontaneous termination of the tachycardia (bottom panel) a pause of 1140 msec occurs before sinus rhythm resumes. The arrows above lead 2 indicate the P waves.

(From Weisfogel, G.M. et al., Am. Heart J. 90:295, 1975).

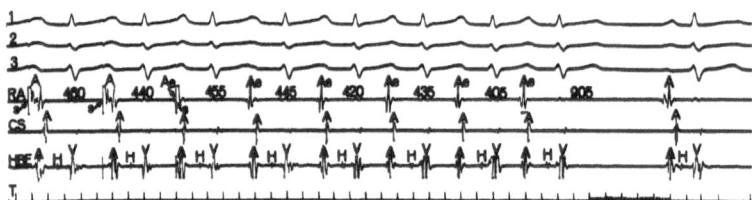

Figure 6. Initiation of sinus node reentrant tachycardia during rapid atrial pacing at a cycle length of 460 msec. Recordings were made from the high right atrium, coronary sinus region and region of the His bundle. The first two atrial complexes are the last in a long series of paced atrial beats. The third atrial complex represents fusion activation between a stimulated and a spontaneously occurring impulse. Upon termination of pacing (starting with the 4th complex) a short run of sinus node reentrant tachycardia occurs. Note similarity of sequence of atrial activation during the tachycardia and sinus rhythm (last beat).

(From Weisfogel G.M. et al., Am. Heart J. 90:295, 1975).

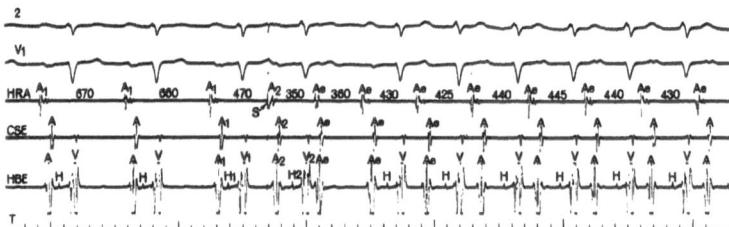

Figure 7. The introduction of a single atrial premature depolarization (A₂) at a coupling interval of 470 msec initiates a sinus node reentrant tachycardia. Note that the first reentrant beat (Ae) is blocked in the A-V node. The sequence of atrial activation during the tachycardia is similar to the sequence during sinus rhythm.

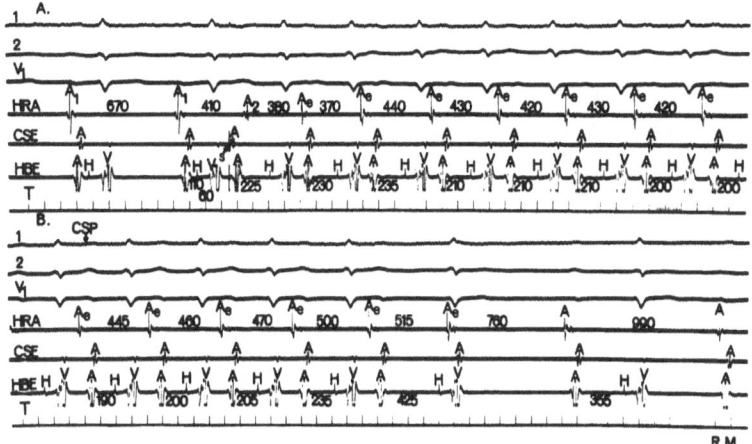

Figure 8. Initiation of sinus node reentrant tachycardia by a single premature atrial depolarization (panel A) and its termination by carotid sinus pressure (CSP) panel B.
(From Weisfogel, G.M. et al., Am. Heart J. 90:295, 1975).

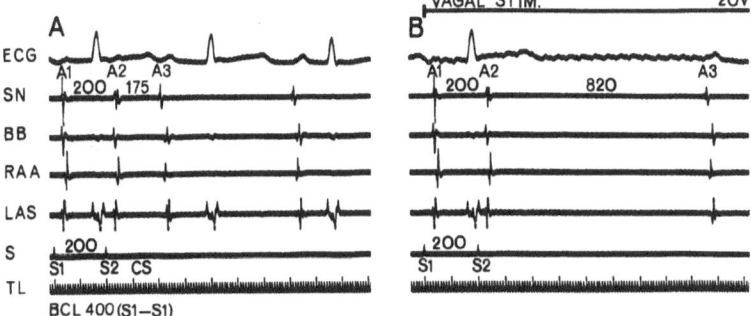

Figure 9. Effect of vagal stimulation on sinus node reentry. Abbreviations same as in Figure 3. A₁ represents the last of a series of basic drive beats from the coronary sinus at a cycle length of 400 msec. A₂ is the premature atrial response also elicited from the coronary sinus at an A₁-A₂ interval of 200 msec. A sinus node reentrant beat (A₃) follows A₂; P wave and sequence of atrial activation are similar to sinus beats (last beat in tracing). In panel B, vagal stimulation at 20 volts prevents the occurrence of sinus node reentry.
(From Paulay, K.L. et al., Circ. Res. 32:323, 1973).

from animal experiments which have shown that the early appearance of A_3 is prevented after crushing the sinus node (Paulay et al., 1974a).

DISCUSSION

Han and co-workers (1968) studied sinus node reentry in isolated rabbit tissue using microelectrode techniques. These investigators suggested that sinus node reentry could occur if: 1) the excitation wave of a premature atrial depolarization failed to engage one margin of the sinus node because of refractoriness at that site, 2) the impulse entering at another

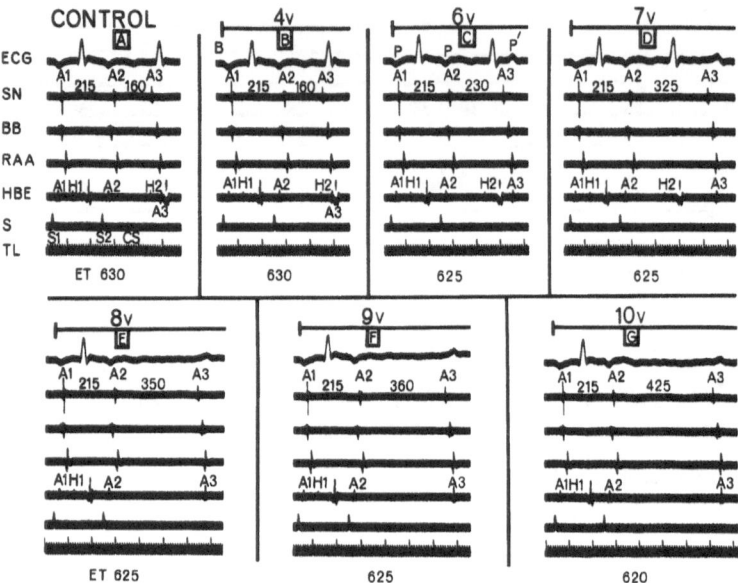

Figure 10. Effects of graded vagal stimulation on the A_2-A_3 interval during coronary sinus stimulation in the dog. In panel A, control data shows that premature stimulation of the coronary sinus at an A_1-A_2 interval of 215 msec is followed in 160 msec by a sinus node reentrant beat (A_3). In panels B to G the effects of graded vagal stimulation on the A_2-A_3 interval are demonstrated. At 4 volts (panel B), the A_2-A_3 interval is unaffected. Between 6 and 20 volts the A_2-A_3 interval progressively increases. The escape time (ET) determined after 10 basic drive beats at all degrees of vagal stimulation was unchanged from control values.
(From Paulay, K.L. et al., Circ. Res. 32:323, 1973).

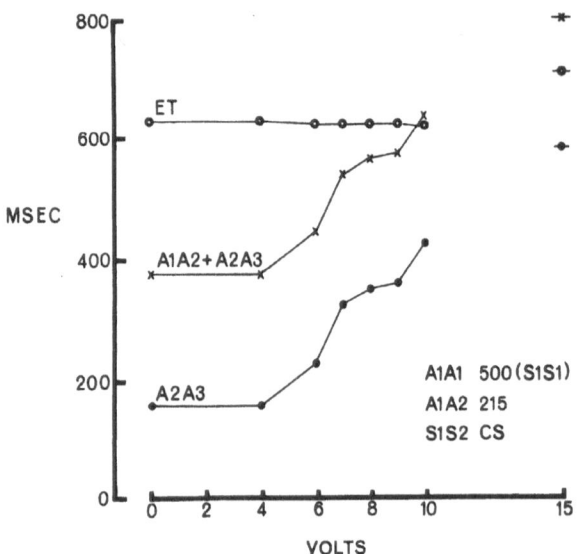

Figure 11. A graphic depiction of data from experiments in Figure 10.
(From Paulay, K.L. et al., Circ. Res. 32:323, 1973).

site traveled slowly throughout nodal tissue and 3) the atrium was excitable when the impulse existed from the sinus node. Direct proof that sinus node reentry exists would require mapping of the reentrant pathway, which, to date, has not been accomplished. We, therefore, must recognize that what we call sinus node reentry is done so on the basis of indirect evidence and therefore alternative explanations must be considered.

Bonke and associates (1971) also studied the phenomenon of sinus node reentry in isolated rabbit tissue. They suggested that the earlier than expected post-extrasystolic response (A_3) may be the result of electronic enhancement of sinus node automaticity caused by the premature atrial impulse (A_2). In their studies, the sum of the pre- and post-extrasystolic intervals (i.e. the A_1-A_3 intervals) were not as abbreviated as found in clinical and intact animal heart studies. Electrotonic enhancement of pacemaker activity may be adequate to explain a single post-extrasystolic response but does not adequately explain sustained accelerated or tachycardic responses. In addition, the concept of electrotonic enhancement of sinus node pacemaker activity appears inconsistent with the effects of graded vagal stimulation. The latter produced progressive increases in the A_2-A_3 interval without affecting sinus node escape time which is a reflection of automaticity.

Another possibility to be considered is that of local reentry occurring at the site of stimulation. This appears unlikely since the origin of what is called sinus node reentrant beats appears to be from the high right atrium with a high to low sequence of atrial activation irrespective of where the premature atrial stimulus is applied (Figures 1, 2). In local reentry, one would expect the origin of A_3 to be at the site of ectopic stimulation.

Sinus node reentry can be distinguished from A-V nodal reentry even though the two phenomena have certain characteristics in common. Similarities include: (1) initiation by single premature atrial depolarizations usually within a well defined coupling (A_1-A_2) zone, (2) variability of atrial cycle length immediately following A_2 and (3) termination by effective vagal stimulation or by single atrial extrasystoles. In A-V nodal reentry (1) the P waves are inverted in leads 2, 3 and aVF, (2) the sequence of atrial activation is from the low to high right atrium and (3) the P wave occurs within the QRS complex whereas in sinus node reentry the P wave generally occurs before the QRS complex. Similar differences also exist between sinus node reentry and reentry utilizing a V-A accessory pathway.

A stimulus induced release of catecholamines accounting for the observed phenomenon seems unlikely since stimulation, even at several times diastolic threshold during the effective refractory period of the atrium failed to elicit the A_3 response. It would appear, therefore, that a propagated atrial response arriving at a critical time in the region of the sinus node is necessary for the phenomenon to occur.

For the most part, sinus node reentry is a laboratory phenomenon. We have observed it in approximately 20% of our clinical cases in which programmed atrial stimulation is performed. It does occur spontaneously but is uncommon and rarely does this arrythmia pose a therapeutic problem of management.

REFERENCES

1. Bonke, F.I.M., Bouman, L.N., Schopman, F.J.G.: Effect of an early atrial premature beat on activity of the sino-atrial node and atrial rhythm in the rabbit. *Circ Res* 29: 704, 1971
2. Han, J., Malozzi, A.M., Moe, G.K.: Sino-atrial reciprocation in the isolated rabbit heart. *Circ Res* 22: 355, 1968
3. Narula, O.S.: Sinus node re-entry. A mechanism for supraventricular tachycardia. *Circulation* 50: 1114, 1974

4. Paulay, K.L., Varghese, P.J., Damato, A.N.: Atrial rhythms in response to an early atrial premature depolarization in man. *Am Heart J* 85: 323, 1973a
5. Paulay, K.L., Varghese, J.P., Damato, A.N.: Sinus node reentry. An in vivo demonstration in the dog. *Circ Res* 32: 455, 1973b
6. Weisfogel, G.M., Batsford, W.P., Paulay, K.L., Josephson, M.E., Ogunkelu, J.B., Akhtar, M., Seides, S.F., Damato A.N.: Sinus node re-entrant tachycardia in man. *Am Heart J* 90: 295, 1975

34

SEQUENCE OF ATRIAL ACTIVATION IN PATIENTS WITH ATRIAL ECHO BEATS*

GÜNTER BREITHARDT AND LUDGER SEIPEL

Experimental studies in the isolated atrium have shown that the sinus node may be a site for reentry (Childers et al., 1973; Han et al., 1968; Paulay et al., 1973a; Strauss and Bigger, 1971; Strauss and Geer, 1977; Wallace and Dagget, 1964). The occurrence of sinus node reentry has also been postulated in man (Brechenmacher and Voegtlin, 1974; Breithardt et al., 1976; Curry and Krikler, 1977; Narula, 1974; Pahlajani et al., 1975; Paritzky et al., 1974; Paulay et al., 1973b, 1975; Wu et al., 1975). Its diagnosis is based on indirect data of which the P wave morphology and the activation sequence of the right atrium during echo beats are the most important. Recent studies have shed some doubt on the reliability of P wave morphology and atrial activation sequence (Waldo, 1977). Therefore, we studied the activation sequence of the right atrium (RA) by use of multiple atrial recordings in patients with atrial echo beats which met the criteria for sinus node reentry.

METHODS

All patients were studied in the non-sedated, postabsorptive state in the catheter laboratory after having given written informed consent. The study was indicated for clinical reasons in all patients. Positioning of electrode catheters and recording of atrial and His bundle electrogram were performed as previously described (Breithardt and Seipel, 1976; Breithardt et al., 1977). Stimulation was done, using the Medtronic Conduction System Analyser (5325). The atrial cycle lengths were measured beat-to-beat by an automatic interval counter designed in collaboration with H. Mescher (IFD, Mülheim/Ruhr, Germany) and printed on a digital printer. The accuracy of measurements could be checked as the RA electrogram and the trigger signal for the interval counter were simultaneously recorded.

In all patients conventional His bundle recordings during spontaneous rhythm, at constant paced cycle lenghts, and during coupled and paired premature atrial stimulation, were done. Sinus node recovery time (SNRT) and sinoatrial conduction time (SACT) were estimated as previously described (Breithardt and Seipel, 1976; Mandel et al., 1971; Narula et al., 1972; Seipel et al., 1974; Strauss et al., 1973). The limitations of the extrastimulus technique for estimation of SACT have previously been discussed in detail (Breithardt and Seipel, 1976; Miller and Strauss, 1974; Ticzon et al., 1975; Strauss et al., 1973; Seipel et al., 1975). The right atrial (RA) intervals, which were automatically measured during premature atrial stimulation, were transferred to a Dietz computer (MINCAL 621) where they were normalized for the spontaneous cycle length and plotted on an oscilloscopic

* Supported in part by the Landesamt für Forschung, Norchkein-Westfalen.

screen for identification of zones of non-reset and reset. SACT was then calculated from responses during the zone of reset.

The atrial intervals were defined as follows:

A_1-A_1: spontaneous cycle length

A_1-A_2: coupling or test interval of the premature stimulus, used for delineation of echo zones

A_2-A_3: return cycle or in case of atrial echo beats (A_E) echo interval;

A_3-A_4: post-return cycle.

The respective stimulated cycles were designated by "S".

In all patients atrial echo beats were carefully searched by premature atrial stimulation. In case of stable and reproducible echoes, endocardial "atrial mapping" was done in the following manner. The tip of a quadripolar electrode catheter was positioned in the right atrial (RA) appendage to ensure a stable position where it adapted an inverted J-shape position. The distal pair of electrodes was used for stimulation. During spontaneous rhythm, the atrial electrogram from the stimulating electrodes could be recorded (compare Figure 2). During stimulation, the recorder was automatically separated from the stimulating electrodes. The proximal pair of electrodes – 6 to 7 cm apart from the tip of the catheter – was used for recording a second high RA electrogram which was used as reference for timing of the other events. Because of the long distance of the proximal electrodes from the tip of the catheter, they were lying in the high RA between the cranial circumference of the RA appendage and the orifice of the vena cava superior. This position seemed to be best suitable for depicting activity from the sinus node region.

For the purpose of atrial mapping, a semi-flexible 4 F bipolar catheter (electrode distance 0.5 cm) was introduced via the right femoral vein for depicting the activation sequence within the RA. Atrial activation during spontaneous rhythm, at basic driven rates and during induced echo beats, was studied consecutively by moving this catheter to different sites within the RA which were localized by biplane fluoroscopy.

The results of analysis of RA activation were graphically documented in a schematic drawing of the RA (Figures 1, 4 and 7). Activation times were referred to the earliest site of activation. As exactly positioning of the recording electrodes is very difficult, only 12 to 15 sites were evaluated in the RA which could clearly be separated. No attempt was made to draw isosynchronic lines because of the relatively small number of activation times.

Ten patients were studied (Table 1). In 8 patients echo beats met the criteria for sinus node reentry (see discussion). Two of these patients complained of intermittent rapid heart action. No arrhythmia could be recorded during long-term ambulatory monitoring In one other patient recurrent atrial tachycardias had been observed for several months. The last patient of this series was studied because of a history of paroxysmal tachycardia which had not yet been electrocardiographically documented.

RESULTS

The clinical data and some electrophysiologic findings in the 10 patients are listed in Table 1. Two patients were studied because of sinus node dysfunction. Sinus node recovery time (SNRT) and sinoatrial conduction time (SACT) were within the limits of normal in

Normal sequence of right atrial activation during sinus rhythm in 10 patients

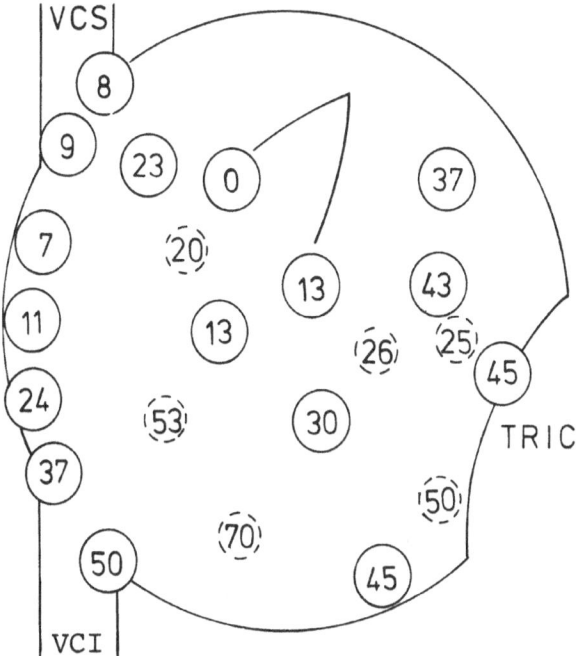

Figure 1. Schematic drawing of the right atrium (RA) showing composite data of endocardial activation times in 10 patients. Mean values of adjacently located sites are indicated; all values in milliseconds. Values are referring to the earliest atrial activation which was recorded in the region of the RA appendage. Values in broken circles represent sites which were posteriorly located. Abbreviations or symbols: vena cava superior = V.C.S.; vena cava inferior = V.C.I.; right atrial appendage =   ; tricuspid orifice = TRIC. See text for further details.

both patients. In one patient who was not suspected to have sinus node dysfunction, a markedly prolonged SNRT was found. The remaining patients were studied for various reasons (Table 1).

In most patients atrial echo beats could be initiated by premature atrial stimulation during spontaneous sinus rhythm. However, as they proved to be more reproducible at basic driven rates, RA mapping was only done under the latter conditions. The absolute width of the echo zone (A_1-A_2) varied between 20 to 80 msec. In most of the patients the lower limit of the echo zone was delineated by the effective refractory period of the RA. The mean echo interval (A_2-A_E) showed large variations between 210 msec and 454 msec (Table 1). Usually only one echo beat was initiated by the premature stimulus. Only rarely several consecutive echo beats were observed. No patient exhibited sustained sinus node tachycardia. Atrial tachycardia degenerating into atrial flutter originated in one patient after application of two premature stimuli (case no. 5). Except for case 9 and 10 (Table 1) the activation sequence was from high to low during echo beats. P waves were positive in lead I and II as far as the morphology of P waves was not obscured by the QRS complex or the T waves.

Table 1. Clinical and electrophysiological data in 10 patients. Abbreviations: m = male, f = female, SB = sinus bradycardia, LBBB = left bundle branch block, RBBB = right bundle branch block, LAH = left axis deviation, AV I° = first degree AV block, fibril. = fibrillation, RAA = right atrial appendage, RA = right atrium, ERP(A) = effective refractory period of the right atrium; SNRT = sinus node recovery time, CSNRT = SNRT after correction for basic cycle length, SACT = sinoatrial conduction time.

Case No	Age	Sex	Diagnosis	A_1A_1	SNRT (CSNRT)	SACT	Place of stimulation	Basic rhythm	Echo zone	ERR(A)	A_2-A_E (mean; range)	Activation sequence
1	65	f	SB, 44 b.p.m. SVEB	785 ± 41	1280 (395)	70	RAA	paired stim. S_1-S_1 600	270–240	220	325 (300–360)	high to low
2	46	m	tachycardia of unknown origin	679 ± 32	925 (246)	103	RAA	paired stim. S_1-S_1 = 600 msec	330–250	190	318 (230–450)	high to low
3	42	f	LBBB (intermitt.)	593 ± 18	856 (263)	91	RAA	paired stim. S_1-A_1 = 600 msec	250–210	200	254 (230–350)	high to low
							low lateral RA	S_1-S_1 = 600 msec	230–200	180	210 (200–220)	low to high
4	69	m	RBBB, LAH AV I°	882 ± 38	1300 (418)	108	RAA low lateral RA	paired stim. S_1-S_1 = 750 msec paired stim. S_1-S_1 = 750 msec	270–220 310–230	210 220	265 (250–270) 320 (310–330)	high to low high to low
5	55	m	SB, 48 b.p.m. SVEB, intermitt. atrial fibril.	1007 ± 60	1300 (293)	115	RAA	paired stim. two premature stimuli S_1-S_1 = 375	S_1-S_2 = 210–220 S_2-S_3 = 170–200	180	atrial tachycardia A-A = 250 to 270	high to low
							low lateral RA	paired, two stimuli S_2-S_3 = 375 msec	S_1-S_2 = 220–210 S_2-S_3 = 180–220	190	atrial tachycardia A-A = 250 to 260	low to high
6	37	m	LBBB	870 ± 45	940 (70)	95	RAA	paired stim. S_1-S_1 = 600 msec	270–240	190	253 (210 to 280)	high to low
							low lateral RA	paired stim. S_1-S_1 = 600 msec	290–240	–	258 (230 to 280)	high to low
7	23	f	tachycardia of unknown origin	1000 ± 56	2481 (1481)	–	RAA	paired stim. S_1-S_1 = 375 msec	320–260	210	379 (360 to 400)	high to low
							low lateral RA	paired stim. S_1-S_1 = 375 msec	310–230	170	454 (400 to 570)	high to low
8	39	m	Carotid sinus syndrome	670 ± 18	900 (230)	126	RAA	paired stim. S_1-S_1 = 600 msec	250–230	200	253 (240 to 270)	high to low
9	22	m	AVN Reentry	800 ± 22	1300 (550)	76	RAA	spontaneous	350–320	290 210	376 (340 to 440) cycle length 500	low to high spontaneous occurrence and cessation, ectopic atrial activation
10	49	m	Ectopic atrial tachycardia	650 ± 7	980 (140)	–		spontaneous				

In one patient (case no. 9) A-V nodal reentrant tachycardias with negative P waves in lead I and II could be produced. Another patient (case no. 10) demonstrated paroxysmal atrial tachycardias at a cycle length of 500 msec with negative P waves in lead I, II and III. The PQ interval during spontaneous sinus rhythm was not significantly different from the one during tachycardia. These episodes could neither be interrupted by high rate atrial stimulation nor by a premature atrial depolarization. The tachycardia always started with an ectopic atrial premature beat. The configuration of P waves and PQ interval of this premature beat was identical to the one of the following beats of the tachycardia which on many occasions ceased spontaneously. Intravenous application of verapamil did not interrupt the tachycardia but only slowed its rate slightly.

ACTIVATION SEQUENCE OF RA DURING SPONTANEOUS SINUS RHYTHM

In order to get some information on the normal sequence of RA activation, the intervals during sinus beats in all 10 patients were composed in Figure 1. Adjacent locations of the recording electrode catheter were identified in the different patients. The mean values of RA activation time at adjacently located sites were then calculated.

The earliest activity was depicted by the reference electrodes in the high RA which were positioned between the cranial basis of the circumference of the RA appendage and the orifice of the vena cava superior. It was followed within 10 msec by the junction between the upper vena cava and the RA and furthermore by the upper two thirds of the lateral aspect of the RA (Figure 1). Activity then proceeded to various parts of the high RA within 10 to 20 msec, and then progressed via the dorso-medial aspects of the RA which is represented by the interatrial septum. The dorso-medial sites nearby the tricuspid orifice were activated as early as 25 msec after the RA appendage whereas the opposite anterior walls were not activated before 30 to 45 msec. At the same time atrial activation was depicted at the lower third of the lateral wall and the region of the orifice of the vena cava inferior. Similarly, the parts of the RA at the lower circumference of the tricuspid orifice were activated relatively late between 45 to 50 msec. Activation sequence in one patient with previously documented atrial fibrillation (case no. 5) was not different from the other cases.

ACTIVATION SEQUENCE OF RA DURING ATRIAL ECHO BEATS

Figure 2A gives a typical example of RA mapping during high RA stimulation from the right atrial appendage at a basic stimulation rate of 80 b.p.m. (S_1-S_1 = 750 msec). At coupling intervals of the premature beat between 270 msec to 220 msec, atrial echo beats with a high-to-low RA sequence could be elicited. The A_2-A_E intervals ranged between 250 msec to 270 msec (mean 265 msec). At the shorter coupling intervals during the echo zone, neither A_2 nor A_E were conducted to the ventricles because of refractoriness of the A-V conduction system. In Figure 2 the latency between S_2 and A_2 is markedly prolonged in comparison with S_1 and A_1. However, this prolongation was no prerequisit for atrial echo beats to occur as they were also observed at coupling intervals without increase in latency (compare the data for low RA stimulation, Figure 3). The sequence of atrial activation of A_E was similar to the one during spontaneous sinus rhythm. This was also

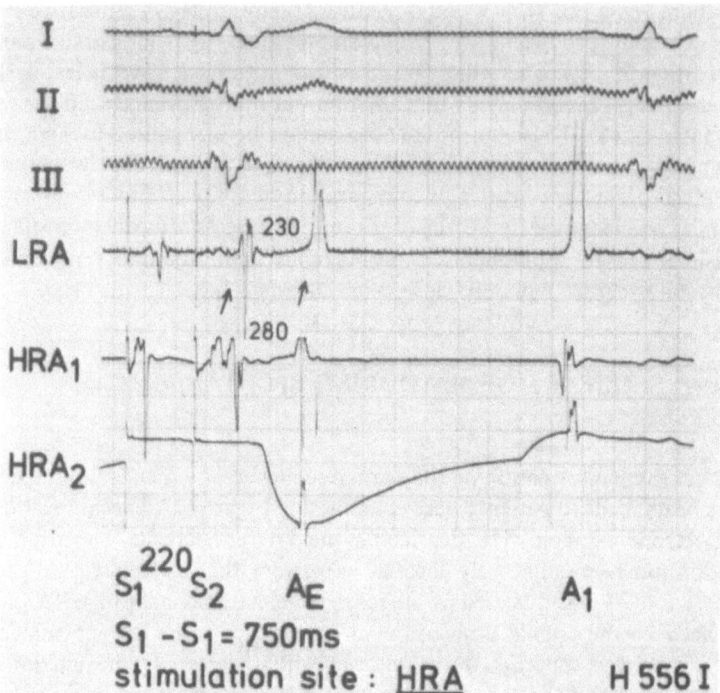

Figure 2a. upper panel: Original registration in Case no. 4 showing lead I, II, and III, low right atrial (LRA) and high right atrial (HRA$_1$ and HRA$_2$) electrograms. QRS complexes show complete right bundle branch block with left axis deviation. HRA$_2$ was recorded via the stimulating electrodes that were disconnected from the recorder during stimulation. Stimulation site: high right atrium. At a basic stimulated cycle length (S$_1$-S$_1$ = 750 msec) a premature stimulus was delivered (S$_1$-S$_2$ = 220 msec). A$_2$ appeared with greater latency (distance between stimulus and atrial electrogram) than A$_1$ because S$_2$ fell within the relative refractory period of the right atrium. Shortly after the premature beat an atrial echo beat (A$_E$) appeared with an echo interval (in HRA) of 280 ms being conducted to the LRA with delay. Activation sequence during spontaneous beats (A$_1$) was from HRA$_1$-HRA$_2$ to LRA. A similar sequence was observed during echo beats (A$_E$). A$_2$ and A$_E$ were not conducted to the ventricles because of refractoriness of the A-V conduction system.

the case when looking at 15 different mapping sites within the RA (Figure 4A). Though there were slight differences in activation time of A$_1$ and A$_E$, there was a fundamental correspondance in activation sequence. The earliest activity of A$_E$ was depicted in the region of the high RA near the atrial appendage.

A similar correspondance between spontaneous atrial activation and activation during echo beats was observed in the remaining cases that were thought to represent sinus node reentry. In all of them the earliest activity of echo beats was depicted in the high RA. In no case any earlier activity could be found outside this region.

In one case (no. 2) the coronary sinus (CS) electrogram was additionally recorded. Again, the sequence of activation of the RA and the arrival of the impulse at the CS was identical during spontaneous and echo beats (Figure 5). In the same patient, some rare variations of this sequence of RA activation were observed at identical sites of stimulation and at identical coupling intervals of the test stimulus. Usually the activation sequence was identical to the one of spontaneous beats (Figure 5, lower panel). However, in a few instances the earliest activity appeared in the CS electrogram (Figure 5, upper panel) suggesting a different site of reentry.

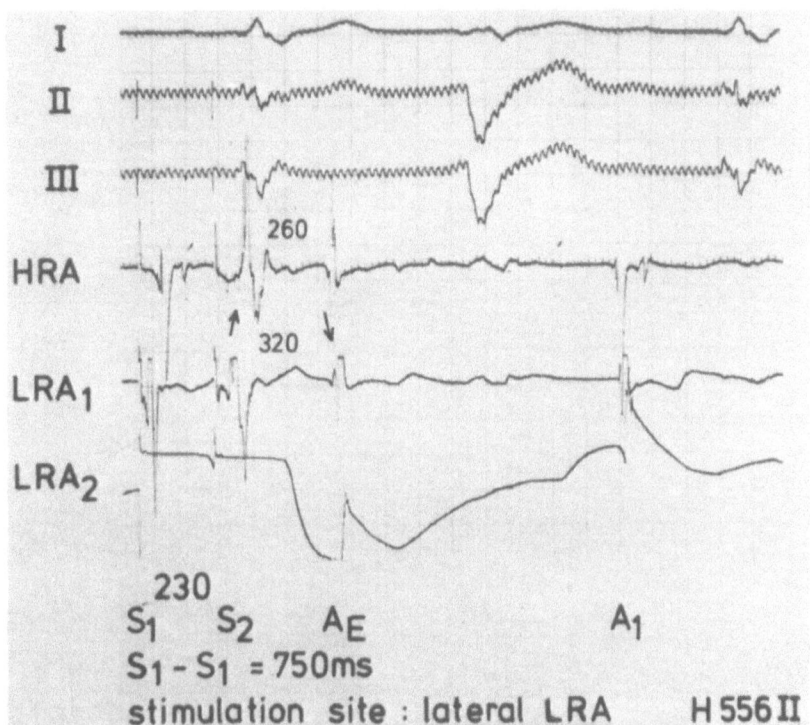

b. middle panel: Stimulation site: low right atrium. Identical notations as in the upper panel. Note that the sequence of atrial electrograms on the recorder has been changed. A premature stimulus with a coupling interval (S_1-S_2) of 230 msec was delivered which was followed within 260 msec (HRA) by an atrial echo beat (A_E) showing identical atrial activation sequence as A_1. There was a slight increase in latency after S_2. A_2 was not conducted to the ventricles, whereas the QRS after A_E showed marked aberrant conduction.

EFFECT OF CHANGE OF STIMULATION SITE ON ACTIVATION SEQUENCE

In five cases premature atrial stimulation was additionally performed at the lateral wall of the low RA. Atrial activity was depicted in the same way as during high RA stimulation. Stimulation was performed either alternatively between high and low RA or low RA stimulation was done after high RA stimulation.

In three cases (no. 4, 6, 7) the activation sequence of echo beats during low RA stimulation was from high to low. Figures 2B and 4B give representative examples. Though activation spread from low to high during premature atrial stimulation (A_2), the echo beat emerged from the high RA travelling downwards. However, in two cases (no. 3, 5) the opposite sequence of RA activation was observed during low RA stimulation (i.e. from low to high). One of these cases (no. 3) had shorter echo intervals ranging from 200 msec to 220 msec during low RA stimulation compared to 230 msec to 350 msec during high RA stimulation. The other case (no. 5) in which two premature atrial stimuli were necessary for induction of echoes, exhibited atrial tachycardias which on several occasions degenerated into atrial flutter.

Figure 6 illustrates the effect of stimulation site on echo zone and echo interval in

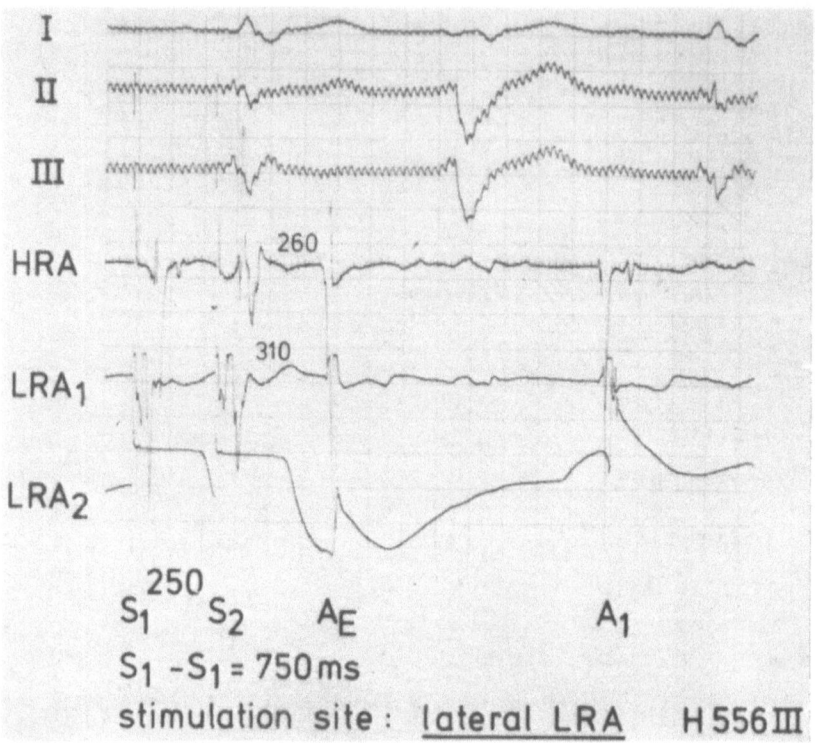

c. lower panel: Identical notations and stimulation site as in middle panel. At a coupling interval (S_1-S_2) of 250 msec there was no increase in latency after S_2. Nevertheless, an echo beat identical to the middle panel was observed.

the three cases with identical sequences of RA activation after both high and low RA stimulation. In one case the test cycles were shorter during low RA stimulation, in one patient they were nearly identical, and in the third patient they were somewhat longer than during high RA stimulation. When looking at the local activity, in two cases the echo intervals were markedly longer after low than after high RA stimulation. In one case they differed only slightly. However, with regard to high RA activity the echo intervals were nearly similar during low and high RA stimulation.

ACTIVATION SEQUENCE OF RA DURING A-V NODAL REENTRY OR ECTOPIC ATRIAL TACHYCARDIA

In one patient with A-V nodal reentrant tachycardia (case no. 9) the sequence of RA activation was from low to high both during single echo beats and during sustained tachycardia. The earliest activity was detected in the low RA near the tricuspid orifice (Figure 7). Activity was then rapidly conducted to the high RA via the interatrial septum. The high RA was activated as early as 5 to 20 msec after the low RA in the vicinity of the A-V junction. The lateral aspects of the RA were activated quite late.

One patient (case no. 10) demonstrated the earliest atrial activity during mapping of

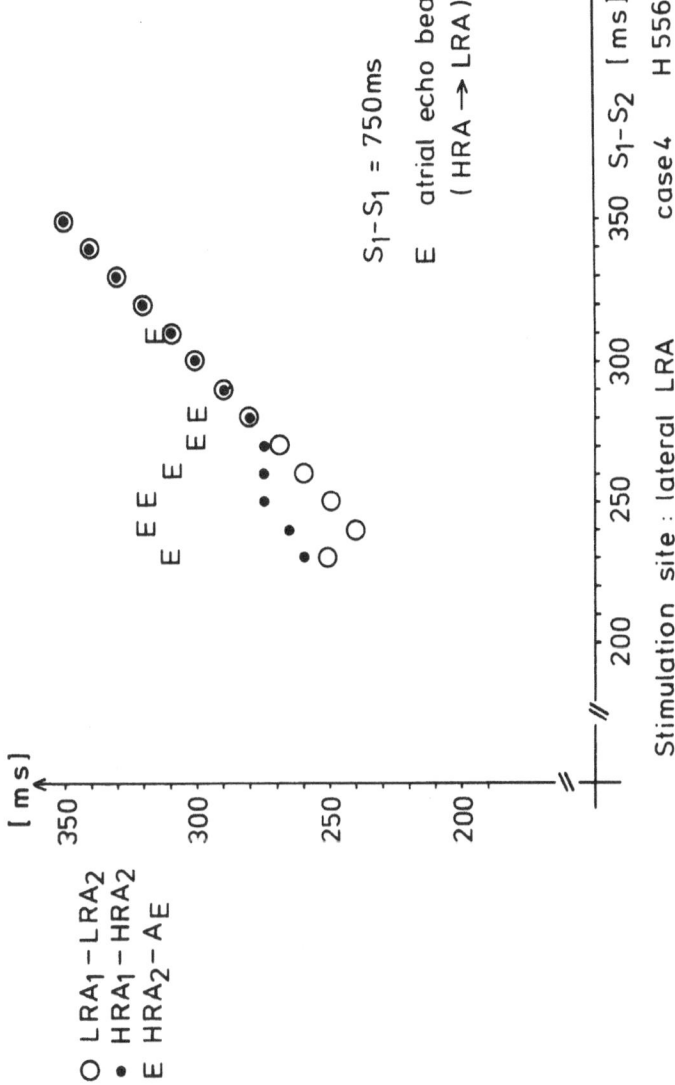

Figure 3. A plot of the interval between the atrial electrograms recorded at LRA and HRA versus the coupling interval of the premature stimulus (S_1-S_2). When the coupling interval is 230–270 msec there is a delay in the conduction of the impulse from the site of stimulation towards the high right atrium, causing that HRA_1-HRA_2 is longer than LRA_1-LRA_2. The atrial echo beats (E) had a more or less equal HRA_2-A_E interval, independent of the coupling interval.

The echo beats showed a HRA LRA sequence.

LRA: low right atrium; HRA: high right atrium; HRA_2-A_E = echo interval.

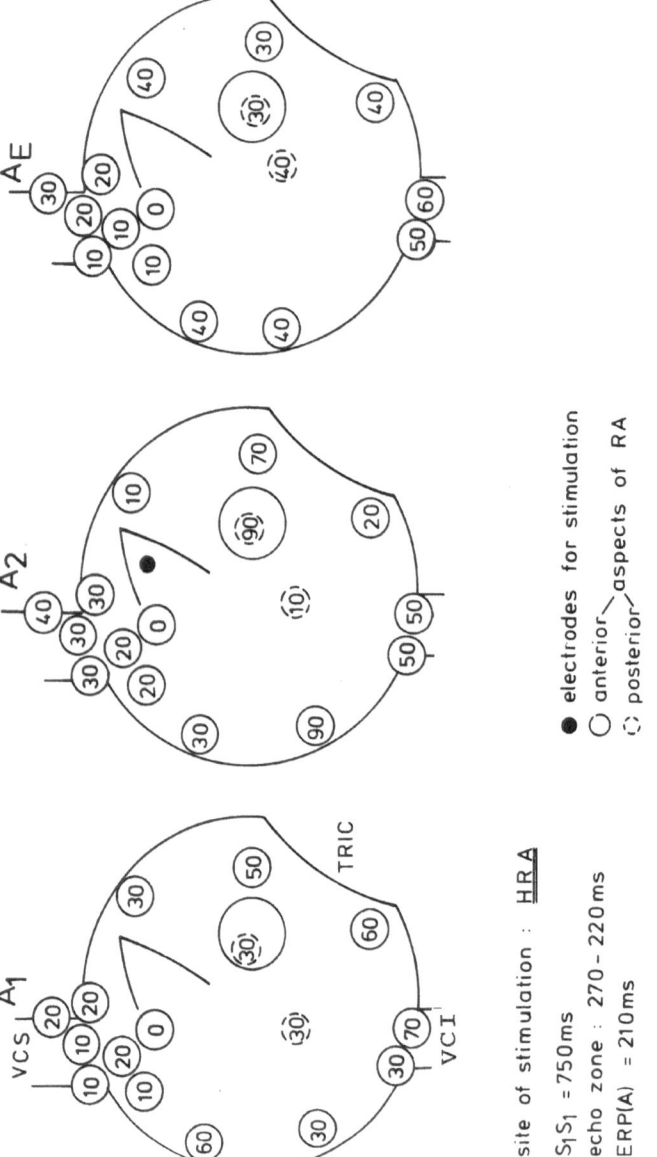

site of stimulation : HRA

$S_1 S_1 = 750$ ms
echo zone : 270 - 220 ms
ERP(A) = 210 ms

● electrodes for stimulation
○ anterior ⎫ aspects of RA
⟨⟩ posterior ⎭

Figure 4A. upper panel: Schematic drawing of the right atrium (RA). Case no. 4. Notations as in Figure 1. During spontaneous sinus rhythm (A_1) earliest activity was depicted in the region of the RA appendage with rapid excitation of all parts of the high RA. Then downward spread of excitation occurred with late arrival at the vena cava inferior. Late excitation was also observed at one site at the upper third of the lateral RA wall (60 msec). During premature depolarization of the RA (A_2) from the RA appendage, there was a different spread of excitation with later excitation of the region of the vena cava superior and some septal sites compared to A_1. During the atrial echo beats (A_E) a pattern of activation similar to the spontaneous rhythm (A_1) was observed with only slight differences as compared to A_1.
ERP(A) = effective refractory period of atrium.

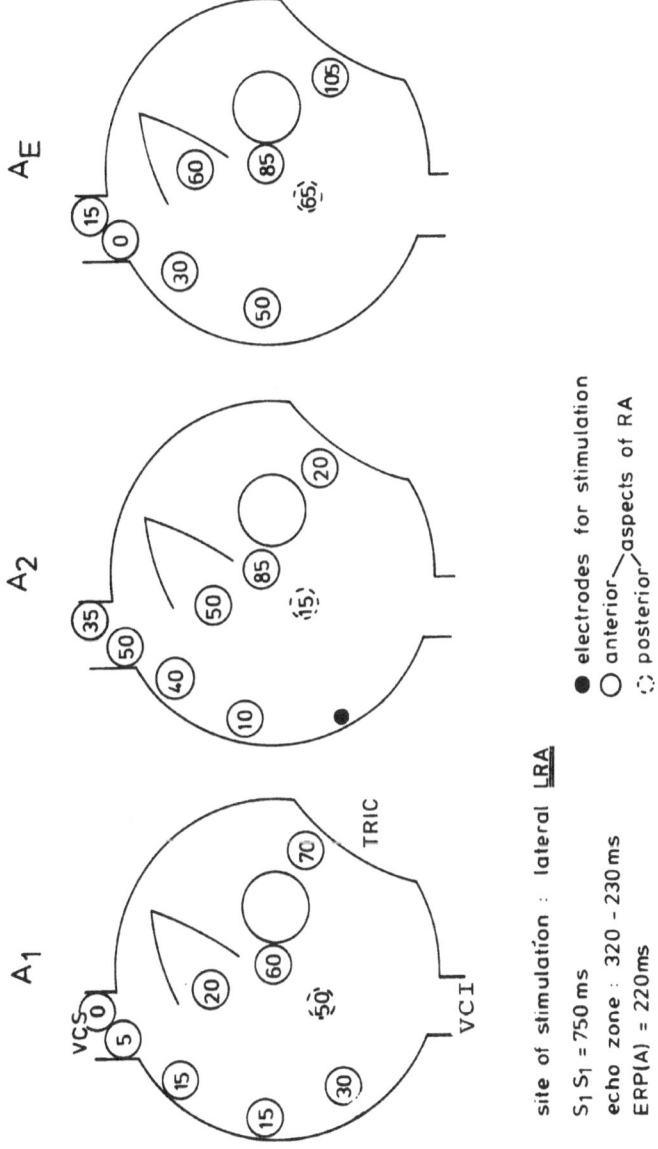

A_1 A_2 A_E

site of stimulation : lateral LRA

$S_1 S_1 = 750$ ms

echo zone : 320 - 230 ms

ERP(A) = 220ms

● electrodes for stimulation

○ anterior ⌒ aspects of RA
⚬ posterior

B. lower panel: Stimulation site was changed to low RA. During the premature depolarization (A_2) the RA was activated from low to high. During the echo beat (A_E) activation again occurred from high to low similar to the spontaneous rhythm.

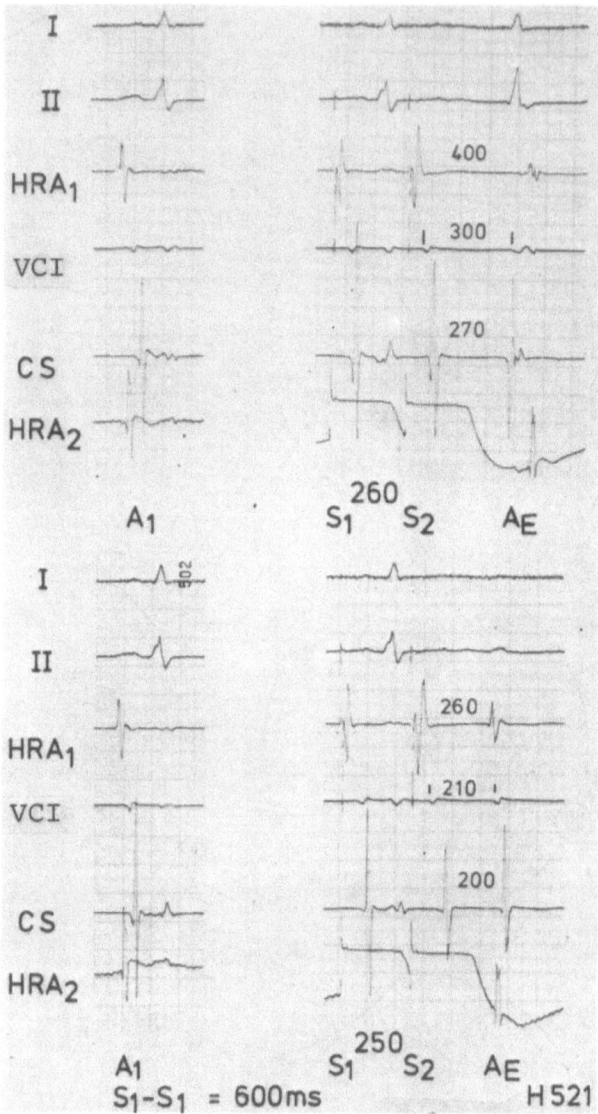

Figure 5. Original registration (case no. 2) showing lead I, II, and electrograms from the high right atrium (HRA₁ and HRA₂), orifice of vena cava inferior (VCI) and coronary sinus (CS). During spontaneous sinus rhythm (left panels) activity spread from HRA to VCI and CS. Atrial echo beats (A$_E$) were initiated at coupling intervals (S₁-S₂) between 330 to 250 msec. Usually a sequence of atrial activation during A$_E$ identical to A₁ was observed (lower right panel). Occasionally a different pattern occurred with earliest activity in CS with spread to VCI and late arrival at HRA. (upper right panel).

tachycardia in the low lateral RA. The left atrium, as recorded from the left pulmonary artery, was activated late. Activity spread upwards and towards the A-V junction. This sequence of activation was thought to be due to an ectopic focus in the lower lateral RA.

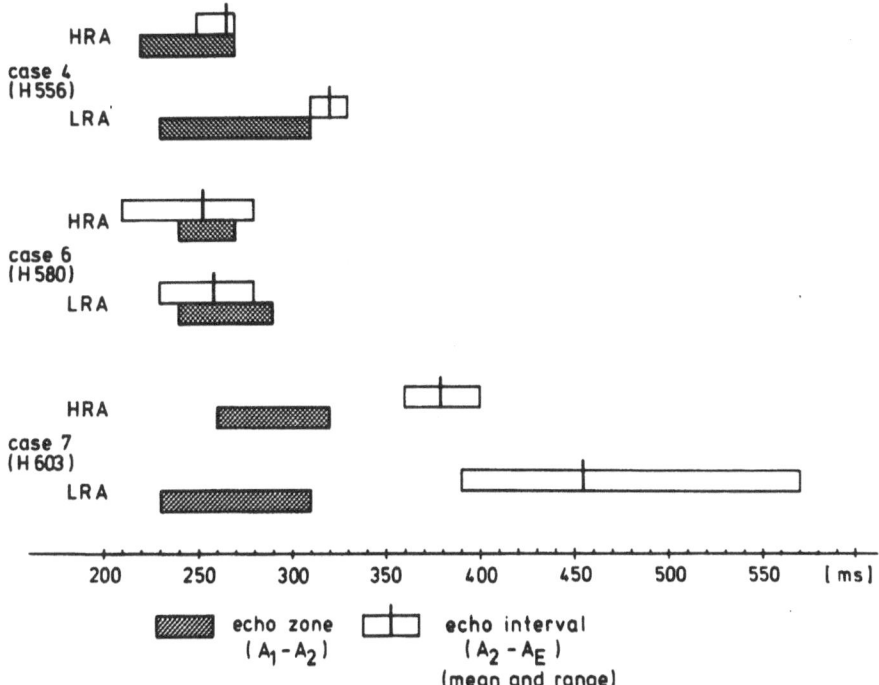

Figure 6. Demonstration of echo zones (A₁-A₂) and echo intervals (A₂-A_E) in 3 cases that exhibited a HRA → LRA sequence of echo beats at two sites of stimulation (high and low RA). See text for further details.

DISCUSSION

Sinus node reentry has been widely accepted as a mechanism of some type of atrial echo beats in man that can be induced by premature atrial depolarization (Brechenmacher und Voegtlin, 1974; Breithardt et al., 1976; Childers et al., 1973; Curry and Krikler, 1977; Han et al., 1968; Narula, 1974; Pahlajani et al., 1975; Paritzky et al., 1974; Paulay et al., 1973b; Wu et al., 1975). Han et al., (1968) suggested that an early premature depolarization may "fail to engage one margin of the sinus node, enter at another site, transverse the relatively refractory nodal tissue so slowly that the atrium has recovered in time to respond again to the emerging response". In man the following criteria have been used for the diagnosis of sinus node reentry (Childers et al., 1973; Narula, 1974; Paritzky et al., 1974; Paulay et al., 1973b, 1975; Wu et al., 1975):

1. Initiation of atrial echo beats by an appropriately timed premature atrial beat outside or independent of the atrial relative refractory period.
2. The echo interval, i.e. the interval between the premature atrial beat (A₂) and the echo beat (A_E) should be shorter than the spontaneous cycle length.
3. The right atrium should be activated during the echo beat from high to low; P wave morphology should be identical to the one of spontaneous sinus beats.
4. The manifestation of sinus node reentry should be independent of A-V nodal delay.
5. If sustained sinus node reentry tachycardia occurs, termination by appropriately timed premature stimuli should be possible.

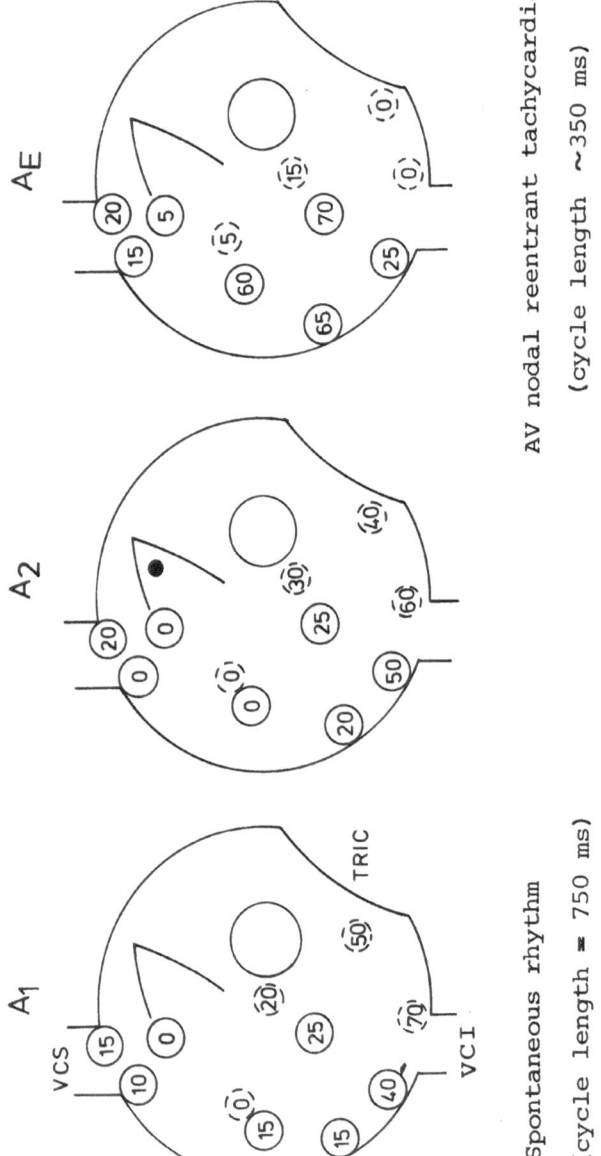

Spontaneous rhythm

(cycle length = 750 ms)

AV nodal reentrant tachycardia

(cycle length ~350 ms)

Figure 7. Schematic drawing of right atrium. Notations as in Figure 1. Stimulation site: high RA. Case no. 9. During spontaneous sinus rhythm sustained A-V nodal reentrant tachycardias were initiated at coupling intervals between 320 to 350 msec. Activation sequence of RA during tachycardia was from low to high with rapid spread to high RA whereas the lateral wall of RA was activated relatively late.

6. Reentry should be reproducible despite a change of right atrial stimulation site.
7. Sinus node entrance block should be excluded. This is possible if the post-return cycle (A_3-A_4) is longer than the spontaneous cycles suggesting reset of the sinus node by the reentrant beat.

Whereas most of these criteria serve to diagnose "reentry" per se, P wave morphology and the activation sequence of the RA by the echo beat are those which are most specifically linked to the diagnosis of the site of reentry. However, recent studies have shed some doubt on the reliability of P wave morphology as a guide to atrial activation sequence, as even activation of the atria from numerous sites in both, right or left atrium can produce positive P waves in lead II, III and aVF which thus mimic those produced by normal sinus rhythm (Mac Lean et al., 1975; Waldo 1977). In view of these limitations of present recording techniques, we started to record atrial activation from numerous sites in patients who met the above-mentioned criteria for sinus node reentry.

Previous studies on atrial activation sequence in man were confined to the registration from a few sites within the RA (Amat-Y-Leon et al., 1976; Massumi et al., 1969) or the investigators were interested in the pattern of retrograde atrial activation (Agha et al., 1976; Amat-Y-Leon, 1976; Gallagher et al., 1976; Grolleau et al., 1970; Tonkin et al., 1975; Svenson et al., 1974). In our study an attempt was made to get a broader spectrum of sites of RA activation. A semi-flexible 4 F bipolar catheter (electrode distance 0.5 cm) was used for endocardial "mapping". Localization of the electrodes was done by biplane fluoroscopy. With respect to the difficulties in differentiating between closely adjacent sites, no attempt was made to record from more than 12 to 15 sites within the RA. As simultaneous registrations from multiple electrodes is difficult in man, the activation sequence of the RA was determined consecutively. Premature atrial stimulation was performed at a basic driven cycle length as echo beats proved to be more reproducible than during spontaneous sinus rhythm. In some cases echo beats could only be initiated at a driven atrial rate. Recently, Strauss and Geer (1977) put forward an explanation for the greater frequency of echo beats at driven atrial rates.

Without a clear picture of what normal activation of the RA is like, demonstration of abnormal sequence is of questionable meaning. Therefore, we first established the normal sequence of endocardial activation of the RA. To exclude individual variabilities and because only a limited number of endocardial sites could be traced in a single patient, the results were combined in a drawing of the activation sequency of all patients (Figure 1). Recently, Boineau et al. (1977) noted in a dog with spontaneous episodes of atrial flutter that the activation sequence of the RA during sinus rhythm was different from that of other dogs without this arrhythmia. We did not notice a similar abnormal activation sequence in one of our patients who had documented atrial fibrillation.

Our data show that the first activity during sinus rhythm is depicted in the high RA. Then there is a rapid spread of activation over the lateral border of the right atrium and the septal aspects whereas the region around the orifice of the vena cava inferior is activated relatively late. These findings are consonant to mapping studies in the isolated atrium which have shown that the spread of activation from the sinus node to the right atrium is not uniform (Boineau et al., 1977; Eyster and Meek, 1916; Holsinger et al., 1968; Puech et al., 1954; Rothberger and Scherf, 1927; Sano and Yamagishi, 1965; Spach et al., 1971). During sinus rhythm, there is preferential atrial activation with rapid spread from the sinus node downwards via the crista terminalis and in septal direction via the anterior internodal tract (Boineau et al., 1977; Hayashi et al., 1974; Spach et al., 1971). This type of preferential conduction is not necessarily based on the existence of specialized internodal tracts, the existence of which has recently been questioned (Janse and Anderson, 1974), but it may readily be explained by the anatomical structure of the atria (Boineau et al., 1977).

During echo beats the activation sequence of the RA was identical in all patients who met the criteria for sinus node reentry. In not one case any activity could be detected that was earlier than the one in the high RA. Thus, these data indicate that the reentry circuit is located in the high RA. However, they do not give any evidence that the sinus node participates in the reentry circuit. A macro-reentry that engages large portions of the RA seems to be improbable. On account of the relatively crude methods used in this study, some uncertainty still remains. For instance, retrograde conduction within a reentry circuit might have occurred in the RA over narrow pathways, which were not detected, or in the left atrium. Then only antegrade conduction from the high to the low RA might have been detected, simulating an atrial activation sequence of sinus beats. Similar observations have recently been reported by Waldo (1977) who suggested the possibility that retrograde conduction, probably via the anterior internodal tract (James, 1963; Meredith and Titus, 1968), might reach the superior aspects of the RA so rapidly that the sequence of atrial activation was in fact from high to low. However, a similar type of retrograde activation of the RA has not been found in previous studies (Amat-Y-Leon et al., 1976; Spach et al., 1971). A further possible mechanism of atrial echo beats might be atrial circus movement. Allessie et al. (1974, 1976, 1977) were able to induce atrial circus movement in isolated segments of the left atrium without apparent anatomic obstacles. However, in case circus movement engaged a larger portion of the RA, we might have been able to record some activity that might indicate retrograde conduction.

Further evidence in support of the assumption that the reentry circuit is located in the high right atrium is provided by the effect of a change of stimulation site. This has not yet been systematically studied in a larger group of patients and no definitive data were given regarding the effect of a change of stimulation site on echo zone and echo interval in the cases reported (Castellanos et al., 1976; Paulay et al., 1973b; Narula, 1974). Weisfogel et al. (1973) reported a wider and later zone for initiation of paroxysmal sinus tachycardia when extra stimuli were given from the high right atrium as compared to the coronary sinus. This is in accordance with the assumption that the greater the distance of the stimulation site from the reentry circuit the earlier the test stimulus must be elicited to arrive in time. Only in one out of three patients with a high-to-low activation sequence at both sites of stimulation the echo zone was as predicted. In the other two patients it was either similar or even somewhat later during low RA stimulation compared to stimulation from the high RA. Several explanations might help to explain this apparent discrepancy between the data and the predicted behaviour. Firstly, the reentry circuit may have been large, including significant parts of the RA, so that the premature impulse might enter the circuit from different directions. This seems less likely since there was no evidence of a large circuit of reentry. Secondly, during stimulation of the low RA at the lateral wall, the impulse might have reached the crista terminalis travelling retrogradely to the high RA with high speed thus obscuring the effect of a more distant site of stimulation. Then, stimulation in the coronary sinus – which we did not do in this study – might have been more effective to show the predicted behaviour. On the other hand, when looking at the respective electrograms, the lengths of the returning echo intervals were well in agreement with the assumption that the reentry circuit was located in the high RA as they were shorter with high RA stimulation compared to low RA stimulation. However, when comparing the high RA electrograms there was no fundamental difference between the two sites of stimulation.

If there is no identical sequence of atrial activation when changing the site of stimulation, this suggests that different sites of reentry exist. This was the case in two patients. In one of them reentry was probably due to atrial vulnerability as two early premature atrial beats were needed to induce atrial tachycardia degenerating into atrial flutter. In the second case, there may have been sinus node reentry during high RA stimulation. Some other site of reentry was manifested when stimulating the low RA. In case no. 2 occassionally different patterns of atrial activation during echo beats were observed. This indicates that multiple sites of reentry may exist as has previously been suggested (Breithardt et al., 1976; Narula, 1974; Wu et al., 1975).

In one patient with A-V node reentry retrograde activation of the RA was fast with rapid spread to the high right atrium. The lateral part of the low right atrium was activated late. This pattern of atrial activation is in contrast to the one during sinus rhythm and has also been described in previous studies (Agha et al., 1976; Amat-Y-Leon et al., 1976; Spach et al., 1971). If only two atrial electrograms (in the high and septal low RA) were recorded – as in previous studies (Amat-Y-Leon et al., 1976) simultaneous activation of both sites would have been detected making the interpretation of atrial activation sequence difficult. In another case, we were able to demonstrate the abnormal activation sequence of the RA during an ectopic atrial rhythm. The order in which the various parts of the RA were activated was characteristic and distinctly different from the one observed when the sinus node was the pacemaker. The sequence of conduction was different from the one noted during A-V nodal reentrant tachycardia. Some data on ectopic atrial rhythms have been reported by Mirowski et al. (1971) and Goldreyer et al. (1973).

The clinical significance of sinus node reentry is still uncertain. No definite data exist on the frequency of spontaneous sinus node reentrant tachycardias. Two of our patients complained of intermittent rapid heart action which could not be documented before the study. However, it remains uncertain whether these episodes were due to sinus node reentry. In most studies no relationship between sinus node dysfunction and sinus node reentry was established (Curry and Krikler, 1977; Breithardt et al., 1976; Narula, 1974; Childers et al., 1973; Paulay et al., 1973b; Wu et al., 1975), though sinus node dysfunction has been found in some cases (Paritzky et al. 1974). The electrophysiologic data of our study support the thesis that sinus node reentry is no manifestation of sinus node dysfunction since both sinus node recovery time (SNRT) and sinoatrial conduction time (SACT) were normal (the upper limit of normal for SNRT after correction for basic cycle length being 525 msec (Narula et al., 1972) and for SACT being 120 msec (Breithardt et al., 1977)). In the case reported by Paritzky et al. (1974) SACT was markedly prolonged (200 msec). Intravenous administration of atropine produced a pronounced shortening of SACT to 70 msec and sustained atrial tachycardia could no longer be elicited. Strauss and Geer (1977) argued that a normal SACT might be a prerequisite for the occurrence of sinus node reentry. Their arguments were based on the theoretical assumption that, provided equal refractory periods of the perinodal tissue, in case of a prolonged SACT large parts of the sinus node may have recovered from antegrade conduction when a premature impulse enters retrogradely. Therefore there may not be enough nodal tissue which is still in a relative refractory state. It will be difficult to prove in man whether these considerations are right. However, the infrequent occurrence of sinus node dysfunction in patients with sinus node reentry should be noted.

Concluding the data presented here give further evidence that atrial echo beats that meet the criteria for sinus node reentry are indeed due to reentrant excitation within the high RA. However, further investigation will be needed, which should be directed to more detailed mapping of atrial excitation in the high RA. The effect of stimulation site on echo zone and echo interval should be tested in every case in order to further define the site of reentry. The effect of drugs might provide further evidence on the location of the reentry circuit (Curry and Krikler, 1977), if drugs are used that act predominantly on the sinus node such as verapamil. A change of vagal tone does not seem to be a reliable criterium as both atrial and intranodal electrophysiologic properties are affected.

In view of the present knowledge on sinus node reentry in man, the question should be raised whether to continue to call it "sinus node" reentry as long as there is no definite proof. We would, therefore, prefer to call it "high right atrial reentry".

REFERENCES

Agha, A.S., Befeler, B., Castellanos, A.M., Sung, R.J., Castillo, C.A., Myerburg, R.J., Castellanos, A.: Bipolar catheter electrograms for study of retrograde atrial activation pattern in patients without pre-excitation syndromes. *Brit Heart J* 38: 641, 1976

Allessie, M.A., Bonke, F.I.M., Schopman, F.J.G.: Circus movement in rabbit atrial muscle as a mechanism of tachycardia. *Circulation Res* 33: 54, 1974

Allessie, M.A., Bonke, F.I.M., Schopman, F.J.G.: Circus movement in rabbit atrial muscle as a mechanism of tachycardia. II. The role of nonuniform recovery of excitability in the occurrence of unidirectional block, as studied with multiple microelectrodes. *Circulation Res* 39: 168, 1976

Allessie, M.A., Bonke, F.I.M., Schopman, F.J.G.: Circus movement in rabbit atrial muscle as a mechanism of tachycardia. III. The "Leading Circle" concept: A new model of circus movement in cardiac tissue without the involvement of an anatomical obstacle. *Circ Res* 41: 9, 1977

Amat-y-Leon, F., Dhingra, A.C., Wu, D.: Catheter mapping of retrograde atrial activation. Observations during ventricular pacing and AV nodal reentrant paroxysmal tachycardia. *Brit Heart J* 38: 355, 1976

Boineau, J.P., Mooney, C.R., Hudson, R.D., Hughes, D.G., Erdin, R.A. Jr., Wylds, A.C.: Observations on re-entrant excitation pathways and refractory period distributions in spontaneous and experimental atrial flutter in the dog. In: Re-entrant arrhythmias. Mechanisms and treatment. Kulbertus, H.E. (ed.), MTP, Lancaster, 1977, p. 72

Bonke, F.I.M., Bouman, L.N. Schopman, F.J.G.: Effect of an early atrial premature beat on activity of the sinoatrial node and atrial rhythm in the rabbit. *Circulation Res* 29: 704, 1971

Brechernmacher, C., Voegtlin, R.: Tachycardie sinusale par réentrée. *Ann Cardiol Angéiol* 25: 535, 1974

Breithardt, G., Seipel, L.: Reaktion des menschlichen Sinusknotens auf frühzeitige Depolarisation: Sinus-knoten-Reentry und Sinusknoten-Eintrittsblock. *Verh Dtsch Ges Kreislaufforschg* 42: 228, 1976

Breithardt, G., Seipel, L.: The effect of premature atrial depolarization of sinus node automaticity in man. *Circulation* 53: 920, 1976

Breithardt, G., Seipel, L., Loogen, F.: Sinus node recovery time and calculated sinoatrial conduction time in normal subjects and patients with sinus node dysfunction. *Circulation* 56, 1977, 43

Castellanos, A., Aranda, J., Moleiro, F., Mallon, S.M., Befeler, B.: Effects of the pacing site in sinus node reentrant tachycardia. *J Electrocardiol* 9: 165, 1976

Childers, R.W., Arnsdorf, M.F., de la Fuente, D.J., Gambetta, M., Svenson, R.: Sinus nodal echoes. Clinical case report and canine studies. *Amer J Cardiol* 31: 220, 1973

Curry, P.V.L., Krikler, D.M.: Paroxysmal reciprocating sinus tachycardia in: Re-entrant arrhythmias. Mechanisms and treatment. Kulbertus, H.E. (ed.), MTP, Lancaster, 1977, p. 39

Eyster, J.A.E., Meek, W.J.: Experiments on the origin and conduction of the cardiac impulse. VI. Conduction of the excitation from the sinoauricular node to the right auricle and atrioventricular node. *Arch Int Med* 18: 775, 1916

Gallagher, J.J., Sealy, W.C., Wallace, A.G.: Correlation between catheter electrophysiological studies and findings on mapping of ventricular excitation in the W.P.W. syndrome. In: The conduction system of the heart, Wellens, H.J.J., Lie, K.I., Janse, M.J. (eds.) Leiden, 1976, p. 588

Geer, M.R., Estrada, E.A., Strauss, H.C.: Sinus node response to early atrial premature depolarizations. *Circulation*, 52: suppl. II–64, 1975

Goldreyer, B.N., Gallagher, J.J., Damato, A.N.: The electrophysiologic demonstration of atrial ectopic tachycardia in man. *Amer Heart J* 85: 205, 1973

Grolleau, R., Dufoix, R., Puech, P., Latour, H.: Les tachycardies par rhythme réciproque dans le syndrome de Wolff-Parkinson-White. *Arch Mal Coeur* 63: 74, 1970

Han, J., Malozzi, A.M., Moe, G.K.: Sino-atrial reciprocation in the isolated rabbit heart. *Circulation Res* 22: 355, 1968

Hayashi, H., Lux, R. Wyatt, R.: Activation sequence in the right atrium of the dog. *Circulation* 50: suppl. III–84, 1974

Holsinger, J.W. Jr., Wallace, A.G., Sealy, W.C.: The identification and surgical significance of the atrial internodal conduction tracts. *Ann Surg* 167: 447, 1968

James, T.N.: The connecting pathways between the sinus node and A-V node and between the right and the left atrium in the human heart. *Amer Heart J* 66: 498, 1963

Janse, M.J., Anderson, R.H.: Specialized internodal atrial pathways – fact or fiction? *Europ J Cardiol* 2: 117, 1974

MacLean, W.A.H., Karp, R.B., Kouchoukos, N.T., James, T.N., Waldo, A.L.: P waves during ectopic atrial rhythms in man. A study utilizing atrial pacing with fixed electrodes. *Circulation* 52: 426, 1975

Mandel, W.J., Hayakawa, H., Danzig, R., Marcus, H.S.: Evaluation of sino-atrial node function in man by overdrive suppression. *Circulation* 44: 59, 1971

Massumi, R.A., Sarin, R.K., Tawakkol, A.A., Rios, J.L., Jackson, H.: Time sequence of right and left atrial depolarization as a guide to the origin of P waves. *Amer J Cardiol* 24: 28, 1969

Meredith, J., Titus, J.L.: Anatomical atrial connections between sinus and A-V node. *Circulation* 37: 566, 1968

Miller, H.C., Strauss, H.C.: Measurement of sinoatrial conduction time by premature atrial stimulation in the rabbit. *Circulation Res* 35: 936, 1974

Mirowski, M., Lau, S.H., Wit, A.L., Steiner, C., Bobb, G.A., Tabatznik, B., Damato, A.N.: Ectopic right atrial rhythms: experimental and clinical data. *Amer Heart J* 81: 666, 1971

Narula, O.S., Samet, P., Javier, R.P.: Significance of the sinus-node recovery time. *Circulation* 45: 140, 1972

Narula, O.S.: Sinus node re-entry. A mechanism for supraventricular tachycardia. *Circulation* 50: 1114, 1974

Pahlajani, D.B., Miller, R.A., Serratto, M.: Sinus node re-entry and sinus node tachycardia. *Amer Heart J* 90: 305, 1975

Paritzky, Z., Obayashi, K., Mandel, W.J.: Atrial tachycardia secondary to sino-atrial node reentry. *Chest* 66: 526, 1974

Paulay, K.L., Varghese, P.J., Damato, A.N.: Sinus node reentry. An in vivo demonstration in the dog. *Circulation Res* 32: 455, 1973a

Paulay, K.L., Varghese, P.J., Damato, A.N.: Atrial rhythms in response to an early atrial premature depolarization in man. *Amer Heart J* 85: 323, 1973b

Paulay, K.L., Weisfogel, B.M., Damato, A.N.: Sinus nodal reentry: the effect of quinidine. *Amer J Cardiol* 33: 617, 1974

Paulay, K.L., Ruskin, J.N., Damato, A.N.: Sinus and atrioventricular nodal reentrant tachycardia in the same patient. *Amer J Cardiol* 36: 810, 1975

Puech, P., Esclavissat, M., Sodi-Pallares, D., Cisneros, F.: Normal auricular activation in the dog's heart. *Amer Heart J* 47: 174, 1954

Rothberger, C., Scherf, D.: Zur Kenntnis der Erregungsausbreitung vom Sinusknoten auf den Vorhof. *Zschr ges exp Med* 53: 792, 1927

Sano, T., Yamagishi, S.: Spread of excitation from the sinus node. *Circulation Res* 16: 423, 1965

Seipel, L., Breithardt, G., Both, A., Loogen, F.: Messung der "sinu-atrialen Leitungszeit" mittels vorzeitiger Vorhofstimulation beim Menschen. *Dtsch med Wschr* 99: 1895, 1974

Seipel, L., Breithardt, G.: Sinusknotenautomatie und sinu-atriale Leitung. *Z Kardiol* 64: 1014, 1975

Spach, M.S., Barr, R.C., Jewett, P.H.: Excitation sequence of the atrium and AV node in isolated hearts of dog and rabbit. *Circulation Res* 29: 156, 1971

Steinbeck, G., Lüderitz, B.: Sinus node recovery time and sinoatrial conduction time. In: Cardiac Pacing. Diagnostic and therapeutic tools. Lüderitz, B. (ed.), Springer, Berlin–New York, 1976, p. 45

Strauss, H.C., Bigger, J.T. Jr.: Slowed conduction, block and reentry in perinodal fibers. *Circulation* 43: suppl. II–74, 1971

Strauss, H.C., Saroff, A.L., Bigger, J.T. Jr., Giardina, E.G.V.: Premature atrial stimulation as a key to the understanding of sinoatrial conduction in man. Presentation of data and critical review of the literature. *Circulation* 47: 86, 1973

Strauss, H.C., Wallace, A.G.: Direct and indirect techniques in the evaluation of sinus node function, in: The conduction system of the heart, Wellens, H.J.J., Lie, K.I., Janse, M.J. (eds.), H.E. Stenfor, Kroese B.V. Leiden, 1976, p. 227

Strauss, H.C., Geer, M.R.: Sinoatrial node re-entry. In: Re-entrant arrhythmias. Mechanisms and treatment. Kulbertus, H.E. (ed.), MTP, Lancaster, 1977, p. 27

Svenson, R.H., Gallagher, J.J., Sealy, W.C., Wallace, A.G.: An electrophysiologic approach to the surgical treatment of the Wolff-Parkinson-White syndrome. Report of two cases utilizing catheter recording and epicardial mapping techniques. *Circulation* 49: 799, 1974

Ticzon, A.R., Strauss, H.C., Gallagher, J.J., Wallace, A.G.: Sinus nodal function in the intact dog heart evaluated by premature atrial stimulation and atrial pacing. *Am J Cardiol* 35: 492, 1975

Tonkin, A.M., Gallagher, J.J., Svenson, R.H., Wallace, A.G., Sealy, W.C.: Antegrade block in accessory pathways with retrograde conduction in reciprocating tachycardia. *Europ J Cardiol* 3: 143, 1975

Waldo, A.L., Cooper, T.B., Mac Lean, W.A.H.: Need for additional criteria for the diagnosis of sinus node reentrant tachycardias. (Editorial) *J Electrocardiol* 10: 103, 1977

Waldo, A.L., MacLean, W.A.H., Karp, R.B., Kouchoukos, T., James, T.N.: Sequence of retrograde atrial activation of the human heart. Correlation with P wave polarity. *Brit Heart J* 39: 634, 1977

Wallace, A.G., Daggett, W.M.: Re-excitation of the atrium. The echo phenomenon. *Amer Heart J* 68, 661
    1964
Weisfogel, G.M., Batsford, W.P., Josephson, M.E., Paulay, K.L., Damato, A.N.: Sinus node re-entrant tachy-
    cardia in man. *Circulation* 48: suppl. IV–122, 1973
Wu, D., Amat-y-Leon, F., Denes, P., Dhingra, R.C., Pietras, R., Rosen, K.M.: Demonstration of sustained
    sinus and atrial re-entry as a mechanism of paroxysmal supraventricular tachycardia. *Circulation* 51: 234,
    1975

P.S.   Shortly after completion of this manuscript a paper on atrial endocardial activation in man appeared
which could not be considered in our paper (Josephson, M.E., Scharf, D.L., Kastor, J.A., Kitchen, J.G.: Atrial
endocardial activation in man. Electrode catheter technique for endocardial mapping. Amer J Cardiol 39:
972, 1977).

35

RE-ENTRY WITHIN THE SINOATRIAL NODE AS DEMONSTRATED BY MULTIPLE MICRO-ELECTRODE RECORDINGS IN THE ISOLATED RABBIT HEART

MAURITS A. ALLESSIE AND FELIX I.M. BONKE

After the possibility of reentry in the sinus node was first suggested by Barker et al. in 1943, in 1960 Hoffman and Cranefield gave a more elaborated concept of sinus node reentry: "If the normally low conduction velocity is further reduced and local blocks are present, the following sequence of events may ensue: Excitation initiated in one part of the node may cause normally propagated activity in the atrium. This atrial activity will rapidly reach and excite some other area of the sinoatrial node. Activity will then spread slowly over some pathways in the node and reexcite the atrial muscle shortly after the end of its effective refractory period. A mechanism of this sort may cause either coupled beats, a doubling of the normal rate, or complete irregularity." In the last years a large number of clinical reports appeared in which a sinus node reentrant mechanism was suggested to underlay atrial echo beats and supraventricular tachycardia in man (Childers et al., 1973; Paulay et al., 1973a; Paritzky et al., 1974; Narula, 1974; Wu et al., 1975; Weisfogel et al., 1975; Pahlajani et al., 1975; Paulay et al., 1975; Dhingra et al., 1975; Curry et al., 1976; Gillette, 1976; Härtel and Hartikainen, 1976; Curry and Krikler, 1977; Strauss and Geer, 1977). However, because of the unavoidable limitations of the methods of investigation which can be used in patients, this hypothesis must be completely based on indirect evidence. Studies on animals in which essentially the same methods are used as in patients, suffer from the same limitations (Wallace and Daggett, 1964; Paulay et al., 1973b, 1974, 1975; Ticzon et al., 1975).

There are only a few studies in which one has tried to demonstrate reentry in the sinus node directly (Han et al., 1968; Bonke et al., 1971; Strauss and Geer, 1977). A conclusive demonstration of sinus node reentry would require many simultaneous recordings of transmembrane potentials at different locations in the sinus node and the adjacent atrial myocardium. Such a high level of resolution has as yet not been achieved. The study that comes closest to the proof that sinus node reentry is possible, unquestionably is that of Han, Malozzi and Moe (1968). With a single microelectrode at hand these investigators have attempted to follow the pathway of the activation wave within and around the sinus node after the induction of an atrial premature beat. In Figure 1 their results are reproduced. The isolated right atrium of the rabbit, drawn schematically in the upper left corner of the figure, was driven at a slightly higher rate than the spontaneous rhythm by basic stimuli (S_1), applied at the atrial roof. After each tenth basic stimulus an early premature stimulus (S_2) was administered at the same site. In their experiment an atrial echo could be produced repeatedly when S_2 was applied about 110 msec after S_1. During the period that reciprocal responses were stable, 18 different fibers, both in the sinus node and in the neighbouring atrial tissue were impaled. This offered the opportunity to compare the time relations between these 18 fibers as well during basic rhythm, the premature beat and the reciprocal response. In the figure, only 5 areas are indicated (Aa, Ab, SNa, SNb, and SNc). Each of these areas include 2 to 4 punctures sites which provided almost

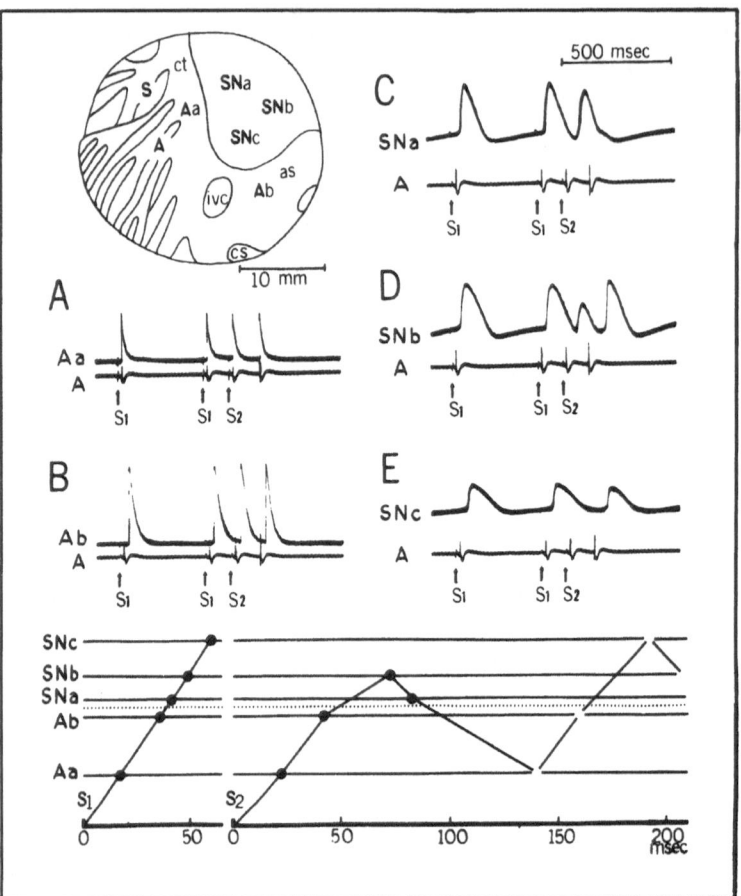

Figure 1. "Mapping" of sinoatrial echoes. Locations of stimulating and recording electrodes are shown in the diagram on the upper left. Anatomical landmarks: ct, crista terminalis; as, atrial septum; ivc, inferior vena cava; cs, coronary sinus. In each record, the upper trace shows transmembrane action potentials recorded at one of areas indicated by Aa, Ab, SNa, SNb, and SNc in the diagram, and the lower trace is a local atrial electrogram recorded at site A. Temporal sequences of these responses are plotted on the bottom graph. Activation time at each of the recording sites was selected at the point of the sharp inflection (from: Han, Malozzi and Moe, Circ. Res. 22: 355–362, 1968, by permission of the American Heart Association, Inc.)

identical temporal patterns. In the ladder diagram at the bottom, the sequence of activation of the different fibers is depicted. During the paced basic rhythm the impulse propagates from the point of stimulation to fibers Aa, Ab, SNa, SNb, and SNc in that order; the retrograde sinoatrial conduction time (measured between the moment of stimulation and the response of fiber SNc) was 60 msec. During the conduction of the premature beat the order of activation of the sinus node fibers had completely changed. Now fiber Snb is activated first (about 75 msec after S$_2$), followed by SNa (85 msec after S$_2$); the area of fiber SNc is not activated at all by the premature impulse (partial sinoatrial entrance block). The impulse leaves the sinus node again somewhere in the area of fiber SNa, and the atrium is reexcited. This echo beat is indicated by open circles in the ladder diagram. Then the impulse invades the sinus node again, namely at the region that not responded primarily to the premature impulse (area SNc). After having induced yet a second response in fiber SNb, the impulse then is extinguished somewhere in the node.

These data of Han, Malozzi and Moe (1968) not only demonstrate functional dissociation in the sinus node, they also strongly suggest the occurrence of a reentrant mechanism within the node. However, because of the limited number of intranodal impalements, the alternative explanation of an extra impulse arising somewhere in the *atrial myocardium* could not be completely excluded.

Later studies of Allessie et al. (1973, 1976, 1977) have shown that circus movement in a small part of the atrial myocardium, without the involvement of the sinus node, indeed can occur. In fact, the responses recorded from the sinus node fibers as given in Figure 1, would be expected if, instead of one premature stimulus (S_2), two closely successive premature stimuli were applied to the atrium. Because the effective refractory period of the sinus node is considerably longer than that of the atrial myocardium, the induction of two or more rapidly succeeding atrial beats will result in different degrees of sinoatrial entrance block.

Figure 2 illustrates that it is not easy to distinguish between these two alternative mechanisms. The figure shows an electrogram recorded from the right atrium and the transmembrane potential of a single sinus node fiber. During spontaneous beating a single premature stimulus was introduced in the atrium (arrow). The three panels (A–C), recorded shortly after each other, show three different responses to this single premature stimulus. In panel A the evoked premature beat was followed by one other, non-stimulated, atrial response. This registration highly resembles the results of Han, Malozzi and Moe (1968). In fact, it is similar to their panel D (compare figure 1). Accordingly, as an isolated observation this response could equally be explained on the basis of sinoatrial reciprocation. However, a short time later panels B and C were recorded. Now the single premature stimulus, applied a little earlier in the cycle, is followed by three, respectively seven atrial discharges. The sinus node fiber responded with only one, respectively three action potentials. This apparent conduction block between the atrium and the sinus node proves that at least the recorded fiber in the sinus node could *not* participate in a reentrant mechanism. For, a continuous propagation of the impulse in a circuitous pathway, requires that each part of the circuit is excited every time the impulse turns around. The beat-to-beat interval of the atrium during the short runs of tachycardia as shown in panels B and C was about 70 msec. This is much too short for the sinus node fibers to recover their excitability and therefore they cannot form part of a circular pathway. Instead, these runs of tachycardia can better be explained by circulating excitation in a small part of the atrial myocardium close to the sinus node. The sinus node then just plays a passive role and behaves as during rapid pacing of the atria; depending on the rate of the tachycardia it shows different degrees of sinoatrial entrance block. In this light it remains uncertain whether the extra response shown in panel A is caused by sinoatrial reciprocation or is based on reentry in the atrial myocardium. With other words, on the basis of the available data, it cannot be decided whether the type of response of the sinus node fiber as shown in panel A is the *cause* of the extra atrial discharge, or just the *result* of it.

To try to solve this problem of "the chicken and the egg", we decided to do an effort to fulfill the criteria for direct demonstration of reentry as expressed by Han, Malozzi and Moe (1968): "Definitive proof of a circuit within the sinus node would require a number of simultaneous impalements of intranodal cells, and a point-to-point demonstration of the course of the activation front during the whole interval between primary and reentrant atrial response."

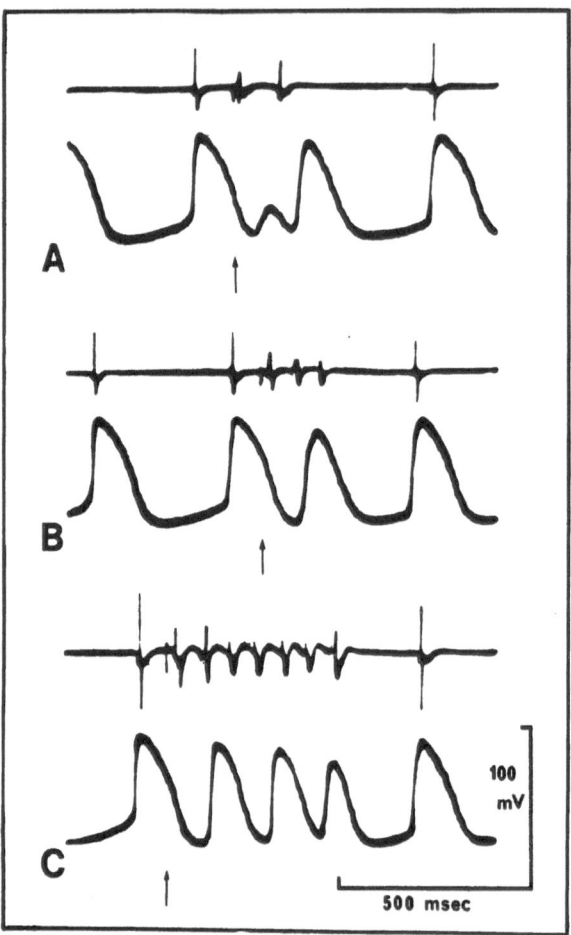

Figure 2. Recordings from a spontaneously beating isolated right atrium of the rabbit. Upper traces: atrium electrogram. Lower traces: transmembrane potential of one fiber in the sinus node. The arrow indicates the moment of premature stimulation. In panel A the premature beat is followed by a single non-stimulated beat, in panel B by two extra beats and in panel C by a series of rapid atrial discharges. The response of the sinus node fiber in panel A is comparable with fiber SNb recorded by Han, Malozzi and Moe (compare with panel D, Figure 1). Note that in panel C the stimulus evokes seven atrial discharges whereas the fiber in the sinus node responds with only three action potentials (from: Bonke, The atrial extrasystole. Thesis, University of Amsterdam, 1968).

In many experiments, we were unable to get stable sinus echoes which would allow this mapping procedure in the sinus node area. In some experiments we were only partly succesful, whereas until now we have done one experiment in which we think we fulfilled the above mentioned criteria for direct demonstration of sinus node reentry. In this communication we will describe only this single, most complete experiment. The study was done on an isolated right atrial preparation of the rabbit. Perfusion system, stimulation and recording techniques, and procedures of data processing were the same as described previously (Bonke et al., 1969, 1971; Allessie et al., 1973, 1976, 1977). The preparation was allowed to beat spontaneously except for the induction of a premature atrial ectopic beat after every 15th spontaneous beat. To study the response of the sinus node to premature

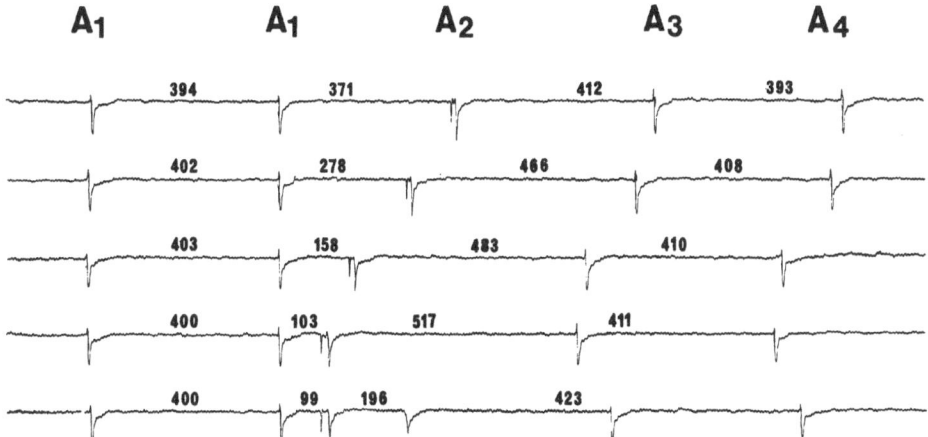

Figure 3. The effect of premature beats of different prematurity on the atrial rhythm. An isolated right atrium of the rabbit was beating spontaneously with an A_1-A_1 interval of about 400 msec. After every 15th spontaneous beat a premature beat was induced by the application of a stimulus on the atrium. The upper trace shows that a late premature beat (A_1-A_2 = 371 msec) is followed by a compensatory pause (A_2-A_3 = 412 msec). When the premature beat is induced earlier in the cycle the A_2-A_3 interval gets longer, but is not compensatory anymore: the sinus rhythm is reset (middle three traces). At a very short A_1-A_2 interval of 99 msec (lower trace) the premature beat is rapidly followed by a second response (A_2-A_3 = 196 msec). It is this second response which forms the subject of the present communication.

stimuli, the moment of the stimulus was varied throughout the spontaneous cycle in steps of 1–5 msec. Figure 3 shows the effect of single stimuli at different degrees of prematurity on the rhythm of the atrium. Premature beats elicited late in the cardiac cycle were followed by a compensatory pause (upper trace). At shorter coupling intervals, the sinus node was captured by the ectopic impulse resulting in an A_2-A_3 interval which was still longer than the normal A_1-A_1 interval, but which was too short to be compensatory (the middle three traces). At so far this response of the sinus node preparation was completely normal. However, when the stimulus was applied very early in the cycle, the ectopic premature beat was followed by yet a second response (see lower trace of Figure 3). This second excitation of the atrium came so early that the sum of the A_1-A_2 (99 msec) and the A_2-A_3 interval (196 msec) was clearly less than the normal A_1-A_1 interval (400 msec). This excludes that this type of response is an interpolated beat. Instead, it was suspected to be based on a reentrant mechanism, either in the atrial myocardium or in the sinus node. In the present experiment, the response shown in the lower trace of Figure 3, was stable during a period of one and a half hour. With the heart beating at a rate of 150/min and the premature stimulus given after every 15th beat we were able to reproduce this response almost a thousand times. This gave us the opportunity not only to map the spread of activation in the right atrium, but also to follow accurately the formation and conduction of the impulse within the sinus node, both during spontaneous beating, the premature ectopic beat, and the extra response.

First, in Figures 4 and 5, the activation of the right atrial myocardium is given. The lower part of Figure 4 shows a sketch of the right atrial preparation in which all the sites of recording are indicated. In total, 32 unipolar electrograms were recorded simultaneously, using a multielectrode template in which the electrodes are positioned in a regular array. In the upper part of Figure 4 the responses of some sites of the atrium to the evoked early

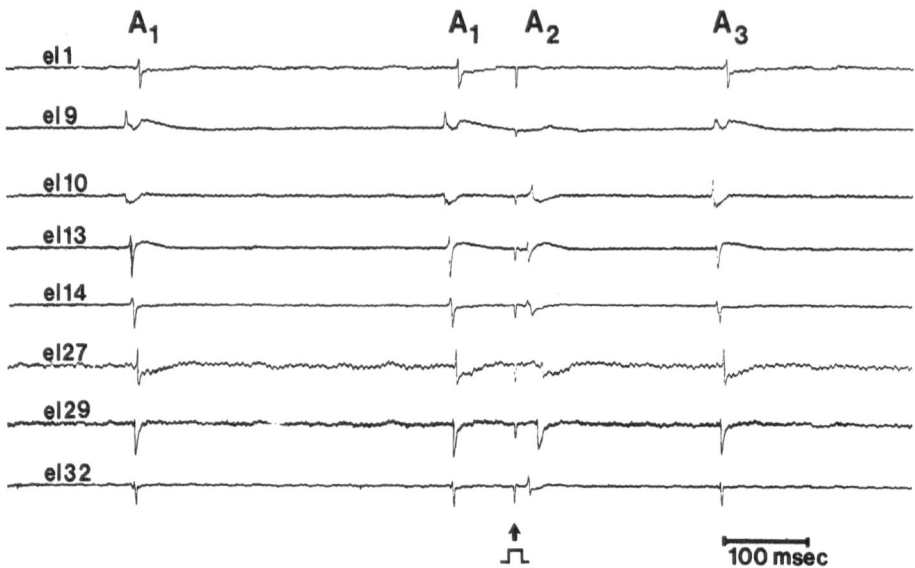

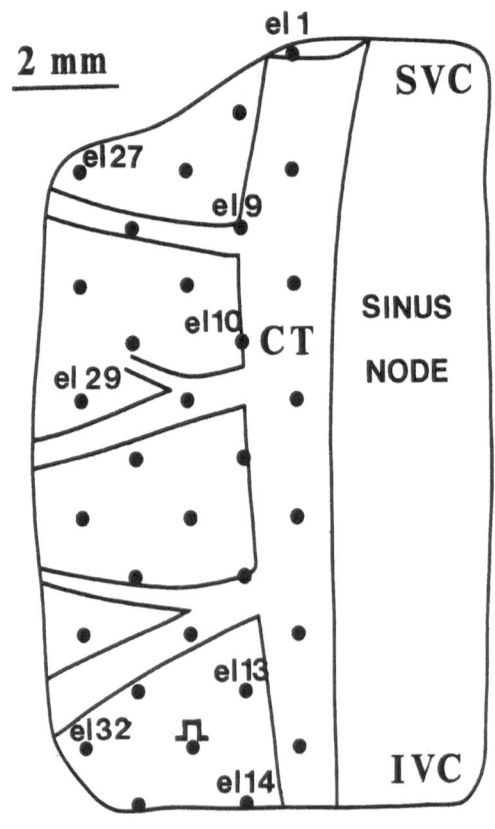

premature beat are shown. From the timing of these selected endocardial electrograms it can already be seen that the excitation during the A_3 response does not differ very much from the spread of activation during normal sinus rhythm (A_1 response). Also the configuration of these complexes recorded during the A_3 response do not differ considerably from those recorded during sinus rhythm. Only at sites close to the sinoatrial border (electrodes, 9, 10, and 13) the configuration of the A_3 complex is slightly different from the A_1 complex. However, at a distance of about 2–3 mm from the sinus node, the shape of the A_3 response was completely identical to that during spontaneous sinus rhythm. Furthermore, it can be seen from these electrograms that a part of the atrium did not respond to the early premature stimulus. So, electrodes 1 and 9 do not show an A_2 response, but only an A_3 response, indicating the occurrence of local intra-atrial conduction block.

In Figure 5, the excitation maps of the right atrial myocardium during sinus rhythm, the ectopic beat and the extra response are given, as they could be reconstructed from the 32 simultaneous surface recordings. During sinus rhythm the activation of the atrium was as could be expected (Sano and Yamagishi, 1965). During the ectopic beat, elicited shortly after the spontaneous beat, the impulse was blocked in the cephalic part of the crista terminalis. This local intra-atrial conduction block can easily be explained, because during our attempts to induce sinus node re-entry, we found that in this particular preparation the refractory period of the upper part of the crista terminalis was relatively long, being in the order of 110 msec. Apparently, the coupling interval of the ectopic beat has been too short for this area to restore its excitability in time. As a consequence, the ectopic premature impulse was blocked in the upper half of the crista terminalis, and the sinus node was invaded exclusively from the lower part. However, as can be seen from the third map of this figure, representing the A_3 response, this occurrence of local intra-atrial conduction block did *not* result in intra-atrial re-entry. By this mapping procedure it could be excluded that a re-entrant mechanism in the atrial myocardium was responsible for the extra response recorded in this preparation. The map of the A_3 response clearly shows that this beat is also emerging from the sinus node. The only difference is that compared with the normal sinus rhythm, the A_3 impulse excited the crista terminalis at a slightly lower level. This might quite well explain the minor differences in configuration between the A_1 and A_3 responses as observed in the electrograms recorded from the crista terminalis (see Figure 4). In general, however, the excitation of the atrium by the A_3 impulse is very similar to the activation pattern during sinus rhythm.

Now, of course, the crucial question that arises is: "What is happening in the sinus node between the invasion of the sino-atrial border by the atrial ectopic beat and the emergence of the A_3 impulse from the sinus node". Is the early A_3 response caused by acceleration or a shift of the sinus node pacemaker? Is this another example of so-called "triggered activity", a phenomenon discussed by Cranefield (this book), or is the A_3 response not the result of disturbed impulse formation, but instead the result of a circulating conduction of the impulse within the sinus node area?

During the one and a half hour that we got stable early A_3 responses in this present

Figure 4. Below: Sketch of the isolated right atrium of the rabbit. SVC = superior vena cava. IVC = inferior vena cava. CT = crista terminalis. The sites of the 32 electrograms recorded simultaneously from the atrium are indicated by black dots. The responses of 8 different locations of the preparation to the same premature stimulus are given in the upper part of the figure. The area of electrodes 1 and 9 do not respond to the premature stimulus. The configuration of the early A_3 responses at electrode 1, 14, 27, 29 and 32 are identical to the complexes recorded during sinus rhythm. At electrodes 9, 10 and 13, located within 2 mm from the sino-atrial border, the configuration of the A_3 response was slightly different from the A_1 responses.

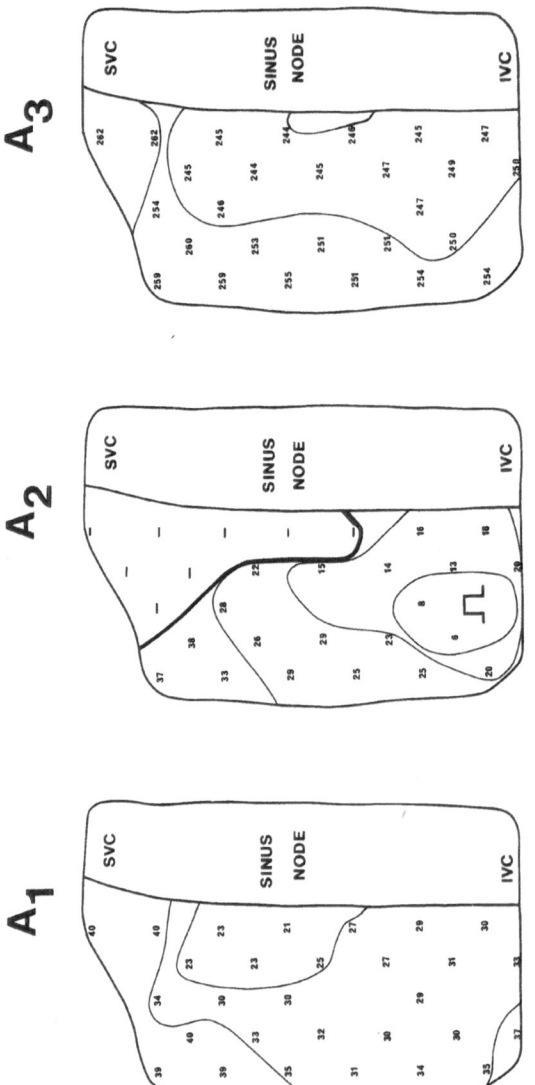

Figure 5. Maps of the spread of activation in the right atrial myocardium during sinus rhythm (A₁), the induction of a premature atrial ectopic beat (A₂) and the early A₃ response which resulted from this ectopic beat. The numbers on the maps indicate the local activation times in msec. During sinus rhythm the moment of earliest discharge in the sinus node is taken as zero reference; the timing during the ectopic beat and the resulting early A₃ response is related to the moment the test stimulus was given. During sinus rhythm there was a normal activation of the preparation. During the ectopic beat the upper part of the crista terminalis showed local intra-atrial conduction-block. The early A₃ response clearly originated from the sinus node region.

experiment, we succeeded to impale with a single microelectrode, 130 fibers in the sinus node region. The site and moment of stimulation and the qualities of the single test stimulus were kept constant during this mapping period. In this way the individual responses of 130 sinus node fibers distributed over the total sinus node area were recorded during normal sinus rhythm, the induction of an early atrial ectopic beat, and the resulting early A_3 response. A reference atrial electrogram was used to relate all measuring points in the sinus node representing successive registrations of the same repetitive event. Figure 6a gives the transmembrane potentials of a selection of 16 sinus node fibers together with the reference atrial electrogram. In Figure 6b, the sites of recording in the sino-atrial region of the 16 fibers are indicated on a sketch of the preparation. During sinus rhythm fibers 5, 6 and 8 were found to be the first from the total population of the 130 impaled fibers to generate an action potential. The moment of activation of these dominant pacemaker fibers has been taken as time zero. For measuring the activation time during the ectopic beat and the A_3 response the moment of the stimulus is taken as zero reference.

During sinus rhythm the impulse, originating in the area of fibers 5, 6 and 8 activates the atrium at the reference electrode after 30 msec. The area of the stimulating electrode, which was positioned at a distance of 2–3 mm from the reference electrode, was excited only a few msec later.

The test stimulus was given with a delay of 83 msec after the local activation of the area of the stimulating electrode by the spontaneous sinus beat.

In the lower part of the node, fibers lying at the sino-atrial border (fibers 16 and 15) were excited by the ectopic impulse, respectively 20 and 30 msec after the stimulus. However, the fibers lying somewhat deeper in the sinus node (fibers 11 to 14) were not able to respond to the premature impulse. In these fibers only electrotonic "humps" of higher or lower amplitude were recorded. Thus from these registrations it follows that the premature ectopic impulse penetrating retrogradely into the sinus node is blocked in the lower part of the node. However, in the upper part of the sinus node such sino-atrial entrance block did *not* occur. There the retrograde activation wave is able to penetrate into the sinus node and although it is conducted slowly it continues to travel from fiber 1 to 2, to 3, to 4 ... etc. After invasion of the sinus node at the upper part, the impulse then travels downwards within the node. In this way also the fibers lying deep in the lower part of the node (fibers 8, 9 and 10) are activated by the retrograde wave front respectively 135, 160 and 168 msec. after the stimulus. The fibers 11 to 14, which earlier exhibited only an electrotonic response, now are truly activated by the impulse coming from the area of fibers 9 and 10. As a result, finally all fibers in the sinus node were activated by the premature impulse, some of them directly, others after a longer or shorter delay because the impulse was travelling slowly and in a roundabout way. This single retrograde activation of the sinus node area lasted more than 200 msec. Fibers 13 and 14 which belonged to the area which was activated the last, were excited 203 and 210 msec after the stimulus. As a result of this slow and circuitous conduction within the sinus node fibers 15 and 16 which already were activated by the premature beat, had restored their excitability at the moment that the adjacent fibers 13 and 14 were excited. As a consequence these fibers were activated for a second time at 225 and 240 msec respectively. This circus movement within the sinus node led to a second activation of the atrium. The reference electrode low on the crista terminalis recorded a second activation at 247 msec after the stimulus. In the meanwhile the impulse also continued to propagate in the sinus node region. Simultaneous with fiber 15, fiber 1 was re-entered (t = 225 msec). From hereon the impulse started a second roundtrip, travelling again from fiber 1 to 2, to 3, to 4 etc. However, now on his

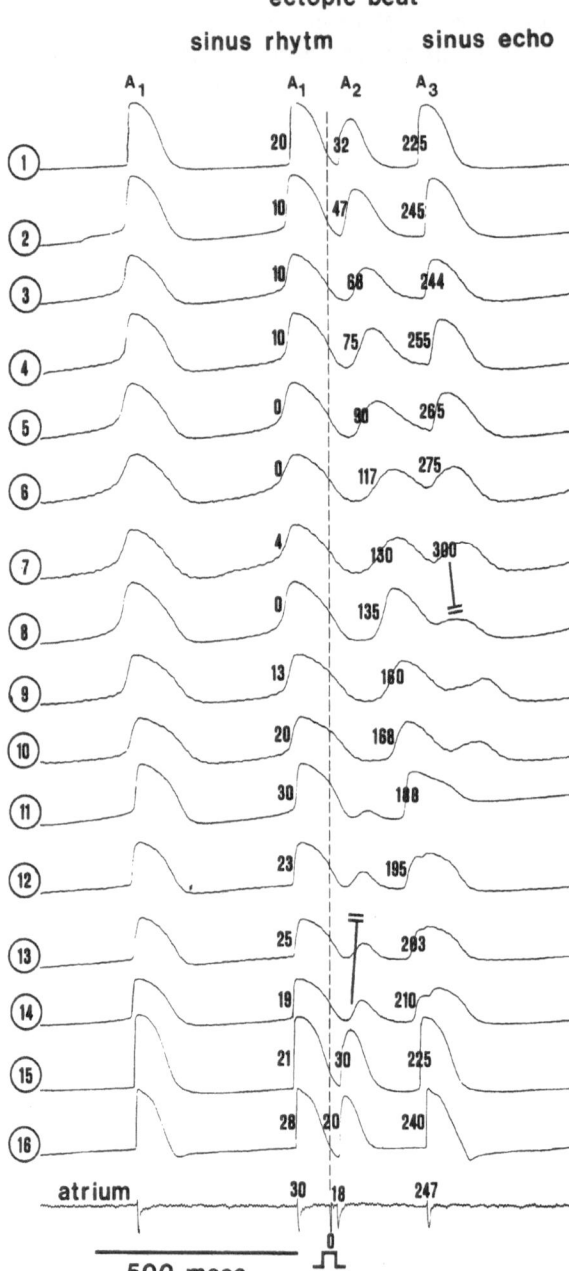

Figure 6a. Transmembrane potentials of 16 different fibers in the sinus node together with a reference atrial electrogram. The different intracellular recordings were not recorded simultaneously but were time aligned using the reference electrogram which showed a constant response. The first two action potentials represent the last two discharges of a series of 15 sinus beats. After the 15th sinus beat an early premature stimulus was applied to the atrium (dotted line). Retrograde invasion of the ectopic beat in the sinus node was blocked in the area of fibers 11–14. However, in the upper part of the node (fibers 1–7) the early premature impulse

second roundtrip the impulse died out somewhere in the area beyond fiber 7 at t = 300 msec. Fibers 8, 9 and 10 only showed electrotonic potentials associated with this blocking impulse. Because of the occurrence of this conduction block no sustained sinus node re-entry took place and only a single sinus echo occurred. In Figure 7 the excitation pattern of the complete right atrial preparation during sinus rhythm, the ectopic beat and the sinus echo is given.

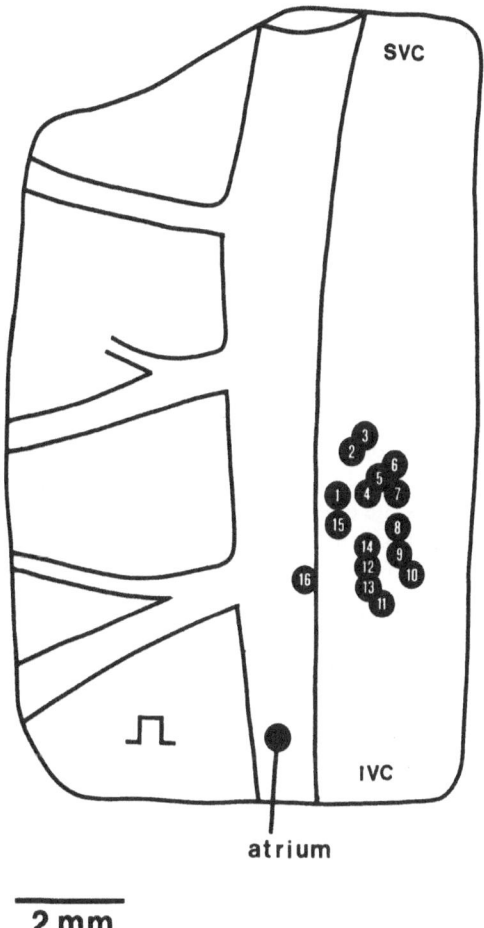

2 mm   Figure 6b

succeeded to penetrate the node. The impulse was conducted along a pathway from fiber 1 to 2 to 3 to 4 to 5 etc. The fibers which initially were not activated directly by the retrograde wavefront (fibers 8–14), now yet were excited in a roundabout way. So, 225 msec after the stimulus, the impulse returned at the site where it entered the node (fibers 1 and 15). Because by this time these fibers had recovered their excitability they were re-excited. Shortly thereafter the impulse left the sinus node again at about the same point where it had entered and the atrium was reexcited also. The reference electrogram shows an activation by this sinus echo at t = 247 msec. Halfway its second roundtrip the impulse died out somewhere in the area of fibers 8–10. This prevented a sustained circus movement within the sinus node and only a single sinus echo resulted.

Figure 6b. Sketch of the isolated atrium of the rabbit on which the sites of the 16 sinus node fibers and the atrial reference electrogram shown in Figure 6a, are indicated.

SINUS RHYTHM ECTOPIC BEAT SINUS ECHO

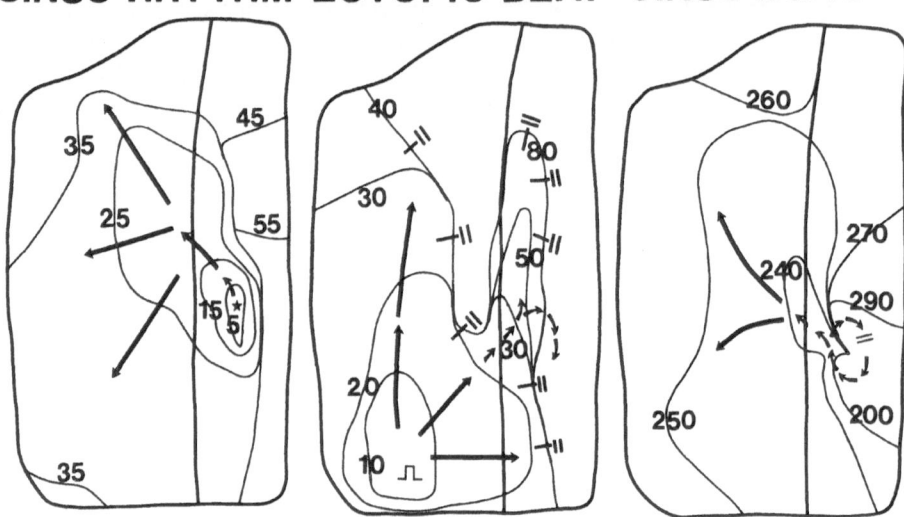

Figure 7. Analysis of the excitation of the sino-atrial preparation during sinus rhythm, the ectopic beat and the resulting sinus echo. See text for discussion.

In summary, during sinus rhythm, there was a completely normal spread of activation from the center of the sinus node to the atrium. (compare Bouman et al. this book). During the ectopic beat intra-atrial conduction block occurred at the higher part of the crista terminalis, resulting in an exclusive invasion of the sinus node at the lower part of the sino-atrial border. From this site of entrance the impulse first moved upward, then turned around in a clockwise direction within the node to reexcite the atrium 240 msec after the stimulus (sinus echo). About halfway its second roundtrip the impulse died out in the node preventing a sustained sinus node re-entrant tachycardia. The diameter of the intranodal circuit in which the impulse circulated for one and a half revolution can be estimated between 1 and 2 mm. The revolution time of the impulse in this circuit was about 200 msec. Thus the average conduction velocity with which the impulse propagated along the circuit must have been in the order of 2–3 cm/sec. It is because of the exceptional situation that a stable sinus echo could be obtained during more than one and a half hour, that this circuit within the sinus node could be directly demonstrated. Although of course it is hazardous to generalize the observations of a single case, at least it proves the *possibility* of sinus node reentry. Whether this mechanism is operational in some types of sustained supra-ventricular tachycardia still remains to be answered.

REFERENCES

Allessie, M.A., Bonke, F.I.M., Schopman, F.J.G.: Circus movement in rabbit atrial muscle as a mechanism of tachycardia. *Circ Res* 33: 54, 1973

Allessie, M.A., Bonke, F.I.M., Schopman, F.J.G.: Circus movement in rabbit atrial muscle as a mechanism of tachycardia. II. The role of nonuniform recovery of excitability in the occurrence of unidirectional block, as studied with multiple microelectrodes. *Circ Res* 39: 168, 1976

Allessie, M.A., Bonke, F.I.M., Schopman, F.J.G.: Circus movement in rabbit atrial muscle as a mechanism of tachycardia. III. The "leading circle" concept: a new model of circus movement in cardiac tissue without the involvement of an anatomical obstacle. *Circ Res* 41: 9, 1977

Barker, P.S., Wilson, F.N., Johnston, F.D.: The mechanism of auricular paroxysmal tachycardia. *Am Heart J* 26: 435, 1943

Bonke, F.I.M., Bouman, L.N., Van Rijn, H.E.: Change of cardiac rhythm in the rabbit after an atrial premature beat. *Circ Res* 24: 533, 1969

Bonke, F.I.M., Bouman, L.H., Schopman, F.J.G.: Effect of an early atrial premature beat on activity of the sinoatrial node and atrial rhythm in the rabbit. *Circ Res* 29: 704, 1971

Bouman, L.H., Mackaay, A.J.C., Bleeker, W.K., Becker, A.E.: Pacemaker shifts in the sinus node. Effects of vagal stimulation, temperature and reduction of extracellular calcium. This book, 1978

Childers, R.W., Arnsdorf, M.F., de la Fuente, D.J., Gambetta, M., Svenson, R.: Sinus nodal echoes. Clinical case report and canine studies. In: *Am J Cardiol* 31: 220, 1973

Cranefield, P.F.: Does spontaneous activity arise from phase 4 depolarization or from triggering? This book, 1978

Curry, P.V.L., Callowhill, E., Krikler, D.M.: Paroxysmal re-entry sinus tachycardia. In: *Brit Heart J* 38: 311, 1976

Curry, P.V.L., Krikler, D.M.: Paroxysmal reciprocating sinus tachycardia. In: Re-entrant Arrhythmias. Mechanisms and Treatment, p. 39. Editor: Kulbertus, H.E. M.T.P. Lancaster, 1977

Dhingra, R.C. Wyndham, C., Amat-y-Leon, F., Denes, P., Wu, D., Rosen, K.M.: Sinus nodal responses to atrial extrastimuli in patients without apparent sinus node disease. *Am J Cardiol* 36: 445–452, 1975

Gillette, P.C.: The mechanisms of supraventricular tachycardia in children. *Circulation* 54: 133–139, 1976

Han, J., Malozzi, A.M., Moe, G.K.: Sino-atrial reciprocation in the isolated rabbit heart. *Circ Res* 22: 355–362, 1968

Härtel, G., Hartikainen, M.: Comparison of verapamil and practolol in paroxysmal supraventricular tachycardia. *Europ J Cardiol* 4/1: 87–90, 1976

Hoffman, B.F., Cranefield, P.F.: Electrophysiology of the heart. McGraw-Hill Book Company, Inc. New York, 1960, p. 124

Narula, O.S.: Sinus node re-entry. A mechanism for supraventricular tachycardia. *Circulation* 50: 1114–1128, 1974

Pahlajani, D.B., Miller, R.A., Serratto, M.: Sinus node re-entry and sinus node tachycardia. *Am Heart J* 90. 305–311, 1975

Paritzky, Z., Obayashi, K., Mandel, W.J.: Atrial tachycardia secondary to sino-atrial node re-entry. *Chest* 66: 526–529, 1974

Paulay, K.L., Varghese, P.J., Damato, A.N.: Atrial rhythms in response to an early atrial premature depolarization in man. *Am Heart J* 85: 323–331, 1973a

Paulay, K.P., Varghese, P.J., Damato, A.N.: Sinus node re-entry. An in vivo demonstration in the dog. *Circ Res* 32: 455–463, 1973b

Paulay, K.P., Weisvogel, G.M., Damato, A.N.: Sinus nodal re-entry. Effect of quinidine. *Am J Cardiol* 33: 617–622, 1974

Paulay, K.P., Damato, A.N.: Effect of digoxin on sinus nodal re-entry in the dog. *Am J Cardiol* 35: 370–375, 1975a

Paulay, K.L., Ruskin, R.N., Damato, A.M.: Sinus and atrioventricular nodal re-entrant tachycardia in the same patient. *Am J Cardiol* 36: 810–816, 1975b

Sano, T., Yamagishi, S.: Spread of excitation from the sinus node. *Circ Res* 16: 423–430, 1965

Strauss, H.C., Geer, M.R.: Sinoatrial node re-entry. p. 27–38. In: Re-entrant Arrhythmias. Mechanisms and Treatment. Editor: Kulbertus, H.E. MTP Lancaster 1977

Ticzon, A.R., Strauss, H.C., Gallagher, J.J., Wallace, A.G.: Sinus nodal function in the intact dog heart evaluated by premature atrial stimulation and atrial pacing. *Am J Cardiol* 35: 492–503, 1975

Weisvogel, G.M., Batsford, W.P., Paulay, K.L., Josephson, M.E., Ogunkelu, J.B., Akhtar, M., Seides, S.F., Damato, A.N.: Sinus node re-entrant tachycardia in man. *Am Heart J* 90: 295–304, 1975

Wu, D., Amat-y-Leon, F., Denes, P., Dhingra, R.C., Pietras, R.J., Rosen, K.M.: Demonstration of sustained sinus and atrial re-entry as a mechanism of paroxysmal supraventricular tachycardia. *Circulation* 51: 234–243, 1975

36

ROLE OF SINUS NODE RE-ENTRY IN THE GENESIS OF SUSTAINED CARDIAC ARRHYTHMIAS

HEIN J.J. WELLENS

In 1972 Narula reported that in the human heart electrically induced atrial premature beats might be followed by atrial complexes showing a configuration and an activation pattern that is the same as in case of spontaneous discharges of the sinus node. He postulated that these atrial complexes were the result of reentry in the region of the sinus node and formulated criteria to be fulfilled for the diagnosis of "sinus node reentry" in the human heart (Narula, 1974). Several authors have reported on this phenomenon subsequently. However till now the exact pathway of the reentry in the sinus node region is never demonstrated and the study of Allessie and Bonke (1978) is the first demonstration in an isolated preparation. The difficulties with intracardiac recordings in delineating the site of impulse formation in the atrium of the intact human heart, have been outlined by Breithardt and Seipel (1978).

SINGLE SINUS NODE RE-ENTRANT BEATS DURING PROGRAMMED ELECTRICAL STIMULATION OF THE HEART

While several authors reported on sinus node re-entry in the human heart little is known on the incidence of this phenomenon in a large series of patients studied by programmed electrical stimulation. The only data are from Dhingra et al. (1975). They reported on an 11% incidence following single atrial test stimuli during sinus rhythm rising to 26% following atrial test stimuli during basic atrial pacing. Sinus node re-entrant beats have been reported in patients with and without heart disease and their diagnostic value as to

Table 1. Classification of patients with tachycardia studied by programmed electrical stimulation of the heart.

		Pts.
Atrial Tachy*		29
Atrial Flutter		40
Paroxysmal AV-Junctional Tachy	AV nodal re-entry	59
	Conc. A.P.	21
	Undetermined	3
Digitalis induced AV-Junctional Tachy		3
Wolff-Parkinson-White Syndrome		144
Other Forms of Pre-excitation		10
Ventricular Tachy		70
	total	379

* Including so called sinus node re-entrant tachycardia.

Abbreviations: Tachy = Tachycardia; Pts = Patients; Conc. A.P. = Concealed Accessory Pathway.

sinus node and/or atrial disease is not clear at the present time. No data are available as to the incidence of sinus node re-entry during programmed electrical stimulation as compared to AV-nodal re-entry.

In our own series of 379 patients studied with programmed electrical stimulation because of symptomatic tachycardia (diagnosis listed in Table 1) one or more sinus node re-entrant beats fulfilling the accepted criteria (Narula, 1974) could be elicited in 37 patients (an incidence of 9.4%) as compared to 111 patients (incidence 28.3%) with one or more AV nodal re-entrant beats. This finding suggests that the phenomenon of sinus node re-entry is less common that AV nodal re-entry in patients suffering from tachycardia and also that sinus node re-entry plays a less important role in the genesis of re-entrant arrhythmias.

OBSERVATIONS ON A POSSIBLE ROLE OF RE-ENTRY IN THE SINUS NODE REGION IN THE GENESIS OF RE-ENTRANT TACHYCARDIA

As shown in Table 2 only three out of seven patients of our own series had tachycardias initiated in the catheterization laboratory that were identical in atrial shape and frequency to the tachycardias clinically registered in these patients (an incidence of less than 1%). In four more patients apart from other tachycardias (which were similar to the ones recorded outside the catheterization laboratory) tachycardias could be initiated during programmed electrical stimulation that seemed to have a part of the sinus node incorporated in their tachycardias circuit. Typical examples of these tachycardias, that can be considered as a fall out of the stimulation study rather than the clinical arrhythmia problem for which they were investigated, are given in Figures 1 and 2. Figure 3 shows a phenomenon which was present in three out of our seven patients with possible sinus node re-entrant tachycardia. As demonstrated in Figure 3 there is alternation in length of subsequent atrial cycles. This phenomenon is highly suggestive for the usage of more than two pathways, during tachycardia (Spurrell et al., 1975; Schlepper, 1977; Amat-y-Leon

Table 2. Data on patients with sinus node re-entrant tachycardia.

Patient	Sex	Age	Diagnosis	Type tachy during PES	Atrial rate during SNR tachy
1	F	48	Mitral stenosis Paroxysmal Tachy	AVN Tachy SNR Tachy*	130/min
2	F	22	WPW type A Paroxysmal Tachy	Reciprocal Tachy incorporating AP SNR Tachy*	170/min
3	M	32	WPW type A Paroxysmal Tachy	SNR Tachy	160/min
4	F	58	Ischaemic HD Paroxysmal Tachy	SNR Tachy	170/min
5	F	61	Ischaemic HD Paroxysmal Tachy	AVN Tachy SNR Tachy*	140/min
6	F	38	Paroxysmal Tachy	Ventricular Tachy AVN Tachy SNR Tachy*	160/min
7	M	42	Paroxysmal Tachy	SNR Tachy	110/min

*In these patients SNR Tachy was only seen during PES. The other type tachycardias in these patients were also recorded outside the catheterisation laboratory.

Abbreviations: PES = Programmed Electrical Stimulation; Tachy = Tachycardia; SNR = Sinusnode Re-entry; WPW = Wolff-Parkinson-White Syndrome; AVN = AV nodal; AP = Accessory Pathway; HD = Heart Disease.

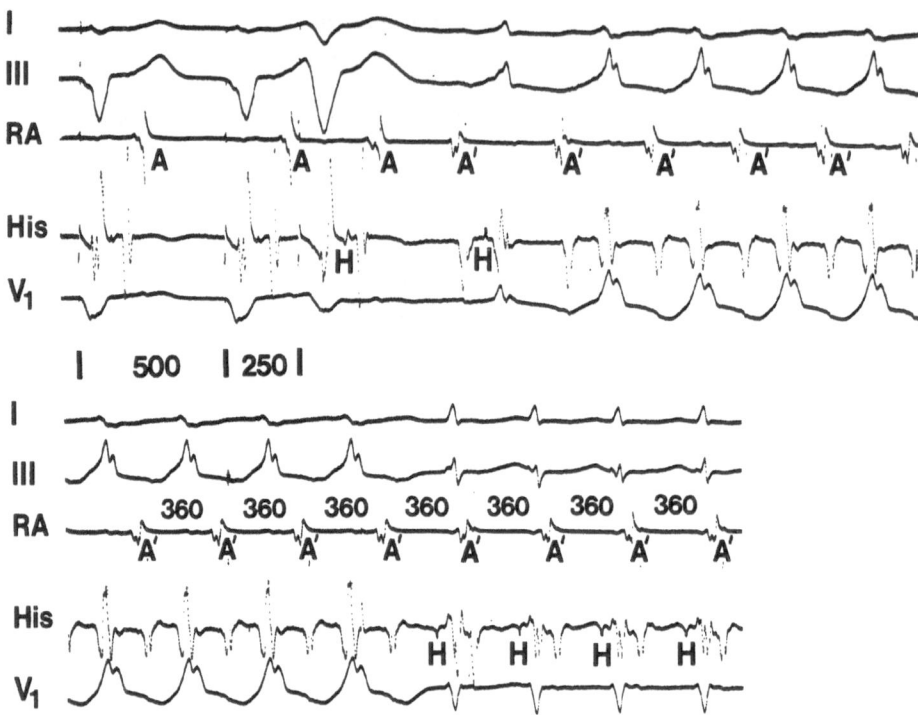

Figure 1. *Upper panel*: Initiation of tachycardia by a single ventricular premature beat during ventricular pacing in a patient with the Wolff-Parkinson-White syndrome type A. Note the high-low sequence of atrial activation during tachycardia with atrial activation preceding ventricular activation. During tachycardia the QRS-complex shows pre-excitation over a left sided accessory pathway (WPW type A).
Lower panel: In the middle of the registration type 2 block occurs in the accessory pathway followed by exclusive AV conduction over the AV node-His pathway.

et al., 1977). This seems to argue against a tachycardia circuit confined to the ordinary atrium but supports the utilization of pathways in a slowly conducting area like the sinus node.

Everybody reporting on sinus node re-entrant tachycardia noted their instable character. Very rarely they present a clinical problem. Frequently the tachycardia terminates spontaneously. If not, carotid sinus massage usually results in slowing in rate followed by termination of tachycardia. This reaction, like the alternation in atrial cycle length (Figure 3) is a strong argument against intra-atrial re-entry.

The effect of both quinidine and digitalis on sinus node re-entry has been studied in the dog heart (Paulay et al., 1974; Paulay and Damato, 1975). Curry and Krikler (1977) reported on the beneficial effect of verapamil in patients with sinus node re-entrant tachycardia. In our series ouabaine was administered to five patients in whom sinus node re-entrant tachycardia could reproducebly be initiated during programmed electrical stimulation. This resulted in all patients in inability to re-initiate tachycardia after ouabaine administration. These observations of the beneficial effect of drugs on this type tachycardia again underscore the labile character of the arrhythmia and the ease of disrupting the delicate electrophysiologic balance required for sustaining tachycardia.

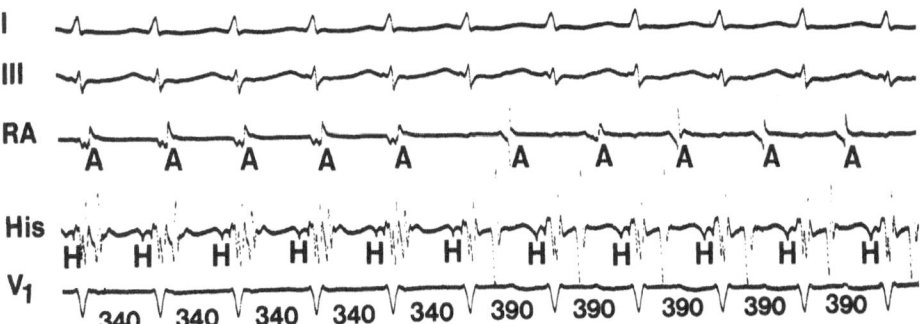

Figure 2. (Same patient as Figure 1). In the middle of the record there is a sudden change in rate during tachycardia with reversal of the sequence of atrial activation. This phenomenon suggests termination of a tachycardia originating high in the right atrium (close to the sinus node region) followed by a tachycardia with antegrade AV conduction over the AV node-His pathway and ventriculo-atrial conduction over an accessory pathway.

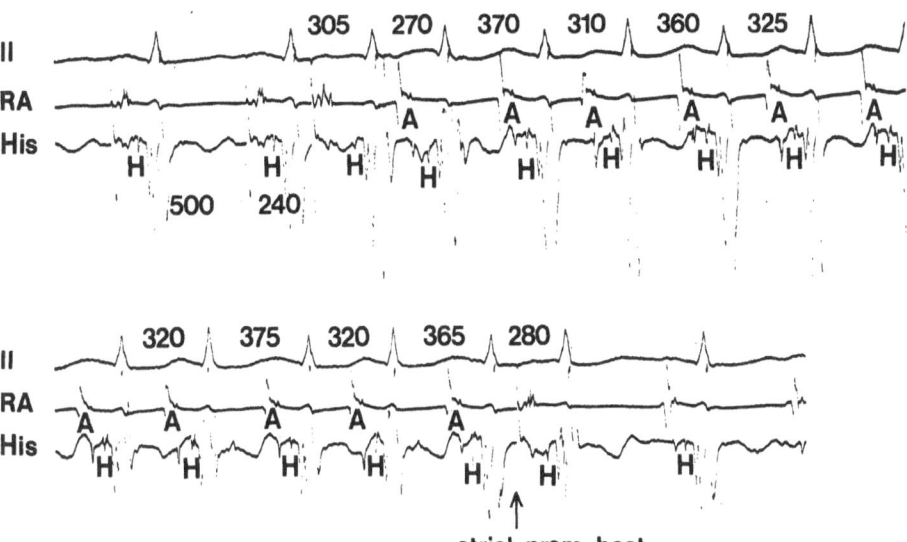

atrial prem. beat

Figure 3. Upper panel: Initiation of tachycardia by an atrial premature beat during atrial pacing. During tachycardia: 1) A high-low sequence of atrial activation is present; 2) There is alternation in length of successive inter-atrial intervals.

Lower panel: Termination of tachycardia by a critically timed atrial premature beat. Note that sequence and timing of atrial activation are similar during tachycardia and sinus rhythm suggesting a site of origin of tachycardia in or close to the sinus node region. Lead II, a high right atrial lead and a Hisbundle lead were recorded simultaneously.

Occasionally one can observe initiation of a re-entrant tachycardia not incorporating the sinus node by a sinus node re-entrant beat (Figure 4). There is the possibility that a single sinus node re-entrant beat acts as the initiating mechanism of more serious arrhythmias like atrial fibrillation. This problem requires further investigation.

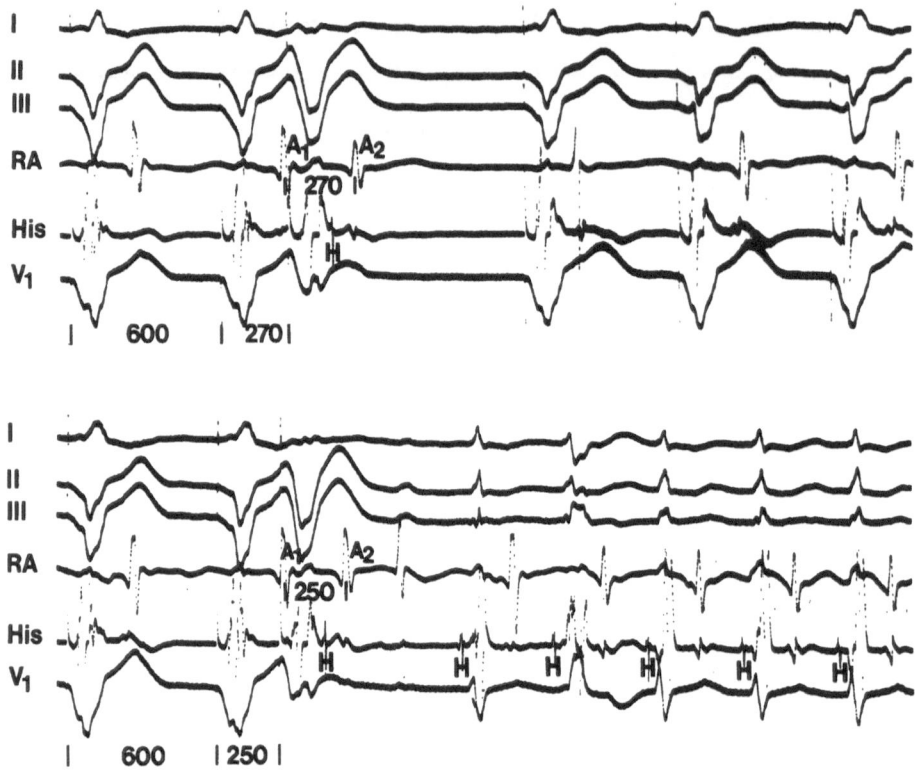

Figure 4. Upper panel: During ventricular pacing with a basic cycle length of 600 msec a ventricular premature beat given after 270 msec is conducted over the accessory pathway towards the atrium.

Lower panel: On shortening the premature beat interval to 250 msec, retrograde atrial activation is followed by an atrial complex showing a high-low atrial activation pattern. This atrial complex initiates a tachycardia with AV conduction over the AV node-His pathway and ventriculo-atrial conduction over the accessory pathway.

REFERENCES

1. Allessie, M.A., Bonke, F.I.M.: Reentry within the sinoatrial node as demonstrated by multiple microelectrode recordings in the isolated rabbit heart. This book, 1978
2. Amat-y-Leon, F., Wyndham, C., Wu, D., Denes, P., Dhingra, R.C., Rosen, K.M.: Participation of fast and slow A-V nodal pathways in tachycardias complicating the Wolff-Parkinson-White syndrome. *Circulation* 55: 663, 1977
3. Breithardt, A., Seipel, L.: Sequence of atrial activation in patients with atrial echo beats. This book, 1978
4. Curry, P.V.L., Krikler, D.M.: Paroxysmal reciprocating sinus tachycardia. In: Re-entrant arrhythmias. Mechanisms and Treatment, edited by H. Kulbertus. MTP Lancaster, 1977, p. 39
5. Dhingra, R.C., Wyndham, C., Amat-y-Leon, F., Denes, P., Wu, D., Rosen, K.M.: Sinus nodal response to atrial extrastimuli in patients without apparent sinus node disease. *Am J Cardiol* 36: 445, 1975
6. Narula, O.S.: Sinus node reentry: mechanism of supraventricular tachycardia (SVT) in man. *Circulation* 46: 11, 1972
7. Narula, O.S.: Sinus node reentry: a mechanism for supraventricular tachycardia. *Circulation* 50: 1114, 1974
8. Paulay, K.L., Weisfogel, G.M., Damato, A.N.: Sinus nodal re-entry. Effect of quinidine. *Am J Cardiol* 33: 617, 1974
9. Paulay, K.L., Damato, A.N.: Effect of digoxin on sinus node re-entry in the dog. *Am J Cardiol* 35: 370, 1975

10. Schlepper, M.: Mechanisms underlying sudden changes in heart rate during paroxysmal supraventricular tachycardia. In: Re-entrant Arrhythmias. Mechanisms and Treatment, edited by H. Kulbertus. MTP Lancaster, 1977, p. 184
11. Spurrell, R.A.J., Krikler, D., Sowton, E.: Two or more intra AV-nodal pathways in association with either a James or Kent extranodal bypass in three patients with paroxysmal supraventricular tachycardia. *Br Heart J* 35: 113, 1973

37

GENERAL CONCLUSIONS

HEIN J. J. WELLENS

1. It is very difficult to prove the occurrence of reentry in the sinus node. The only study in which the reentry path in the sinus node was mapped, was by Allessie and Bonke (1978, in this book) on the isolated right atrium of the rabbit. Intracardiac recordings in patients are prone to changes in configuration and amplitude due to respiration, rate, location of the electrodes, etc. and are certainly not full proof for identification of the sinus node as the area of reentry.

2. In cases of sustained atrial tachycardia the phenomenon of slowing of the rate during carotid sinus massage was accepted as suggestive for the incorporation of the sinus node or part of the sinus node in a reentry circuit. The finding of alternation in the A-A interval during atrial tachycardia requires further study as to its value in pointing to involvement of the sinus node in a reentry circuit.

3. Sustained reentry in the area of the sinus node is rare as demonstrated by the fact that the total number of cases diagnosed as such by the participants of the workshop, was less than fifty. During stimulation studies in the catheterisation laboratory a single re-entrant beat in the "high right atrial" area is common (figures were quoted by the participants in the workshop ranging from 5–30%) but not as common as reentry in the AV node.

4. Sustained reentry in the sinus node region is seldom a therapeutic problem. Drugs reported to be favorable for the termination or prevention of reentrant tachycardias are verapamil, quinidine and digitalis.

5. It is not believed that the phenomenon of sinus node reentry is diagnostic for disease in the region of the sinus node. The role of reentry in the sinus node region as mechanism for more serious atrial arrhythmias, like atrial fibrillation, needs further study.

LITERATURE REFERENCE LIST

Abbott, J.P., Kunkel, F., Hirschfeld, D.S., Scheinmann, M.M., Effects of cardiac pacing and heart rate acceleration on exercise-induced symptoms in patients with sick sinus syndrome. Circulation *49 and 50*, 111–9, 1974.

Abrams, W.B., Davies, R.O., The antiarrhythmic mechanisms of beta-adrenergic blocking agents. In: Cardiac Arrhythmias. Editors: Dierfuss, L.S., Likoff., W., Grune and Stratton, New York, 1973, p. 517

Agha, A.S., Befeler, B., Castellanos, A.M., Sung, R.J., Castillo, C.A., Myerburg, R.J., Castellanos, A., Bipolar catheter electrograms for study of retrograde atrial activation pattern in patients without pre-excitation syndromes. Br. Heart J. *38*, 641, 1976.

Allessie, M.A., Bonke, F.I.M., Lammers, W.J.E.P., The effects of carbamylcholine, adrenaline, ouabain, quinidine, and verapamil on circus movement tachycardia in isolated segments of rabbit atrial myocardium. In: Reentrant Arrhythmias: Mechanisms and Treatment. Editor: Henri E, Kulbertus/MTP Press, Lancaster, U.K. (1977) Chapter 5, p. 63.

Allessie, M.A., Bonke, F.I.M., Schopman, F.J.G., Circus movement in rabbit atrial muscle as a mechanism of tachycardia. III. The "Leading circle" concept: a new model of circus movement in cardiac tissue without the involvement of an anatomical obstacle. Circ. Res. *41*, 9, 1977.

Allessie, M.A., Bonke, F.I.M., Schopman, F.J.G., Circus movement in rabbit atrial muscle as a mechanism of tachycardia. II. The role of nonuniform recovery of exitability in the occurrence of unidirectional block, as studied with multiple microelectrodes. Cir. Res. *39*, 168, 1976.

Allessie, M.A., Bonke, F.I.M., Schopman, F.J.G., Circus movement in rabbit atrial muscle as a mechanism of tachycardia. Circ. Res. *33*, 54, 1974.

Amat-y-Leon, F., Dhingra, R.C., Wu, D., Catheter mapping of retrograde atrial activation. Observations during ventricular pacing and AV nodal reentrant paroxismal tachycardia. Br. Heart J. *38*, 355, 1976.

Amat-y-Leon, F., Wu, D., Dhingra, R.C., Denes, P., Wyndham, R., Simpson, R., Rosen, K.M., Electrophysiological mechanisms of supraventricular tachyarrhythmia in patients with sinus node disease. Circulation *56* (suppl. III), 106, 1977

Amat-y-Leon, F., Wyndham, C., Wu, D., Denes, P., Dhingra, R.C., Rosen, K.M., Participation of fast and slow A-V nodal pathways in tachycardias complicating the Wolff-Parkinson-White syndrome. Circulation 55:663, 1977

Amory D.A., West, T.C., Chronotropic response following direct electrical stimulation of the isolated sinoatrial node: a pharmacologic evaluation. J. Pharmacol. Exp. Ther. *137*, 14, 1962.

Anderson, R.H., Janse, M.J., van Capelle, F.J.L., Billette, J., Becker, A.E., Durrer, D., A combined morphologic and electrophysiologic study of the atrioventricular node of the rabbit heart. Circ. Res. *35*, 909, 1974.

Anderson, R.H., Wenink, A.C.G., Becker, A.E., Janse, M.J., The development of the cardiac specialized tissue. In: The Conduction System of the Heart. Structure, Function, and Clinical Implications. Editors: Wellens, H.J.J., Lie, K.I., and Janse, M.J., H.E. Stenfert Kroese, Leiden, 1976, p. 1–28.

Anderson, R.H., Wenink, A.C.G., Losekoot, R.G., Becker A.E., Congenitally complete heart block – Developmental aspects. Circulation 56, 90, 1977

Angelakos, E.T., Regional distribution of catecholamines in the dog heart. Circ. Res. *16*, 39, 1965.

Angelakos, E.T., Fuxe, K., Torchiana, M.L., Chemical and histochemical evaluation of the distribution of catecholamines in the rabbit and guinea pig hearts. Acta Physiol. Scand. *59*, 184, 1963.

Angus, J.A., Richmond, D.R., Dhumma-Upakorn, P., Cobbin, L.B., Goodman, A.H., Cardiovascular action of verapamil in the dog with particular reference to myocardial contractility and atrioventricular conduction. Cardiovasc. Res. *10*, 623, 1976.

Arguss, N.S., Rosin, E.Y., Adolph, A.J., Fowler, N.O., Significance of chronic sinus bradycardia in elderly people. Circulation *46*, 924, 1972.

Aschoff, L., Referat über die Herzstörungen in ihren Beziehungen zu den spezifischen Muskelsystems des Herzens. Verh. Dtsch. Path. Ges. *14*, 3, 1910.

Babskii, E.B., Berdiaev, S.J., Khorunchi, V.A., Manganese ion action on the automaticity of frog cardiac pacemakers. Doklad. Acad. Sci. (U.S.S.R.), *209*, 996, 1972.

Balke, B., Ware, R.W., An experimental study of physical fitness of air force personnel. U.S. Armed Forces Med. J. *10*, 675, 1959.

Barker, P.S., Wilson, F.N., Johnson, F.D., The mechanism of auricular paroxysmal tachycardia. Am. Heart J. *26*, 435, 1943.

Berks, J.B., Bosman, C.K., Cochrane, J.W.C., Congenital cardiac arrhythmias. Lancet *2*, 531, 1964.

Bashour, T., Hemb, R., Wickramesekaran, R., Strauss, H.C., Bigger, J.T. Jr., An unusual effect of atropine on overdrive suppression. Circulation *48*, 911, 1973.

Bassingthwaighte, J. B., Reuter, H., Calcium movements and excitation-contraction coupling in cardiac cells. In: Electrical phenomena in the heart. Editor: de Mello, W.C., Academic Press, New York - London, 1972, p. 353.

Bath, J.C.L., Treatment of cardiac arrhythmias in unanesthetized patients. Role of adrenergic beta-receptor blockade. Am. J. Cardiol. *18*, 415, 1966.

Bayer, R., Kalusche, D., Kaufmann, R., Mannhold, R., Inotropic and electrophysiological actions of verapamil and D 600 in mammalian myocardium. III. Effects of the optical isomers on transmembrane action potentials. Nauny-Schmiedeberg's Arch. Pharm. *290*, 81, 1975.

Becker, A.E., Anderson, R.H., Morphology of the human atrioventricular junctional area. In: The Conduction System of the heart. Structure, Function, and Clinical Implications. Editors: Wellens, H.J.J., Lie, K.I., and Janse, M.I., H.E. Stenfert Kroese, Leiden, 1976, p. 263–266.

Beeler, G.W., Reuter, H., Reconstruction of the action potential of ventricular myocardial fibers. J. Physiol. *268*, 177, 1977.

Beeler, G.W., Reuter, H., Membrane calcium current in ventricular myocardial fibres. J. Physiol. (Lond.) *207*, 191, 1970.

Beiser, G.D., Epstein, S.E., Stampfer, M., Goldstein, R.E., Impaired heart rate response to sympathetic nerve stimulation in patients with cardiac decompensation. Circulation *38*, VI–40, 1968.

Belz, G.G., Bender, F., Therapie der Herzrhythmusstörungen mit Verapamil. Gustav Fischer Verlag, Stuttgart, 1974.

Bencosme, S.A., Berger, J.M., Specific granules in mammalian and non-mammalian vertebrate cardiocytes. Methods Achiev. Exp. Pathol. *5*, 173, 1971.

Bender, F., Isoptin zur Behandlung der tachykarden Form des Vorhofflatterns. Med. Klin. *62*, 634, 1967.

Benditt, D.G., Strauss, H.C., Scheinmann, M.M., Behar, U.S., Wallace, A.G., Analysis of secondary pauses following termination of rapid atrial pacing in man. Circulation *43*, 436, 1976.

Bennett, G., Leblond, C.P., Haddad, A., Migration of glycoprotein from the golgi apparatus to the surface of various cell types as shown by radioauthography after labelled fucose injection into rats. J. Cell Biol. *60*, 258, 1974.

Berger, J.M., Rona, G., Functional and fine structural heterogeneity of atrial cardiocytes. Methods Achiev. Exp. Pathol. *5*, 540, 1971.

Berger, W.K., Correlation between the ultrastructure and function of intercellular contacts. In: Electrical phenomena in the heart. Editor: de Mello, W.C., Academic Press, New York-London, 1972, p. 63.

Berkowitz, W.D., Wit, A.L., Lau, S.H., Steiner, C., Damato, A.N., The effects of propranolol in cardiac conduction. Circulation *40*, 855, 1969.

Bigger, J.T., A simple, rapid method for the diagnosis of first-degree sinoatrial block in man. Am. Heart J. *87*, 731, 1974.

Bigger, J.T., The sick sinus syndrome. Prac. Cardiol. *3*, 66, 1977.

Bigger, J.T., Strauss, H.C., The evaluation of sinoatrial node function in man. Med. Coll. Virg. Quart. *9*, 79, 1973.

Bigger, J.T., Strauss, H.C., Digitalis toxicity: drug interaction promoting toxicity and the management of toxicity. Sem. Drug Treatment *2*, 147, 1972.

Birkhead, J.S., Vaughan Williams, E.M., Dual effects of disopyramide on atrial and atrioventricular conduction and refractory periods. Br. Heart J. *39*, 657, 1977.

Blair, D.M., Davies, F., Observations on the conducting system of the heart. J. Anat. *69*, 303, 1935.

Blanquet, P.R., Ultrahistochemical study on the ruthenium red surface staining. II. Nature and affinity of the electron dense marker. Histochemistry *47*, 175, 1976.

Bleeker, W.K., Mackaay, A.J.C., Masson-Pevet, M., Bouman, L.N., Functional and morphological organization of the rabbit sinoatrial node. Submitted for publication, 1978.

Bleifeld, W. Rupp, M., Fleischmann, D., Effert, S., Syndrom des kranken Sinusknotens ("Sick-Sinus"- Syndrom). Dtsch. Med. Wochenschr. *99*, 795, 1974.

Blömer, H., Wirtzfeld, A., Delius, W., Sebening, H., Das Sinusknoten-Syndrom. Z. Kardiol. *64*, 697, 1975.

Bremmer, F., Fry, C.H., McGuigan, J.A.S., Action of ouabain on Na-free contraction in mammalian ventricular muscle. J. Physiol. *268*, 30, 1977.

Boakes, R.J., Bramwell, G.J., Briggs, I., Candy, J.M., Tempesta, E., Localization with pontamine sky blue of neurones in the brainstem responding to microiontophoretically applied compounds. Neuropharmacology *13*, 475, 1974.

Bogusch, G., Enzymatic digestion and urea extraction on leptomeric structures and normomeric myofibrils in heart muscle cells. J. Ultrastuct. Res. *55*, 245, 1976.

Boineau, J.P., Mooney, C.R., Hudson, R.D., Hughes, D.G., Erdin, R.A.Jr., Wylds, A.C., Observations on reentrant excitation pathways and refractory period distributions in spontaneous and experimental atrial flutter in the dog. In: Reentrant Arrhythmias, Mechanisms and Treatment. Editor: H.E. Kulbertus, MTP, Lancaster, 1977, p. 72.

Bojsen-Möller, F., Tranum-Jensen, J., Rabbit heart nodal tissue, sinoatrial ring bundle and atrioventricular connexions identified as a neuromuscular system. J. Anat. *112*, 367, 1972.

Bojsen-Möller, F., Tranum-Jensen, J., Whole-mount demonstration of cholinesterase-containing nerves in the right atrial wall, nodal tissue, and atrioventricular bundle of the pig heart. J. Anat. *108*, 375, 1971.

Bompiani, G.D., Rouiller, C., Hatt, P.Y., Le tissu de conduction du coeur chez le rat. Etude au microscope électronique. I. Le tronc commun du faisceau de His et les cellules claires de l'oreillette droite. Arch. Mal. Cœur *52*, 1257, 1959.

Bond, R.C., Engel, T.R., Schaal, S.F., Effect of digitalis on sinoatrial conduction in man (abstr.) Am. J. Cardiol. *33*, 128, 1974.

Bonke, F.I.M., The sinoatrial node function. In: Cardiac Pacing. Diagnostic and Therapeutic Tools. Editor: B. Lüderitz. Springer Verlag, Berlin-Heidelberg-New York, 1976, p. 5.

Bonke, F.I.M., Passive electrical properties of atrial fibers in the rabbit heart. Pflügers Arch. *339*, 1, 1973.

Bonke, F.I.M., Electrotonic spread in the sinoatrial node of the rabbit heart. Pflugers Arch. *339*, 17, 1973.

Bonke, F.I.M., Bouman, L.N., van Rijn, H.E., Change of cardiac rhythm in the rabbit after an atrial premature beat. Circ. Res. *24*, 533, 1969.

Bonke, F.I.M., Bouman, L.N., Schopman, F.J.G., Effect of an early atrial premature beat on activity of the sinoatrial node and atrial rhythm in the rabbit. Circ. Res. *29*, 704, 1971.

Bouman, L.N., De werking van de nervus vagus op de prikkelvorming in de sino-auriculaire knoop. Thesis 1965.

Bouman, L.N., Gerlings, E.D., Biersteker, P.A., Bonke, F.I.M., Pacemaker shift in the sino-atrial node during vagal stimulation. Pflügers Arch. *302*, 255, 1968.

Bouman, L.N., van der Westen, H.M., Pacemaker shift in the sinoatrial node induced by a change of temperature. Pflügers Archiv. *318*, 262, 1970.

Boura, A.L.A., Green, A.F., The actions of bretylium: adrenergic neurone blocking and other effects. Br. J. Pharmacol. *14*, 536, 1959.

Bozler, E., The initiation of impulses in cardiac muscle. Am. J. Physiol. *138*, 273, 1943.

Brady, A.J., Hecht, J., On the origin of the heart beat. Am. J. Med. *17*, 110, 1954.

Brandfonbrener, M., Landowne, M., Shock, N.W., Changes in cardiac output with age. Circulation *12*, 557, 1955.

Branton, D., Fracture faces of frozen membranes. Proc. Nat. Acad. Sci. U.S.A. *55*, 1948, 1966.

Branton, D., Bullivant, S., Gilula, N.B., Karnovsky, M.J., Moor, A., Mühlethaler, K., Northcote, D.H., Packer, L., Satir, B., Satir, P., Speth, V., Staehlin, L.A., Steer, R.L., Weinstein, R.S., Freeze-etching nomenclature. Science *190*, 54, 1975.

Brasil, A., Autonomic sinoatrial block. A new disturbance of the heart mechanism. Arq. Bras. Cardiol. *8*, 159, 1955.

Brechenmacher, C., Voegtlin, R., Tachycardie sinusale par réentrée. An Cardiol. Angéiol. *23*, 535, 1974.

Breithardt, G., Seipel, L., The effect of premature atrial depolarization on sinus node automaticity in man. Circulation *53*, 920, 1976.

Breithardt, G., Seipel, L., Reaktion des menschlichen Sinusknotens auf frühzeitige Depolarisations: Sinus knoten-Reentry und Sinusknoten-Eintrittsblock. Verh. Dtsch. Ges. Kreislaufforsch. *42*, 228, 1976.

Breithardt, G., Seipel, L., The influence of drugs on sinoatrial conduction time in man. In: Cardiac Pacing, Diagnostic and Therapeutic Tools. Editor: B. Lüderitz, Springer Verlag Berlin-Heidelberg-New York, 1976, p. 58.

Breithardt, G., Seipel, L., Both, A., Loogen, F., The effect of atropine on calculated sinoatrial conduction time in man. Eur. J. Cardiol. *4*, 49, 1976.

Breithardt, G. Seipel, L., Höhfeld, E., Both, A., Loogen, F., Pharmakologische Beeinflussung der "sinu-atrialen Leitungszeit" und der Sinusknotenautomatie beim Menschen. Z. Kardiol. *64*, 895, 1975.

Breithardt, G., Seipel, L., Loogen, F., Sinus node recovery time and calculated sinoatrial conduction time in normal subjects and patients with sinus node dysfunction. Circulation *56*, 43, 1977.

Breithardt, G., Seipel, L., Wiebringhaus, E., Loogen, F., Effect of verapamil on sinus node in patients with normal and abnormal sinus node function. Circulation *54*, suppl. II, 19, 1976.

Brodsky, M., Wu, D., Denes, P., Kanakis, G., Rosen, K.M., Arrhythmias documented by 24-hour continuous electrocardiographic monitoring in 50 male medical students without apparent heart disease. Am. J. Cardiol. *39*, 390, 1977.

Bronk, D.W., Ferguson, L.K., Solandt, D.Y., Inhibition of cardiac acceleratory impulses by the carotid sinus. Proc. Soc. Exp. Biol. Med. *31*, 579, 1934.

Brooker, G., Oscillation of cyclic adenosine monophosphate concentration during the myocardial contraction cycle. Science *182*, 933, 1973.

Brooks, C.McC., Lu, H.H., The sinoatrial pacemaker of the heart. Springfield, Ill. 1972. (Charles C. Thomas) p. 109–110.

Brown, H.F., Clark, A., Noble, S.J., Identification of the pacemaker current in frog atrium. J. Physiol. *258*, 521, 1976.

Brown, H.F., Clark, A., Noble, S.J., Analysis of pacemaker and repolarisation currents in frog atrium. J. Physiol. *258*, 547, 1976.

Brown, H.F., Giles, W., Noble, S.J., Voltage clamp of from sinus venosus. J. Physiol. (Lond.) *258*, 78 (abstract), 1976.

Brown, H.F., Giles, W.R., Noble, S.J., Cholinergic inhibition of frog sinus venosus. J. Physiol. *267*, 38, 1977.

Brown, H.F., Giles, W.R., Noble, S.J., Membrane currents underlying rhythmic activity in frog sinus venosus. J. Physiol. (Lond.), 271, 783, 1977.

Brown, H.F., Noble, S.J., Membrane currents underlying delayed rectification and pacemaker activity in frog atrial muscle. J. Physiol. (Lond.) *204*, 717, 1969.

Brown, A.M., Walker Jr., J.L., Sutton, R.B., Increase chloride conductance as the proximate cause of hydrogen ion concentration effects in Aplysia neurons. J. Gen. Physiol. *56*, 559, 1970.

Brittinger, D.W., Schwarzbeck, A., Wittenmeier, K.W., Twittenhoff, W.D., Stegaru, B., Huber, W., Ewald, R.W., van Henning, G.E., Fabricius, M., Strauch, M., Klinisch-experimentelle Untersuchungen über die blutdrucksenkende Wirkung von verapamil. Dtsch. Med. Wschr. 95, 1871, 1970.

Burgen, A., Terroux, K., On the negative inotropic effect in the cat's auricle. J. Physiol. (Lond.) *120*, 449, 1953.

Burnstock, G., Iwayama, T., Fine-structure identification of autonomic nerves and their relation to smooth muscle. Prog. Brain Res. *34*, 389, 1971.

Butterworth, K. R., Mann, M., The release of adrenaline and noradrenaline from the adrenal gland of the cat by acetylcholine. Br. J. Pharmacol. *12*, 422, 1957.

Carlsson, A., Rosengren, E., Bertler, A., Nilsson, J., Effect of reserpine on the metabolism of catecholamines. In: Psychotropic Drugs. Editors: Garattini, S., Ghetti, V., Elseviér Publishing Co., Amsterdam, 1957, p. 363.

Carmeliet, E.E., Chloride ions and the membrane potential of Purkinje fibers. J. Physiol. (Lond.) *156*, 375, 1961.

Carmeliet, E.E., Verdonck, F., Reduction of potassium permeability by chloride substitution in cardiac cells. J. Physiol. (Lond.) *265*, 193, 1977.

Castellanos, A., Aranda, J., Moleiro, F., Mallon, S.M., Befeler, B., Effects of the pacing site in sinus node reentrant tachycardia. J. Electrocardiol. *9*, 165, 1976.

Chadda, K.D., Banka, V.S., Bodenheimer, M.M., Helfant, R.H., Corrected sinus node recovery time. Experimental physiologic and pathologic determinants. Circulation *51*, 797, 1975.

Chai, C.Y., Wang, H.H., Hoffman, B.F., Wang, S.C., Mechanisms of bradycardia induced by digitalis substances. Am. J. Physiol. *212*, 26, 1967.

Challice, C.E., Studies on the microstucture of the heart. I. The sinoatrial node and the sinoatrial ring bundle. J. roy. Micr. Soc. *85*, 1, 1966.

Challice, C.E., Functional morphology of the specialized tissues of the heart. Methods Achiev. exp. Pathol. *5*, 121, 1971.

Cheng, Y.P., The ultrastructure of the rat sinoatrial node. Acta anat. Nipponica *46*, 339, 1971.

Chiba, S., Effects of verapamil on the blood-perfused, isolated atrium preparation of the dog heart. Jpn. Heart J. *16*, 709, 1975.

Chiba, T., Electron microscopic and histochemical studies on the synaptic vesicles in mouse vas deferens and atrium after 5-hydroxydopamine administration. Anat. Rec. *176*, 35, 1973.

Childers, R.W., Classification of cardiac arrhythmias. Med. Clin. North Am. *60*, 3, 1976.

Childers, R.W., Arnsdorf, M.F., de la Fuente, D.J., Gambetta, M., Svenson, R., Sinus nodal echoes. Clinical case report and canine studies. Am. J. Cardiol. *31*, 220, 1973.

Christoffersen, G.R.J., Skibsted, L.H., Calcium ion activity in physiological salt solutions: influences of anions substituted for chloride. Comp. Biochem. Physiol. *52*, 317, 1975.

Chuquimia, R., Vasquez, M., Qureshi, T., Khan, M., Towne, W.D., Narula, O.S., Effect of propranolol on sinus node recovery time and sinoatrial conduction time. Clin. Res. *25*, 212A, 1977.

Cochrane, D.E., Douglas, W.W., Mouri, T., Nakazato, Y., Calcium and stimulus-secretion coupling in the adrenal medulla: contrasting stimulating effects of the ionophores X-537A and A23187 on catecholamine output. J. Physiol. *252*, 363, 1975.

Cohen, I., Daut, J., Noble, D., An analysis of the actions of low concentrations of ouabain on membrane currents in Purkinje fibers. J. Physiol. (Lond.) *260*, 75, 1976.

Cohn, A.E., Lewis, T., Auricular fibrillation and complete heart block: A description of a case of Adams-Stoke syndrome including the postmortem examination. Heart *4*, 15, 1912.

Cohn, A.E., Lewis, T., Auricular fibrillation and complete heart block. A description of a case of Adams-Stokes syndrome including the postmortem examination. Heart *4*, 15, 1913.

Colborn, G.L., Carsey, E.Jr., Electron microscopy of the sinoatrial node of the squirrel monkey (saimiri sciureus). J. Mol. Cell Cardiol. *4*, 525, 1972.

Conde, C., Leppo, J., Lipski, J., Stimmel, B., Litwak, R., Donoso, E., Dack, S., Effectiveness of pacemaker treatment in the bradycardiatachycardia syndrome. Am. J. Cardiol. *32*, 209, 1973.

Copen, D.L., Cirillo, D.P., Vassalle, M., Tachycardia following vagal stimulation. Am. J. Physiol. *215*, 696, 1968.

Corday, E., Bazika, V., Lang, T.W., Pappelbaum, S., Gold, H., Berstein, H., Detection of phantom arrhythmias and evanescent ECG abnormalities. JAMA *193*, 417, 1965.

Coumel, Ph., Supraventricular Tachycardias. In: Cardiac Arrhythmias: the modern electrophysiological approach. Editors: Krikler, D.M., Goodwin, J.F. Saunders, W.B. London, Philadelphia and Toronto, 1975, Chapter 5.

Coumel, Ph., Attuel, P., Flammang, D., The role of the conduction system in supraventricular tachycardias. In: The Conduction System of the Heart. Structure, Function, and Clinical Implications. Editors: Wellens, H.J.J., Lie, K.I., and Janse, M.J., H.E. Stenfert Kroese, Leiden, 1976, Chapter 24, p. 424.

Covell, J.W., Chidsey, C.A., Braunwald, E., Reduction of the cardiac responses to postganglionic sympathetic nerve stimulation in patients with cardiac decompensation. Circ. Res. *19*, 51, 1966.

Cranefield, P.F., Action potentials, after-potentials and arrhythmias. Circ. Res. *41*, 415, 1977.

Cranefield, P.F., The conduction of the cardiac impulse. The slow response and cardiac arrhythmias. Mount Kosco, Futura Publishing Co., 1975.

Cranefield, P.F., Greenspan, K. The role of oxygen uptake of quiescent cardiac muscle. J. Gen. Physiol. *44*, 235, 1960.

Crook, B.R.M., Cashman, P.M.M., Stott, F.D., Raftery, E.B., Tape monitoring of the electrocardiogram in ambulant patients with sinoatrial disease. Br. Heart J. *35*, 1009, 1973.

Crook, B., Kitson, D., McComish, M., Jewitt, D., Indirect measurement of sinoatrial conduction time in patients with sinoatrial disease. Br. Heart J. *39*, 771, 1977.

Csapo, G., Personal communication (1976)

Curry, P.V.L., Fundamentals of arrhythmias: modern methods of investigation. In: Cardiac Arrhythmias: the modern electrophysiological approach. Editors: Krikler, D.M., Goodwin, J.F.. Saunders, W.B., London, 1975, p. 39.

Curry, P.V.L., Callowhill, E., Krikler, D.M., Paroxysmal reentry sinus tachycardia. Br. Heart J. *38*, 311, 1976.

Curry, P.V.L., Krikler, D.M., Significance of cycle length alternation during drug treatment of supraventricular tachycardia (abstr.) Br. Heart J. *38*, 882, 1976.

Curry, P.V.L., Krikler, D.M., Paroxysmal reciprocating sinus tachycardia. In: Reentrant Arrhythmias, Mechanisms and Treatment. Editor: H.E. Kulbertus, MTP Lancaster, 1977, p. 39.

Cushny, A.R., Matthews, S.A., On the effects of electrical stimulation of the mammalian heart. J. Physiol. *21*, 213, 1897.

Dahlström, A., Fuxe, K., Mya-Tu, M., Zetterström, B.E.M., Observations on adrenergic innervation of dog heart. Am. J. Physiol. *209*, 689, 1965.

Dauchot, P., Gravenstein, J.S., Effects of atropine on the electrocardiogram in different age groups. Clin. Pharmacol. Ther. *12*, 274, 1971.

Davies, M.J., Pomerance, A., Quantitative study of aging changes in the human sinoatrial node and internodal tracts. Br. Heart J. *34*, 150, 1972.

Davis, L.D., Effect of changes in cycle length on diastolic depolarization produced by ouabain in canine Purkinje fibers. Circ. Res. *32*, 206, 1973.

Davis, L.D., Temte, J.V., Effects of propranolol in the transmembrane potentials of ventricular muscle and Purkinje fibers of the dog. Circ. Res. *22*, 661, 1968.

Dean, P.M., Exocytosis modelling: an electrostatic function for calcium in stimulus-secretion coupling. J. Theor. Biol. *54*, 289, 1975.

De Bold, A.J., Bencosme, S.A., Studies on the relationship between the catecholamine distribution in the atrium and the specific granules present in atrial muscle cells. 2. Studies on the sedimentation pattern of atrial noradrenaline and adrenaline. Cardiovasc. Res. *7*, 364, 1973.

Deck, K.A., Dehnungseffekte am spontanschlagenden, isolierten Sinusknoten. Pflügers Arch. ges. Physiol. *280*, 120, 1964.

Deck, K.A., Kern, R., Trautwein, W., Voltage clamp technique in mammalian cardiac fibres. Pflügers Arch. *280*, 50, 1964.

DeHaan, R.L., DeFelice, L.J., Oscillatory properties and excitability of the heart cell membrane. In: Periodicities in Chemistry and Biology. Editor: H. Eying, Academic Press, 1977.

DeHaan, R.L., Gottlieb, S.H., The electrical activity of embryonic chick heart cells isolated in tissue culture singly or interconnected cell shiets. J. Gen. Physiol. *52*, 643, 1968.

Del Castillo, J., Katz, B., The membrane potential changes in frog's heart produced by inhibitory nerve impulses. Nature, *175*, 1035, 1955.

Del Castillo, J., Katz, B., Changes in end-plate activity produced by presynaptic polarization. J. Physiol. (Lond.) *124*, 586, 1954.

Delius, W., Wirtzfeld, A., Significance of the sinus node recovery time. In: Cardiac Pacing. Diagnostic and Therapeutic Tools. Editor: B. Lüderitz, Springer Verlag Berlin-Heidelberg-New York, 1976, p. 25.

Delius, W., Wirtzfeld, A., Sebening, H., Blömer, H., Bedeutung der Sinusknotenerholungszeit beim Sinusknotensyndrom. Dtsch. Med. Wochenschr. *100*, 2305, 1975.

de Mello, W.C., Some aspects of the interrelationship between ions and electrical activity in specialized tissue of the heart. In: The specialized tissues of the heart. Editors: Paes de Carvalho, A., de Mello, W.C., Hoffman, B.F., Elsevier Publishing Co., Amsterdam, 1961, p. 95.

de Mello, W.C., Role of chloride ions in cardiac action and pacemaker potentials. Am. J. Physiol. *205*, 567, 1963.

Demoulin, J.-C., Kulbertus, H.E., Pathological correlates of atrial arrhythmias. In: Reentrant Arrhythmias. Mechanisms and Treatment. Editor: Kulbertus, H.E., MTP Press, Lancaster, 1977, p. 99.

Denes, P., Delon, W., Dhingra, R.C., The effects of cycle length on cardiac refractory periods in man. Circulation *49*, 32, 1974.

Denes, P., Dhingra, R.C., Wu, D., Chuquimia, R., Amat-y-Léon, F., Wyndham, C., Rosen, K.M., Chronic HV interval in patients with bifascicular block, right bundle branch block and left anterior hemiblock. Clinical, electrocardiographic, and electrophysiologic correlations. Am. J. Cardiol. *35*, 23, 1975.

DeSilva, R.A., Shubrocks, S.J., Mitral valve prolaps with atrioventricular and sinoatrial node abnormalities of long duration. Am. Heart J. *93*, 772, 1977.

Devine, C.E., Somlyo, A.V., Sarcoplasmic reticulum and excitation-contraction coupling in mammalian smooth muscles. J. Cell Biol. *52*, 690, 1972.

Dewey, M.M., The structure and function of the intercalated disc in vertebrate cardiac muscle. In: Comparative physiology of the heart. Editor: McCann, F.V., Experientia, Suppl. *15*, 10, 1969.

Dewey, M.M., Barr, L., Intercellular connection between smooth muscle cells: the nexus. Science N.Y. *137*, 670, 1962.

Dhingra, R.C., Amat-y-Leon, F., Wyndham, C., Deedwania, P.C., Wu, D., Denes, P., Rosen, K.M., Clinical significance of prolonged sinoatrial conduction time. Circulation *55*, 8, 1977.

Dhingra, R.C., Amat-y-Leon, F., Wyndham, C., Denes, P., Wu, D., Miller, R.H., Rosen, K.M., Electrophysiologic effects of atropine on sinus node and atrium in patients with sinus nodal disfunction. Am. J. Cardiol. *38*, 848, 1976.

Dhingra, R.C., Amat-y-Leon, F., Wyndham, C., Denes, P., Wu, D., Pouget, J.M., Rosen, K.M., Electrophysiologic effects of atropine on human sinus node and atrium. Am. J. Cardiol. *38*, 429, 1976.

Dhingra, R.C., Amat-y-Leon, F., Wyndham, C., Wu, D., Denes, P., Rosen, K.M., The electrophysiological effects of ouabain on sinus node and atrium in man. J. Clin. Invest. *56*, 555, 1975.

Dhingra, R.C., Deedwania, P.C., Cummings, J.M., Amat-y-Léon, F., Wu, D., Denes, P., Rosen, K.M., Electrophysiologic effects of lidocaine on sinus node and atrium in patients with and without sinoatrial dysfunction. Circulation, in press.

Dhingra, R.C., Denes, P., Wu, D., Chuquimia, R., Amat-y-Léon, F., Wyndham, C., Rosen, K.M., Syncope in patients with chronic bifascicular block. Significance causative mechanisms, and clinical implication. Ann. Intern. Med. *81*, 302, 1974.

Dhingra, R.C., Denes, P., Wu, D., Chuquimia, R., Amat-y-Léon, F., Wyndham, C., Rosen, K.M., Chronic right bundle branch block and left posterior hemiblock. Clinical, electrophysiologic and prognostic observations. Am. J. Cardiol. *35*, 23, 1975.

Dhingra, R.C., Denes, P., Wu, D., Wyndham, C., Amat-y-Léon, F., Towne, W.D., Rosen, K.M., Prospective observations in patients with chronic bundle branch block and marked HV prolongation. Circulation *53*, 600, 1976.

Dhingra, R.C., Rosen, K.M., Rahimtoola, S.H., Normal conduction intervals and responses in sixty-one patients using His bundle recording and atrial pacing. Chest *64*, 55, 1973.

Dhingra, R.C., Wyndham, C., Amat-y-Léon, F., Denes, P., Wu, D., Rosen, K.M., Sinus nodal responses to atrial extrastimuli in patients without apparent sinus node disease. Am. J. Cardiol. *36*, 445, 1975.

Dighton, D.H., Sinus bradycardia. Autonomic influences and clinical assessment. Br. Heart J. *36*, 791, 1974.

Dighton, D.H., Sinoatrial block. Autonomic influences and assessment. Br. Heart J., *37*, 321, 1975.

Dimich, I., Steinfeld, L., Richman, R., Lasser, R., Treatment of recurrent paroxysmal ventricular tachycardia. Am. Heart J. *79*, 811, 1970.

Disertori, M., Molinis, G., Lanzetta, T., Antonini, L., Furlanello, F., Effetti del Verapamil sulla funzione sinusale e sulla conduzione atrio-ventricolare, lungo le vie normali ed anormali, in pazienti con preesistenti alterazioni della eccito-conduzione. G. Ital. Cardiol. *6*, 300, 1976.

Douglas, W.W., Stimulus-secretion coupling: the concept and clues from chromaffin and other cells. Br. J. Pharmacol. *34*, 451, 1968.

Dreifuss, J.J., Girardier, L., Forssmann, W.G., Etude de la propagation de l'excitation dans le ventricule de rat au moyen de solutions hypertoniques. Pflügers Arch. *292*, 13, 1966.

Dudel, J., Trautwein, W., Der Mechanismus der automatischen rhythmischen Impulsbildung der Herzmuskelfaser. Pflügers Arch. *267*, 553, 1958.

Dudel, J., Trautwein, W., Elektrophysiologische Messungen zur Strophanthin-wirkung am Herzmuskel. Naunyn-Schmiedeberg's Arch. Exp. Pathol. Pharmacol. *239*, 393, 1953.

Dulhunty, A.F., Franzini-Armstrong, C., Caveolae as specialized structural components of the surface membrane of skeletal muscle. Fed. Proc. *33*, 401, 1974.

Eccles, J.C., Hoff, H.E., Rhythm of heart beat: II. Disturbance of rhythm produced by late premature beats. Proc. R. Soc. Lond. (Biol.) *115*, 327, 1934.

Eckberg, D.L., Drabinsky, M., Braunwald, E., Defective cardiac parasympathetic control in patients with heart disease. New Engl. J. Med. *285*, 877, 1971.

Eggleton, G.P., Eggleton, P., Hill, A.V., The coefficient of diffusion of lactic acid through muscle. Proc. Roy. Soc.: ser. B., *103*, 620, 1928.

Ehinger, B., Falck, B., Persson, H., Sporrong, B., Adrenergic and cholinesterase-containing neurons of the heart. Histochemie *16*, 197, 1968.

Ellestad, M.H., Stress testing: principles and practice. F.A. Davis, publishing company.Philadelphia, Penn., 1975, p. 38.

Ellison, J.P., The adrenergic cardiac nerves of the cat. Am. J. Anat. *139*, 209, 1974.

Engel, T.R., Bond, R.C., Schaal, S.F., First-degree sinoatrial heart block: sinoatrial block in the sick sinus syndromes. Am. Heart J. *91*, 303, 1976.

Engel, T.R., Meister, S.G., Feitosa, G.S. Fisher, H.A., Frankl, W.S., Appraisal of sinus node artery disease. Circulation *52*, 286, 1975.

Engel, T.R., Schaal, S.F., Digitalis in the sick sinus syndrome. The effects of digitalis on sinoatrial automaticity and atrioventricular conduction. Circulation *48*, 1201, 1973.

Engelmann, T.W., Über den Ursprung der Herzbewegung und die physiologischen Eigenschaften der grossen Herznerven des Frosches. Arch. f.d. ges. Physiol. *65*, 109, 1897.

Eriksson, A., Thornell, L.E., Stigbrand, T., Ultrastructural and biochemical observations on cytoplasmic filaments of heart Purkinje fibers. J. Ultrastruct. Res. *54*, 481, 1976.

Eyster, J.A.E., Evans, J.S., Sino-auricular heart block: with report of a case in man. Arch. Intern. Med. *10*, 832, 1915.

Eyster, J.A.E., Meek, W.J., Experiments on the origin and conduction of the cardiac impulse. VI. Conduction of the excitation from the sino-auricular node to the right auricle and atrioventricular node. Arch. Intern. Med. *18*, 775, 1916.

Eyster, J.A.E., Meek, W.J., The point of primary negativity in the mammalian heart and the spread of negativity to other regions. Heart *5*, 119, 1914.

Ezerman, E.B., Ishikawa, H., Differentiation of the sarcoplasmic reticulum and T-system in developing chick skeletal muscle in vitro. J. Cell Biol. *35*, 405, 1967.

Farqhar, M.G., Palade, G.E., Junctional complexes in various epithelia. J. Cell Biol. *17*, 375, 1963.

Ferrer, M.I., The sick sinus syndrome, Mount Kisco, Futura Publishing Co., New York 1974.

Ferrer, M.I., The sick sinus syndrome, Circulation *47*, 635, 1973.

Ferrer, M.I., The sick sinus syndrome in atrial disease. JAMA. *206*, 645, 1968.

Ferrier, G.R., Moe, G.K., Effect of calcium on acetylstrophanthidin-induced transient depolarizations in canine Purkinje tissue. Circ. Res. *33*, 508, 1973.

Ferrier, G.R., Saunders, J.H., Mendez, C., A cellular mechanism for the generation of ventricular arrhythmias by acetylstrophantidin. Circ. Res. *32*, 600, 1973.

Fleischmann, P., Interpolation of atrial premature beats of infra-atrial origin due to concealed AS conduction. Am. Heart J. *66*, 309, 1963.

Fleischmann, P., Sinoatrial node entrance block (letter). Circulation *47*, 210, 1973.

Fisch, C., Greenspan, K., Knobel, S.B., Feigenbaum, H., Effect of digitalis on conduction of the heart. Prog. Cardiovasc. Dis. *6*, 343, 1964.

Forssmann, W.G., Girardier, L., A study of the T-system in rat heart. J. Cell Biol. *44*, 1, 1970.

Fozzard, H.A., Lee, C.O., Influence of changes in external potassium and chloride ions on membrane potential and intracellular potassium ion activity in rabbit ventricular muscle. J. Physiol. *256*, 663, 1976.

Franzini-Armstrong, C., Membrane particles and transmission at the triad. Fed. Proc. *34*, 1382, 1975.

Fraser, G.R., Froggat, P., James, T.N., Congenital deafness associated with electrocardiographic abnormalities, fainting attacks and sudden death: a recessive syndrome. Quart. J. Med. *33*, 361, 1964.

Furchgott, R.F., De Gubaroff, T., Grossman, A., Release of autonomic mediators in cardiac tissue by suprathreshold stimulation. Science *129*, 328, 1959.

Gaffney, T.E., Kahn, J.B., Van Maanen, E.F., Acheson, G.H., A mechanism of the vagal effect of cardiac glycosides. J. Pharmacol. Exp. Ther. *122*, 423, 1958.

Gallagher, J.J., Sealy, W.C., Wallace, A.G., Correlation between catheter electrophysiological studies and findings on mapping of ventricular excitation in the W.P.W.-syndrome. In: The Conduction System of the Heart. Structure, Function, and Clinical Implications. Editors: Wellens, H.J.J., Lie, K.I., Janse, M.J., H.E. Stenfert Kroese, Leiden, 1976, p. 588.

Gallo, P., A study on the topographical and quantitative relations between capillaries and fibres of the conduction system of the heart and on their functional significance. Cardiologica (Basel) *29*, 241, 1956.

Garvey, H.L., The mechanism of action of verapamil on the sinus and AV nodes. Eur. J. Pharmacol. *8*, 159, 1969.

Gaskell, W.H., On the innervation of the heart with especial reference to the heart of the tortoise. J. Physiol. (Lond.) *4*, 43, 1884.

Geer, M.R., Estrada, E.A., Strauss, H.C., Sinus node response to early atrial premature depolarizations. Circulation *52*, suppl. II, 64, 1975.

Geer, M.R., Wagner, G.S., Waxman, M., Wallace, A.G., Chronotropic effect of acetylstrophanthidin infusion into the canine sinus nodal artery. Am. J. Cardiol. *39*, 684, 1977.

George, C.F., Conolly, M.E., Briant, F., Dollery, C.T., Intravenously administered isoproterenol sulfate: dose-response curves in man. Arch. Intern. Med. *30*, 361, 1972.

George, W.J., Wilkerson, R.D., Kadowitz, P.J., Influence of acetylcholine on contractile force and cyclic nucleotide levels in the isolated perfused rat heart. J. Pharmacol. Exp. Ther. *184*, 228, 1973.

Gettes, L.S., Reuter, H., Slow recovery from inactivation of inward currents in mammalian myocardial fibres. J. Physiol. (Lond.) *240*, 703, 1974.

Giles, W., Tsien, R.W., Effects of acetylcholine on membrane currents in frog atrial muscle. J. Physiol. (Lond.) *246*, 64, 1975.

Giles, W., Noble, S.J., Changes in membrane currents in bullfrog atrium produced by acetylcholine. J. Physiol. *261*, 103, 1976.

Gillette, P.C., The mechanisms of supraventricular tachycardia in children. Circulation *54*, 133, 1976.

Gillis, R.A., Cardiac sympathetic nerve activity: changes induced by ouabain and propranolol. Science *166*, 508, 1969.

Glauert, A.M., Glauert, R.H., Araldite as an embedding medium for electron microscopy. J. Biophys. Biochem. Cytol. *4*, 191, 1958.

Gleichmann, U., Seipel, L., Loogen, F., Der Einfluss von Antiarrhythmika auf die intrakardiale Erregungsleitung (His-Bündel-Elektrographie) und Sinusknotenautomatie beim Menschen. Dtsch. Med. Wschr. *98*, 1487, 1973.

Glick, G., Braunwald, E., Relative roles of the sympathetic and parasympathic nervous system in the reflex control of the heart. Circ. Res. *16*, 363, 1965.

Glitsch, H.G., Reuter, H., Scholz, H., The effect of the internal sodium concentration on calcium fluxes in isolated guinea-pig auricles. J. Physiol, (Lond.) *209*, 25, 1970.

Goldberg, J.M., Intra-SA-nodal pacemaker shifts induced by autonomic nerve stimulation in the dog. Am. J. Physiol. *229*, 1116, 1975.

Goldberg, N.D., Haddox, M.K., Hartle, D.K., Hadden, J.W., In: Proceedings of the fifth international congress on Pharmacology. Editors: Maxwell, R.A., Achson, G.H., Karger, Basel, 1973, p. 146.

Goldberg, A.N., Moran, J.F., Resnekov, L.. Multistage electrocardiographic tests. Am. J. Cardiol. *26*, 84, 1970.

Goldreyer, B.N., Sinus node dysfunction: a physiologic consideration of arrhythmias involving the sinus node. In: Complex electrocardiography 2. Cardiovascular Clinics. Vol. *6*, I. Editor: Fisch, C., publ.: Davis, F.A. Co., Philadelphia, 1974. p. 180.

Goldreyer, B.N., Damato, A.N., Sinoatrial-node entrance block. Circulation *44*, 789, 1971.

Goldreyer, B.N., Gallagher, J.J., Damato, A.N., The electrophysiologic demonstration of atrial ectopic tachycardia in man. Am. Heart J. *85*, 205, 1973.

Goldstein, R.E., Beiser, D.G., Stampfer, M., Epstein, S.E., Impairment of autonomically mediated heart rate control in patients with cardiac dysfunction. Circ. Res. *36*, 571, 1975.

Goodman, D.J., Rosen, R.M., Ingham, R., Rider, A.K., Harrison, D.C., Sinus node function in the denervated human heart. Effect of digitalis. Br. Heart J. *37*, 612, 1975.

Gossrau, R., Histochemische, fluoreszenzmikroskopische und experimentelle Untersuchungen am Reizleitungssystem von Goldhamster, Maus und Ratte. Histochemie *26*, 44, 1971.

Greengard, P., Possible role for cyclic nucleotides and phosphorylated membrane proteins in postsynaptic actions of neurotransmitters. Nature *260*, 101, 1976.

Greenspan, A.M., Morad, M., Electromechanical studies on the inotropic effects of acetyl-strophanthidin in ventricular muscle. J. Physiol. (Lond.). *253*, 357, 1975.

Greenwood, R.S., Finkelstein, D., Sinoatrial heart block. Springfield, Ill., 1964 (Charles C. Thomas).

Grendahl, H., Miller, M., Sivertssen, E., Registration of sinus node recovery time in patients with sinus rhythm and in patients with dysrhythmias. Acta Med. Scand. *197*, 403, 1975.

Grolleau, R., Dufoix, R., Puech, P., Latour, H., Les tachycardies par rhyme réciproque dans le syndrome de Wolff-Parkinson-White. Arch. Mal. Cœur *63*, 74, 1970.

Grossman, A. Furchgott, R.F., The effects of various drugs on calcium exchange in the isolated guinea-pig left auricle. J. Pharmacol. Exp. Ther. *145*, 162, 1964.

Gupta, P.K., Lichstein, E., Chadda, K.D., Badui, E., Appraisal of sinus nodal recovery time in patients with sick sinus node syndrome. Am. J. Cardiol. *34*, 265, 1974.

Gurtner, H.P., Lenzinger, H.R., Dolder, M., Clinical aspects of sick sinus syndrome. In: Cardiac Pacing, Diagnostic and Therapeutic Tools. Editor: B. Lüderitz, Springer Verlag Berlin-Heidelberg-New York, 1976, p. 12.

Hagiwara, S., Toyama, K., Hayashi, H., Mechanisms of anion and cation permeations in the resting membranes of a barnacle muscle fiber. J. Gen. Physiol. *57*, 408, 1971.

Hamlin, R.L., Smith, C.R., Smetzer, D.L., Sinus arrhythmia in the dog. Am. J. Physiol. *210*, 321, 1966.

Han, J., Malozzi, A.M., Moe, G.K., Sinoatrial reciprocation in the isolated rabbit heart. Circ. Res. *22*, 355, 1968.

Harary, I., Farley, B., In vitro studies on single beating heart cells. Exp. Cell Res. *29*, 451, 1963.

Harris, E.J., Hutter, O.F., The action of acetylcholine on the movement of potassium ions in the sinus venosus of the heart. J. Physiol. *133*, 588, 1956.

Hartel, G., Talvensaari, T., Treatment of sinoatrial syndrome with permanent cardiac pacing in 90 patients. Acta Med. Scand. *198*, 341, 1975.

Härtel, G., Hartikainen, M., Comparison of verapamil and practolol in paroxysmal supraventricular tachycardia. Eur. J. Cardiol. Vol. 4, *1*, 87, 1976.

Hashimoto, K., Kimura, T., Kubota, K., Study of the therapeutic and toxic effects of ouabain by simultaneous observations on the excised and blood-perfused sinoatrial node and papillary muscle preparations and in the in situ heart of dogs. J. Pharmacol. Exp. Ther. *186*, 463, 1973.

Hashimoto, K., Kubota, K., Positive chronotropic effect of ouabain in the excised and blood-perfused canine SA node preparation of the dog. Naunyn-Schiedeberg's Arch. Pharmacol. *281*, 357, 1974.

Hashimoto, K., Moe, G.K., Transient depolarizations induced by acetylstrophanthidin in specialized tissue of dog atrium and ventricle. Circ. Res. *32*, 618, 1973.

Hauswirth, O., Noble, D., Tsien, R. W., Separation of the pacemaker and plateau components of delayed rectification in cardiac Purkinje fibers. J. Physiol. (Lond.) *255*, 211, 1972.

Hayashi, K., An electron microscopy study on the conduction system of the cow heart. Jpn. Circ. J. *26*, 765, 1962.

Hayashi, S., Electron microscopy of the heart conduction system of the dog. Arch. Histol. Jpn. *33*, 67, 1971.

Hayashi, H., Lux, R., Wyatt, R., Activation sequence in the right atrium of the dog. Circulation 50, suppl. III, 84, 1974.

Hayashi, S., Oga, K., Otsuka, N., The fine structure of nerve endings in the sinus node of the canine heart. J. Electron Microsc. *19*, 176, 1970.

Heuser, J.E., Reese, T.S., Evidence of recycling of synaptic vesicle membrane during transmitter release at the frog neuromuscular junction. J. Cell Biol. *57*, 351, 1973.

Hewlett, A.W., Digitalis heart block. JAMA *48*, 47, 1907.

Heymans, C., Bouckaert, J.J., Regniers, P., Sur le mécanisme réflexe de la bradycardie provoquée par les digitaliques. Arch. Intern. Pharmacodyn. *44*, 31, 1932.

Higgins, C.B., Vatner, S.F., Braunwald, E., Parasympathetic control of the heart. Pharmacol. Rev. *25*, 119, 1973.

Hirschfeld, D.S., Peters, R., Kunkel, F., Scheinmann, M.M., Sinoatrial conduction time (SACT) and abnormal perinodal refractoriness in patients with sinus node disease (SND). Circulation *52*, II-112, 1975.

Hodgkin, A.L., Horowicz, P., The influence of potassium and chloride ions on the membrane potential of single muscle fibres. J. Physiol. *148*, 127, 1959.

Hoffman, B.F., Cranefield, P.F., In: Electrophysiology of the heart, McGraw-Hill, New York, 1960.

Hoffman, B.F., Singer, D.H., Effects of digitalis on electrical activity of cardiac fibers. Prog. Cardiovasc. Dis. *7*, 226, 1964.

Hogan, P., Albuquerque, E., The pharmacology of batrachotoxin. Effects on the heart Purkinje fibers. J. Pharmacol. Exp. Ther. *176*, 529, 1971.

Holden, W., McAnullty, J., Rahimtoola, S., Inadequate heart rate response to exercise in the sick sinus syndrome. Circulation *53 and 54*, II-146, 1976.

Holder, M.S., Anolik, M.A., Vassalle, M., Positive chronotropic effect of vagus on sinus node. Arch. Sci. Biol. *55*, 103, 1971.

Holsinger, J.W.Jr., Wallace, A.G., Sealy, W.C., The identification and surgical significance of the atrial internodal conduction tracts. Ann. Surg. *167*, 447, 1968.

Howell, W.H., Duke, W.W., The effect of vagus inhibition on the output of potassium from the heart. Am. J. Physiol. *21*, 51, 1908.

Howitt, G., Husaim, M., Rowlands, D.J., Logan, W.F.W.E., Shanks, R.G., Evans, M.G., The effect of the dextro isomer of propranolol in sinus rate and cardiac arrhythmias. Am. Heart J. *76*, 736, 1968.

Howse, H.D., Ferrans, V.J., Hibbs, R.G., A comparative histochemical and electro-microscopic study of the surface coatings of cardiac muscle cells. J. Mol. Cell. Cardiol. *1*, 157, 1970.

Hudson, R.E.B., The human pacemaker and its pathology. Br. Heart J. *22*, 153, 1960.

Huet, M., Benchimol, S., Castonguay, Y., Cantin, M., Ultrastructural cytochemistry of atrial muscle cells, III. Reactivity of specific granules in man. Histochemistry *41*, 87, 1974.

Husaini, M.H., Kvasnicka, J., Rydén, L., Holmberg, S., Action of Verapamil on sinus node, atrioventricular and intraventricular conduction. Br. Heart J. *35*, 734, 1973.

Hutter, O.F., Noble, D., The chloride conductance of frog skeletal muscle. J. Physiol. (Lond.) *151*, 89, 1960.

Hutter, O.F., Noble, D., Anion conductance of cardiac muscle. J. Physiol. *157*, 335, 1961.

Hutter, O.F., Trautwein, W., Vagal and sympathetic effects on the pacemaker fibers in the sinus venosus of the heart. J. Gen. Physiol. *39*, 715, 1956.

Hutter, O.F., Trautwein, W. Effect of vagal stimulation on the sinus venosus of the frog's heart. Nature (Lond.) *176*, 512, 1955.

Iijima, T., Tai ra, N., Modification by manganese ions and Verapamil of the response of the atrioventricular node to norepinephrine. Eur. J. Pharmacol. *37*, 55, 1976.

Ijpeij, D., Kerkhof, P.L.M., Bobbert, A.C., Muscle length and neuromuscular transmission in the frog. Pflügers Arch. *347*, 309, 1974.

Ikemoto, Y., Goto, M., Nature of the negative inotropic effect of acetylcholine on the myocardium. An elucidation on the bullfrog atrium. Proc. Jpn. Acad. *51*, 501, 1975.

Irisawa, A., The fine structure of the sinoatrial node of the rabbit heart. Abstract. In: the 8th Natl. Mtg. of the Intr. Study Group for Research in Cardiac Metabolism, 1976, p. 151.

Irisawa, H., Electrical activity of rabbit sinoatrial node as studied by a double sucrose gap method. In: Symposium and Colloquium on the electrical field of the heart. Editor: P. Rijlant, Bruxelles, Presses Academiques Européennes, 1972.

Irisawa, H., Noma, A., Contracture and hyperpolarization of the rabbit sinoatrial node cell in Na-depleted solution. Jpn. J. Physiol. *26*, 133, 1976.

Irisawa, H., Seyama, I., Noma, A., Resting and action potentials of rabbit sinoatrial node cells. In: Developmental and physiological correlates of cardiac muscle. Editors: Liebermann, M., Shano, T., Raven Press, New York, 1975, p. 287.

Isa, L., Matturi, L., Rossi, L., Contributo iso-citologico al riconoscimento delle connessioni internodali atriali. G. Ital. Cardiol. *6*, 1024, 1976.

Isaacson, R., Boucek, R.J., The atrioventricular conduction tissue of the dog. Histochemical properties; influence of electric shock. Am. Heart J. *75*, 206, 1968.

Isenberg, G., Is potassium conductance of cardiac Purkinje fibers controlled by (Ca^{++})? Nature *253*, 273, 1975.

Ishikawa, H., Yamada, E., Differentiation of the sarcoplasmic reticulum and T-system in developing mouse cardiac muscle. In: Developmental and physiological correlates of cardiac muscle. Editors: Lieberman, M., Sano, T., Raven Press, New York, 1975, p. 21.

Ito, M., Arita, M., Saeki, K., Tanoué, M., Fukushima, I., Yanaga, T., Mashiba, H., Functional properties of sinocaval conduction. Jpn. J. Physiol. *17*, 174, 1967.

Iversen, L., Catecholamine uptake processes. Br. Med. Bull. *29*, 130, 1973.

Jacobowitz, D., Histochemical studies on the relationship of chromaffin cells and adrenergic nerve fibers to the cardiac ganglia of several species. J. Pharmacol., Exp. Ther. *158*, 227, 1967.

James, T.N., Pulse and impulse in the sinus node. Henry Ford Hosp. Med. J. *15*, 275, 1967.

James, T.N., Anatomy of the human sinus node. Anat. Rec. *141*, 109, 1961.

James, T.N., Myocardial infarction and atrial arrhythmias. Circulation *24*, 761, 1961.

James, T. N., The connecting pathways between the sinus node and AV node and between the right and the left atrium in the human heart. Am. Heart J. *66*, 498, 1963.

James, T.N., Nadeau, R.A., The chronotropic effect of digitalis studied by direct perfusion of the sinus node. J. Pharmacol. Exp. Ther. *139*, 42, 1963.

James, T.N., Sherf, L.N., Fine, G., Morales, A.R., Comparative ultrastructure of the sinus node in man and dog. Circulation *34*, 139, 1966.

Jamieson, J.D., Palade, G.E., Specific granules in atrial muscle cells. J. Cell Biol. *23*, 151, 1964.

Janse, M.J., Anderson, R.H., Specialized internodal atrial pathways – fact or fiction? Eur. J. Cardiol. *2*, 117, 1974.

Jennings, R.B., Ganote, C.E., Structural changes in myocardium during acute ischemia. Circ. Res. *34–35. Suppl. III*, 156, 1974.

Jordan, J.L., Yamaguchi, I., Mandel, W.J., The sick sinus syndrome: pathophysiology, significance and treatment. Cardiol. Dig. *12*, 11, 1977.

Jordan, J., Yamaguchi, I., Mandel, W.J., Characteristics of sinoatrial conduction in patients with coronary artery disease. Circulation *55*, 569, 1977.

Jordan, J., Yamaguchi, I., Mandel, W.J., Studies on the mechanism of sinus node dysfunction in the sick sinus syndrome. Circulation *54*, suppl. II, 230, 1976.

Jordan, J., Yamaguchi, I., Mandel, W.J., McCullen, A.E., Comparative effects of overdrive on sinus and subsidiary pacemaker function. Am. Heart J. *93* 367, 1977.

Jose, A.D., Effect of combined sympathetic and parasympathetic blockade on heart rate and cardiac function in man. Am. J. Cardiol. *18*, 476, 1966.

Jose, A.D., Collison, D., The normal range and determinants of the intrinsic heart rate in man. Cardiovasc. Res. *4*, 160, 1970.

Jose, Taylor, R.R., Autonomic blockade by propranolol and atropine to study intrinsic myocardial function in man. J. Clin. Invest. *48*, 2019, 1969.

Josephson, M.E., Scharf, D.L., Kastor, J.A., Kitchen, J.G., Atrial endocardial activation in man. Electrode catheter technique for endocardial mapping. Am. J. Cardiol. *39*, 972, 1977.

Jung, L., Tagand, R., Pierre, M., Sur le trajet des éléments cardio-accélérateurs contenus dans le cordon vagosympathique du chien. Compt. Rend. Soc. Biol. *117*, 441, 1934.

Kao, C., Tetrodotoxin, saxitoxin, and their significance in the study of excitation phenomena. Pharmacol. Rev. *18*, 997, 1966.

Kaplin, B.M., Langendorf, R., Lev, M., Pick, A., Tachycardia-bradycardia syndrome (so-called: Sick sinus syndrome). Pathology, mechanisms and treatment. Am. J. Cardiol. *31*, 497, 1973.

Karnovsky, M.J., The ultrastructural basis of capillary permeability studied with peroxidase as tracer. J. Cell Biol. *35*, 213, 1967.

Katz, A.M., Contractile proteins of the heart. Physiol. Rev. *50*, 63, 1970.

Katz, L.N., Pick, A., The arrhythmias. In: Clinical Electrocardiography, Part I, Lea and Febiger, Philadelphia, 1956.

Kawamura, K., Sino-atrial node and atrio-ventricular node. In: Conduction system (in Japanese). Editor: Sano, T., Igaku Shoin Co., Tokyo, 1974, p. 22.

Kawamura, K., Electron microscope studies on the cardiac conduction system of the dog. II. The sino-atrial and atrioventricular nodes. Jpn. Circ. J. *25*, 973, 1961.

Kawamura, K., Hayashi, K., Electron microscope study of the cardiac conduction system. Jpn. Circ. J. *30*, 149, 1966.

Kawamura, K., James, T.N., Comparative ultrastructure of cellular junctions in working myocardium and the conduction system under normal and pathologic conditions. J. Mol. Cell. Cardiol. *3*, 31, 1971.

Keith, A., Flack, M., The form and nature of the muscular connections between the primary division of the vertebrate heart. J. Anat. and Physiol. *41*, 172, 1907.

Kikuchi, S., The structure and innervation of the sinuatrial node of the mole heart. Cell Tissue Res. *172*, 345, 1976.

Kirshner, N., Function and organization of chromaffin vesicle. Life Sci. *14*, 1153, 1974.

Klein, H.O., Singer, D.H., Hoffman, B.F., Effects of atrial premature systoles on sinus rhythm in the rabbit. Circ. Res. *32*, 480, 1973.

Koch, W., Weitere Mitteilungen über den Sinusknoten des Herzens. Verh. Dtsch. Path. Ges. *13*, 85, 1909.

Koelle, G.B., The histochemical identification of acetylcholinesterase in cholinergic, adrenergic and sensory neurons. J. Pharmacol. Exp. Ther. *114*, 167, 1955.

Kohlhardt, M., Bauer, B., Krause, H., Fleckenstein, A., Differentiation of the transmembrane Na and Ca channels in mammalian cardiac fibers by the use of specific inhibitors. Pflügers Arch. *335*, 309, 1972.

Kohlhardt, M., Figulla, H.-R., Tripathi, O., The slow membrane channel as the predominant mediator of the excitation process of the sinoatrial pacemaker cell. Basic Res. Cardiol. *71*, 17, 1976.

Konisai, T., Electrophysiologic consideration on sick sinus syndrome. Jpn. Circ. J. *40*, 194, 1976.

Kreitner, D., Evidence for the existence of a rapid sodium channel in the membrane of rabbit sinoatrial cells. J. Mol. Cell. Cardiol. *7*, 655, 1975.

Krikler, D., Verapamil in cardiology. Eur. J. Cardiol. *2*, 3, 1974.

Krikler, D.M., Curry, P V.L., Attuel, P., Coumel, Ph., "Incessant" tachycardias in WPW syndrome. I. Initiation without antecedent extrasystoles or PR lengthening, with reference to reciprocation after shortening of cycle length. Br. Heart J. *38*, 885, 1976.

Krueger, E., Unna, K., Comparative studies on the toxic effects of digitoxin and ouabain in cats. J. Pharmacol. Exp. Ther. *76*, 282, 1942.

Kulbertus, H.E., De Leval-Rutten, F., Demoulin, J.C., Sinoatrial disease: a report on 13 cases. J. Electrocardiol. *6*, 303, 1973.

Kulbertus, H.E., De Leval-Rutten, F., Mary, L., Casters, P., Sinus node recovery time in the elderly. Br. Heart. J. *37*, 420, 1975.

Ladle, R.O., Walker, J.L., Intracellular chloride activity in frog heart. J. Physiol. (Lond.) *251*, 549, 1975.

Lange, G., Action of driving stimuli from intrinsic and extrinsic sources on in situ cardiac pacemaker tissues. Circ. Res. *17*, 449, 1965.

Langendorf, R., Lesser, M.E., Plotkin, P., Levin, B.D., Atrial parasystole with interpolation: Observations on prolonged sinoatrial conduction. Am. Heart J. *63*, 649, 1962.

Langer, G.A., Coupling calcium in mammalian ventricle: its source and factors regulating its quantity. Cardiovasc. Res. *Suppl. I*, 71, 1971.

Langer, G.A., Ion fluxes in cardiac excitation and contraction and their relation to myocardial contractility. Physiol. Rev. *48*, 708, 1968.

Laslett, E.E., Syncopal attacks, associated with prolonged arrest of the whole heart. Quart. J. Med. *2*, 347, 1909.

Lawson, W.H., Elastic tissue staining; modification of Weigert-Sheridan method. J. Tech. Meth. *16*, 42, 1936.

Lederer, W.J., Tsien, R.W., Transient inward current underlying arrhythmogenic effects of cardiotonic steroids Purkinje fibers. J. Physiol. (Lond.) (In press).

Lederer, W.J., Tsien, R.W., Transient inward current underlying strophanthidin's enhancement of pacemaker activity in Purkinje fibers. J. Physiol. (Lond.) *249*, 40, 1975.

Lee, B.B., Mandl, G., Stean, J.P.B., Microelectrode tip position marking in nervous tissue: a new dye method. Electroencephalogr. Clin. Neurophysiol. *27*, 610, 1969.

Lee, F.L., The relation between norepinephrine content and response to sympathetic nerve stimulation of various organs of cats pretreated with reserpine. J. Pharmacol. Exp. Ther. *156*, 137, 1967.

Lee, K.S., Klaus, W., The subcellular basis for the mechanism of inotropic action of cardiac glycosides. Pharmacol. Rev. *23*, 193, 1971.

Lefkowitz, R.J., O'Hara, D.S., Warshaw, J., Binding of catecholamines to receptors of the sinoatrial node. Circ. Res. *17*, 460, 1965.

Legato, M.J., Ultrastructural characteristics of the rat ventricular cell grown in tissue culture, with special reference to sarcomerogenesis. J. Mol. Cell. Cardiol. *4*, 299, 1972.

Legato, M.J., Langer, G.A., The subcellular localization of calcium ion in mammalian myocardium. J. Cell Biol. *41*, 401, 1969.

Lemberg, L., Castellanos, A., Arcebal, A.G., The use of propranolol in arrhythmias complicating acute myocardial infarction. Am. Heart J. *80*, 479, 1970.

Lenfant, J., Analyse des propriétés de la membrane myocardique sino-auriculaire: genèse de l'activité spontanée. Thesis, Poitiers, 1972.

Lenfant, J., Mironneau, J., Aka, J.K., Analyse des propriétés de la membrane myocardique sinoauriculaire; genèse de l'activité spontanée. C.R. Acad. Sci. Paris *273*, 1729, série D, 1971.

Lenfant, J., Mironneau, J., Aka, J.K., Activité répétitive de la fibre sino-auriculaire de grenouille: analyse des courants membranaires responsables de l'automatisme cardiaque. J. Physiol. (Paris) *64*, 5, 1972.

Lenfant, J., Mironneau, J., Cargouil, Y., Galand, G., Analyse de l'activité électrique spontanée du centre de l'automatisme cardiaque de lapin par les inhibiteurs de perméabilités membraires. C.R. Acad. Sci. *266*, 901, 1968.

Lev, M., Aging changes in the human sinoatrial node. J. Gerontol. *9*, 1, 1954.

Lev, M., Bharati, S., Lesions of the conduction system and their functional significance. In: Pathology Annual. Editor: Sommers, S.C., Appleton-Century-Crofts, New York, 1974, pp. 157–207.

Levine, S.A., Observations on sino-auricular heart block. Arch. Intern. Med. (Chicago) *17*, 153, 1916.

Lewis, Th., Oppenheimer, B.S., Oppenheimer, A., The site of origin of the mammalian heart beat; the pacemaker in the dog. Heart *2*, 147, 1910.

Lewis, Th., Meakings, J., White, P.D., The excitatory process in the dog's heart. Philos. Trans. R. Soc. *205*, 375, 1914.

Limas, C.J., Calcium-binding sites in rat myocardial sarcolemma. Arch. Biochem. Biophys. *179*, 302, 1977.

Lipsius, S., Vassalle, M., Effects of ionic changes and glucosides on sinus node action potentials. Fed. Proc. *35*, 319, 1976.

Livengood, D.R., Kusano, K., Modulation of the crustacean heart rate by an electrogenic Na-pump. Neurobiology of Invertebrates, Tohany, 1971, *213*, 1973.

Loeb, J.M., Vassalle, M., The positive chronotropic action of the vagus nerve on the heart. Fed. Proc. *35*, 446, 1976.

Loewenstein, W.R., Permeable junctions. Cold Spring Harbor. Symp. Quant. Biol. *40*, 49, 1976.

Lorber, V., Bertaud, W.S., Cellular surfaces of amphibian atrial muscle. J. Cell. Sci. *9*, 427, 1971.

Lown, B., In: 14th Hahnemann symposium on mechanisms and therapy of cardiac arrhythmias. Editors: Dreifus, L., Likoff, W., Moyer, J., Philadelphia, Grune Stratton, 1966, p. 185.

Lown, B., Wyatt, N.F., Levine, H.D., Paroxysmal atrial tachycardia with block. Circulation *21*, 129, 1960.

Lu, H.H., Shifts in pacemaker dominance within the sinoatrial region of cat and rabbit hearts resulting from increase of extracellular potassium. Circ. Res. *26*, 339, 1970.

Lu, W.-H., McC. Brooks, C., Role of calcium in cardiac pacemaker cell action. Bull., N.Y. Acad. Med. *45*, 100, 1969.

Lu, H.H., Lange, G., McC. Brooks, C., Factors controlling pacemaker action in cells of the sinoatrial node. Circ. Res. *17*, 460, 1965.

Lucchesi, B.R., Hardman, H.F., The influence of dichlor-isoproternenol (DCl) and related compounds upon ouabain and acetylstrophantidin induced cardiac arrhythmias. J. Pharmacol. Exp. Ther. *132*, 372, 1961.

Lüderitz, B., Steinbeck, G., The use of programmed rate related premature stimulation in managing tachyarrhythmias. In: Cardiac Pacing, Diagnostic and Therapeutic Tools. Editor: B. Lüderitz, Springer Verlag Berlin-Heidelberg-New York, 1976, p. 227.

Luft, J.H., Ruthenium red and violet. II. Fine structural localization in animal tissues. Anat. Rec. *171*, 369, 1971.

Luft, J.H., Improvement in epoxy resin embedding methods. J. Biophys. Biochem. Cytol. *9*, 409, 1961.

Lüttgau, H.C., Niedergerke, R., The antagonism between Ca and Na ions on the frog's heart. J. Physiol. *143*, 486, 1958.

McAllister, R.E., Noble, D., Tsien, R.W., Reconstruction of the electrical activity of cardiac Purkinje fibers. J. Physiol. *251*, 1, 1975.

McDonald, T.F., Trautwein, W. The potassium current underlying delayed rectification in cat ventricular muscle. J. Physiol. 274, 217, 1978.

McDonald, T.F., Nawrath, H., Trautwein, W., Membrane currents and tension in cat ventricular muscle treated with cardiac glycosides. Circ. Res. *37*, 674, 1975.

Mc Ewen, L.M., The effect on the isolated rabbit heart of vagal stimulation and its modification by cocaine, hexamethonium and ouabain. J. Physiol. *131*, 678, 1956.

McGuigan, J.A.S., Some limitations of the double sucrose gap, and its use in a study of the slow outward current in mammalian ventricular muscle. J. Physiol. *240*, 775, 1974.

Mackenzie, J., The cause of heart irregularity in influenza. Br. Med. J. *2*, 1411, 1902.

McLain, P.L., Kruse, T.K., Redick, T.F., The effect of atropine on digitoxin bradycardia in cats. J. Pharmacol. Exp. Ther. *139*, 42, 1963.

Mc Lean, W.A.H., Karp, R.B., Kouchoukos, N.T., James, T.N., Waldo, A.L., P waves during ectopic atrial rhythms in man. A study utilizing atrial pacing with fixed electrodes. Circulation *52*, 426, 1975.

McNutt, N.S., Ultrastructure of intercellular junctions in adult and developing cardiac muscle. Am. J. Cardiol. *25*, 169, 1970.

McNutt, N.S., Fawcett, D.W., The ultrastructure of the cat myocardium. J. Cell. Biol. *42*, 46, 1969.

McNutt, N.S., Weinstein, R.S., The ultrastructure of the nexus. A correlated thin-section and freeze-cleave study. J. Cell. Biol. *47*, 666, 1970.

Mackawa, M., Nohara, Y., Kawamura, K., Hayashi, K., Electron microscope study of the conduction system in mammalian hearts. In: Electrophysiology and ultrastructure of the heart. Editors: Sano, T., Mizuhira, V., Matsuda, K., Bunkodo, Tokyo, 1967, p. 41.

Mandel, W.J., Hayakawa, H., Allen, H.N., Danzig, R., Kermaier, A.I., Assessment of sinus node function in patients with sick sinus node syndrome. Circulation *46*, 761, 1972.

Mandel, W.J., Hayakawa, H., Danzig, R., Marcus, H.S., Evaluation of sinoatrial node function in man by overdrive suppression. Circulation *44*, 59, 1971.

Mandel, W.J., Laks, M.M., Overview of the sick sinus syndrome. Chest *66*, 223, 1974.

Mandel, W.J., Laks, M.M., Obayashi, K., Sinus node function: evaluation in patients with and without sinus node disease. Arch. Intern. Med. *135*, 386, 1975.

Margolis, J.R., Strauss, H.C., Miller, H.C., Gilbert, M., Wallace, A.G., Digitalis and the sick sinus syndrome. Clinical and electrophysiologic documentation of a severe toxic effect on sinus node function. Circulation *52*, 162, 1975.

Mascher, D., Peper, K., Two components of inward current in myocardial muscle fibers. Pflügers Arch. *307*, 190, 1969.

Masini, G., Dianda, R., Analysis of the interpolation phenomenon in man evaluated by premature atrial stimulation Cardiovasc. Res. *11*, 334, 1977.

Masini, G., Dianda, R., Rilievi clinici ed elettrofisiologici in pazienti con bradicardia sinusale. G. Ital. Cardiol. *7*, 325, 1977.

Masini, G., Dianda, R., Grazina, A., Analysis of sinoatrial conduction in man using premature atrial stimulation. Cardiovasc. Res. *9*, 498, 1975.

Masson-Pevet, M., Jongsma, H.J., Bruijne de, J., Collagenase – and trypsin – dissociated heart cells: a comparative ultrastructural study. J. Mol. Cell. Cardiol. *8*, 747, 1976.

Massumi, R.A., Sarin, R.K., Tawakkol, A.A., Rios, J.L., Jackson, H., Time sequence of right and left atrial depolarization as a guide to the origin of P waves. Am. J. Cardiol. *24*, 28, 1969.

Mazel, P., Holland, W.C., Acetylcholine and electrolyte metabolism in the various chambers of frog and turtle heart. Circ. Res. *6*, 684, 1958.

Mazet, F., Cartaud, J., Freeze-fracture studies of frog atrial fibres. J. Cell. Sci. *22*, 427, 1976.

Medvedowsky, J.L., Barney, C., Delaage, M., Nicolai, P., Chostakoff, F., Étude de la fonction sinusale. Arch. Mal. Cœur *68*, 225, 1975.

Mendez, C., Aceves, J., Mendez, R., Inhibition of adrenergic cardiac acceleration by cardiac glycosides. J. Pharmacol. Exp. Ther. *131*, 191, 1961.

Meek, W.J., Eyster, J.A.E., The effect of vagal stimulation and of cooling on the location of the pacemaker within the sino-auricular node. Am J. Physiol. *34*, 368, 1914.

Meredith, J., Titus, J.L., Anatomical atrial connections between sinus and AV node. Circulation *37*, 566, 1968.

Metzger, A.L., Goldberg, A.N., Hunter, R.L., Sick sinus node syndrome as the presenting manifestation of reticulum cell sarcoma. Chest *60*, 602, 1971.

Miki, Y, Rothberger, C.J., Experimentelle Untersuchungen über die Pause nach Vorhofextrasystolen. Z. ges. exp. Med. *30*, 347, 1922.

Miller, H.C., Strauss, H.C., Measurement of sinoatrial conduction time by premature atrial stimulation in the rabbit. Circ. Res. *35*, 935, 1974.

Mirowski, M., Lau, S.H., Wit, A.L., Steiner, C., Bobb, G.A., Tabatznik, B., Damato, A.N., Ectopic right atrial rhythms: experimental and clinical data. Am. Heart J. *81*, 666, 1971.

Miyagishima, Y., Studies on catecholamine (CA) of the heart – fluorescence histochemical method. Jpn. Circ. J. *39*, 361, 1975.

Mobley, B.A., Page, E., The surface area of sheep cardiac Purkinje fibers. J. Physiol. *220*, 547, 1972.

Moe, G.K., Farah, A.E., Digitalis and allied cardiac glycosides. In: The pharmacological basis of therapeutics. Editors: Goodman, L.S., Gilman, A., Macmillan Publishing Co., Inc., New York, (5th edition), 1975, p. 660.

Moor, H., Mühlethaler, K., Fine structure of frozen-etched yeast cells. J. Cell Biol. *17*, 609, 1963.

Moss, A.J., Davis, R.J., Brady-tachy syndrome. Prog. Cardiovasc. Dis. *16*, 439, 1974.

Muir, A.R., Further observations on the cellular structure of cardiac muscle. J. Anat. *99*, 27, 1965.

Muir, A.R., The effects of divalent cations on the ultrastructure of the perfused rat heart. J. Anat. *101*, 239, 1967.

Nadeau, R.A., James, T.N., Antagonistic effects on the sinus node of acetylstrophantidin and adrenergic stimulation. Circ. Res. *13*, 388, 1963.

Narula, O.S., Sinus node reentry: mechanism of supraventricular tachycardia (SVT) in man (abstr.). Circulation *46, Suppl. II*, 11, 1972.

Narula, O.S., Sinus node reentry. A mechanism for supraventricular tachycardia. Circulation *50*, 1114, 1974.

Narula, O.S., Disorders of sinus node function: electrophysiologic evaluation. In: His bundle electrocardiography & clinical electrophysiology. Editor: Narula, O.S., Publ.: F.A. Davis, Philadelphia, 1975, p. 275.

Narula, O.S., Cohen, L.S., Scherlag, B.J., Samet, P., Lister, J.W., Hildner, F.J., Localization of AV conduction defects in man by recordings of the His bundle electrogram. Am. J. Cardiol. *25*, 228, 1970.

Narula, O.S., Samet P., Javier, R.P., Significance of the sinus node recovery time. Circulation *45*, 140, 1972.

Nawrath, H., Does cyclic GMP mediate the negative inotropic effect of acetylcholine in the heart. Nature *267*, 72, 1977.

Neuss, H., Nowak, F., Schlepper, M., Changes of conduction properties of anomalous pathways in cases with WPW syndrome "overdrive suppression" of conductivity. Z. Kardiol. *62*, 489, 1973.

Neuss, H., Schlepper, M., Der Einfluss von Verapamil auf die atrioventrikuläre Überleitung. Verh. Dtsch. Ges. Kreisl. Forschg. *37*, 433, 1971.

New, W., Trautwein, W., The ionic nature of slow inward current and its relation to contraction. Pflügers Arch. *334*, 24, 1972.

Nielsen, K.C., Owman, Ch., Difference in cardiac adrenergic innervation between hibernators and non-hibernating mammals. Acta physiol. scand., *Suppl. 316*, 1, 1968.

Nies, A.S., Shand, D.G., Clinical pharmacology of propranolol. Circulation *52*, 6, 1975.

Nilsson, E., Sporrong, B., Electron microscopic investigation of adrenergic and non-adrenergic axons in the rabbit SA node. Z. Zellforsch. *111*, 404, 1970.

Noble, D., The initiation of the heart beat. Oxford University Press, 1975.

Noble, D., Tsien, R.W., The kinetics and rectifier properties of the slow potassium current in cardiac Purkinje fibers. J. Physiol. *195*, 185, 1968.

Noble, D., Tsien, R.W., Outward membrane currents activated in the plateau range of potentials in cardiac Purkinje fibers. J. Physiol. *200*, 205, 1969.

Noble, D., Tsien, R. W., Reconstruction of the repolarization process in cardiac Purkinje fibers based on voltage clamp measurements of membrane current. J. Physiol. *200*, 233, 1969.

Noble, S.J., Potassium accumulation and depletion in frog atrial muscle. J. Physiol. *258*, 578, 1976.

Noma, A., Mechanisms underlying cessation of rabbit sinoatrial node pacemaker activity in high potassium solutions. Jpn. J. Physiol. *26*, 619, 1976.

Norma, A., Irisawa, H., Electrogenic sodium pump in rabbit sinoatrial node cell. Pflügers Arch. *351*, 177, 1974.

Noma, A., Irisawa, H., Contribution of an electrogenic sodium pump to the membrane potential in rabbit sinoatrial node cells Pflügers Arch. *358*, 289, 1975.

Norma, A., Irisawa, H., Membrane currents in the rabbit sinoatrial node cell as studied by the double micro-electrode method. Pflügers Arch. *364*, 45, 1976.

Noma, A., Irisawa, H., Effects on Na^+ and K^+ on the resting membrane potential of the rabbit sinoatrial node cell. Jpn. Physiol. 25, 287, 1975.

Noma, A., Irisawa, H., A time- and voltage-dependent potassium current in the rabbit sinoatrial node cell. Pflügers Arch. *366*, 251, 1976.

Noma, A., Irisawa, H., Effects of calcium ion on the rising phase of the action potential in rabbit sinoatrial node cells. Jpn. J. Physiol. *26*, 93, 1976.

Noma, A., Irisawa, H., The effect of sodium on the initial phase of the sino-atrial pacemaker action potentials in rabbits. Jpn. J. Physiol. *24*, 617, 1974.

Noma, A., Yanagihara, K., Irisawa, H., Inward current of the rabbit sinoatrial node cell. Pflügers Arch. 372, 43, 1977.

Obayashi, K., Nagasawa, K., Mandel, W.J., Vyden, J. K., Cardiovascular effects of the new antiarrhythmic agent verapamil. Am. J. Cardiol. *35*, 161, 1975.

Ochi, R., The slow inward current and the action of manganese ions in guinea-pig's myocardium. Pflügers Arch. *316*, 81, 1970.

Okada, T., Konishi, T., Effects of verapamil on SA and AV nodal action potentials in the isolated rabbit heart. Jpn. Circ. J. *39*, 913, 1975.

Okimoto, T., Ueda, K., Kamata, C., Yoshida, H., Ohkawa, S., Hirooka, K., Kuwajima, I., Sugiura, J., Murakami, M., Matsuo, H., Sinus node recovery time and abnormal postpacing phase in the aged patients with sick sinus syndrome. Jpn. Heart J. *17*, 290, 1976.

Oliphant, L.W., Loewen, R.D., Filament systems in Purkinje cells of the sheep heart: possible alterations of myofibrillogenesis. J. Mol. Cardiol. *8*, 679, 1976.

Opitz, H., Weiss, E., Quantitative Untersuchungen der inotropen Vaguswirkung auf den isolierten Kaninchen-Vorhof. Pflügers Arch. *267*, 600, 1958.

Orci, L., Amherdt, M., Malaisse-Lagae, F., Rouiller, Ch., Reynold, A.E., Insulin release by emiocytosis: demonstration with freeze-etching technique. Science *179*, 82, 1973.

Paes de Carvalho, A., The two components of the cardiac action potential. p. 71. In: Research in Physiology, a liber memoralis in honour of C.McC. Brooks. Editors: Kao, F.F., Koizumi, K., Vassalle, M., Publ.: Aulo Guggi, Bologna, 1971, p. 71.

Paes de Carvalho, A., Cellular electrophysiology of the atrial specialized tissues. In: The specialized tissues of the heart. Editors: Paes de Carvalho, A., de Mello, W.C., Hoffman, B.F., Elsevier publishing company, Amsterdam, 1961, p. 115.

Paes de Carvalho, A., Hoffman, B.F., De Paula Carvalho, M., Two components of the cardiac action potential. I. Voltage-time course and the effect of acetylcholine on atrial and nodal cells of the rabbit heart. J. Gen. Physiol. *54*, 607, 1969.

Paes de Carvalho, A., de Mello, C.W., Hoffman, B.F., Electrophysiological evidence for specialized fiber types in rabbit atrium. Am. J. Physiol. *196*, 483, 1959.

Pahlajani, D.B., Miller, R.A., Serratto, M., Sinus node reentry and sinus node tachycardia. Am. Heart J. *90*, 305, 1975.

Pape, C., Küber, W., van Smekal, P., Morphometrie am Reizzleitungssystem und Arbeitsmyokard des Kalbherzens. Beitr. Pathol. *140*, 23, 1969.

Papka, R.E., Studies of cardiac ganglia in pre- and postnatal rabbits. Cell Tissue Res. *175*, 17, 1976.

Paritzky, Z., Obayashi, K., Mandel, W.J., Atrial tachycardia secondary to sinoatrial node reentry. Chest *66*, 526, 1974.

Pasmooij, J.H., Van Enst, G.C., Bouman, L.N., Allessie, M.A., Bonke, F.I.M., The effect of heart rate on the membrane responsiveness of rabbit atrial muscle. Pflügers Arch. *366*, 223, 1976.

Patten, B.M., Development of the sinoventricular conduction system. Univ. Mich. Med. Bull. *22*, 1, 1956.

Paulay, K.L., Damato, A.N., Effect of digoxin on sinus nodal reentry in the dog. Am. J. Cardiol. *35*, 370, 1975.

Paulay, K.L., Damato, A.N., Comparison of atrial and ventricular drive on sinus nodal function in dog. Am. J. Cardiol. *31*, 41, 1973.

Paulay, K.L., Ruskin, J.N., Damato, A.N., Sinus and atrioventricular nodal reentrant tachycardia in the same patient. Am. J. Cardiol. *36*, 810, 1975.

Paulay, K.L., Varghese, P.J., Damato, A.N., Sinus node reentry. An in vivo demonstration in the dog. Circ. Res. *32*, 455, 1973.

Paulay, K.L., Varghese, P.J., Damato, A.N., Atrial rhythms in response to an early atrial premature depolarization in man. Am. Heart J. *85*, 323, 1973.

Paulay, K.L., Weisfogel, B.M., Damato, A.N., Sinus nodal reentry: the effect of quinidine, Am. J. Cardiol. *33*, 617, 1974.

Pollack, G.H., AV nodal transmission: a proposed electromechanical mechanism. J. Electrocardiol. *7*, 245, 1974.

Pollack, G.H., Intercellular coupling in the atrioventricular node and other tissues of the rabbit heart. J. Physiol. *255*, 275, 1976.

Pollack, G.H., Cardiac pacemaking: an obligatory role of catecholamines? A possible mechanism underlaying spontaneous pacemaking can be deduced from several recent clues. Science *196*, 731, 1977.

Pollen, D.W., Scott, A.C., Wallace, W.F.M., A comparison of the direct effects of d/l and d-propranolol in the electrical and mechanical behavior of isolated frog ventricle. Cardiovasc. Res. *3*, 7, 1969.

Prokopczuk, A., Lewartowski, B., Czarnecka, M., On the cellular mechanism of the inotropic action of acetylcholine on isolated rabbit and dog atria. Pflügers Arch. *339*, 305, 1973.

Puech, P., Esclavissat, M., Sodi-Pallares, D., Cisneros, F., Normal auricular activation in the dog's heart. Am. Heart J. *47*, 174, 1954.

Radford, D.J., Julian D.G., Sick sinus syndrome: experience of a cardiac pacemaker clinic. Br. Med. J. *3*, 504, 1974.

Rasmussen, K., Chronic sinoatrial heart block. Am. Heart J. *81*, 38, 1971.

Rayns, D.G., Simpson, F.O., Ledingham, J.M., Ultrastructure of desmosomes in mammalian intercalated disc; appearances after lanthanum treatment. J. Cell Biol. *42*, 322, 1969.

Reiffel, J.A., Bigger, J.T., Giardina, E.G.V., "Paradoxical" prolongation of sinus nodal recovery time after atropine in the sick sinus syndrome. Am. J. Cardiol. *36*, 98, 1975.

Reiffel, J.A., Bigger, J.T., Konstam, M.A., The relationship between sinoatrial conduction time and sinus cycle length during spontaneous sinus arrhythmia in adults. Circulation *50*, 924, 1974.

Reiffel. J. A., Reid, D.S., Bigger, J.T., Holter monitoring and functional testing for sinus node dysfunction. Circulation Suppl. *52*/II, 111, 1975.

Repke, K., Metabolism of cardiac glycosides. In: Proceedings of the First International Pharmacological Meeting, Stockholm, Pergamon Press, New York, vol. 3, 1961, p. 17.

Repke, K., Schön, R., Henke, W., Schönfeld, W., Streckenbach, B., Dittrich, F., Experimental and theoretical examination of the flip-flop model of (Na, K) – ATPase function. Ann. N.Y. Acad. Sci. *242*, 203, 1974.

Reuter, H., Localization of BETA adrenergic receptors, and effects of noradrenaline and cyclic nucleotides on action potentials, ionic currents and tension in mammalian cardiac muscle. J. Physiol. *242*, 429, 1974.

Reuter, H., Über die Wirkung von Adrenalin auf den cellulären Ca-Umsatz des Meerschweinchenvorhofs. Arch. Pharmakol. Exp. Pathol. *251*, 401, 1965.

Reuter, H., Divalent cations as charge carriers in excitable membranes. Prog. Biophys. Mol. Biol. *26*, 1, 1973.

Reuter, H., Exchange of calcium ions in the mammalian myocardium. Mechanisms and physiological significance. Circ. Res. *34*, 599, 1974.

Reuter, H., Beeler, G.W. Jr., Calcium current and activation of contraction in ventricular myocardial fibers. Science, N.Y. *163*, 399, 1969.

Reuter, H., Scholz, H., A study of the ion selectivity and the kinetic properties of the calcium dependent slow inward current in mammalian cardiac muscle. J. Physiol. *264*, 17, 1977.

Reuter, H., Seitz, H., The dependence of calcium efflux from cardiac muscle on temperature and external ion composition. J. Physiol. (Lond.) *195*, 451, 1968.

Revel, J.P., Karnovsky, M.J., Hexagonal array of subunits in intercellular junctions of the mouse heart and liver. J. Cell. Biol. *33*, C7, 1967.

Reynolds, E.S., The use of lead citrate at high pH as an electron opaque stain in electron microscopy. J. Cell Biol. *17*, 208, 1963.

Rhodin, J.A.G., Del Missier, P., Reid, L.C., The structure of the specialized impulse conduction system of the steer heart. Circulation *24*, 349, 1961.

Rich, J.M., Meisner, M.H., Fontana, M.E., Wooley, C.F., Electrophysiologic stress tests in man: sinoatrial node suppression and recovery (abstr.). J. Lab. Clin. Med. *78*, 805, 1971.

Richardson, K.C., Electron microscope identification of autonomic nerve endings. Nature *210*, 756, 1966.

Rios, J.C., Bashour, T., Cheng, T.O., Motomiya, T., Atrial pacing in sick sinus node syndrome (abstr.). Circulation *45–46, Suppl. II*, 122, 1972.

Robb, J.S., Kaylor, C.T., Turman, W.G., A study of specialized heart tissue at various stages of development of the human fetal heart. Am. J. Med. *5*, 324, 1948.

Robb, J.S., Petri, R., Expansions of the atrioventricular system in the atria. In: The specialized tissues of the heart. Editors: Paes de Carvalho, A., de Mello, W.C., Hoffman, B.F., Elsevier publishing company, Amsterdam 1961, p. 1.

Rockseth, R., Hatle, L., Prospective study on the occurrence and management of chronic sinoatrial disease, with follow-up. Br. Heart J. *36*, 582, 1974.

Rosen, K.M., Barwolf, G., Ehsaui, A., Rahimtoola, S.H., Effects of lidocaine and propranolol in the normal and anomalous pathways in patients with pre-excitation. Am. J. Cardiol. *30*, 801, 1972.

Rosen, K.M., Loeb, H.S., Sinno, M.Z., Rahimtoola, S.H., Gunnar, R.M., Cardiac conduction in patients with symptomatic sinus node disease. Circulation *43*, 836, 1971.

Rosen, K.M., Wit, A.L., Hoffman, B.F., Electrophysiology and pharmacology of cardiac arrhythmias. VI. Cardiac effects of verapamil. Am. Heart J. *89*, 665, 1975.

Rosen, M.R., Gelband, H., Hoffman, B.F., Correlation between effects of ouabain on the canine electrocardiogram and transmembrane potentials of isolated Purkinje fibers. Circulation *47*, 65, 1973.

Rosen, M.R., Gelband, H., Merker, C., Mechanisms of digitalis toxicity: effects of ouabain on phase four of canine Purkinje fiber transmembrane potentials. Circulation *47*, 681, 1973.

Rosenbleuth, A., Transmission of nerve impulses at neuroeffector junctions and peripheral synapses. The Technology Press of Massachussets Institute of Technology and John Wiley and Sons, New York, 1950, p. 96.

Ross, G., Jorgensson, C.R., Cardiovascular action of ipoveratril. J. Pharmacol. Exp. Ther. *158*, 504, 1967.

Rostgaard, J., Behnke, O., Fine structural localization of adenine nucleoside phosphatase activity in the sarcoplasmic reticulum of striated muscle. In: Intracellular Transport, Academic Press, 1966, p. 103.

Rothberger, C., Scherf, D., Zur Kenntnis der Erregungsausbreitung vom Sinusknoten auf den Vorhof. Z. ges. exp. Med. *53*, 792, 1927.

Rougier, O., Vassort, G., Garnier, D., Gargouil, Z.M., Coraboeuf, E., Existence and role of a slow inward current during the frog atrial action potential. Pflügers Arch. *308*, 91, 1969.

Rougier, O., Vassort, G., Stämpfli, R., Voltage clamp experiments on frog atrial heart muscle fibers with the double sucrose gap technique. Pflügers Arch. ges. Physiol. *301*, 91, 1968.

Rubenstein, J.J., Schulman, C.L., Yurchak, P.M., DeSanctis, R.W., Clinical spectrum of the sick sinus syndrome. Circulation *46*, 5, 1972.

Ruska, H., In: International symposium on electrophysiology of the heart. Editors: Taccardi, B., Marchetti, G., Pergamon Press, New York, 1965, p. 1.

Rydén, L., Saetre, H., The haemodynamic effects of verapamil. Eur. J. Clin. Pharmacol. *3*, 153, 1971.

Rylant, P., Ablation et greffe intracardiaque du noeud de Keith-Flack (sinus) chez le chien. Arch. Int. Physiol. Biochim. *26*, 113, 1965.

Saetersdal, T.S., Myklebust, R., Berg Justesen, N.-P., Ultrastructural localization of calcium in the pigeon papillary muscle as demonstrated by cytochemical studies and X-ray microanalysis. Cell Tissue Res. *155*, 57, 1974.

Sano, T., Yamagishi, S., Spread of excitation from the sinus node. Circ. Res. *16*, 423, 1965.

Sandoval, I.V., Cuatrecasas, P., Opposing effects of cyclic AMP and cyclic GMP on protein phosphorylation in tubulin preparations. Nature *262*, 511, 1976.

Saroff, A. L., Strauss, H.C., Bigger, J.T., Steiner, C., Giardina, E.G., Evaluation of sinus node function in patients with sinus bradycardia. Circulation *43–44*, Suppl. II, 97, 1971.

Schamroth, L., Immediate effect of intravenous propranolol on various cardiac arrhythmias. Am. J. Cardiol. *18*, 438, 1966.

Schamroth, L., Krikler, D.M., Garrett, C., Immediate effects of intravenous verapamil in cardiac arrhythmias. Br. Med. J. *1*, 660, 1972.

Scheinmann, M.M., Kunkel, F.W., Peters, R.W., Hirschfeld, D.S., Schoenfeld, P.L., Abbott, J.A., Modin, G., Atrial pacing in patients with sinus node dysfunction. Am. J. Med. *61*, 641, 1976.

Scheinmann, M.M., Kunkel, F.W., Peters, R.W., Schoenfeld, P.L., Abbott, J.A., Sinoatrial function and atrial refractoriness in patients with sick sinus syndrome. Circulation *48*, Suppl. IV, 215, 1973.

Scheinmann, M.M., Peters, R.W., Hirschfeld, D.S., Abbott, J.A., Kunkel, F.W., The sick sinus and ailing atrium. West. J. Med. *121*, 473, 1974.

Scheinmann, M.M., Strauss, H.C., Abbott, J.A., Evans, G.T., Peters, R.W., Benditt, D.G., Wallace, A.G., Electrophysiologic testing in patients with sinus pauses and/or sinoatrial exit block.   Eur. J. Cardiol., (in press).

Scheinmann, M.M., Strauss, H.C., Evans, G.T., Ryan, C., Massie, B., Wallace, A.G., Adverse effects of sympatholytic agents in patients with hypertension and sinus node dysfunction. Am. J. Med., (in press).

Scher, A. M., Rodrigues, M.I., Lukane, J., Young, A.C., The mechanism of atrioventricular conduction. Circ. Res. *7*, 54, 1959.

Scherf, D., The mechanisms of sinoatrial block. Am. J. Cardiol. *23*, 769, 1969.

Scherlag, B.J., Abelleira, J.L., Narula, O.S., Samet, P., The differential effects of ouabain on sinus. AV-nodal, His bundle and idioventricular rhythms. Am. Heart J. *81*, 227, 1971.

Scherlag, B.J., Lau, S.H., Helfant, R.H., Berkowitz, W.D., Stein, E., Damato, A.N., Catheter technique for recording His bundle activity in man. Circulation *39*, 13, 1969.

Schiebler, T.H., Doer, W., Orthologie des Reizleitungssystems. In: Das Herz des Menschen. Editors: Bargman, W., Doer, W., Thieme, Stuttgart, 1963.

Schiebler, T.H., Starck, M., Caesar, R., Die Stoffwechselsituation des Reizleitungssystems. Klin. Wschr. *34*, 181, 1956.

Schlepper, M. Mechanisms underlying sudden changes in heart rate during paroxysmal supraventricular tachycardia. In: Re-entrant Arrhythmias. Mechanisms and Treatment. Editor: H. Kulbertus, MTP Lancaster, 1977, p. 184.

Schmahl, F.W., Betz, E., Die Wirkung von α-Isopropyl-α-(N-methyl-N-homoveratryl)-γ-aminopropyl-3, 4-dimethoxyphenylacetonnitrile auf die Durchblutung von Myokard, Leber, Niere, Skeletmuskulatur und Gehirn der Katze, Arzneim. Forsch. *14*, 1159, 1964.

Schreurs, A.W., Meijer, A.A., Bouman, L.N., Bonke, F.I.M., Micromanipulator with an electrode driver used for micro-electrode work. Pflügers Arch. *346*, 163, 1974.

Schwarz, F., Thormann, J., Zimmerman, H., Vagaler Einfluss auf Sinusknotenfrequen/ und AV-Überleitung bei hypersensitivem Karotissinus Reflex und "Sick-Sinus-Syndrom". Schweiz. Med. Wochenschr. *105*, 240, 1975.

Seides, S.F., Josephson, M.E., Batsford, W.P., Weisfogel, G.M., Lau, S.H., Damato, A.N., The electrophysiology of propranolol in man. Am. Heart J. *88*, 733, 1974.

Seifen, E., Schaer, H., Marshall, J.M., Effect of calcium on the membrane potentials of single pacemaker fibers in isolated rabbit atria. Nature *202*, 1223, 1964.

Seipel, L., Both, A., Breithardt, G., Gleichmann, U., Loogen, F., Action of antiarrhythmic drugs on His bundle electrogram and sinus node function. Acta Cardiol. (Brux.), Suppl. *18*, 251, 1974.

Seipel, L., Breithardt, G., Sinus recovery time after disopyramide phosphate. Am. J. Cardiol. *37*, 1118, 1976.

Seipel, L., Breithardt, G., Sinusknotenautomatie und   sinu-atriale Leitung. Z. Kardiol. *64*, 1014, 1975.

Seipel, L., Breithardt, G.; Both, A., Loogen, F., Diagnostische Probleme beim Sinusknotensyndrom. Z. Kardiol. *64*, 1, 1975.

Seipel, L., Breithardt, A., Both, A., Loogen, F., Messung der sinuatrialen Leitungszeit mittels vorzeitiger Vorhofstimulation beim Menschen. Dtsch. Med. Wschr. *99*, 1895, 1974.

Seipel, L., Breithardt, G., Döhring, H.P., Die Wirkung von Atenolol auf Sinusknoten und intrakardiale Erregungsleitung beim Menschen im Vergleich zu Propranolol. Z. Kardiol. *66*, 719, 1977.

Seyama, I., Characteristics of the rectifying properties of the sinoatrial node cell of the rabbit. J. Physiol. *255*, 379, 1976.

Seyama, I., The effect of anions on the membrane properties of sinoatrial node cell of the rabbit. J. Physiol. Soc. Jpn. *39*, (in press).

Shinebourne, E., White, R., and Hamer, J., A qualitative distinction between the beta-receptor-blocking and local anesthetic actions of antiarrhythmic agents. Circ. Res. *24*, 853, 1969.

Short, D.S., The syndrome of alternating bradycardia and tachycardia. Br. Heart J. *16*, 208, 1954.

Sigurd, B. Jensen, G., Meibom, J., Sandoe, E., Adams-Stokes-syndrome caused by sinoatrial block. Br. Heart J. *35*, 1002, 1973.

Simon, M., Conversion of guanosine 3′, 5′-monophosphate to adenosine 3′, 5′-monophosphate in frog myocardial tissue. Biochem. Biophys. Res. Commun. *68*, 1219, 1976.

Simonin, P., Niederhauser, H.U., Duchosal, P.W., Contribution de l'exploration électrique endocavitaire à l'étude de la dysrhythmie auriculaire. Arch. Mal. Cœur *69*, 341, 1976.

Simpson, F.O., Rayns, D.G., Ledingham, J.M., The ultrastructure of ventricular and atrial myocardium. In: Ultrastructure of the mammalian heart. Editors: Challice, C.E., Viràgh, S., Academic Press, 1973, p. 1.

Small, J.V., Sobieszek, A., Studies on the function and composition of the 10 nm (100 A) filaments of vertebrate smooth muscle. J. Cell. Sci. *23*, 243, 1977.

Smith, T.W., Haber, E., Digitalis (First of four parts). N. Eng. J. Med. *289*, 945, 1973.

Smith, T.W., Haber, E., Digitalis (Second of four parts). N. Engl. J. Med. *289*, 1010, 1973.

Smith, T.W., Willerson, J.T., Suicidal and accidental digoxin ingestion: report of five cases with serum digoxin level correlations. Circulation *44*, 29, 1971.

Smith, U., Smith, D.S., Winkler, H., Ryan, J.W., Exocitosis in adrenal medulla demonstrated by freeze-etching. Science *179*, 79, 1973.

Smithen, C.S., Balcon, R., Sowton, E., Use of bundle of His potentials to assess changes in atrio-ventricular conduction produced by a series of beta-adrenergic blocking agents. Br. Heart J. *33*, 955, 1971.

Sommer, J.R., Johnson, E.A., Cardiac Muscle. A comparative study of Purkinje fibers and ventricular fibers. J. Cell Biol. *36*, 497, 1968.

Sommer, J.R., Johnson, E.A., Comparative ultrastructure of cardiac cell membrane specializations. A review. Am. J. Cardiol. *25*, 184, 1970.

Sommer, J.R., Waugh, R.A., The ultrastructure of the mammalian cardiac muscle cell – with special emphasis on the tubular membrane systems. Am. J. Pathol. *82*, 192, 1976.

Sowton, E., Hendrix, G., Roy, P., Ten-year survey of treatment with implanted cardiac pacemaker. Br. Med. J. *3*, 155, 1974.

Spach, M.S., King, T.D., Barr, R.C., Boaz, D.E., Morrow, H.N., Herman-Giddens, S., Electrical potential distribution surrounding the atria during depolarization and repolarization in the dog. Circ. Res. *24*, 857, 1969.

Spach, M.S., Lieberman, M., Scott, J.C., Barr, R.C., Johnson, E.A., Kootsey, J.M., Excitation sequences of the atrial septum and AV node in isolated hearts of the dog and rabbit. Circ. Res. *29*, 156, 1971.

Spellberg, R.D., Familial sinus node disease. Chest *60*, 246, 1971.

Sperelakis, N., Electrical properties of embryonic heart cells. In: Electrical Phenomena in the Heart. Editor: de Mello, W.C., Academic Press, New York, 1972, p. 1–61.

Spurgeon, H.A., Priola, D.V., Montoya, P., Weiss, G.K., Alter, W.A., III, Catecholamines associated with conductile and contractile myocardium of normal and denervated dog hearts. J. Pharmacol. Exp. Ther. *190*, 466, 1974.

Spurr, A.R., A low viscosity epoxy resin embedding medium for electron microscopy. J. Ultrastruct. Res. *26*, 31, 1969.

Spurrell, R.A.J., Krikler, D., Sowton, E., Two or more intra AV-nodal pathways in association with either a James or Kent extranodal bypass in three patients with paroxysmal supraventricular tachycardia. Br. Heart J. *35*, 113, 1973.

Steinbeck, G., Körber, H.J., Lüderitz, B., Die Bestimmung der sinuatrialen Leitungszeit beim Menschen durch gekoppelte atriale Einzelstimulation. Klin. Wschr. *52*, 1151, 1974.

Steinbeck, G., Körber, H.J. Lüderitz, B., Untersuchungen zur Sinusknotenfunktion beim Bradykardie-Tachykardie-Syndrom. Verh. Dtsch. ges. Inn. Med. *80*, 1126, 1974.

Steinbeck, G., Lüderitz, B., Störungen der Sinusknotenfunktion, Diagnostik und klinische Bedeutung. Dtsch. med. Wschr. *102*, 35, 1977.

Steinbeck, G., Lüderitz, B., Comparative study of sinoatrial conduction time and sinus node and sinus node recovery time. Br. Heart J. *37*, 956, 1975.

Steinbeck, G., Lüderitz, B., Sinus node recovery time and sinoatrial conduction time. In: Cardiac Pacing. Diagnostic and Therapeutic Tools, Editor: Lüderitz, B. Springer Verlag, Berlin-Heidelberg-New York, 1976, p. 45.

Steinbeck, G., Naumann d'Alnoncourt, C., Lüderitz, B., Digitalis und Sinusknotenfunktion. Z. Kardiol., Suppl. 3, 135, 1976.

Stern, S., Eisenberg, S., The effect of propranolol (Inderal) on the electrocardiogram of normal subjects. Am. Heart J. *77*, 192, 1969.

Stock, J.P.P., Beta-adrenergic blocking drugs in the clinical management of cardiac arrhythmias. Am. J. Cardiol. *18*, 44, 1966.

Strauss, H.C., Bigger, J.T., Slowed conduction, block and reentry in perinodal fibers. Circulation 43, Suppl. II, 74, 1971.

Strauss, H.C., Bigger, J.T., Electrophysiological properties of the rabbit sinoatrial perinodal fibers. Circ. Res. *31*, 490, 1972.

Strauss, H.C., Bigger, J.T., Saroff, A.L., Giardina, E.G.V., Electrophysiologic evaluation of sinus node function in patients with sinus node dysfunction. Circulation *53*, 763, 1976.

Strauss, H.C., Geer, M.R., Sinoatrial node reentry. In: Reentrant Arrhythmias. Mechanisms and Treatment. Editor: H.E. Kulbertus, MTP Lancaster, 1977, p. 27.

Strauss, H.C., Gilbert, M., Svenson, R.H., Miller, H.C., Wallace, A.G., Electrophysiologic effects of propranolol on sinus node function in patients with sinus node dysfunction. Circulation *54*, 452, 1976.

Strauss, H.C., Prystowsky, E.N., Scheinmann, M.M., Sinoatrial and atrial electrogenesis. Prog. Cardiovasc. Dis. *19*, 385, 1977.

Strauss, H.C., Saroff, A.L., Bigger, J.T., Giardina, E.G.V., Premature atrial stimulation as a key to the understanding of sinoatrial conduction in man. Circulation *47*, 86, 1973.

Strauss, H.C., Scheinmann, M.M., Evans, G.T., Bashore, T., Wallace, A.G., Electrophysiologic effects of disopyramide in patients with sinus node dysfunction. Circulation *54*, *Suppl. II*: 17, 1976.

Strauss, H.C., Wallace, A.G., Direct and indirect techniques in the evaluation of sinus node function. In: The Conduction System of the Heart. Editors: Wellens, H.J.J., Lie, K.I., and Janse, M.J., Stenfert Kroese, Leiden, 1976, p. 227.

Strauss, H.C., Wallace, A.G., Premature atrial stimulation for evaluation of sinoatrial conduction in man. In: Cardiac Pacing. Diagnostic and Therapeutic Tools. Editor: Lüderitz, B., Springer Verlag, Berlin-Heidelberg-New York, 1976, p. 33.

Stretton, A.O.W., Kravits, E.A., Intracellular dye injection: the selection of procion yellow and its application in preliminary studies of neuronal geometry in the lobster nervous system. In: Intracellular staining in neurobiology. Editors: Kater, S.B., Nicholson, C., Springer Verlag, Berlin-Heidelberg-New York, 1973, p. 21.

Sulze, W., Ein Beitrag zur Kenntnis des Erregungsablaufs im Säugetierherzen. Z. für Biol. *60*, 495, 1913.

Svenson, R.H., Gallagher, J.J., Sealy, W.C., Wallace, A.G., An electrophysiologic approach to the surgical treatment of the Wolff-Parkinson-White syndrome. Report of two cases utilizing catheter recording and epicardial mapping techniques. Circulation *49*, 799, 1974.

Szekely, P., Jackson, F., Wynne, N.A;, Vohra, J.K., Batson, G.A., Dow, W.I.M., Clinical observations on the use of propranolol in disorders of cardiac rhythm. Am. J. Cardiol. *18*, 426, 1966.

Szekeres, L., Papp, G.J., Experimental cardiac arrhythmias and antiarrhythmic drugs. Budapest, Akademiai, Kiado, 1971.

Tarr, M., Two inward currents in frog atrial muscle. J. Gen. Physiol. *58*, 55, 1971.

Ten Eick, R.E., Hoffman, B.F., Chronotopic effect on cardiac glycosides in dogs, cats, and rabbits. Circ. Res. *25*, 365, 1969.

Ten Eick, R., Nawrath, H., McDonald, T.F., Trautwein, W., On the mechanism of the negative inotropic effect of acetylcholine. Pflügers Arch. *361*, 207. 1976.

Teo, T.S., Wang, J.H., Mechanisms of activation of a cyclic adenosine 3'5'-monophosphate phosphodiesterase from bovine heart by calcium ions. Identification of the protein activator as a Ca^{2+} binding protein J. Biol. Chem. *248*, 5950, 1973.

Thaemert, J.C., Atrioventricular node innervation in ultrastructural three dimensions. Am. J. Anat. *128*, 239, 1970.

Thames, M.D., Kontos, H.A., Mechanisms of baroreceptor-induced changes in heart rate. Am. J. Physiol. *218*, 251, 1970.

Thornell, L.E., Evidence of an imbalance in synthesis and degradation of myofibrillar proteins in rabbit Purkinje fibers. J. Ultrastruct. Res. *44*, 85, 1973.

Thornell, L.E., Distinction of glycogen and ribosome particles in cow Purkinje fibers by enzymatic digestion en bloc and in sections. J. Ultrastruct. Res. *47*, 153, 1974.

Ticzon, A.R., Strauss, H.C., Gallagher, J.J., Wallace, A.G., Sinus nodal function in the intact dog heart evaluated by premature atrial stimulation and atrial pacing. Am. J. Cardiol. *35*, 492, 1975.

Toda, N., West, T.C., Interaction between Na, Ca, Mg, and vagal stimulation in the S-A node of the rabbit. Am. J. Physiol. *212*, 424, 1967.

Toda, N., West, T.C., Interactions of K, Na, and vagal stimulation in the S-A node of the rabbit. Am. J. Physiol. *212*, 416, 1967.

Toda, N., Electrophysiological effects of sodium ions on the membrane potential of the sino-atrial node in response to sympathetic nerve stimulation. J. Physiol. *196*, 677, 1968.

Toda, N., Electrophysiological effects of potassium and calcium ions in the sinoatrial node in response to sympathetic nerve stimulation. Pflügers Arch. *310*, 45, 1969.

Toda, N., Shimamoto, K., The influence of sympathetic stimulation on transmembrane potentials in the SA node. J. Pharmacol. Exp. Ther. *159*, 298, 1968.

Toda, N., West, T.C., The influence of ouabain on cholinergic responses in the sino-atrial node. J. Pharmacol. Exp. Ther. *153*, 104, 1966.

Tonkin, A.M., Gallagher, J.J., Svenson, R.H., Wallace, A.G., Sealy, W.C., Antegrade block in accessory pathways with retrograde conduction in reciprocating tachycardia. Eur. J. Cardiol. *3*, 143, 1975.

Torii, H., Electron microscope observations of the SA and AV nodes and the Purkinje fibers of the rabbit. Jpn. Circ. J. *26*, 39, 1962.

Tranum-Jensen, J., The ultrastructure of the sensory end-organs (baroreceptors) in the atrial endocardium of young mini-pigs. J. Anat. *119*, 255, 1975.

Tranum-Jensen, J., The fine structure of the atrial and atrio-ventricular (AV) junctional specialized tissues of the rabbit heart. In: The Conduction System of the Heart. Structure, Function and Clinical Implications. Editors: Wellens, H.J.J., Lie, K.I. and Janse, M.J., Stenfert Kroese, Leiden, 1976, pp. 55-81.

Tranum-Jensen, J., Bojsen-Möller, F., The ultrastructure of the sinoatrial ring bundle and of the caudal extension of the sinus node in the right atrium of the rabbit heart. Z. Zellforsch. *138*, 97, 1973.

Tranzer, J.P., Thoenen, H., An electron microscopic study of selective, acute degeneration of sympathetic nerve terminals after administration of 6-hydroxy-dopamin. Experientia *24*, 155, 1968.

Tranzer, J.P., Thoenen, H., Ultramorphologische Veränderungen der Sympathischen Nervenendigungen der Katze nach Vorbehandlung mit 5- and 6-Hydroxydopamin. Naunyn-Schmiedeberg's Arch. Pharmakol. Exp. Pathol. *257*, 343, 1967.

Tranzer, J.P., Thoenen, H., Electronmicroscopic localization of 5-hydroxydopamine (3,4,5-trihydroxy-phenyl-ethylamine), a new "false" sympathetic transmitter. Experientia *23*, 743, 1967.

Trautwein, W., Dudel, J., Hemmende und "erregende" Wirkungen des Acetylcholin am Warmblüterherzen. Zur Frage der spontanen Erregungsbildung. Pflügers Arch. *266*, 653, 1958.

Trautwein, W., Membrane currents in cardiac muscle fibers. Physiol. Rev. *53*, 793, 1973.

Trautwein, W., Dudel, J., Zum Mechanismus der Membranwirkung des Acetylcholin an der Herzmuskelfaser. Pflügers Arch., *266*, 324, 1958.

Trautwein, W., Zink, K., Über Membran- und Aktionspotentiale einzelner Myokardfasern des Kalt- und Warmblütherzens. Pflügers Arch. ges. Physiol. *256*, 68, 1952.

Trautwein, W., Kassebaum, D.G., On the mechanism of spontaneous impulse generation in the pacemaker of the heart. J. Gen. Physiol. *45*, 317, 1961.

Trautwein, W., Uchizono, K., Electron microscopic and electrophysiologic study of the pacemaker in the sinoatrial node of the rabbit heart. Z. Zellforsch. Mikrosk. Anat. *61*, 96, 1963.

Trinci, G., Cellule cromaffini e "mastzellen" nella regione cardiaca dei mammiferi. Mem. Reale Accad. Sci. Ist. Bologna *4*, 191, 1907.

Truex, R.C., Structural basis of atrial and ventricular conduction. Cardiovasc. Clin. *6*, 1, 1974.

Truex, R.C., The sinoatrial node and its connections with the atrial tissues. In: The Conduction System of the Heart. Structure, Function and Clinical Implications. Editors: Wellens, H.J.J., Lie, K.I., Janse, M.J., Stenfert Kroese, Leiden, 1976, p. 209.

Truex, R.C., Smythe, M.Q., Taylor, M.J., Reconstruction of the human sinoatrial node. Anat. Rec. *159*, 371, 1967.

Tuganowski, W., Krause, M., Korczak, K., The effect of diputyryl 3′5′-cyclic AMP on the cardiac pacemaker arrested with reserpine and alpha-methyl-tyrosine. Naunyn-Schmiedeberg's Arch. Pharmacol. *280*, 63, 1973.

Turner, J.R.B., Propranolol in the treatment of digitalis-induced and digitalis-resistant tachycardias. Am. J. Cardiol. *18*, 450, 1966.

Ueda, K., Kamata, C., Matsuo, H., Ohkawa, S., Okimoto, T., Sugiura, M., A Study on sinoatrial conduction in the aged. Jpn. Heart J. *18*, 143, 1977.

Ushiyama, J., Brooks, C.M., Intercellular stimulation and recording from single cardiac cells in the rabbit atrium. J. Electrocardiol. *7(2)*, 119, 1974.

Van Mierop, L.H.S., Gessner, I.H., The morphologic development of the sinoatrial node in the mouse. Am. J. Cardiol. *25*, 204, 1970.

Van Mierop, L.H.S., Patterson, P.R., Reynolds, R.W., Two cases of congenital asplenia with isomerism of the cardiac atria and the sinoatrial nodes. Am. J. Cardiol. *13*, 407, 1964.

Van Mierop, L.H.S., Wiglesworth, F.W., Isomerism of the cardiac atria in the asplenia syndrome. Lab. Invest. *11*, 1303, 1962.

Vassalle, M., Generation and conduction of impulses in the heart under physiological and pathological conditions. Pharmacol. Ther. B. *3*, 1, 1977.

Vassalle, M., Analysis of cardiac pacemaker potential using a "voltage clamp" technique. Am. J. Physiol. *210*, 1335, 1966.

Vassalle, M., Cardiac pacemaker potentials at different extra- and intra-cellular K-concentrations. Am. J. Physiol. *208*, 770, 1965.

Vassalle, M., Mandel, W.J., Holder, M.S., Catecholamine stores under vagal control. Am. J. Physiol. *218*, 115, 1970.

Vassort, G., Rougier, O., Garnier, D., Sauviat, M.P., Coraboef, E., Gargouïl, Y.-M., Effects of adrenaline on membrane inward currents during the cardiac action potential. Pflügers Arch. *309*, 70, 1969.

Vatner, S.F., Higgins, C.B., Franklin, D., Braunwald, E., Autonomic components of reflex tachycardia induced by hypotension. Physiologist *15*, 294, 1972.

Vaughan-Williams, E.M., Mode of action of beta-receptor antagonists on cardiac muscle. Am. J. Cardiol. *18*, 399, 1966.

Vincenzi, F.F., West, T.C., Release of autonomic mediators in cardiac tissue by direct subthreshold electrical stimulation. J. Pharmacol. Exp. Ther. *141*, 185, 1963.

Viràgh, S., Challice, C.E., Variations in filamentous and fibrillar organization and associated sarcolemmal structures, in cells of the normal mammalian heart. J. Ultrastruct. Res. *28*, 321, 1969.

Viràgh, S., Challice, C.E., Origin and differentiation of cardiac muscle cells in the mouse. J. Ultrastruct. Res. *42*, 1, 1973.

Viràgh, S., Challice, C.E., The impulse generation and conduction system of the heart. In: Ultrastructure of the mammalian heart. Editors: Challice, C.E., Viràgh, S., Academic Press, 1973, p. 43.

Viràgh, S., Porte, A., Structure fine du tissu vecteur dans le cœur de rat. Z. Zellforsch. *55*, 263, 1961.

Viràgh, S., Porte, A., Le nœud de Keith et Flack et les différentes fibres auriculaires du cœur de rat. Etude au microscope optique et électronique. CR acad. Sci. (Paris) *251,* 2086, 1960.

Viràgh, S., Porte, A., The fine structure of the conducting system of the monkey heart (Macaca mulatta). I. The sinoatrial node and the inter-nodal connections. Z. Zellforsch. *145,* 191, 1973.

Viràgh, S., Porte, A., On the impulse conducting system of the monkey heart (Macaca mulatta). II. The atrioventricular node and bundle. Z. Zellforsch. *145,* 363, 1973.

Vitek, M., Trautwein, W., Slow inward current and action potential in cardiac Purkinje fibers. Pflügers Arch. *323,* 204, 1971.

Wagner, J., Schümann, H.J., Görlitz, B.D., Änderung der Toxizität des Calciumantagonisten Verapamil durch Brenzkatechinaminverarmung. Arzneim. Forsch./Drug Res. *27,* 558, 1977.

Waldo, A.L., Cooper, T.B., Mac Lean, W.A.H., Need for additional criteria for the diagnosis of sinus node reentrant tachycardias. (Editorial) J. Electrocardiol. *10,* 103, 1977.

Waldo, A.L., Mac Lean, W.A.H., Karp, R.B., Kouchoukos, T., James, J.N., Sequence of retrograde atrial activation of the human heart. Correlation with P wave polarity. Br. Heart J. *39,* 634, 1977.

Wallace, A.G., Daggett, W.M., Re-excitation of the atrium. The echo phenomenon. Am. Heart J. *68,* 661, 1964.

Walker, J.L., Ladle, R.O., Frog heart intracellular potassium activities measured with potassium microelectrodes. Am. J. Physiol. *225,* 263, 1973.

Wan, S.H., Lee, G.S., Toh, C.C.S., The sick sinus syndrome. A Study of 15 cases. Br. Heart J. *34,* 942, 1972.

Ward, O.C., A new familial cardiac syndrome in children. J. Irish Med. Assoc. *54,* 103, 1964.

Weibel, E.R., Kistler, G.S., Walter, F.S., Practical stereological methods for morphometric cytology. J. Cell Biol. *30,* 23, 1966.

Weidmann, S. Effect of current flow on the membrane potential of cardiac muscle. J. Physiol. *115,* 227, 1951.

Weidmann, S., The effect of cardiac membrane potential on the rapid availability of the sodium carrying system. J. Physiol. (Lond.) *127,* 213, 1955.

Weingart, R., The actions of ouabain on intercellular coupling and conduction velocity in mammalian ventricular muscle. J. Physiol. (Lond.) *264,* 341, 1977.

Weisfogel, G.M., Batsford, W.P., Paulay, K.L., Josephson, M.F., Ogunkelu, J.B., Akhtar, M., Seides, S.F., Damato, A.N., Sinus node reentrant tachycardia in man. Am. Heart J. *90,* 295, 1975.

Wellens, H.J.J., Electrical stimulation of the heart in the study and treatment of tachycardia. H.E. Stenfert Kroese BV, Leiden, 1971.

Wellens, H.J.J., Cats, V.M., Düren, D.R., Symptomatic sinus node abnormalities following lithium carbonate therapy. Am. J. Med. *59,* 285, 1975.

Wenckebach, K.F., Ueber die Dauer der kompensatorischen Pause nach Reizung der Vorkammer des Saugetierherzens. Arch. Anat. Physiol. 57, 1903.

Wenckebach, K.F., Arrhythmia of the heart. A physiological and clinical study. Translated by T. Snowball. William Green & Sons, Edinburgh and London, 1904.

Wenckebach, K.F., Beiträge zur Kenntnis der menschlichen Herztätigkeit. Arch. Anat. Physiol. 297, 1906.

Wenink, A.C.G., Development of the human cardiac conducting system. J. Anat. *121,* 617, 1976.

West, T.C., Electrophysiology of the sinus node. In: Electrical phenomena in the heart. Editor: de Mello, Academic Press, New York, 1972.

West, T.C., Ultramicroelectrode recording from the cardiac pacemaker. J. Pharmacol. Exp. Ther. *115,* 283, 1955.

West, T.C., Effects of chronotropic influences on subthreshold oscillations in the sinoatrial node. In: The Specialized Tissues of the Heart. Editors: Paes de Carvalho, A., de Mello, W.C., and Hoffman, B.F., Elsevier Publishing Company, Amsterdam-London-New York-Princeton, 1961, p. 81.

West, T.C., Electrophysiology of the sinoatrial node. In: Electrical Phenomena in the Heart. Editor: de Mello, W.C., Academic Press, New York-London, 1972, p. 191.

West, T.C., Landa, J., Transmembrane potentials and contractility in the pregnant rat uterus. Am. J. Physiol. *187,* 333, 1956.

Wilkens, L.A., Electrophysiological studies of the heart of bivalve molluscs. Modiolus demissus. I. Ionic basis of the membrane potential. J. Exp. Biol. 56, 273, 1972.

Winegrad, S., Autoradiographic studies of intracellular calcium in frog skeletal muscle. J. Gen. Physiol. 48, 455, 1965.

Winegrad, S., Studies of cardiac muscle with a high permeability to calcium produced by treatment with ethylenediaminetetraacetic acid. J. Gen. Physiol. 58, 71, 1971.

Wit, A.L., Cranefield, P.F., Triggered activity in cardiac muscle fibers on the simian mitral valve. Circ. Res. 38, 85, 1976.

Wit, A.L., Cranefield, P.F., Triggered and automatic activity in the canine coronary sinus. Circ. Res. 41, 415, 1977.

Wit, A.L., Cranefield, P.F., Effect of verapamil on the sinoatrial and atrioventricular nodes of the rabbit and the mechanisms by which it arrests reentrant atrioventricular nodal tachycardia. Circ. Res. 35, 413, 1974.

Wollenberger, A., The role of cyclic AMP in the adrenergic control of the heart. In: Contraction and relaxation in the myocardium. Editor: Nayler, W.G., Academic Press, New York, 1975.

Wollenberger, A., Babskii, G.B., Krause, E.G., Genz, S., Blohn, D., Bogdanova, E.V., Cyclic changes in levels of cyclic AMP and cyclic GMP in frog myocardium during the cardiac cycle. Biochem. Biophys. Res. Commun. 55, 446, 1973.

Woodbury, J.W., Brady, A.J., Intracellular recording from moving tissue with a flexibly mounted ultra microelectrode. Science, 123, 100, 1956.

Woodcock, C.L.F., Bell, P.R., A method for mounting 4 μ resin sections routinely for ultra thin sectioning. J. Roy. Micr. Soc. 3/4, 485, 1967.

Wu, D., Amat-y-Leon, F., Denes, P., Dhingra, R.C., Pietras, R.J., Rosen, K.M., Demonstration of sustained sinus and atrial reentry in a mechanism of paroxysmal supraventricular tachycardia. Circulation 51, 234, 1975.

Yabek, S.M., Jarmakani, J.M., Roberts, N.K., Sinus node function in children. Factors influencing its evaluation. Circulation 53, 28, 1976.

Yamagishi, S., Sano, T., Effect of temperature on pacemaker activity of rabbit sinus node. Am. J. Physiol. 212, 829, 1967.

Yamagishi, S., Sano, T., Effect of tetrodoxin on the pacemaker action potential of the sinus node. Proc. Jpn. Acad. 42, 1194, 1966.

Yamagishi, Y., Fujiwara, M., Toda, N., Effects of catecholamines injected into sinoatrial nodal cells on their electrical activity. Jpn. J. Pharmacol. 24, 383, 1974.

Yamaguchi, I., Mandel, W.J., The effect of stimulation site on electrophysiologic features of the sinus node. Am. J. Cardiol. 41, 374, 1978.

Yamaguchi, I., Mandel, W.J., Electrophysiological effects of atrial premature depolarizations on sinus node function. J. Appl. Physiol., (in press).

Yamauchi, A., Electron microscopic observations on the development of SA and AV nodal tissues in the human embryonic heart. Z. Anat. Entw. Gesch. 124, 562, 1965.

Yamauchi, A., Ultrastructure of the innervation of the mammalian heart. In: Ultrastructure of the mammalian heart. Editors: Challice, C.E., Viràgh, S., Academic Press, 1973, p. 127.

Yamauchi, A., Yokota, R., Fujimaki, Y., Reciprocal synapses between cholinergic axons and small granule-containing cells in the rat cardiac ganglion. Anat. Rec. 181, 195, 1975.

Ypey, D.L., Feedback in isotonic muscle contraction on neuromuscular impulse transmission in the frog. Pflügers Arch. 355, 291, 1975.

Zipes, D.P., Fischer, J.C., Effects of agents which inhibit the slow channel on sinus node automaticity and atrioventricular conduction in the dog. Circ. Res. 34, 184, 1974.

INDEX